Springer Series in Statistics

Advisors:
P. Bickel, P. Diggle, S. Fienberg, U. Gather,
I. Olkin, S. Zeger

For other titles published in this series, go to
http://www.springer.com/692

Mark J. van der Laan • Sherri Rose

Targeted Learning

Causal Inference for Observational and Experimental Data

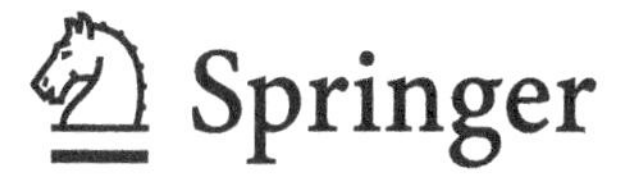

Mark J. van der Laan
Division of Biostatistics
University of California
Berkeley
Berkeley California
USA
laan@berkeley.edu

Sherri Rose
Division of Biostatistics
University of California
Berkeley
Berkeley California
USA
sherri@berkeley.edu

ISSN 0172-7397
ISBN 978-1-4419-9781-4 e-ISBN 978-1-4419-9782-1
DOI 10.1007/978-1-4419-9782-1
Springer New York Dordrecht Heidelberg London

Library of Congress Control Number: 2011930854

Printed on acid-free paper

Springer is part of Springer Science+Business Media (www.springer.com)

To Martine, Laura, Lars, and Robin
To Burke, Pop-pop, Grandpa, and Adrienne

Foreword

Targeted Learning, by Mark J. van der Laan and Sherri Rose, fills a much needed gap in statistical and causal inference. It protects us from wasting computational, analytical, and data resources on irrelevant aspects of a problem and teaches us how to focus on what is relevant – answering questions that researchers truly care about.

The idea of targeted learning has its roots in the early days of econometrics, when Jacob Marschak (1953) made an insightful observation regarding policy questions and structural equation modeling (SEM). While most of his colleagues on the Cowles Commission were busy estimating each and every parameter in their economic models, some using maximum likelihood and some least squares regression, Marschak noted that the answers to many policy questions did not require such detailed knowledge – a combination of parameters is all that is necessary and, moreover, it is often possible to identify the desired combination without identifying the individual components. Heckman (2000) called this observation "Marschak's Maxim" and has stressed its importance in the current debate between experimentalists and structural economists (Heckman 2010). Today we know that Marschak's Maxim goes even further – the desired quantity can often be identified without ever specifying the functional or distributional forms of these economic models.

Until quite recently, however, Marschak's idea has not attracted the attention it deserves. For statisticians, the very idea of defining a target quantity not as a property of a statistical model but by a policy question must have sounded mighty peculiar, if not heretical. Recall that policy questions, and in fact most questions of interest to empirical researchers, invoke causal vocabulary laden with notions such as "what if," "effect of," "why did," "control," "explain," "intervention," "confounding," and more. This vocabulary was purged from the grammar of statistics by Karl Pearson (1911), an act of painful consequences that has prevented most data-driven researchers from specifying mathematically the quantities they truly wish to be targeted. Understandably, seeing no point in estimating quantities they could not define, statisticians showed no interest in Marschak's Maxim.

Later on, in the period 1970–1980, when Donald Rubin (1974) popularized and expanded the potential-outcome notation of Neyman (1923) and others and causal vocabulary ascended to a semilegitimate status in statistics, Marschak's Maxim met with yet another, no less formidable, hurdle. Rubin's potential-outcome vocabulary, while powerful and flexible for capturing most policy questions of interest, turned out to be rather inept for capturing substantive knowledge of the kind carried by structural equation models. Yet this knowledge is absolutely necessary for turning targeted questions into estimable quantities. The opaque language of "ignorability," "treatment assignment," and "missing data" that has ruled (and still rules) the potential-outcome paradigm is not flexible enough to specify transparently even the most elementary models (say, a three-variable Markov chain) that experimenters wish to hypothesize. Naturally, this language could not offer Marschak's Maxim a fertile ground to develop because the target questions, though well formulated mathematically, could not be related to ordinary understanding of data-generating processes.

Econometricians, for their part, had their own reasons for keeping Marschak's Maxim at bay. Deeply entrenched in the quicksands of parametric thinking, econometricians found it extremely difficult to elevate targeted quantities such as policy effects, traditionally written as sums of products of coefficients, to a standalone status, totally independent of their component parts. It is only through nonparametric analysis, where targeted quantities are defined procedurally by transformational operations on a model (as in $P(y \mid do(x))$; Pearl 2009), and parameters literally disappear from existence, that Marschak's Maxim of focusing on the whole without its parts has achieved its full realization.

The departure from parametric thinking was particularly hard for researchers who did not deploy diagrams in their toolkit. Today, as shown in Chap. 2 of this book, students of graphical models can glance at a structural equation model and determine within seconds whether a given causal effect is identified while paying no attention to the individual parameters that make up that effect. Likewise, these students can write down an answer to a policy question (if identified) directly in terms of probability distributions, without ever mentioning the model parameters. Jacob Marschak, whom I had the great fortune of befriending a few years before his death (1977), would have welcomed this capability with open arms and his usual youthful enthusiasm, for it embodies the ultimate culmination of his maxim in algorithmic clarity.

Unfortunately, many economists and SEM researchers today are still not versed in graphical tools, and, consequently, even authors who purport to be doing nonparametric analysis (e.g., Heckman 2010) are unable to fully exploit the potentials of Marschak's Maxim. Lacking the benefits of graphical models, nonparametric researchers have difficulties locating instrumental variables in a system of equations, recognizing the testable implications of such systems, deciding if two such systems are equivalent, if two counterfactuals are independent given another, whether a set of measurements will reduce bias, and, most importantly, reading the causal and counterfactual information that such systems convey (Pearl 2009, pp. 374–380).

Targeted learning aims to fill this gap. It is presented in this book as a natural extension to the theory of structural causal models (SCMs) that I introduced in Pearl (1995) and then in Chaps. 3 and 7 of my book *Causality* (Pearl 2009). It is a simple and friendly theory, truly nonparametric, yet it subsumes and unifies the potential outcome framework, graphical models, and structural equation modeling in one mathematical object. The match is perfect.

I will end this foreword with a description of a brief encounter I recently had with another area in dire need of targeted learning. I am referring to the analysis of mediation, also known as "effect decomposition" or "direct and indirect effects" (Robins and Greenland 1992; Pearl 2001).

The decomposition of effects into their direct and indirect components is of both theoretical and practical importance, the former because it tells us "how nature works" and the latter because it enables us to predict behavior under a rich variety of conditions and interventions. For example, an investigator may be interested in assessing the extent to which an effect of a given exposure can be reduced by weakening one specific intermediate process between exposure and outcome. The portion of the effect mediated by that specific process should then become the target question for mediation analysis.

Despite its ubiquity, the analysis of mediation has long been a thorny issue in the social and behavioral sciences (Baron and Kenny 1986; MacKinnon 2008) primarily because the distinction between causal parameters and their regressional surrogates have too often been conflated. The difficulties were amplified in nonlinear models, where interactions between pathways further obscure their distinction. As demands grew to tackle problems involving categorical variables and nonlinear interactions, researchers could no longer define direct and indirect effects in terms of sums or products of structural coefficients, and all attempts to extend the linear paradigms of effect decomposition to nonlinear systems, using logistic and probit regression, produced distorted results (MacKinnon et al. 2007). The problem was not one of estimating the large number of parameters involved but that of combining them correctly to capture what investigators mean by direct or indirect effect (forthcoming, Pearl 2011).

Fortunately, nonparametric analysis permits us to define the target quantity in a way that reflects its actual usage in decision-making applications. For example, if our interest lies in the fraction of cases for which mediation was *sufficient* for the response, we can pose that very fraction as our target question, whereas if our interest lies in the fraction of responses for which mediation was *necessary*, we would pose this fraction as our target question. In both cases we can dispose of parametric analysis altogether and ask under what conditions the target question can be identified/estimated from observational or experimental data.

Taking seriously this philosophy of "define first, identify second, estimate last" one can derive graphical conditions under which direct and indirect effects can be identified (Pearl 2001), and these conditions yield (in the case of no unmeasured confounders) simple probability estimands, called mediation formulas (Pearl 2010b), that capture the effects of interest. The mediation formulas are applicable to both continuous and categorical variables, linear as well as nonlinear interactions, and, moreover, they can consistently be estimated from the data.

The derivation of the mediation formulas teaches us two lessons in targeted learning. First, when questions are posed directly in terms of the actual causal relations of interest, simple probability estimands can be derived while skipping the painful exercise of estimating dozens of nonlinear parameters and then worrying about how to combine them to answer the original question.

Second, and this is where targeted learning comes back to parametric analysis, the expressions provided by the mediation formulas may demand a new parameterization, unrelated to the causal process underlying the mediation problem. It is this new set of parameters, then, that need to be optimized over while posing the estimation accuracy of the mediation formula itself as the objective function in the maximum likelihood optimization. Indeed, in many cases the structure and dimensionality of the mediation formula would dictate the proper shaping of this reparametrization, regardless of how intricate the multivariate nonlinear process is that actually generates the data.

I am very pleased to see the SCM serving as a language to demonstrate the workings of targeted learning, and I am hopeful that readers will appreciate both the transparency of the model and the power of the approach.

Los Angeles, January 2011 *Judea Pearl*

Foreword

Mark J. van der Laan and Sherri Rose both describe their "journey" to this wonderful book in their preface. As an epidemiologist, I too have a journey with respect to this book. In 2001, I approached Mark about collaborating with me on a very difficult project. I brought with me my applied training in "traditional" statistical applications that I had learned as a master's student and over many years as a practicing epidemiologist. During our discussions, Mark opened up a new world for me regarding how one uses statistical methods to answer causal questions. I have spent the years since then continuing to collaborate with Mark on questions related to the epidemiology of aging and the effects of air pollution on children's respiratory health. I have learned a great deal (conditioned, of course, by my somewhat limited background in formal mathematics and statistics) about these approaches and their tremendous value as tools for the formulation of hypotheses and the design and analysis of observational data. My collaboration with Mark has radically changed my approach to teaching master's and doctoral students in epidemiology about the theoretical concepts related to epidemiological studies and their analysis.

Having made this journey myself along with many of my students, I want to share some of my excitement about this book with scientists from all disciplines who conduct studies in the hopes that many of them will use this book to take a journey of their own.

For those who are faint of heart when it comes to more in-depth biostatistical treatises, do not fear; the authors' clear writing and extremely helpful examples will carry you along the way or allow you to skip over fine details without missing the forest for the trees. What I have tried to do in this foreword is to provide a preview to each introductory chapter in the hopes that these previews will stimulate the reader's interest in seeing what van der Laan and Rose have to say.

To quote the authors, Chap. 1 *"was intended to motivate the need for causal inference, highlight the troublesome nature of the traditional approach to effect estimation, and introduce important concepts such as the data, model, and target parameter.*" They have achieved their goal with clear exposition, easily understood examples, and well-defined notation. The chapter should be accessible to anyone with a basic course in biostatistics and some practical experience. The case for an alternative approach to traditional parametric statistical models and modeling has a strong logic behind it, and the reader is primed to open herself to learning how to see things in a different light. That light has three important elements. (1) Those who carry out observational studies need to be absolutely clear about what they actually know about the distributions that generate their observed data. (2) Statistical models, at their heart, are models for the true data-generating distribution that produced the observed data. (3) The parameters of interest in observational studies are not simply the regression coefficients in front of an exposure (or treatment) variable; instead, they are expressions of a specific research question.

Chapter 2 takes the reader from nonparametric structural equation models through counterfactuals, the definition of the parameter of interest, and the problem of estimation. It asks more of the nonstatistician reader than does Chap. 1: (1) familiarity with basic concepts of causal graphs, although this is not absolute, since the basic concepts are presented in a lucid but abbreviated manner; and (2) patience to stick with the notation and the logic that is built into it. If the reader brings these requisites, particularly the second one, the presentation is logical and lucid, with simple examples to guide the way. It is easy to miss the forest for the trees in the chapter on the first read; therefore, several reads will be needed. For those who have patience for only one read, several important messages are encoded in the jargon; look for them. (1) Uncertainty (unmeasured or mismeasured exogenous variables, also known as unmeasured confounders) is integral to the data-generating distribution and all attempts to define a parameter of interest must be prepared to make assumptions of more or less strength about them. (2) "Models" are statistical models augmented with nontestable assumptions that encode assumptions that make identifiability possible. (3) Target parameters can have statistical and causal interpretations, the major distinction being that causal interpretations are based on models that must encode some untestable assumptions. One brief comment for nonstatisticians, particularly epidemiologists: failure of the positivity assumption across any stratum of covariates makes statistical (and thereby causal) inference a fantasy. Pay close attention!

"Since a parametric statistical model is wrong...we want an estimator that is able to learn from the data using the true knowledge represented by the actual statistical model..." for the unknown data-generating distribution. So begins Chap. 3 and the exploration of "super learning." However, how are we to know which estimator to use a priori? This chapter takes the reader through the answers to a series of questions related to how we find the "best" estimator of the true target parameter, given our limited knowledge about the true data-generating distribution for our data as represented by the statistical model. The questions are simple and the answers complicated. However, the concept is clear: Having defined our data, model and target parameter, we need to "learn" from our data what the *"maximally unbiased and semiparametric efficient normally distributed estimator"* of our target parameter is. What do van der Laan and Rose mean by "learn" from the data, and what is a

super learner? “Learning,” in this context, is being open to the possibility that your favorite parametric model (e.g., logistic regression), or semiparametric model in the more frequent use of the term (e.g., Cox proportional hazards model), just does not represent any of the possible data-generating distributions from which your data could have been derived. In other words, you made a bad guess! “Learning” is the process that attempts to provide the best estimate of our target parameter from a library of guesses. What is the best? It is the estimator that is closest to that which we would have derived had we known the true data-generating distribution. What is the library of guesses? It is the collection of “models” that we think might be consistent with the true data-generating function. What is the super learner? It is the loss-function-based tool that allows us to obtain the best prediction of our target parameter based on a weighted average of our guesses. Thus, we “learn” what our data have to say about this parameter based on the true knowledge that we have about the data and any causal assumptions that we made to assure identifiability!

Chapter 4 provides an introduction to targeted maximum likelihood estimators (TMLEs). The key message is that a TMLE is a semiparametric method that provides an optimal tradeoff between bias and variance in the estimation of the target parameter (e.g., difference between treated and untreated in the example in the chapter). The introductory material of the chapter expresses these ideas clearly and concisely. The highlight of the chapter is Sect. 4.2, which is a step-by-step example based on real data that illustrates the TMLE. The example is linked to the more detailed theoretical presentation in the next chapter. The sections on the TMLE in randomized controlled trials and observational studies are particularly relevant for epidemiologists. Chapter 5 provides the theoretical support for the implementation described in Chap. 4 and really is targeted at statisticians. Nonstatisticians will just need to follow along, perhaps reading only the gray summary boxes, to get the general idea.

Chapter 6 provides comparisons between TMLEs and other estimators. Some of the material requires statistical knowledge that is beyond many epidemiologists. However, the tables provide summaries that contain the take-away messages. The conclusions about the desirability of unbiased efficient estimators is obvious. However, the authors highlight one important property of the TMLE that is particularly desirable – good performance with respect to bias and efficiency in finite samples.

The remaining chapters in the book delve into additional data structures, parameters, and methodological extensions of the TMLE. You may wish to jump immediately to the chapters relevant to your work, such as case-control data, genomics, censored data, or longitudinal data, once you have a firm understanding of the core material presented in Part I. Readers who plan to implement these methods will benefit from reading all of the chapters in Part II, which include: continuous outcomes, direct effects, marginal structural models, and the positivity assumption. However, there are two chapters that warrant careful reading by everyone. Chapter 8 deals with estimation of direct effects when covariates are hypothesized as causal intermediates and distinguishes the assumptions for this estimation from the situation where covariates are considered confounders. The key concepts are found in the gray box at the end of Sect. 8.2 and the first paragraph of the discussion. Investigators who carry out observational studies need to pay special heed to these concepts. Chapter 10 deals with the concept of positivity – the concept, to quote the authors, that *"[t]he identifiability of causal effects requires sufficient variability in treatment or exposure assignment within strata of confounders."* This is a concept that is all but ignored in most published epidemiologic studies. The introductory material states the issues clearly and identifies the choices one has when faced with this problem. This chapter provides methods to address the problem and is a must read!

In summary, this book should be on the shelf of every investigator who conducts observational research and randomized controlled trials. The concepts and methodology are foundational for causal inference and at the same time stay true to what the data at hand can say about the questions that motivate their collection. The methods presented provide the tools to remain faithful to the data while providing minimally biased and efficient estimators of the parameters of interest. To my epidemiologic colleagues, the message is: the parameters of exposure that interest us are not simply regression coefficients derived from statistical models whose relevance to the data-generating distribution is unknown! This book really does provide *super learning*!

Berkeley, January 2011 *Ira B. Tager*

Preface

The statistics profession is at a unique point in history. The need for valid statistical tools is greater than ever; data sets are massive, often measuring hundreds of thousands of measurements for a single subject. The field is ready for a revolution, one driven by clear, objective benchmarks under which tools can be evaluated.

Statisticians must be ready to take on this challenge. They have to be dynamic and thoroughly trained in statistical concepts. More than ever, statisticians need to work effectively in interdisciplinary teams and understand the immense importance of objective benchmarks to evaluate statistical tools developed to learn from data. They have to produce energetic leaders who stick to a thorough a priori road map, and who also break with current practice when necessary.

Why do we need a revolution? Can we not keep doing what we have been doing? Sadly, nearly all data analyses are based on the application of so-called parametric (or other restrictive) statistical models that assume the data-generating distributions have specific forms. Many agree that these statistical models are wrong. That is, everybody knows that linear or logistic regression in parametric statistical models and Cox proportional hazards models are specified incorrectly. In the early 1900s, when R.A. Fisher developed maximum likelihood estimation, these parametric statistical models were suitable since the data structures were very low dimensional. Therefore, saturated parametric statistical models could be applied. However, today statisticians still use these models to draw conclusions in high-dimensional data and then hope these conclusions are not too wrong.

It is too easy to state that using methods we know are wrong is an acceptable practice: it is not!

The original purpose of a statistical model is to develop a set of realistic assumptions about the probability distribution generating the data (i.e., incorporating background knowledge). However, in practice, restrictive parametric statistical models are essentially always used because standard software is available. These statistical models also allow the user to obtain p-values and confidence intervals for the target parameter of the probability distribution, which are desired to make sense out of data. Unfortunately, these measures of uncertainty are even more susceptible to bias than the effect estimator. We know that for large enough sample sizes, every study, including one in which the null hypothesis of no effect is true, will declare a statistically significant effect.

Some practitioners will tell you that they have extensive training, that they are experts in applying these tools and should be allowed to choose the statistical models to use in response to the data. Be alarmed! It is no accident that the chess computer beats the world chess champion. Humans are not as good at learning from data and are easily susceptible to beliefs about the data.

For example, an investigator may be convinced that the probability of having a heart attack has a particular functional form – a function of the dose of the studied drug and characteristics of the sampled subject. However, if you bring in another expert, his or her belief about the functional form may differ. Or, many statistical model fits may be considered, dropping variables that are nonsignificant, resulting in a particular selection of a statistical model fit. Ignoring this selection process, which is common, leaves us with faulty inference.

With high-dimensional data, not only is the correct specification of the parametric statistical model an impossible challenge, but the complexity of the parametric statistical model also may increase to the point that there are more unknown parameters than observations. The true functional form also might be described by a complex function not easily approximated by main terms.

For these reasons, allowing humans to include only their true, realistic knowledge (e.g., treatment is randomized, such as in a randomized controlled trial, and our data set represents n independent and identically distributed observations of a random variable) is essential. That is, instead of assuming misspecified parametric or heavily restrictive semiparametric statistical models, and viewing the (regression) coefficients in these statistical models as the target parameters of interest, we need to define the statistical estimation problem in terms of nonparametric or semiparametric statistical models that represent realistic knowledge, and in addition we must define the target parameter as a particular function of the true probability distribution of the data. This changes the game in a dramatic way relative to current practice; one starts thinking about real knowledge in terms of the underlying experiment that generated the data set and what the real questions of interest are in terms of a feature of the data-generating probability distribution.

The concept of a statistical model is very important, but we need to go back to its true meaning. We need to be able to incorporate true knowledge in an effective way. In addition, we need to develop and use data-adaptive tools for all parameters of the data-generating distribution, including parameters targeting causal effects of interventions on the system underlying the data-generating experiment. The latter typically represent our real interest. We are not only trying to sensibly observe, but also to learn how the world operates.

What about machine learning, which is concerned with the development of blackbox algorithms that map data (and few assumptions) into a desired object? For example, an important topic in machine learning is prediction. Here the goal is to map the data, consisting of multiple records with a list of input variables and an output variable, into a prediction function that can be used to map a new set of input variables into a predicted outcome. Indeed, this is in sharp contrast to using misspecified parametric statistical models. However, the goal is often a whole prediction function, and the machines are tailored to fit this whole prediction function. As a consequence, these methods are too biased (and not grounded by efficiency theory) for a particular effect of interest. Typical complexities in the data such as missingness or censoring have also received little attention in machine learning. In addition, statistical inference in terms of assessment of uncertainty (e.g., confidence intervals) is typically lacking in this field.

Even in machine learning there is often unsupported devotion to beliefs, in this case, to the belief that certain algorithms are superior. No single algorithm (e.g., random forests, support vector machines, etc.) will always outperform all others in all data types, or even within specific data types (e.g., SNP data from genomewide association studies). One cannot know a priori which algorithm to choose. It's like picking the student who gets the top grade in a course on the first day of class.

The tools we develop must be grounded in theory, such as an optimality theory, that shows certain methods are more optimal than others and, in addition, should be evaluated with objective benchmark simulation studies. For example, one can compare methods based on mean squared error with respect to the truth. It is not enough to have tools that use the data to fit the truth well. We also require an assessment of uncertainty (e.g., confidence intervals), the very backbone of statistical learning. That is, we cannot give up on the reliable assessment of uncertainty in our estimates.

Examples of new methodological directions in statistical learning satisfying these requirements include (1) the full generalization and utilization of cross-validation as an estimator selection tool so that the subjective choices made by humans are now made by the machine and (2) targeting the fitting of the probability distribution of the data toward the target parameter so that the mean squared error of the substitution estimator of the target parameter with respect to the target parameter is optimized. Important and exciting statistical research areas where new developments are taking place in response to the nonvalidity of the previous generation of tools are: adaptive designs in clinical trials and observational studies, multiple and group sequential testing, causal inference, and Bayesian learning in realistic semiparametric statistical models, among others.

Statisticians cannot be afraid to go against standard practice. Remaining open to, interested in, and a developer of newer, sounder methodology is perhaps the one key thing each statistician can do. We must all continue learning, questioning, and adapting as new statistical challenges are presented.

The science of learning from data (i.e., statistics) is arguably the most beautiful and inspiring field – one in which we try to understand the very essence of human beings. However, we should stop fooling ourselves and actually design and develop powerful machines and statistical tools that can carry out specific learning tasks. There is no better time to make a truly meaningful difference.[1]

[1] A version of this content originally appeared in the September 2010 issue of *Amstat News*, the membership magazine of the American Statistical Association (van der Laan and Rose 2010).

The Journey

Mark: I view targeted maximum likelihood estimation (TMLE), presented in this book, as the result of a long journey, starting with my Ph.D. research up to now. We hope that the following succinct summary of this path towards a general toolbox for statistical learning from data will provide the reader with useful perspective and understanding.

During my Ph.D. work (1990–1993) under the guidance of Dr. Richard Gill, I worked on the theoretical understanding of the maximum likelihood estimator for semiparametric statistical models, with a focus on the nonparametric maximum likelihood estimator of the bivariate survival distribution function for bivariate right-censored survival times and a nonparametric statistical model for the data-generating distribution. This challenging bivariate survival function estimation problem demonstrated that the nonparametric maximum likelihood estimator easily fails to be uniquely defined, or fails to approximate the true data-generating distribution for large sample sizes. That is, for realistic statistical models for the data-generating distribution, and even for relatively low-dimensional data structures, the maximum likelihood estimator is often ill defined and inconsistent for target parameters, and regularization through smoothing or stratification is necessary to repair it. It also demonstrated that, for larger dimensional data structures, the repair of maximum likelihood estimation in nonparametric statistical models through smoothing comes at an unacceptable price with respect to finite sample performance.

Right after completing my Ph.D., I met Dr. James M. Robins, whose research focused on estimation with censored data and, in particular, estimation of causal effects of time-dependent treatment regimens on an outcome of interest based on observing replicates of high-dimensional longitudinal data structures in the presence of informative missingness and dropout and time-dependent confounding of the treatment. This was an immensely exciting time, and a whole new world opened up for me. Instead of working on toy extractions of real-world problems, Robins and his colleagues worked on solving the actual estimation problems as they occur in practice, avoiding convenient simplifications or assumptions. The work of Robins' group made clear that statistical learning was far beyond the world of standard software and the corresponding practice of statistics based on restrictive parametric statistical models, and also far beyond the world of maximum likelihood estimation for semiparametric statistical models.

Concepts such as coarsening at random, orthogonal complement of the nuisance tangent space of a target parameter, estimating functions for the target parameter implied by the latter, double robustness of these estimating functions and their corresponding estimators, locally efficient estimators of the target parameter, and so on, became part of my language. As a crown on our collaborations, in 2003 we wrote a book called *Unified Methods for Censored Longitudinal Data and Causality*. This book provided a comprehensive treatment of the estimating equation methodology for estimation of target parameters of the data-generating distribution in semiparametric statistical models, demonstrated on complex censored and longitudinal (causal inference) data structures.

From a person trying to repair maximum likelihood estimation, I had become a proponent for estimating equation methodology, a methodology that targets the parameter of interest instead of the maximum likelihood estimation methodology, which aims to estimate the whole distribution of the data. When writing the book in 2003, some nonnatural hurdles occurred and we proposed no solutions for them. To start with, the optimal estimating function for the target parameter might not exist since the efficient influence curve, though a function of the distribution of the data on the unit, cannot necessarily be represented as an (estimating) function in the target parameter of interest and a variation-independent nuisance parameter. If we ignored this first hurdle, we were still left with the following hurdles. Estimators defined by a solution of an estimating equation (1) might not exist, (2) might be nonunique due to the existence of multiple solutions, (3) are not substitution estimators and thus do not respect known statistical model constraints, and (4) are sensitive to how the nuisance parameter (that the estimating function depends on) is estimated, while a good fit of the nuisance parameter itself is not a good measure for its role in the mean squared error of the estimator of the target parameter.

These hurdles, which also affect the practical performance and robustness of the estimators, made it impossible to push this impressive estimating equation methodology forward as a general statistical tool to replace current practice. It made me move back towards substitution estimators using methods based on maximizing or minimizing an empirical criterion such as the maximum likelihood estimator, and plugging in the resulting estimator in the target parameter mapping that maps a probability distribution of the data into the desired target parameter.

Specifically, additional research we conducted in 2003 proposed a unified loss-based learning methodology (van der Laan and Dudoit 2003). The methodology was based on defining a (typically infinite-dimensional) parameter of the probability distribution of the data as a minimizer of the expectation of a loss function (e.g., log-likelihood or squared error loss function) and the aggressive utilization of cross-validation as a tool to select among candidate estimators. The loss function for the desired part of the probability distribution of the data was also allowed to be indexed by an unknown nuisance parameter, thereby making this methodology very general, including prediction or density estimation based on general censored data structures.

The general theoretical optimality result for the cross-validation selector among candidate estimators generated a new concept called "loss-based super learning," which is a general system for fitting an infinite-dimensional parameter of the probability distribution of the data that allows one to map a very large library of candidate estimators into a new improved estimator. It made it clear that, given some global bounds on the semiparametric statistical model, humans should not choose the estimation procedure for fitting the probability distribution of the data, or a relevant part thereof, but an a priori defined estimator (i.e., the super learner) should fully utilize the data to make sound informed choices based on cross-validation. That is, the theory of super learning allows us to build machines that remove human intervention as much as possible.

Even though the theory teaches us that the super learner of the probability distribution does make the optimal bias–variance tradeoff with respect to the probability distribution as a whole (i.e., with respect to the dissimilarity between the super learner and the truth, as implied by the loss function), it is too biased for low-dimensional target features of the probability distribution, such as an effect of a variable/treatment/exposure on an outcome. The super learner is instructed to do well estimating the probability distribution, but the super learner was not told that it was going to be used to evaluate a one-dimensional feature of the probability distribution such as an effect of a treatment. As a consequence, the substitution estimator of a target parameter obtained by plugging in the super learner into the target parameter mapping is too biased.

By definition of an efficient estimator, it was clear that the efficient influence curve needed to play a role for these substitution estimators to become less biased and thereby asymptotically linear and efficient estimators of the target parameter. But how? The current literature on efficient estimation had used the efficient influence curve as an estimating function (van der Laan and Robins 2003), and one either completely solved the corresponding estimating equation or one used the first step of the Newton–Raphson method for solving the estimating equation (e.g., Bickel et al. 1997) in case one already had a root-n-consistent initial estimator available. A new way of utilizing the efficient influence curve within the framework of loss-based learning needed to be determined.

The super learner had to be modified so that its excess bias was removed. The idea of the two-stage targeted maximum likelihood estimator was born: (1) use, for example, the super learner as the initial estimator, (2) propose a clever parametric statistical working model through the super learner, providing a family of candidate fluctuations of the super learner and treating the super learner as fixed offset, (3) choose the fluctuation that maximizes the likelihood (or whatever loss function was used for the super learner), and (4) iterate so that the resulting modified super learner solves the efficient influence curve estimating equation. This resulted in the original TMLE paper with Daniel B. Rubin (van der Laan and Rubin 2006), which provides a general recipe for defining a TMLE for any given data structure, semiparametric statistical model for the probability distribution, and target parameter mapping, and thereby served as the basis of this book.

TMLEs can also be represented as loss-based learning. Here, the loss function is defined as a targeted version of the loss function used by the initial estimator, where the nuisance parameter of this targeted loss function plays the role of the unknown fluctuation parameters in the TMLE steps. TMLEs are a special case of loss-based learning.

TMLEs solved the above mentioned remaining issues that the estimating equation methodology suffered from: a TMLE does not require that the efficient influence curve be an estimating function, a TMLE solves the efficient influence curve estimating equation but is not defined by it (just like a maximum likelihood estimator solves a score equation but is uniquely defined as a maximum of the log-likelihood), a TMLE is a substitution estimator and thus respects the global constraints of the statistical model, a TMLE naturally integrates loss-based super learning (i.e., generalized machine learning based on cross-validation) and can utilize the same loss function to select among different TMLEs indexed by different nuisance parameter estimators that are needed to carry out the targeting update step. That is, even the choice of nuisance parameter estimator can now be tailored toward the target parameter of interest (van der Laan and Gruber 2010). Finally, under conditions that allow efficient estimation of the target parameter, a TMLE is an asymptotically efficient substitution estimator. □

Sherri: My methodological contributions have largely focused on adapting TMLE for case-control studies. Additionally, I've spent significant time with Mark formulating a general framework for teaching TMLE, with comprehensive notation and language, in a way that is accessible for researchers and students in fields such as epidemiology.

I received my B.S. in statistics in 2005 with the goal of going to graduate school for a career in medical research. Thus, I thought this meant I would be an "applied" statistician using existing tools. Then I took one of Mark's upper division courses during the first year of my Ph.D. program at UC Berkeley. Even though I didn't immediately understand all of the technical aspects of what he was teaching, the concepts made complete sense. I contacted him and projects took off immediately.

My point in this addendum to Mark's journey is that you need not be a fully trained theoretical statistician to start understanding and using these methods. The work is driven by real-world problems, and thus is immediately applicable in practice. It is *theoretical* because new methods needed to be developed based on efficiency theory, but it is also very *applied*. You see this in the many examples that permeate this text. We don't present anything that isn't based on a real data set that we've encountered. In short, this book is not meant to sit on a shelf. □

The book: The book itself also went through a journey of its own. We started seriously writing for the book in January 2010 and for many months went back and forth debating the level we were trying to target. Should we generate a textbook that was more like an epidemiology text and would be broadly accessible to a greater number of applied readers with less formal statistical training? Should we develop a purely theoretical text that would mostly be of interest to a certain subset of statisticians? Ultimately, we struck a level that is somewhere in between these two extremes. Since there is no other book on targeted learning, we could not escape the inclusion of statistical formalism. However, we also did not want to lose all accessibility for nontheoreticians.

This led to a book that begins with six chapters that should be generally readable by most applied researchers familiar with basic statistical concepts and traditional data analysis. That is not to say many topics won't be new and challenging, but these chapters are peppered with intuition and explanations to help readers along. The book progresses to more challenging topics and data structures, and follows a recognizable pattern via a road map for targeted learning and the general description of each targeted estimator. Thus, applied readers less interested in *why* it works and more interested in implementation can tease out those parts. Yet, mathematicians and theoretical statisticians will not get bored, as extensive rigor is included in many chapters, as well as a detailed appendix containing proofs and derivations.

Lastly, this book is unique in that it also contains wonderful contributions from multiple invited authors, yet it is not a traditional edited text. As the authors of *Targeted Learning*, we have spent significant time crafting and reworking each of the contributed chapters to have consistent style, content, format, and notation as well as a familiar road map. This yields a truly cohesive book that reads easily as one text. □

Intended Readership

We imagine a vast number of readers will be graduate students and researchers in statistics, biostatistics, and mathematics. This book was also written with epidemiologists, medical doctors, social scientists, and other applied researchers in mind. The first six chapters of the book, which comprise Part I, are a complete introduction to super learning and TMLE, including related concepts necessary to understand and apply these methods. Part I is designed to be accessible on many levels, and chapters that deal with more advanced statistical concepts feature guides that direct the reader to key information if they'd rather skip certain details. Additionally, these chapters could easily be used for a one-semester introductory course. The remaining chapters can be digested in any order that is useful to the reader, although we attempted to order them according to ease and subject matter. Parts II–IX handle more complex data structures and topics, but applied researchers will immediately recognize these data problems from their own research (e.g., continuous outcomes, case-control studies, time-dependent covariates, HIV data structures).

Outline

Introduction. The book begins with an introduction written by Richard J.C.M. Starmans titled "Models, Inference, and Truth: Probabilistic Reasoning in the Information Era." This introduction puts the present state of affairs in statistical data analyis in a historical and philosophical perspective for the purpose of clarifying, understanding, and accounting for the current situation and to underline the relevance of topics addressed by TMLE for both the philosophy of statistics and the epistemology/philosophy of science. It identifies three major developments in the history of ideas that provide a context for the emergence of the probabilistic revolution and it discusses some important immanent developments in the history of statistics that have led to the current situation or at least may help to understand it.

Part I – Targeted Learning: The Basics

The chapters in Part I of the book can stand alone as material for a complete introductory course on super learning and TMLE in realistic nonparametric and semiparametric models. They cover essential information crucial to understanding this methodology, encapsulated in the convenient road map for targeted learning. We present in detail the TMLE of an additive causal effect of treatment on a binary or continuous outcome based on observing n independent and identically distributed random variables defined by the following type of experiment: randomly sample a subject from a population, measure baseline covariates, subsequently assign a treatment, and finally measure an outcome of interest. This TMLE is demonstrated in the estimation of the effect of vigorous exercise on survival in an elderly cohort.

Chapter 1. This chapter introduces the open problem of targeted statistical learning. We discuss, in general terms, the traditional approach to effect estimation as well as the concepts of data, data-generating distribution, model, and the target parameter of the data-generating distribution. We also motivate the need for estimators that are targeted and present the road map for targeted learning that will be explained in depth in Chaps. 2–5.

Chapter 2. In this chapter, readers will learn about structural causal models (SCMs), causal graphs, causal assumptions, counterfactuals, identifiability of the target parameter, and interpretations of the target parameter (i.e., causal or purely statistical). This material is essential background before moving on to the estimation steps in the road map for targeted learning. The chapter is based on the methods pioneered by Judea Pearl and are given thorough treatment in the recently published second edition of *Causality* (Pearl 2009).

Chapter 3. The first step in the TMLE is an initial estimate of the data-generating distribution P_0, or the relevant part Q_0 of P_0 that is needed to evaluate the target parameter. Estimation of Q_0 incorporating the flexible ensemble learner super learner is presented in this chapter. Cross-validation is an essential component of super learning and is also presented. Simulation studies and multiple data analysis examples illustrate the advantages of super learning.

Chapters 4 and 5. In these two chapters, the TMLE methodology is presented in detail, including a conceptual overview, implementation, and theory. TMLE is a two-step procedure where one first obtains an estimate of the relevant portion Q_0 of P_0. The second stage updates this initial fit in a step targeted toward making an optimal bias–variance tradeoff for the parameter of interest (i.e., target parameter), instead of the overall density P_0. It does this by proposing a parametric submodel through the initial fit of Q_0, and estimating the unknown parameter of this submodel that represents the amount of fluctuation of the initial fit. The submodel typically depends on a fit of a nuisance parameter such as a treatment or censoring mechanism. Finally, one evaluates the target parameter of this TMLE fit of Q_0, which is called the TMLE of the target parameter. The TMLE of the target parameter is double robust and can incorporate data-adaptive likelihood-based estimation procedures to estimate Q_0 and the nuisance parameter. Inference (i.e., confidence intervals) and interpretation are also explained, concluding the road map for targeted learning.

Chapter 6. The many attractive properties of TMLE include the fact that it produces well-defined, loss-based, consistent, efficient substitution estimators of the target parameter. These topics are explained in depth, and the TMLE is compared to other estimators of a target parameter of the data-generating distribution, with respect to these properties.

Part II – Additional Core Topics

Part II delves deeper into some core topics: the choice of submodel and loss function that defines the TMLE, causal parameters defined by marginal structural working models, and an in-depth coverage of methods dealing with violations of the positivity assumption. It focuses on experiments involving the measurement of baseline covariates, a treatment, possibly an intermediate random variable, and a final outcome.

Chapter 7. The TMLE of a parameter of a data-generating distribution, known to be an element of a semiparametric statistical model, involves constructing a parametric statistical working model through an initial density estimator with parameter ϵ representing an amount of fluctuation of the initial density estimator, where the score of this fluctuation model at $\epsilon = 0$ equals or spans the efficient influence curve/canonical gradient. The latter constraint can be satisfied by many parametric fluctuation models, since it represents only a local constraint of its behavior at zero fluctuation. However, it is very important that the fluctuations stay within the semiparametric statistical model for the observed data distribution, even if the parameter can be defined on fluctuations that fall outside the assumed observed data model. In particular, in the context of sparse data, a violation of this property can heavily affect the performance of the estimator. We demonstrate this in the context of estimation of a causal effect of a binary treatment on a continuous outcome that is bounded. It results in a TMLE that inherently respects known bounds and, consequently, is more robust in sparse data situations than the TMLE using a naive fluctuation model. The TMLE is based on a quasi-log-likelihood loss function and a logistic regression fluctuation model.

Chapter 8. In this chapter we consider estimation of a direct effect of treatment on an outcome in the presence of an intermediate variable. The causal model, the direct effect, the estimand defined by the identifiability result for the direct effect, and the TMLE of the target parameter are presented. As an illustration we estimate the direct effect of gender on salary in a gender-inequality study. It is shown that the same TMLE can be used to estimate the estimand defined by the identifiability result for the causal effect of a treatment on an outcome among the treated within an appropriate (different) causal model.

Chapter 9. One is often interested in assessing how the effect of a treatment is modified by some baseline covariates. For this purpose, we present marginal structural models that model the causal effect of treatment as a function of such effect modifiers. The TMLE of the unknown coefficients in the marginal structural model is presented. The marginal structural models are used as working models to define the desired effect modification parameters, so that they do not make unrealistic assumptions in the causal model and thereby on the data-generating distribution. As an example, we assess the effect of missing doses on virologic failure as a function of the number of months of past viral suppression in an HIV cohort.

Chapter 10. The estimand that is defined by the identifiability result for the causal quantity of interest defines the target parameter of the data-generating distribution. The definition of the estimand itself often requires a particular support condition, which is called the positivity assumption. For example, the estimand that defines the additive causal effect of treatment on an outcome is only defined if for each value of the covariates (representing the confounders) there is a positive probability on both treatment and control. This chapter provides an in-depth discussion of the positivity assumption, and the detrimental effect of the practical or theoretical violation of this assumption on the statistical inference, due to the sparse-data bias induced by this violation. In addition, this chapter presents a parametric bootstrap-based diagnostic tool that allows one to diagnose this sparse-data bias. Its performance is demonstrated on simulated data sets and in assessing the effect of a mutation in the HIV virus on drug resistance in an HIV data application. Finally, the chapter presents common approaches to dealing with positivity violations and concludes with the presentation of a systematic general approach.

Part III – TMLE and Parametric Regression in Randomized Controlled Trials

Part III still considers an experiment that generates baseline covariates, treatment, and a final outcome, as highlighted in Parts I and II, but it delves deeper into the special case where treatment is randomized. In this case, the TMLE is always consistent and asymptotically linear, thereby allowing the robust utilization of covariate information. We demonstrate that a TMLE that uses as initial estimator a maximum likelihood estimator according to a parametric regression model does not update the initial estimator, proving a remarkable robustness property of maximum likelihood estimation in randomized controlled trials (RCTs). In addition, we show how the fit of the parametric regression model (i.e., the initial estimator in the TMLE) can be optimized with respect to the asymptotic variance of the resulting TMLE, thereby guaranteeing improvement over existing practice.

Chapter 11. The TMLE of a causal effect of treatment on a continuous or binary outcome in an RCT is presented. It is shown that the TMLE can be based on a maximum likelihood estimator according to a generalized linear working model, where the maximum likelihood estimation fit is inputted in the target parameter mapping defined by the so-called g-formula for the desired causal effect.

Chapter 12. As in Chap. 11, the TMLE in this chapter is based on a parametric regression model, but the coefficients of the initial estimator in the TMLE are fitted so that the resulting TMLE has minimal asymptotic variance. This results in a TMLE that is guaranteed to outperform current practice (i.e., unadjusted estimator), even if the parametric model is heavily misspecified. Other estimators presented in the literature are also discussed, and a simulation study is used to evaluate the small sample performance of these estimators.

Part IV – Case-Control Studies

The data-generating experiment now involves an additional complexity called biased sampling. That is, one assumes the underlying experiment that randomly samples a unit from a target population, measures baseline characteristics, assigns a treatment/exposure, and measures a final binary outcome, but one samples from the conditional probability distribution, given the value of the binary outcome. One still wishes to assess the causal effect of treatment on the binary outcome for the target population. The TMLE of a causal effect of treatment on the binary outcome based on such case-control studies is presented. Matched case-control studies are considered as well. It is also shown how to apply super learning to risk prediction in a nested case-control study.

Chapter 13. Case-control study designs are frequently used in public health and medical research to assess potential risk factors for disease. These study designs are particularly attractive to investigators researching rare diseases, as they are able to sample known cases of disease, vs. following a large number of subjects and waiting for disease onset in a relatively small number of individuals. Our proposed case-control-weighted TMLE for case-control studies relies on knowledge of the true prevalence probability, or a reasonable estimate of this probability, to eliminate the bias of the case-control sampling design. We use the prevalence probability in case-control weights, and our case-control weighting scheme successfully maps the TMLE for a random sample into a method for case-control sampling.

Chapter 14. Individually matched case-control study designs are commonly implemented in the field of public health. While matching is intended to eliminate confounding, the main *potential* benefit of matching in case-control studies is a gain in efficiency. This chapter investigates the use of the case-control-weighted TMLE to estimate causal effects in matched case-control study designs. We compare the case-control-weighted TMLE in matched and unmatched designs in an effort to determine which design yields the most information about the causal effect. In many practical situations where a causal effect is the parameter of interest, researchers may be better served using an unmatched design.

Chapter 15. Using nested case-control data from a large Kaiser Permanente database, we generate a function for mortality risk prediction with super learning. The ensemble super learner for predicting death (risk score) outperformed all single algorithms in the collection of algorithms, although its performance was similar to several included algorithms. Super learner improved upon the worst algorithms by 17% with respect to estimated risk.

Part V – RCTs with Survival Outcomes

In Part V we consider the following experiment: one randomly samples a unit from a target population, measures baseline characteristics, randomly assigns a treatment, and follows the subject to the minimum of dropout, the time to event of interest, and time to the end of study. The dropout time is allowed to be affected by the baseline covariates. We present the TMLE of the causal effect of treatment on survival, and we also consider effect modification by discrete baseline factors.

Chapter 16. In most RCTs, the primary outcome is a time-to-event outcome that may not be observed due to dropout or end of follow-up. The dropout or right censoring time may depend on the baseline characteristics of the study subject. The TMLE of a causal effect of treatment on the survival function of such a time-to-event outcome requires estimation of the conditional failure time hazard as a function of time, treatment, and the baseline covariates. The super learner of this hazard function is presented and is demonstrated with a lung cancer RCT.

Chapter 17. The TMLE of a causal effect of treatment on a survival function in an RCT is presented. This requires an update of the initial estimator of the conditional hazard function (e.g., super learner), where the update relies on an estimator of the right censoring mechanism and the treatment assignment mechanism (where the latter is known in an RCT). The statistical properties of the TMLE are discussed showing that it provides a superior alternative to current practice in terms of unadjusted Cox proportional hazards estimators or multiple imputation (maximum likelihood estimation)-based estimators.

Chapter 18. It is often of interest to assess if the causal effect of treatment on survival is modified by some baseline factors. In this chapter, we define the appropriate causal model and the target parameters that quantify effect modification by a discrete baseline factor. We present the TMLE of these effect modification parameters. The TMLE is demonstrated on an HIV clinical trial to assess effect modification by gender and by baseline CD4 in an HIV study. The results are contrasted with current practice, demonstrating the great utility of targeted learning.

Part VI – C-TMLE

Collaborative TMLE (C-TMLE) provides a further advance within the framework of TMLE by tailoring the fit of the nuisance parameter required in the TMLE-step for the purpose of the resulting TMLE of the target parameter. That is, the C-TMLE introduces another level of targeting beyond a regular TMLE. This part demonstrates the C-TMLE for the causal effect of treatment on an outcome, including time-to-event outcomes that are subject to right censoring. Simulation studies as well as data analyses are provided to demonstrate the practical utility of C-TMLE.

Chapter 19. The C-TMLE of the additive causal effect of treatment on an outcome is presented, allowing an a priori-specified algorithm to decide what covariates to include in the treatment mechanism fit, where the decisions are based on a loss-function that measures the fit of the corresponding TMLE instead of the fit of the treatment mechanism itself. The TMLE and C-TMLE are compared in simulation studies. The C-TMLE is also applied to assess the effect of all mutations in the HIV virus on drug-resistance, controlling for the history of the patient, dealing with the many strong correlations between mutations resulting in practical violations of the positivity assumption.

Chapter 20. The C-TMLE of the causal effect of treatment on a survival time that is subject to right censoring is developed. A simulation study is used to evaluate its practical performance in the context of different degrees of violation of the positivity assumption.

Chapter 21. This chapter uses simulation studies proposed in the literature to evaluate a variety of estimators for estimating the mean of an outcome under missingness, and the additive effect of treatment when treatment is affected (i.e., confounded) by baseline covariates. These simulations are tailored to result in serious practical violations of the positivity assumption, causing a lot of instability and challenges for double robust efficient estimators such as the TMLE. These simulations have been extensively debated in the literature. This chapter includes TMLE and C-TMLE in the debate. We contrast the C-TMLE to the TMLE and other estimators, showing that the C-TMLE is able to deal with sparsity (i.e., violations of positivity) in a sensible and robust way, while still preserving the optimal asymptotic properties of TMLE.

Part VII – Genomics

In Part VII we consider the experiment in which one randomly samples a unit from a target population, one measures a whole genomic profile on the unit, beyond other baseline characteristics, one possibly measures a treatment, and one measures a final outcome. In such studies one is often interested in assessing the effect of each genomic variable on the outcome or on the effect of the treatment. TMLE targets the effect of each genomic variable separately, contrary to current practice in variable importance analysis. These genomic variables are often continuous, so that one needs to define an effect of a continuous marker on the outcome of interest. For that purpose we employ semiparametric regression models. The TMLE of the effect measures defined by these semiparametric regression models are presented, and demonstrated in genomic data analyses.

Chapter 22. The TMLE for assessing the effect of biomarkers is presented and compared with other methods for variable importance analysis, such as random forest, in a comprehensive simulation study, and a breast cancer gene expression study.

Chapter 23. We present the TMLE and C-TMLE for assessing the effect of a marker on a quantitative trait, across a very large number of markers along the whole genome. Simulations and genomic data analyses are used to demonstrate the TMLE and C-TMLE.

Part VIII – Longitudinal Data Structures

In Part VI, we consider experiments that generate the full complexity of current day longitudinal data structures: one randomly samples a unit from a target population, measures baseline characteristics, and at regular or irregular monitoring times collects measurements on time-dependent treatments or exposures, time-dependent covariates, and intermediate outcomes, until the minimum of right-censoring or time to the event of interest. Observing such longitudinal data structures on a unit allows the identification of causal effects of multiple time point treatment regimens as well as individualized treatment rules. In this part, we demonstrate the roadmap for addressing the scientific questions of interest and the corresponding TMLE for three such longitudinal case studies. Technically-inclined readers may first wish to read the longitudinal sections of Appendix A before digesting these chapters.

Chapter 24. A longitudinal HIV cohort is presented and three scientific questions of interest are formulated. The road map is applied. It starts out with the definition of the causal model, the definition of the target causal parameters that represent the answers to the scientific questions, and the identifiability result resulting in the estimand of interest. The statistical model and the estimand/target parameter of the data-generating distribution define the estimation problem. Different methods for estimation are reviewed and presented: maximum likelihood estimation, inverse probability of censoring weighted estimation (IPCW), targeted maximum likelihood estimation, and inefficient practically appealing TMLEs referred to as IPCW reduced-data TMLEs.

Chapter 25. A longitudinal study is presented which involves the follow up of women going through an in vitro fertilization (IVF) program. One is interested in assessing the probability of success of a complete IVF program. The road map is applied as in all chapters. The TMLE of the probability of success of a complete IVF program is developed, and applied to the study. Simulations are also presented.

Chapter 26. In this chapter, targeted maximum likelihood learning is illustrated with a data analysis from a longitudinal observational study to investigate the question of “when to start” antiretroviral therapy to reduce the incidence of AIDS defining cancer in a population of HIV infected patients. Two treatment rules are considered: (1) start when CD4 count drops below 350, and (2) start when CD4 count drops below 200. The TMLE of the corresponding causal contrast is developed and applied to the database maintained by Kaiser Permanente.

Part IX – Advanced Topics

We deal with the following explicit questions. Is the utilization of machine learning in the TMLE a concern for establishing asymptotic normality? Can we develop a TMLE for group sequential adaptive designs in which the treatment assignment probabilities are set in response to the data collected in previously observed groups? What are the asymptotics of this TMLE for such a complex experiment in which all subjects are correlated due to treatment assignment being a function of the outcomes of previously observed subjects? Does sequential testing still apply? Since Bayesian learning is nontargeted and suffers from the same drawbacks as maximum likelihood based estimation, can we employ the principles of TMLE to construct a targeted Bayesian learning method?

Chapter 27. The cross-validated TMLE (CV-TMLE) is presented where asymptotic linearity and efficiency can be established under minimal conditions. A formal theorem is presented for the CV-TMLE of the additive causal effect, demonstrating that it is able to fully utilize all the machine learning power in the world while still allowing, and, in fact, enhancing, valid statistical inference.

Chapter 28. It is shown that the TMLE procedure naturally lends itself to targeted Bayesian learning in which a prior probability distribution on the target parameter of interest is mapped into a posterior distribution of the target parameter of interest. The frequentist properties of the mean and spread of the posterior distribution are established showing that the proposed procedure is completely valid: the mean of the posterior distribution is a double robust efficient estimator of the target parameter, and the posterior distribution yields valid credible intervals.

Chapter 29. We consider targeted group sequential adaptive designs that adapt the randomization probabilities in response to all the data collected in previous stages. The TMLE of the desired causal effect of the treatment is developed and presented. Asymptotics of the TMLE are based on martingale central limit theorems. It is shown that sequential testing can still be naturally embedded in such adaptive group sequential designs.

Part X – Appendices

Part X consists of two appendices providing important supplementary material in support of the central text. The core of the first appendix is a theoretical guide covering essential topics, derivations, and proofs. This is followed by a brief introduction to R code for super learning and TMLE. Additional R code is available on the book's website: www.targetedlearningbook.com.

Appendix A. This appendix provides a succinct but comprehensive review of the empirical process, asymptotic linearity, influence curves, and efficiency theory. This theory establishes the theoretical underpinnings of TMLE, C-TMLE, and CV-TMLE. In addition, Appendix A provides a generic approach that allows one to compute a TMLE on a new estimation problem in terms of the definition of the data structure, data-generating distribution, the statistical model, and the target parameter mapping that maps a probability distribution in its target parameter value. The TMLE for general longitudinal data structures is presented. A variety of examples are used to demonstrate the power of this generic machinery for computing a TMLE. Appendix A can be used to teach an advanced class about the theory of estimation and, in particular, of TMLE.

Appendix B. This brief appendix provides R code and links to R code for each of the implementations of the TMLE as presented in this book.

Acknowledgements

This book reflects the greater effort of a large team of people, without whom it would not have been completed. We thank the following students for their work on these methods: Laura Balzer, Katie Benton, Jordan Brooks, Paul Chaffee, Iván Díaz Muñoz, Susan Gruber, Sam Lendle, Kristin E. Porter, Stephanie Sapp, Boriska Toth, Catherine Tuglus, and Wenjing Zheng. We also thank our colleagues, many of whom contributed a chapter in this book, for their contributions to and discussions on these methods, as well as their vital collaborative efforts: Ben Arnold (UC Berkeley), David R. Bangsberg (Harvard), Oliver Bembom (AdBrite), Marco Carone (UC Berkeley), Antoine Chambaz (Université Paris Descartes), Jack Colford (UC Berkeley), Steven G. Deeks (UCSF), Victor De Gruttola (Harvard), W. Jeffrey Fessel (Kaiser Permanente), Bruce Fireman (Kaiser Permanente), Alan E. Hubbard (UC Berkeley), Nicholas P. Jewell (UC Berkeley), Kelly L. Moore (Jewish Home), Torsten B. Neilands (UCSF), Romain S. Neugebauer (Kaiser Permanente), Michelle Odden (UCSF), Judea Pearl (UCLA), Maya L. Petersen (UC Berkeley), Eric C. Polley (NCI), Art Reingold (UC Berkeley), Elise D. Riley (UCSF), Michael Rosenblum (Johns Hopkins), Daniel B. Rubin (FDA), Robert W. Shafer (Stanford), Jasjeet S. Sekhon (UC Berkeley), Michael J. Silverberg (Kaiser Permanente), Greg Soon (FDA), Richard J.C.M. Starmans (Universiteit Utrecht), Ori M. Stitelman (UC Berkeley), Ira B. Tager (UC Berkeley), Thamban Valappil (FDA), Hui Wang (Stanford), Yue Wang (Novartis), and C. William Wester (Vanderbilt).

Much of the content presented in this book has been taught by Mark in multiple upper-division biostatistics courses at UC Berkeley (e.g., PH240B, PH243D, PH243A, and PHC246A). The authors would like to thank the students in these courses, as their questions guided the format of this text. We thank Maya L. Petersen and Ira B. Tager for many insightful discussions on content and organization for Part I of the book. We also thank our thorough and patient copyeditor Glenn Corey, who took our manuscript to the next level. Computing is a central component of the work we do, and thus we thank our systems administrator Burke J. Bundy.

Berkeley, January 2011

Mark J. van der Laan
Sherri Rose

Contents

List of Contributors

Mark J. van der Laan
University of California, Berkeley, Division of Biostatistics and Department of Statistics, 101 Haviland Hall, #7358, Berkeley, CA 94720, USA, e-mail: laan@berkeley.edu

Sherri Rose
University of California, Berkeley, Division of Biostatistics, 101 Haviland Hall, #7358, Berkeley, CA 94720, USA, e-mail: sherri@berkeley.edu

---

Antoine Chambaz
Université Paris Descartes, MAP5 UMR CNRS 8145, 45, rue des Saints-Pères, 75270 Paris cedex 06, France, e-mail: antoine.chambaz@parisdescartes.fr

Victor De Gruttola
Harvard School of Public Health, Department of Biostatistics, 655 Huntington Avenue, Boston, MA 02115, USA, e-mail: degrut@hsph.harvard.edu

Iván Díaz Muñoz
University of California, Berkeley, Division of Biostatistics, 101 Haviland Hall, #7358, Berkeley, CA 94720, USA, e-mail: ildiazm@berkeley.edu

Bruce Fireman
Kaiser Permanente Division of Research, 2000 Broadway, Oakland, CA 94612, USA, e-mail: Bruce.Fireman@nsmtp.kp.org

Susan Gruber
University of California, Berkeley, Division of Biostatistics, 101 Haviland Hall, #7358, Berkeley, CA 94720, USA, e-mail: sgruber@berkeley.edu

Alan E. Hubbard
University of California, Berkeley, Division of Biostatistics, 101 Haviland Hall, #7358, Berkeley, CA 94720, USA, e-mail: hubbard@berkeley.edu

Nicholas P. Jewell
University of California, Berkeley, Division of Biostatistics and Department of Statistics, 101 Haviland Hall, #7358, Berkeley, CA 94720, USA, e-mail: jewell@berkeley.edu

Kelly L. Moore
Jewish Home, 302 Silver Avenue, San Francisco, CA 94112, USA, e-mail: kellylmoore1@gmail.com

Romain Neugebauer
Kaiser Permanente Division of Research, 2000 Broadway, Oakland, CA 94612, USA, e-mail: romain.s.neugebauer@kp.org

Judea Pearl
University of California, Los Angeles, Computer Science Department, 4532 Boelter Hall, Los Angeles, CA 90095, USA, e-mail: judea@cs.ucla.edu

Maya L. Petersen
University of California, Berkeley, Division of Epidemiology and Division of Biostatistics, 101 Haviland Hall, #7358, Berkeley, CA 94720, USA, e-mail: mayaliv@berkeley.edu

Eric C. Polley
National Cancer Institute, Biometric Research Branch, Division of Cancer Treatment and Diagnosis, 6130 Executive Plaza, Rockville, MD 20852, USA, e-mail: eric.polley@nih.gov

Kristin E. Porter
University of California, Berkeley, Division of Biostatistics, 101 Haviland Hall, #7358, Berkeley, CA 94720, USA, e-mail: kristinporter@berkeley.edu

Michael Rosenblum
Johns Hopkins Bloomberg School of Public Health, Department of Biostatistics, 615 N. Wolfe Street, Baltimore, MD 21230, USA, e-mail: mrosenbl@jhsph.edu

Daniel B. Rubin
Food and Drug Administration, Center for Drug Evaluation and Research, Office of Biostatistics, 10903 New Hampshire Avenue, Silver Spring, MD 20993, USA, e-mail: daniel.rubin@fda.hhs.gov

Jasjeet S. Sekhon
University of California, Berkeley, Travers Department of Political Science, 210 Barrows Hall, #1950, Berkeley, CA 94720, USA, e-mail: sekhon@berkeley.edu

Michael J. Silverberg
Kaiser Permanente Division of Research, 2000 Broadway, Oakland, CA 94612, USA, e-mail: michael.j.silverberg@kp.org

Richard J.C.M. Starmans
Universiteit Utrecht, Department of Information and Computing Sciences, Buys Ballot Laboratory, Princetonplein 5, De Uithof, 3584 CC Utrecht, The Netherlands, e-mail: starmans@cs.uu.nl

Ori M. Stitelman
University of California, Berkeley, Division of Biostatistics, 101 Haviland Hall, #7358, Berkeley, CA 94720, USA, e-mail: ostitelman@berkeley.edu

Ira B. Tager
University of California, Berkeley, Division of Epidemiology, 101 Haviland Hall, #7358, Berkeley, CA 94720, USA, e-mail: ibt@berkeley.edu

Catherine Tuglus
University of California, Berkeley, Division of Biostatistics, 101 Haviland Hall, #7358, Berkeley, CA 94720, USA, e-mail: ctuglus@berkeley.edu

Hui Wang
Stanford School of Medicine, Department of Pediatrics, 300 Pasteur Drive, Stanford, CA 94305, USA, e-mail: hwangui@stanford.edu

Yue Wang
Novartis Pharmaceuticals Corporation, Integrated Information Sciences IHC Franchise, One Health Plaza, East Hanover, NJ 07936, USA, e-mail: wangyue@gmail.com

C. William Wester
Vanderbilt University School of Medicine, 2525 West End Avenue, Suite 750, Nashville, TN 37203, USA, e-mail: william.wester@vanderbilt.edu

Wenjing Zheng
University of California, Berkeley, Division of Biostatistics, 101 Haviland Hall, #7358, Berkeley, CA 94720, USA, e-mail: wzheng@stat.berkeley.edu

Abbreviations and Notation

Frequently used abbreviations and notation are listed here.

TMLE	Targeted maximum likelihood estimation/estimator
C-TMLE	Collaborative targeted maximum likelihood estimation/estimator
SL	Super learner
SCM	Structural causal model
MLE	Maximum likelihood substitution estimator of the g-formula *Not to be confused with nonsubstitution estimators using maximum likelihood estimation. MLE has been referred to elsewhere as g-computation*
IPTW	Inverse probability of treatment-weighted/weighting
A-IPTW	Augmented inverse probability of treatment-weighted/weighting
IPCW	Inverse probability of censoring-weighted/weighting
A-IPCW	Augmented inverse probability of censoring-weighted/weighting
RCT	Randomized controlled trial
MSE	Mean squared error
SE	Standard error
i.i.d.	Independent and identically distributed
O	Observed ordered data structure
W	Vector of covariates
A	Treatment or exposure
Y	Outcome
Y_1, Y_0	Counterfactual outcomes with binary A
C	Censoring
P_0	True data-generating distribution; $O \sim P_0$
P	Possible data-generating distribution
P_n	Empirical probability distribution; places probability $1/n$ on each observed $O_i, i \ldots, n$
p_0	True density of data-generating distribution P_0
p	Possible density of data-generating distribution P_0

Uppercase letters represent random variables and lowercase letters are a specific value for that variable. $P_0(O = o)$ for a particular value o of O can be defined as a probability if O is a discrete random variable, or we can use the concept of probability density if O is continuous. For simplicity and the sake of presentation, we will often treat O as discrete so that we can refer to $P_0(O = o)$ as a probability. For a simple example, suppose our data structure is $O = (W, A, Y) \sim P_0$. Thus, for each possible value (w, a, y), $P_0(w, a, y)$ denotes the probability that (W, A, Y) equals (w, a, y).

$\mathcal{M}$	Statistical model; the set of possible probability distributions for P_0
$P_0 \in \mathcal{M}$	P_0 is known to be an element of the statistical model $\mathcal{M}$

In this text we often use the term *semiparametric* to include both nonparametric and semiparametric. When semiparametric excludes nonparametric, and we make additional assumptions, this will be explicit. A *statistical model* can be augmented with additional nonstatistical (causal) assumptions providing enriched interpretation. We refer to this as a *model* (see $\mathcal{M}^F$ and $\mathcal{M}^{F*}$).

$X = (X_j : j)$	Set of endogenous variables, $j = 1, \ldots, J$
$U = (U_{X_j} : j)$	Set of exogenous variables
$P_{U,X}$	Probability distribution for (U, X)
$Pa(X_j)$	Parents of X_j among X
f_{X_j}	A function of $Pa(X_j)$ and an endogenous U_{X_j} for X_j
$f = (f_{X_j} : j)$	Collection of f_{X_j} functions that define the SCM
$\mathcal{M}^F$	Collection of possible $P_{U,X}$ as described by the SCM; includes nontestable assumptions based on real knowledge; $\mathcal{M}$ augmented with additional nonstatistical assumptions known to hold
$\mathcal{M}^{F*}$	Model under possible additional causal assumptions required for identifiability of target parameter
$P \to \Psi(P)$	Target parameter as mapping from a P to its value
$\Psi(P_0)$	True target parameter
$\hat{\Psi}(P_n)$	Estimator as a mapping from empirical distribution P_n to its value
$\psi_0 = \Psi(P_0)$	True target parameter value
ψ_n	Estimate of ψ_0

Consider $O = (L_0, A_0, \ldots, L_K, A_K, L_{K+1}) \sim P_0$.

L_j	Possibly time-varying covariate at $t = j$; alternate notation $L(j)$
A_j	Time-varying intervention node at $t = j$ that can include both treatment and censoring
$Pa(L_j)$	$=(\bar{A}_{j-1}, \bar{L}_{j-1})$
$Pa(A_j)$	$=(\bar{A}_{j-1}, \bar{L}_j)$
$P_{L_j,0}$	True conditional distribution of L_j, given $Pa(L_j)$, under P_0
P_{L_j}	Conditional distribution of L_j, given $Pa(L_j)$, under P
$P_{L_j,n}$	Estimate of conditional distribution $P_{L_j,0}$ of L_j
$P_{A_j,0}$	True conditional distribution of A_j, given $Pa(A_j)$, under P_0
P_{A_j}	Conditional distribution of A_j, given $Pa(A_j)$, under P
$P_{A_j,n}$	Conditional distribution of A_j, given $Pa(A_j)$, under P_n

$\Psi(Q_0)$	Alternate notation for true target parameter where it only depends on P_0 through Q_0
g_0	Treatment/exposure/censoring mechanism
g_n	Estimate of g_0
g	Possible treatment mechanism
ϵ	Fluctuation parameter
ϵ_n	Estimate of ϵ
H^*	Clever covariate
H_n^*	Estimate of H^*
$L(O, \bar{Q})$	Example of a loss function where it is a function of O and $\bar{Q}$; alternate notation $L(\bar{Q})(O)$ or $L(\bar{Q})$
$D(\psi)(O)$	Estimating function of the data structure O and parameters; shorthand $D(\psi)$
$D^*(\psi)$	Estimating function implied by efficient influence curve
$D^*(P_0)(O)$	Efficient influence curve; canonical gradient; shorthand $D^*(P_0)$ or $D^*(O)$
$IC(O)$	Influence curve of an estimator, representing a function of O

In several chapters we focus on a simple data structure $O = (W, A, Y) \sim P_0$. In this example, the following specific notation definitions apply:

$Q_{Y,0}$	True conditional distribution of Y given (A, W)
Q_Y	Possible conditional distribution of Y given (A, W)
$Q_{Y,n}$	Estimate of $Q_{Y,0}$
$\bar{Q}_0$	Conditional mean of outcome given parents; $E_0(Y \mid A, W)$
$\bar{Q}$	Possible function in the parameter space of functions that map parents of the outcome into a predicted value for the outcome
$\bar{Q}_n$	Estimate of $\bar{Q}_0$
$\bar{Q}_n^0$	Initial estimate of $\bar{Q}_0$
$\bar{Q}_n^1$	First updated estimate of $\bar{Q}_0$
$\bar{Q}_n^k$	kth updated estimate of $\bar{Q}_0$
$\bar{Q}_n^*$	Targeted estimate of $\bar{Q}_0$ in TMLE procedure; $\bar{Q}_n^*$ may equal $\bar{Q}_n^1$
$Q_{W,0}$	True marginal distribution of W
Q_W	Possible marginal distribution of W
$Q_{W,n}$	Estimate of $Q_{W,0}$
Q_0	$= (\bar{Q}_0, Q_{W,0})$
Q_n	Estimate of Q_0
Q_n^*	Targeted estimate of Q_0
Q	Possible value of true Q_0
$\Psi(Q_0)$	Alternate notation for true target parameter when it only depends on P_0 through Q_0
$\Psi(Q_0)_{RD}$	Additive causal risk difference; $E_0Y_1 - E_0Y_0 = E_W[E_0(Y \mid A = 1, W) - E_0(Y \mid A = 0, W)]$

Models, Inference, and Truth: Probabilistic Reasoning in the Information Era

Richard J.C.M. Starmans

Targeted maximum likelihood estimation (TMLE) strongly criticizes current practice in statistical data analysis as pervasively manifest in the sciences, medicine, industry, and government, if not in all segments of society. For the most part, analyses conducted in these fields rely heavily on incorrectly specified parametric models with assumptions that do not use realistic background knowledge and in no way contain the (optimal approximation of the) data-generating function. Especially in large and complex, highly dimensional data sets this may cause biased estimators, uninterpretable coefficients, and, in the end, wrong results. In addition, TMLE challenges the customary approaches to statistical learning, as developed in the field of computational intelligence (machine learning, data mining, knowledge discovery in databases), which usually do not treat missing or censored data in a statistically sound way, neglect the importance of confidence intervals, and are often not rooted in efficiency theory whatsoever. They are also habitually unnecessarily biased because the algorithms are not targeted but developed to fit the full (prediction) distribution. And all too often the choice of algorithms is determined by subjective, human preferences, rather than by objective and rational criteria.

From a methodological point of view TMLE establishes a new "learning from data" paradigm by offering *an integrative approach to data analysis or statistical learning*. It combines mathematical statistics with techniques derived from the field of computational intelligence to overcome the drawbacks of current approaches to statistical data analysis or learning, providing analysts and scientists with a sound research methodology, enabling them to cope with increasingly complicated, high-dimensional data structures, which are currently prevalent in the sciences, industry, government, and health care.

First and foremost, TMLE reassigns to the very concept of *estimation*, canonical as it has always been in *statistical inference*, the leading role in any theory of or approach to "learning from data," whether it deals with establishing causal relations, classifying or clustering, time series forecasting, or multiple testing. This remark may seem rather trivial from a statistical perspective, but it is far from insignificant from a historical and philosophical point of view and – perhaps more importantly

– will appear to be even crucial in understanding the situation in research practice today. Secondly, TMLE reaffirms or rather *reestablishes* the concept of a *statistical model* in a prudent and parsimonious way, allowing humans to include only their *true*, realistic knowledge (e.g., data are randomized, representing n independent and identically distributed observations of a random variable) in the model. Rather than assuming misspecified parametric or highly restrictive semiparametric statistical models, TMLE defines the statistical estimation problem in terms of non-parametric or semiparametric statistical models that represent realistic knowledge, i.e., knowledge in terms of the underlying experiment that generated the data at hand. Thirdly, TMLE *rethinks* the relation between research questions and analysis by adhering to estimating equation methodology. The obvious methodological maxim that the analysis must "be guided by" the research problem should not prevent the researcher from relating the question of interest in the analysis to features of the data-distributing function. TMLE defines the target parameter as a particular function of the *true probability distribution* of the data and estimates the target parameter accordingly with a plug-in estimator; it refrains from estimating the entire probability distribution. Finally, TMLE integrates statistics and computational intelligence techniques by the development of the super learning theory, which unintentionally and ironically helps to restore the old ideal of artificial intelligence (AI) by further reducing human intervention in the very process of automatic reasoning. It therefore marks an important step in the convergence between the world of algorithms of computer science (including AI) on the one hand and the world of mathematical statistics on the other.

Clearly, controversy and debate are not unusual in science, and many disciplines lack uniformity or even embrace a pluralism of methods or paradigms. In this respect, the current situation in statistical data analysis seems rather peculiar. From a foundational perspective the field consists of several competing schools with sometimes incompatible principles, approaches, or viewpoints. Simultaneously, the burgeoning statistical textbook market offers many primers and even advanced studies that wrongly suggest a uniform and united field with foundations that are fixed and on which full agreement has been reached, while we rather experience a striking piece of philosophical eclecticism.

Against the background of this somewhat paradoxical situation we will reflect on TMLE in this philosophical essay. Indeed, there are many important implications, not only for the philosophy of statistics in particular but also for the epistemology/philosophy of science in general. Obviously, in exploring these we must restrain ourselves. TMLE is a rather new, rapidly developing field, and there are many ramifications in philosophy, only a few of which can be touched upon here. We will put the present state of affairs in a *historical and philosophical perspective* so as *to clarify, understand,* and *account for* the current situation in statistical data analysis and to underline the relevance of topics addressed by TMLE for both the philosophy of statistics and the epistemology/philosophy of science. This historical and philosophical perspective involves:

- taking an *externalist* stance and identifying three major developments in the history of ideas that provide a context for the emergence of the probabilistic revolution and define the arena where it receives its relevance;
- taking an *internalist* stance and identifying some major immanent developments in the history of statistics that have led to the current situation or at least may help to understand it;
- providing a prelude to a *conceptual analysis* of some key notions, focusing on the nature and status of the very concepts of *statistical model* and *probability distribution*, on the role of *statistical inference* and *estimation*, and on the notion of *truth* and its relation to *reality*.

This approach unavoidably implies deftly navigating between the Scylla of the archaeologist and the Charybdis of the futurologist, thus trying to avoid both plain historical excursions and mere speculation. But it also means dragging the concepts at stake into the philosophical triangle, built up by the notions of reality, thoughts, and language, and evoking classical questions like: *What is reality? Does it exist mind-independently? Do we have access to it? If yes, how? Can we make true statements about it? If yes, what is truth and how is it connected to reality?* These questions, which are pivotal in the philosophy of the empirical sciences, will appear to be of equal relevance here. Answering these questions always involves taking or at least considering certain philosophical positions, and it is shown that specific philosophical ideas, embraced by the main protagonists who shaped the field of statistics can help to account for the current state of affairs.

Informational Metaphysics and the Science of Data

No doubt this is the information era and our exploration only gets its full relief against a background where *the concept of information* dominates our entire world(view). It plays a fundamental role in all the sciences and therefore in epistemology as well. Some philosophers even stipulate its *metaphysical* importance. For example, when the digital revolution was barely launched, the American philosopher, mathematician, and founder of cybernetics Norbert Wiener (1894–1964) postulated in a famous quote from 1961 that the concept of information is more fundamental than matter and energy. In his renowned "It from Bit" doctrine, the physicist John Archibald Wheeler (1911–2008) did more or less the same, claiming that all things in nature have an immaterial source and explanation and are essentially information-theoretic in origin.

Unsurprisingly, such informational descriptions of reality have been embraced by many antimaterialist philosophers, suffering under the yoke of the currently prevailing naturalism or physicalist reductionism. And they were a prelude to the modest rise of the current *informational metaphysics* in which man inhabits an information space, his mind is regarded as an information-processing system, physical reality is presented as a massive computer, and physical processes are regarded as calculations or state transitions. But these considerations on information are also warranted by current foundational research in the various empirical sciences. Here information and information processes are essential, underlie many theories, and are formalized and simulated from different perspectives and with different objectives. Salient examples, which have also proved their relevance in contemporary philosophy of science, are mainly found in mathematics (classical information theory of Shannon), computer science (Kolmogorov complexity), physics (Gibbs entropy), biology (DNA coding) and economics (game theory). It goes without saying that the very idea of semantic information, which dominates the humanities, can easily be added to this list as well.

Philosophers disagree whether a unified theory of information, covering all these approaches and perspectives, is feasible or even desirable. However, as a starting point for our conceptual analysis, and to proceed in a more down-to-earth way, we adhere to the traditional point of view that information is just *data plus interpretation*, or at least presupposes a *concept of data*, a "medium," that should be considered at a symbolic, semiotic, or physical/acoustic level and that is assumed to represent, enable, convey, or even materialize information. This shifts the focus in a conceptual analysis to the nature and status of these data, and especially to their relationship with reality, from which – in one way or another – they have been "taken," or from which they have been generated, or which they are supposed to represent, access, encrypt, simulate, replace, or perhaps even build up, depending on the philosophical position one is willing to embrace. These data must be collected, stored, and analyzed, and they give rise to at least three fundamental questions:

- How do the phenomena in all their complexity and dynamics, and their postulated underlying structures and mechanisms relate to variation, change, relationships, and hidden patterns in data?
- How can complex analyses and manipulations of data, and computational models based on these manipulations, yield reliable knowledge of reality?
- How can systems that store and manipulate data to change or control reality be validated in the sense that it is evaluated whether they helped to create the proposed changes?

Both statistics and computer science scrutinize these interrelated questions, where the division of tasks is not always clear in advance. For a long time both have been continuing their own institutionalized role despite some recent rapprochements between the statistics and the computational intelligence community. Yet from an external or *functional* perspective they both build up – each in their own way – a "science of data" and are together eligible for the title "Queen and Servant of Science," a label once famously assigned by E.T. Bell to mathematics in general.

Both help the aforementioned information-oriented disciplines with their keen interest in informational descriptions of nature to answer these questions, laying (or at least partially explaining) the foundations on which these sciences can build. Interestingly, it appears that the analyses that are performed (in answering these questions) are usually *intrinsically probabilistic*, i.e., they are based on or derived from probability theory and statistics. In manipulating these data, all aforementioned information-oriented sciences perform probabilistic reasoning; their key notions are probabilistic, and their research methods, indeed entire theories if not the underlying wordview are probabilistic.

When the probabilistic revolution emerged in the late nineteenth century, this transition became recognizable in old, established sciences like physics (kinetic gas theory, the statistical mechanics of Boltzmann, Maxwell, and Gibbs), but especially in new emerging disciplines like the social sciences (Quetelet and later Durkheim), biology (evolution, genetics, zoology), agricultural science, and psychology. Biology even came to maturity due to its close interaction with statistics. Today, this trend has only further strengthened, and as a result there is a plethora of fields of application of statistics ranging from biostatistics, geostatistics, epidemiology, and econometrics to actuarial science, statistical finance, quality control, and operational research in industrial engineering and management science. Probabilistic approaches have also intruded upon many branches of computer science; most noticeably they dominate AI, having supplanted the once mighty logical tradition in this field. Indeed, all too often scientific reasoning seems nearly synonymous with probabilistic reasoning. It therefore comes as no surprise that in contemporary philosophy of science, the "probabilistic approach" strongly dominates when it comes to the aforementioned classical questions regarding reality, knowledge, and truth. This is reflected in the following list of key issues and controversies, deemed relevant in and consistently addressed by the vast majority of contemporary textbooks in this field:

- The scientific realism debate, the Quine–Duhem thesis/underdetermination;
- The structure of scientific theories;
- The search for unity of science;
- Rationality and progress in science;
- (Bayesian) confirmation theory;
- The role of causality, models of explanation, and natural laws;
- Evolution of scientific practices/dissemination of knowledge.

It would demand another couple of essays to demonstrate how these key issues in the philosophy of science are all dominated or at least influenced by probabilistic approaches, incorporating probability theory or statistics. As a result, many classical questions brought forward in epistemology, regarding reality, truth, and obtaining knowledge, can only be dealt with or interpreted in a probabilistic way. In view of the fact that *scientific inference increasingly depends on probabilistic reasoning and that statistical analysis is not as well founded as might be expected*, the issue addressed in this essay is of crucial importance for epistemology, especially for those who want to safeguard the rationality of science and pursue truth in an era where scientism seems dominant and many people believe that science is the only valid source of knowledge.

However, before these speculations on the metaphysics of information could be launched, and before the new science of data could address the questions listed above, an even more essential revolution was needed, invoking a change in worldview, a new view of reality. This happened in the nineteenth century when a historicizing of the world took place, when 2000 years of substance thinking came under pressure, and when, according to the philosopher Ian Hacking, an "erosion of determinism" became visible. In this process the concepts of variation and change played a pivotal role, after they went through an emancipation process that took about 2500 years.

From Parmenides to Pearson

For a long time the related concepts of variation and change had a rather pejorative connotation in philosophy and science. It all began with the ancient Greek philosophers, who sought an explanation for the different aspects of change: change of location (motion), growth and decay, change in quality and quantity. Its existence was often denied or deemed impossible and reduced to nonchange. Variation was regarded as a deviation from a rule or standard, which at best should be explained. Both were indications of imperfection and unpredictability.

The Eleatic philosopher Parmenides was the most radical advocate of the immutability of being. Backed by the famous paradoxes of his apprentice Zeno, he argued that motion was impossible on logical and metaphysical grounds. Changes are nothing but effects on the senses; reality is unified, indivisible, and unchangeable. Plato pursued this idea from Parmenides and placed against the imaginary world of phenomena a "real" transcendental world, timeless and unchanging. Atomists like Leucippus and Democritus did not deny the reality of perception, but tried to reduce change to nonchange. Movement, growth and decay, and changes in quantity and quality were considered nothing more than a rearrangement of elementary particles. Aristotle disputed both the atomists and Plato by respectively introducing the potential being and his hylomorphism, where form and matter are bound together and the essential forms lay hidden in the things themselves. But although he was a biologist par excellence, Aristotle also struggled with the variation in the sublunary world. The variety and changeability of matter constituted an obstacle to formulating laws and raised serious problems for his axiomatic-deductive ideal of knowledge. Put roughly, despite the work of Heraclitus, and due to the vision of the aforementioned thinkers and especially the influence of Aristotle's substance thinking, the notions of variation and change long remained problematic in the Western history of ideas.

In the seventeenth century, many "dynamic" theories such as Descartes' vortex theory and Leibniz's monadology were proposed, but, especially owing to the development of calculus by Newton and Leibniz, science finally got a grip on the phenomenon of change. However, variation in nature remained problematic, even after the general acceptance of classical mechanics and the improvement of measurement techniques. Pierre-Simon Laplace (1749–1827) developed his famous error function, in this context a noteworthy, perhaps ominous, name. In his celestial mechanics he "explained" the deviations from the planetary orbits, showing they were normally distributed, and thus he "rescued" the deterministic worldview, of which he was the principal exponent. Laplace's student Adolphe Quetelet (1796–1874) took a significant step forward by applying the normal distribution to human qualities: he introduced his abstraction of "l'homme moyen," claiming the mean to be the "essence." He did not deny the relevance of spread and variation, but these "deviations" were bound to the Procrustean bed of the normal distribution; they had to be corrected or at least restrained.

The volatility of (living) nature and her many appearances were thus an obstacle to a deterministic world in which causal laws prevail, and they foiled a mathematical approach to the phenomena. Even great pioneers of statistics like Laplace and Quetelet could bring only limited change, notwithstanding straightforward application of Queteletian ideas by physicists (statistical mechanics). The conceptual breakthrough came no earlier than with the theory of evolution of Wallace and Darwin. Aristotelian essentialism and the alleged invariability of species were replaced by the idea that variation is inherent in nature and that the Earth has a long history of genesis and change. The implications were soon understood by Darwin's cousin Francis Galton (1822–1911), an amateur scientist who privately funded numerous studies and was an indefatigable advocate for the application of mathematics to the study of living nature. However, he had to leave the decisive step in this emancipation process of the concepts of variation and change to his protégé Karl Pearson (1857–1936), eminent statistician and influential philosopher in his time. Before we show how Pearson put the crown on this process, we must emphasize two things.

Firstly, the process whereby variation and change were no longer treated in a pejorative way was not only recognizable in animate nature and a prerequisite for the rise of mathematical statistics. In fact, it was not exclusively attributable to biology/evolutionism either but shows its many faces in nineteenth century philosophy. For example, the "historicizing of the world" was reflected in Hegel's idealistic dialectics, and afterward in the materialist dialectics of Feuerbach and Marx. The reinforcement of Heraclitean, antisubstance philosophy was recognizable in the process thinking of Henri Bergson and Alfred N. Whitehead. Herbert Spencer and others made a first move toward evolutionary ethics. Also, the decline of concepts like determinism and essentialism should be viewed in this light. Especially the strong indeterminism of leading pragmatist philosopher C.S. Peirce influenced the intellectual climate in this respect. The list could easily be extended. Secondly, it goes without saying that ever since this change in worldview, anyone who wanted to approach reality *from a scientific point of view and represent it in a formal way* had to do justice to the new situation, treating variation and change in a nonpejorative way and act accordingly in answering the key questions mentioned in the introduction: *What is reality? Does it exist mind-independently? Do we have access to it? If yes, how? Can we make true statements about it? If yes, what is truth and how is it connected to reality?* The next section shows that Pearson was the first statistician who faced this challenge and proposed answers to all these questions.

The Pearsonian Philosophy

Galton convinced Pearson that animate nature indeed allowed for a mathematical treatment without deprecatory interpretations of deviations, error functions, etc. Pearson did justice to the complex reality by identifying variation not in errors, but in the phenomena themselves (encoded in data), and by not trying to reduce this variation to the normal distribution but by considering all kinds of (classes of) probability distributions. Variability manifests itself in a point cloud of measurements, and Pearson essentially looked for the best fitting "model," the function that best described the mechanism that generated the data. As such he was the first one to give probability distributions a fundamental role in science, and he opened the door to inferential statistics.

A crucial first step was Pearson's work on skewed distributions. Studying large numbers (biometric) data collected at the Galton laboratory, he realized that many phenomena were not normal but intrinsically skewed and could be described using four parameters (mean, standard deviation, skewness, and kurtosis) and be classified in families of (skewed) distributions. According to Pearson, the unity of the sciences could be found in this constructive, albeit very labor-intensive, methodology. He therefore employed large groups of women (the "calculatores") in a studio, calculating the four parameters of huge numbers of data files.

In philosophical terms, Pearson was influenced by Ernst Mach's phenomenalism, an extremely empiricist doctrine that states that reality consists of elements (colors, vibrations, times) emerging in streams of sense data or immediate sensations. These are supposed to be neutral (neither mental nor material), and both physical objects and content of the mind are constructed from these sensations. Science has primarily a "think-economic" function, describing and summarizing these streams as economically as possible and refraining from postulating nonverifiable theoretical constructs. Newtonian notions such as force and attraction found no favor with Ernst Mach, who tried to rewrite classical mechanics in a "sound," phenomenalistic way. Unsurprisingly, Mach rejected causal explanations as well.

One of Pearson's main achievements, his contribution to the correlation and regression analysis, should be viewed in this light. Along with Bertrand Russell he became the main anticausalist at the beginning of the twentieth century. Science is all about correlations; causality should be radically eliminated from science and could at best be relegated to metaphysics. But Pearson also had an *idealistic* view of reality and regarded science mainly as a classification and analysis of the content of the mind. Because of these philosophical principles, which were for the most part already apparent in *The Grammar of Science* of 1892, Pearson saw the world on another level of abstraction, where data, variation in data, data-generating mechanisms, and parameters of distributions encode or build up reality: they replaced the alleged materialist physical reality rather than representing it. Interpreting his probability distributions in an almost Pythagorean way, the clouds of measurements were the objects of science, and the (concept of) reality was replaced by the probability distribution, or rather the four parameters. It was an abstract world, but "observable," close to the data, accessible, knowledgeable through observation, and essentially a summary of the data. Insofar as he had a concept of *statistical inference*, it was mainly based on the idea of goodness-of-fit testing. Still, Pearson's distributions were much more than a purely mathematical notion; they were the crown of the emancipation process sketched above. Therefore its importance truly exceeds the history of statistics.

Material Eliminativism vs. Common Sense

By replacing the materialist world with that of a probability distribution and by taking a strong anticausalist stance, Pearson contributed notably to a third major development in the history of ideas, brought forward in this essay, whose relevance for the current situation in statistical data analysis can hardly be overemphasized. This trend, or rather tension, has a long and impressive history in Western thought, starting with the pre-Socratics and reaching a (temporary) peak, showing its many faces in contemporary science. Gradually the worldview being developed in philosophy and science became more abstract and less tangible. It seems far removed from our daily experiences, intuitive concepts, commonsense notions, and the natural categories we use to understand ourselves, our situatedness, and the contingencies of being.

Already around 600 BC Ionian and Dorian philosophers advocated a strong reductionism, distancing itself from everyday perceptions and reducing the multiplicity of phenomena to first principles or primary elements. Thales' solution (water) and that of Heraclitus (fire) still had some graphic "imagery," but Anaximander appealed to the abstract concept of "apeiron," or the fundamental indeterminate. As has been stated before, Eleatan philosopher Parmenides denied the variability of being and thus the primacy of the senses; the Pythagoreans put the reality of numbers and numerical relations above alleged material and observable objects. Plato combined the two ideas in his theory and had little admiration for science that focused on the phenomena. The atomists, and in their wake, Epicurus distinguished between "primary" (shape, size, location) and "secondary" (color, taste, sound) properties. It was above all Aristotle who in a way championed commonsense thinking because he put the "essential forms" in phenomena, took great interest in the analysis of ordinary language, and at times showed a fundamentally empirical attitude.

The problem emerged differently in the eighteenth century, when Scottish philosopher Thomas Reid took a position against the rationalist philosopher Descartes and the empiricist philosophers Locke, Berkeley, and Hume. Encouraged by the successes of science in understanding the "outside world," these famous predecessors and contemporaries of Reid started to investigate the "inner world" with emphasis on perception, mental representations, and the development of "theories of ideas." Reid criticized them because in his opinion all, each in their own way, wrongly "placed" perceptions and mental representations between the objects in reality and the subjects who perceive reality, making an unnecessary rift between subject and object, inner and outer world, resulting in paradoxes, solipsism, or skepticism. Some distrusted the senses, or at least a portion of the sensory input (Descartes), or labeled experiences of color, taste, and sound as "secondary" to real or "primary" qualities of the world (Locke). Others claimed that material objects do not exist independently of the mind (Berkeley) or are in fact not knowable (Hume). At best, reality was hidden behind a "veil of perception." Reid defended a direct realism with an external world that is knowable; rather than closing the road to our ideas "outside," it opens it correctly. God has given mankind a number of valid mechanisms for acquiring knowledge, such as the principle of induction and the ability to see some obvious truths. Our *sensus communis* is not only a precondition for reasoning, but also a sufficiently reliable basis for philosophical analysis.

Immanuel Kant came up with a "solution" or rather a compromise. In a sense, he created a gap by postulating a true but inaccessible noumenal reality and a knowable phenomenal reality, formed by the knowing subject itself with *Anschauungsformen* of time and (Euclidean) space, and categories such as causality, necessity, modality, and other "conditions" for having an experience at all. Yet it is the phenomenal world that is actually being studied in the natural sciences, and consequently the aforementioned "commonsense" categories are necessarily valid, enabling purely "synthetic a priori knowledge." Kant's solution soon proved to be problematic. In the nineteenth century, non-Euclidean geometry was developed, at the turn of the 20th century the theory of relativity made absolute time and space problematic if not untenable, and shortly thereafter the famous Copenhagen interpretation of quantum mechanics cracked our intuitive notion of causality as a Kantian building block of reality.

Indeed a dualism seems manifest between the intuitive environment of phenomena, with its experiences (perceptions, impressions, sensations) and its (postulated) material objects on the one hand and the scientific worldview on the other hand, offering us abstract, often mathematical, models, representations of the "real" world, that are supposed to lie behind these experiences, to cause or to explain these. Many believe that our experiences and intuitive concepts, commonsense notions, and natural categories (in the Aristotelian or Kantian sense) are no longer a reliable basis for scientific theories, describing the underlying mechanisms, abstract principles, and laws that govern the "real" world, as described by the language and nomenclature of science. In the course of time, many of these intuitive concepts and commonsense notions have been banned or received a specific abstract or mathematical interpretation. This concerns concepts like space, time, motion, causality, and intentionality, but also the notions of meaning, spirit, free will, personal identity, and consciousness.

Notorious in this respect are the views of philosopher and neuroscientist Paul Churchland, who radically rejects a tradition that is sometimes pejoratively referred to as "folk psychology." It exploits the idea that people typically try to understand, explain, and predict the behavior of themselves and others in terms of (causally relevant) factors such as motives, intentions, beliefs, and commitments. Churchland argues for a radical "eliminative materialism" in relation to these propositional attitudes and suggests that the whole idea of folk psychology, including the concept of consciousness, wrongly approaches the human mind and its internal processes.

Likewise, he regrets the concerns of philosophers and AI researchers with language and its assumed significance for the mind and for reasoning! Developments in neuroscience, he believes, will lead to the elimination of these errors, which according to Churchland's scientific worldview are equally relevant as the eighteenth-century phlogiston theory of Stahl to modern chemistry or medieval ideas about witchcraft to contemporary psychology. The extreme and very controversial view expressed by Churchland is in no way the general opinion. In fact we experience an ongoing dualism, a debate that is far from being passé and continues to be fueled by developments in philosophy (e.g., the scientific realism debate) and the sciences.

It is not a mere choice between folk psychology and abstraction or a simple black-and-white dichotomy. History shows that not only intuitive notions or (allegedly) vague metaphysical concepts such as Bergson's élan vital, Whitehead's organism, or Heidegger's dark neologisms fall prey to "elimination." Highlights in the history of science have also been targeted. We already referred to Ernst Mach discrediting Newtonian notions of force and attraction. Conversely, many commonsense concepts appear persistent and vital. In fact, current AI research on the "thinking" machine, automatic reasoning, and knowledge representation is a shining counterexample. According to "Strong AI" man builds machines "in his own image," or is inspired by (our knowledge of) human cognition. Even stronger, the most fundamental concept in computing, the Turing machine was based on this idea! AI designs working artifacts but takes into account the human mind, including concepts such as intelligence, reasoning, consciousness, and the role that language and knowledge, belief, and uncertainty play in this respect. Natural concepts and categories that we use to understand ourselves and our environment are not suppressed at all but used in intelligent systems for knowledge representation and reasoning with it. Many subfields in AI, especially those of symbolic AI, successfully combat this eliminativism, starting with McCarthy's seminal work in 1953 on Programs with Common Sense, Pat Hayes' Naïve Physics Manifesto, and the field of qualitative reasoning and reaching a peak in current multiagent research, where autonomous agents are supposed to have high-level cognitive functions and reason with beliefs, intentions, and desires and are even supposed to express emotions – indeed a straightforward implementation of folk psychology.

Returning to statistics, we have already stated that Pearson made a vital contribution to this debate, and although causality would make a big revival in statistics after Pearson, his Pythagorean view of the world as a probability distribution stands firmly today. In the next sections it is shown that the tension sketched above even intensified after Pearson throughout the development of 20th-century statistics and continues to cast its shadows on statistics today. The general problem for (philosophy of) statistics is clear: How can intuitive notions on reasoning, risk, odds, uncertainty, chance, or confidence – which are crucial in the world we experience and from which we want to obtain knowledge – be covered, represented, or harmonized with or replaced by notions from mathematical probability and statistics: significance level, likelihood, testing, confidence intervals and effect size, parameter estimation, power, and type 1 and type 2 errors. Is convergence or alignment possible? Unsurprisingly, in the many disciplines concerned with probabilistic reasoning this has been debated. Are humans intuitive statisticians like the psychologist C.R. Peterson claimed in the sixties, or did famous experiments conducted by Kahneman and Tversky prove the opposite? Or should we perhaps pay more attention to the strenuous objections of L.J. Cohen, who scorned what he called the "Pascalian" tradition? Statisticians themselves have been playing their part in this debate, and the success of the so-called Bayesian paradigm in AI and epistemology is largely attributable to this issue. The allegory of the thinking machine in AI is exploited not only in symbolic AI (knowledge representation), but even in subsymbolic AI, where probabilistic reasoning has achieved immense success (e.g., in Bayesian belief networks and learning), and in this respect it brought statistics and computer science closer together. This issue will be pursued a little further in a later section.

The Fisherean Turn: Estimation, Models and Causality

Pearson's extreme phenomenalism prevented him from establishing relations other than correlative ones and made him reluctant to accept any concept of reality or model that went far beyond the data. In fact, Pearson considered the statistical distribution as describing the actual collection of data, a large but finite subset of the set of all possible measurements that could only be measured in an ideal situation. As long as the subset was big enough, the computed parameters would be the same as those of the entire collection. Probability should not be related to some obscure, abstract underlying reality, beyond phenomena.

Ronald A. Fisher (1890–1962), on the other hand, was not constrained by Machean doctrines and looked deeper into the Pythagorean universe. For him reality was an abstract mathematical distribution rather than a sparse, "think-economic" description of the data at hand. These data were just a random sample, having a distribution of their own. Truth didn't collapse with the data, but it could only be estimated. As such, evaluation criteria were needed based on the characteristics of the sampling distribution. Fisher famously came up with criteria that, although altered by his descendants, are persistent in current practice: unbiasedness, consistency, and efficiency. In this way he could prove Pearson "wrong" on many occasions.

He also made a big step forward in the development of the idea of significance testing, which was in some primitive form already recognizable with John Arbuthnot in the eighteenth century and which went no further with Pearson than the idea of goodness of fit. Fisher achieved this by nearly single-handedly developing concepts like p-values, significance level, degrees of freedom, and especially a clear distinction between sample and population. The latter was necessary to create the very idea of estimation, which obtained a central place in statistical inference due to Fisher. He also worked on well-founded notions of randomization and random samples, unlike Pearson, who rather relied on large amounts of data collected at the Galton laboratory by convenience sampling. Thus Fisher made a definitive step toward inferential statistics. He also reinstated the concept of causality in science by giving it a central place in his methodology.

In fact, Fisher did what Pearson initiated but failed to accomplish: establishing a new statistical methodology, the core of which still stands today. The analysis of variance offered a framework for experimental design, and his maximum likelihood estimation has dominated scientific reasoning up to the present and has gained an unprecedented popularity. His criteria for the assessment of estimators marked the rise of efficiency theory and provided him with the tools to vigorously attack the Pearsonian bastion. Last but not least we must emphasize another great achievement that is largely attributable to Fisher: the whole idea of a statistical model. Just like the notion of estimation, this concept was determined by the underlying philosophy regarding reality and knowledge. The conception of a statistical model as a collection of probability distributions containing the data-generating function that could only be estimated based on statistics with a distribution of its own was a Fisherean concept; it was not explicitly part of the Pearsonian philosophy.

No doubt Pearson and Fisher were antipodes, and this also became apparent in their contributions to biology: Pearson being a biometrician, Fisher a mendelian. Both camps were involved in vicious ideological clashes for decades. Many would be inclined to agree that in answering the epistemic key questions Fisher was an improvement on Pearson in many ways, and indeed he has changed the face of statistics considerably. However, he did not refute or sweep the Pearsonean philosophy away. In fact, it could be argued that Pearson's statistical ideas are still influential and have even enjoyed a revival in recent decades in computational intelligence approaches like data mining.

This field has many powerful techniques and an underlying methodology that rather show a greater affinity with the heritage of Pearson than demonstrate a continuation of Fisher's work. Algorithms such as association rules, decision trees, and tree induction have taken over the donkey work of Pearson's calculatores. These techniques certainly do perform probabilistic reasoning based on large amounts of data; how the data have been collected and the underlying mechanism that would have generated them may seem less important. This applies to the relationship between sample and population too; in computational intelligence, this is more like Pearson than Fisher. Even more important is the role of estimation, which is in many computational intelligence techniques no longer the guiding principle or key notion in statistical inference, and the same applies to corresponding assessment criteria from efficiency theory. Pearsonian goodness of fit, cross validation, and all kinds of notions of similarity and measures for predictive success are dominant.

We therefore will defend the claim that the first factor responsible for the current situation in statistical data analysis can be traced back to the contrast between Pearson and Fisher. More precisely, the fact that several elements from both philosophies coexist while being mutually exclusive is of prime importance; the different answers they gave to the epistemic key questions resound in their views on models, reality, inference, and truth.

Hypothesis Testing: The Fisher–Neyman/Pearson Controversy

Fisher's contribution to statistics was even more controversial, and his legacy contributed largely to the current situation. The reason for this was that many of his ideas and concepts were canonized and applied before they were fully developed, agreed upon, and understood. For example, significance testing was, according to Fisher, a weak argument, only to be applied in randomized experiments and powerful in a series of tests. Significance did not imply rejection once and for all, and insignificance didn't imply unimportance in the "substantial" domain.

Ironically, the confusion was partly due to one of Fisher's magnificent performances, his *Statistical Methods for Research Workers* (1925). In fact, this was the first genuine methodology handbook in history. He accomplished what philosophers like Aristotle, Francis Bacon, and, in the nineteenth century, J.S. Mill and Herschel had tried but failed to achieve. It contained no hard mathematics or proofs, but practical advice and techniques to be applied by nonmathematicians and practitioners: biologists, agricultural scientists, psychologists, and social scientists working in the field. But Fisher was often quite unclear about the precise interpretation of concepts like significance level, rejection and confirmation, proof, and truth.

Be that as it may, the social sciences, and especially psychology, which had just emerged from a period dominated by positivism, were eager to enhance their scientific status and desperately looking for a logic of scientific inference. This involved drawing conclusions from data in many ways: confirming or rejecting hypotheses concerning the "real" world, manipulating measured variables, hypothesizing about latent constructs or unmeasured variables, dealing with positive and negative evidence, "deriving" statistical laws in the Queteletian way, etc. It seemed that the recipes could all be found in Fisher's book. Sometimes chasing low p-values (including the celebration of significance and not reporting nonsignificance) seemed the royal, if not the only, road to truth.

But the whole idea of Fisherian significance testing came under real attack by peers like Jerzy Neyman (1894–1981) and Egon Pearson (1895–1980), Karl Pearson's son. Impressed as they both were with Fisher's maximum likelihood estimation and his concept of a statistical model, they could not approve Fisher's arbitrary criteria for a test statistic and rejection area. They argued that testing a hypothesis only made sense if one confronted the hypothesis with a set of alternative hypotheses, that one should consider two types of error that are usually of unequal importance (type 1 and type 2 errors), which gave rise to their famous theory on statistical power and related ideas on effect size and calculations of sample size. Neyman and Pearson gave hypothesis testing a central place in inferential statistics, next to estimation. Fisher didn't accept the criticism, overemphasizing the differences between significance testing and hypothesis testing. According to Neyman they were conceptually similar, he only intended to improve on Fisher. Again two schools seemed to emerge. Analogous problems could be formulated with respect to confidence intervals, which were also not acknowledged by Fisher, who experimented with his own ideas on interval estimation, the so-called fiducial probabilities, that would find little support.

In fact, there were many more (philosophically inspired) controversies between both Fisher and Neyman, that cannot be dealt with here. Both were frequentists at heart, but Neyman took a behavioristic stance and accused Fisher of using concepts that could not be dealt with in a decent frequentist way, making references to epistemic connotations, sometimes even acting in a semi-Bayesian way. In those days this was a serious indictment. Still, today no definite synthesis has been achieved and as such the controversy between Fisher and Neyman/Pearson may be regarded as the second factor in the history of statistics that influenced current practice. Again elements of both statistical traditions are concurrently applied in practice and sometimes used in a rather odd, ecumenist way.

Bayesianism, Indirect Probability, Knowledge Representation

The third immanent development in the history of statistics that must be identified is no less dominant than the previous one, and has everything to do with the tension or dualism between scientific worldview and commonsense worldview that we sketched in our discussion of material eliminativism. Also, Pearson's successors Fisher and Neyman contributed to this tension, albeit in a different way.

Many concepts related to probability, estimation, and testing introduced by both are notoriously difficult to interpret and are far removed from our intuitive notions about knowledge, uncertainty, truth, and reasoning: significance, *p*-values, degrees of freedom, confidence intervals, and effect size. An interpretation is often only possible with a frequentist approach to the concept of probability. For example, confidence intervals serve well as an effect size but are notoriously difficult to interpret and in a way presuppose a frequentist view on probability. That is precisely the problem, because ever since the emergence of probability in the seventeenth century, it has been clear that probability expresses not only regularity in the long run but also has epistemic and doxastic connotations that must be accounted for.

In addressing the interpretation of probability we unavoidably enter the realm that is arguably the most important theme in the philosophy of probability in the twentieth century, giving rise to many different approaches: frequentist (John Venn, Richard von Mises), logical (John Keynes), propensity (Karl Popper, inspired by C.S. Peirce), and subjective and objective Bayesian (Jimmy Savage, Bruno de Finetti, and Harold Jeffreys). Bayesianism can be traced back to the eighteenth century, building upon the work of Thomas Bayes (1702–1761) on inverse probabilities and on Laplace's epistemic notion of probability. It led to a paradigm that attacked the inconveniences, paradoxes, and alleged shortcomings of mainstream, "frequentist" statistics and has been flourishing especially outside statistics as a dominant paradigm for probabilistic reasoning, with applications ranging from AI, decision theory, and epidemiology to formal epistemology and even theology, where Richard Swinburne used Bayesian methods to make the existence of God more plausible.

It is highly questionable whether Bayes would have recognized himself in modern Bayesianism, but he did give an impetus to it in his famous posthumously published paper on indirect probability, sometimes referred to as the probability of causes. In the seventeenth century Jacob Bernoulli had advocated direct probability, that is – somewhat anachronistically put – assigning a probability to a sample based on a known distribution at the population level. Bayes asked the reversed question: how to draw conclusions about a population based on available evidence. He achieved this by applying conditional probabilities in his inversion rule. Thus he became the first to link the philosophical concept of induction (addressed by philosophers like Bacon and Hume) to probability or, rather, statistics.

Fisher and Neyman had little in common except a shared hatred of Bayesianism and subjectivist statistics. Initially, their dominance prevented the breakthrough of this paradigm. But the development went steadily on with the work of Jimmy Savage, Bruno de Finetti, and Harold Jeffreys in decision theory, but especially due to computational progress in the 1990s and in particular in the project of AI. In this field, which is focused on high-level cognitive functions using human categories, Bayesianism is in many ways attractive: knowledge and belief and their associated concepts can be directly represented in an object language rather than informally in a metalanguage. One can make probability statements about propositions, theories, and hypotheses instead of assigning probabilities to subsets of events. The whole idea of reasoning with new knowledge is of course encrypted in a straightforward way using posterior distributions and a straightforward application of Bayes' rule. One can also express different degrees of confidence or belief in alternative hypotheses or theories, thus avoiding the problems related to naive Popperian falsificationism, that troubled early Fisherian significance testing, but even the more advanced Neyman–Pearson approach.

Indeed, the differences with traditional "statistical" knowledge representation and reasoning are considerable. For example, the interval estimators of de Finetti and Savage are very different from Neyman's confidence bounds. The maximum likelihood estimation procedure is not comparable with the "update mechanism" of the posterior distribution. Truth is no longer a fixed, but unknown, parameter because the parameter now has a distribution. Put roughly, the case has not been settled, and, for example, in fields like decision theory and epidemiology, classical and Bayesian approaches are concurrently applied, while many of the concepts are inconsistent or incompatible.

Beyond Parametric Statistics and Maximum Likelihood Estimation: A Pragmatist Perspective

Finally, we must distinguish a fourth trend. The great popularity of maximum likelihood estimation and parametric statistics could not conceal its limitations; objections were raised by mathematicians, but were also expressed by (nonmathematical) workers in the field, which traditionally have played an important role in the history of statistics. Sometimes the conditions for application could not be met sometimes application did not lead to useful knowledge. As a result, complementary or even alternative approaches to parametric statistics, and even inferential statistics, were proposed.

In the 1930s many nonparametric techniques were developed, starting with the work of the chemist Frank Wilcoxon, the mathematician Henry Mann, and many others working on distribution-free tests. Today they still have a modest but solid place in the toolkit of the statistical analyst. More important was the work of John Tukey, whose exploratory data analysis evolved from a complement of inferential statistics to a real alternative one, at least according to some. Data were analyzed with a minimum of theoretical ballast, searching for patterns, finding hypotheses, and focusing on data inspection and data visualization. In particular, the notion of a model as introduced by Fisher, and the associated conception of truth are no longer cherished. Intended or not, Tukey was and is often cited as a protagonist of George Box's view that models are by definition wrong, and may legitimately depend on speculative assumptions or wild guesses that may lead to something.

This popular view on models has also been exploited in another important development that does not build upon the maximum likelihood estimation approach and its assumptions: the advent of computer-intensive techniques (e.g., resampling) and especially the many machine learning techniques that have been developed since the 1980s, including ensemble learning, where multiple models are used to acheive better predictive success. As has been argued previously, the philosophical underpinning is Pearsonian, rather than Fisherian! Be that as it may, practice shows that these techniques were unable to displace the parametric tradition, do sometimes complement it, but at any rate are part of the toolbox/statistical packages.

Leaving the internalist perspective for a moment, it must be said that the underlying philosophy of Tukey and computational intelligence research is in the current era epistemologically justified and even seems to be encouraged. The age of all-encompassing and foundational epistemology ended in the 1960s. Thomas Kuhn emphasized the importance of the social and historical context of science, Paul Feyerabend attacked the standard view on science as a rational process, and Bruno Latour even advocated purely descriptive approaches. Pluralism and relativism go hand in hand. Postmodern thinkers like Richard Rorty even claimed that science and its models didn't "mirror nature" anymore and had lost their proverbial representative function. Of course, the latter philosopher can be considered postmodern or even antiscientific, but this cannot be said of another philosophical movement, which it may also be claimed endorsed the current situation: the pragmatism movement that arose in the nineteenth century with the work of C.S. Peirce and William James. It is still vital today, has many faces, and is strongly antifoundationalist in particular with respect to the concept of truth. Pragmatists refrain from a correspondence theory or coherence theory of truth but interpret truth as something that works in practice and that makes a difference in real life. For example, Peirce considered science the result of two human interests: the removal of irritation caused by doubt and imperatives to act decisively. It is not surprising that a pragmatist approach to truth and science is appreciated by statisticians, who naturally seek to identify differences and have always worked together with researchers on real-world problems. Generally speaking, a pragmatic view seems to tolerate, up to a point, the present situation in data analysis with respect to models, inference and truth. But it may not justify a gross oversimplification that relegates all theoretical and fundamental principles to the background, especially if these theoretical considerations prove themselves relevant in practice, making a difference! Still, pragmatism reinforces the need for empirical evaluation, ranging from the ancient replication experiments to calls for serious benchmarks, well-defined competitions, or other empirical validation procedures.

Conclusion

In this chapter, we have traversed, with seven-mile steps, the history of ideas and highlighted crucial developments in statistics as well. What conclusions can be drawn with respect to the current situation in statistical data analysis and how should TMLE be viewed from this historical/philosophical perspective? Obviously, in this exploratory essay we have only touched upon a few key issues and the most pressing challenges for the philosophy of statistics and epistemology.

Taking an externalist stance, we first sketched three aspects of the pervasiveness of information: its metaphysical implications and foundational role in the sciences, its appearance at the "level" of data and the need for a science of data, incorporating statistics and computer science, and, finally, the probabilistic turn in the sciences and the problems it poses for epistemology. No doubt the integration, also at the foundational level, of statistics and computational intelligence is one of the challenges for contemporary philosophy of statistics. In this respect TMLE takes an important step with the super learning methodology as it integrates the full range of machine learning techniques (including intensive cross-validation to select the initial estimators) into a statistical framework based on estimation as the key notion of inference and confidence intervals, firmly rooted in efficiency theory. In addition, the general problem that statistical analysis is not as well founded as we would like, given its crucial importance for epistemology, marks a related but distinct major task for the philosophy of statistics. TMLE may shed new light on this issue because it rethinks crucial concepts like estimation, models, truth, and causation. TMLE reassigns to the concept of estimation, which in some ways had lost its crucial place in probabilistic reasoning, the leading role in any theory of/approach to "learning from data", preserving the log-likelihood as the principal criterion in estimation, and renewing Fisherian statistics. It also reestablishes the concept of a model in a parsimonious way. Models should only contain the genuine background knowledge of the agent, not speculative assumptions or wild guesses that may lead to something. It does not stick to the popular interpretation of models as mere representations of "something" in which truth is regarded as an unnecessary and even obsolete concept, bound to be eliminated with Occam's razor. On the contrary, truth is a prerequisite for meaningful use of models. It relates to fixed, but unknown, parameters, that are to be estimated. It therefore needs neither the pragmatist stance, identifying truth with "what makes a difference in reality" or "what works in practice," nor a conventionalist or constructivist position. No doubt its place in the current scientific realism debate is certainly something worth exploring. Also noticeable is the concept of causality, abandoned by Pearson, reinstated by Fisher, but still highly problematic in probabilistic reasoning. Analogous to the, in our view, regrettable methodological gap between the ideal of internal vs. external validity, probabilistic reasoning sometimes seems divided by communities working on confounding or on estimation. In TMLE causal inference takes place within the "extended" model, i.e., the statistical model expanded with possible additional nontestable causal assumptions, under which the targeted parameter can be interpreted as a causal parameter. Be that as it may, epistemology should realize that dealing with foundational problems like these, requires close collaboration with statistics and its philosophy. Paradoxically, the strong emphasis on probabilistic reasoning in epistemology has seldom led to a comparable interest in immanent developments in statistics. Admittedly, the Bayesian paradigm has been embraced canonized, if not overemphasized, but more important contributions to statistics are largely neglected. For example, Pearson seems now a forgotten philosopher, whose name is often not even mentioned in mainstream textbooks on the philosophy of science. Furthermore, because TMLE has been developed and applied in large-scale empirical domains and has to deal with real-life questions emerging there, it may well complement the much used isolated "toy examples" that have long been dominant in epistemology.

The second major development concerned the emancipation process of variation and change as fundamental or essential characteristics of reality and the fact that science must do justice to this in modeling reality. Paradoxically and ironically, more than 2500 years after Parmenides, variation and chance remain problematic because, due to progress in science (better instruments for measurement) and computer science (better techniques for data management, storage, and retrieval), variation and change can be identified easier: more subjects, variables ranging over larger intervals, longitudinal data, and especially more variables, resulting in high-dimensional data sets. The end of this is still nowhere in sight! Fisher did his famous studies on crop variation at the Rothamsted Experimental Station with only a few independent variables. A misspecified model could do less harm than in a situation with thousands of variables, where error is propagated and increased through the analysis, indeed a notorious aspect of the curse of dimensionality. TMLE states that questions about our infinite-dimensional, semiparametric Pythagorean universe are not well addressed by parametric models. It pleas for utilizing methods specially designed to estimate a relatively small-dimensional, precisely specified parameter within a realistic semiparametric model that is identifiable from the data. The point is that likelihood-based estimators generally are aimed at estimating the density of the distribution of the data themselves, seeking a bias–variance tradeoff that is optimal for the whole density. Clearly the variance of an optimally smoothed density estimator is typically much larger than the variance of a smooth (pathwise-differentiable) parameter of the density estimator. As a result, substitution estimators based on density estimators involving an optimal (e.g., likelihood-based) bias–variance tradeoff (for the whole density) are usually unnecessarily biased relative to their variance as they are not targeted toward the parameter of interest. The ideal method to deal with variation and change would incorporate this and would also be entirely a priori specified without relying on ad hoc specifications, have attractive statistical properties, and be computationally feasible.

The third development we sketched concerned the tension between our commonsense notions and natural categories on the one hand and the scientific worldview and nomenclature on the other. We stated that there is no simple opposition between Reid's *sensus communis* and "folk psychology" on the one hand and eliminativism on the other. Indeed, all key problems in the philosophy of statistics can be viewed against this background. Of course, it would require a detailed study to find out how nomenclature developed or used in TMLE (e.g., nuisance parameter, bias–variance tradeoff, loss-based super learning) is related to specific issues in the substantial domain. Here we restrict ourselves to three aspects, the first of which addresses the issue of personal or subjective elements in inference. In a way these are always manifest. Fisher had to choose the test statistic and statistical model, Neyman had to decide upon a set of rival hypotheses, and the Bayesians had to come up with suitable prior distributions. TMLE further reduces subjectivity in a different way. It restores the old ideal of AI, contributing to automatic reasoning by reducing the role of human intervention without appealing to "Fingerspitzengefühl" or skillful art. Another aspect concerns the fact that the research question, an important aspect of the substantial domain, should be related to properties of the data-generating distribution, which of course highly affects the interpretation of coefficients. A coefficient in a parametric model typically fails to represent the research question, even in the unrealistic scenario that the model is correct, and lacks any commonsense interpretation if the parametric model is misspecified. TMLE decouples the choice of model from the definition of the target parameter that represents the research question, thereby allowing the researcher's world and knowledge to be translated into a realistic (and thereby semiparametric) model and representative commonsense target parameter. A third aspect involves the "two-layer" knowledge representation in TMLE, first the statistical model, representing true realistic knowledge in a parsimonious way, second the "extended" model, i.e., the statistical model expanded with possible additional nontestable causal assumptions, under which the targeted parameter can be interpreted as a causal parameter.

We also took an internalist stance, sketching four developments in the history of statistics, that all left their mark in research practice but are quite different with respect to such notions as models, inference, and truth. We then outlined various aspects of TMLE, showing that there can be no question of a forced marriage with the existing tradition or a mere addition to the "toolkit." TMLE establishes a new "learning from data" paradigm by offering an integrative approach to data analysis or statistical learning, which in many ways marks a break with the past. In a sense, TMLE builds on and renews the Fisherian tradition, but it also dismantles the parametric bastion that has emerged from this tradition and its alleged universal applicability. The persistent debate between classical and Bayesian statistics has many aspects that are less relevant from the perspective of TMLE since they both are not targeted, facing analogous problems in high-dimensional data sets. Regarding the computational and nonparametric tradition, TMLE shows that a pragmatic view on knowledge and the use of a variety of intelligent computational techniques entail neither relativism nor a statistically less fundamental methodology.

Scientific debates as we have outlined are not solved "ex cathedra," certainly not by philosophical considerations. Whether or not theories are successful is determined by many factors, externalist as well. But a revolution is primarily fought in the streets, and in this respect a new "TMLE version" of "statistical methods for research workers" would be a good start. Education is vital: people are inclined to keep working in the tradition where they were raised, and use the same software they have always used. Our historical and philosophical perspective was aimed not only at clarifying, understanding, and accounting for the current situation in statistical data analysis but also at relating topics addressed by TMLE in both the philosophy of statistics and the epistemology/philosophy of science. Any epistemologist who considers information processes to be fundamental, who wants to do justice to variation and change in reality, and who addresses the tension between a scientific worldview and common sense can hardly neglect debates about immanent trends in statistics and the key problems they pose for the philosophy of statistics. This applies even more if one takes the view that any interesting concept in epistemology and science can only be genuinely developed by considering real-life problems occurring in large-scale knowledge domains. The associated methodology for probabilistic reasoning should be from the same mold.

Part I
Targeted Learning: The Basics

Chapter 1
The Open Problem

Sherri Rose, Mark J. van der Laan

The debate over hormone replacement therapy (HRT) has been one of the biggest health discussions in recent history. Professional groups and nonprofits, such as the American College of Physicians and the American Heart Association, gave HRT their stamp of approval 15 years ago. Studies indicated that HRT was protective against osteoporosis and heart disease. HRT became big business, with millions upon millions of prescriptions filled each year. However, in 1998, the Heart and Estrogen-Progestin Replacement Study demonstrated increased risk of heart attack among women with heart disease taking HRT, and in 2002 the Women's Health Initiative showed increased risk for breast cancer, heart disease, and stroke, among other ailments, for women on HRT. Why were there inconsistencies in the study results?

Mammography gained relatively widespread acceptance as an effective tool for breast cancer screening in the 1980s. While there was still debate, several studies, including the Health Insurance Plan trial and the Swedish Two-County trial, demonstrated that mammography saved lives. This outweighed the minimal evidence against mammography. Thus, in 2009, many medical practitioners and nonprofits were surprised by the new recommendations from the U.S. Preventive Services Task Force. Among women without a family history, mammography was now only recommended for women aged 50 to 74. The previous guidelines started at age 40. Why was there a seemingly sudden paradigm shift?

A political scientist examines the effect of butterfly ballots in an election, which may in turn change local election laws. A group of economists studies the effect of microlending on the local economy in rural areas of Africa in hopes of promoting greater adoption of this practice. Public health policy decisions regarding how frequently to perform gynecological exams await the completion of several new investigations. The question then becomes, how does one translate the results from these studies, how do we take the information in the data, and draw effective conclusions?

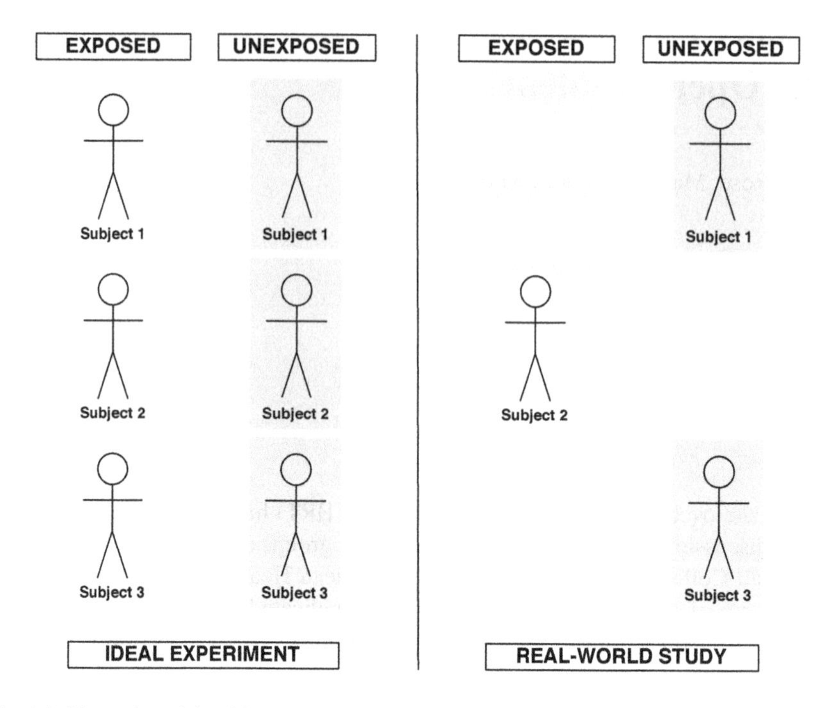

Fig. 1.1 Illustration of the "ideal experiment" vs. studies conducted in the real world

1.1 Learning from Data

One of the great open problems across many diverse fields of research has been obtaining causal effects from data. Data are typically sampled from a population of interest since collecting data on the entire population is not feasible. Frequently, the researcher is not interested in merely studying association or correlation in this sample data; she wants to know whether a treatment or exposure causes the outcome in the population of interest. If one can show that the treatment or exposure causes the outcome, we can then impact the outcome by intervening on the treatment or exposure.

Just what type of studies are we conducting? The often quoted "ideal experiment" is one that cannot be conducted in real life. Let us say we are interested in studying the causal effect of a toxin on death from cancer within 5 years. In an ideal experiment, we intervene and set the exposure to *exposed* for each subject. All subjects are followed for 5 years, where the outcome under this exposure is recorded. We then go back in time to the beginning of the study, intervene, and set all subjects to *not exposed* and *follow them under identical conditions* until the end of the study, recording the outcome under this exposure. As noted, we obviously cannot administer such a study since it is not possible to go back in time.

However, let's assume in principle there is a system where this ideal experiment could have been conducted. This experiment generates random variables. Say the experiment is that we sample a subject (i.e., draw a random variable) from a population and take several measurements on this subject. This experiment is repeated multiple times until we have sampled an a priori specified number (representing the sample size) of subjects. These random variables also have a true underlying probability distribution. Our observed data are realizations of these random variables. If we were to conduct our repeated experiment again, we would observe different realizations of these random variables.

Any knowledge we have about how these observed data were generated is referred to as a model. For example, it might be known that the data consist of observations on a number of independent and identically distributed (i.i.d.) random variables. What does i.i.d. mean? We are repeatedly drawing random variables from the same probability distribution, but each draw is mutually independent from all others. A common toy example used in statistics texts is the roll of a fair die. Say the experiment is to roll a die. We perform this experiment six times, each time rolling it following the same procedure (e.g., shaking). If we roll the die six times, we will see one set of realizations of these random variables, e.g., we observe a 1, 5, 3, 6, 2, and then a 5. Each roll of the die (i.e., each experiment) is independent from the previous roll. The observed unit in many cases may be the individual, where we sample repeatedly individual subjects from a population of interest. However, the observed unit can also be a household of individuals or a community of people.

So, our data are i.i.d. random variables, but the probability distribution of the random variable is typically completely unknown. This is also information we incorporate into our model. We will refer to this as a nonparametric model for the probability distribution of the random variable. (Do note, however, that assuming the data vector is i.i.d. in our nonparametric model is a real assumption, although one we will always make in this book.) Our model should always reflect true knowledge about the probability distribution of the data, which may often be a nonparametric model, or a semiparametric model that makes some additional assumptions. For example, perhaps it is known that the probability of death is monotonically increasing in the levels of exposure, and we want to include this information in our model.

The knowledge we have discussed thus far regarding our model pertains to our observed data and what we call the statistical model. The statistical model is, formally, the collection of possible probability distributions. The model may also contain extra information in addition to the knowledge contained in the statistical model. Now we want to relate our observed data to a causal model. We can do this with additional assumptions, and we refer to a statistical model augmented with these additional causal assumptions as the model for the observed data. These additional assumptions allow us to define the system where this ideal experiment could have been conducted. We can describe the generation of the data with nonparametric structural equations, intervene on treatment or exposure and set those values to *exposed* and *not exposed*, and then see what the (counterfactual) outcomes would have been under both exposures. This underlying causal model allows us to define a causal effect of treatment or exposure.

One now needs to specify the relation between the observed data on a unit and the full data generated in the causal model. For example, one might assume that the observed data corresponds with observing all the variables generated by the system of structural equations that make up the causal model, up till background factors that enter as error terms in the underlying structural equations. The specification of the relation between the observed data and this underlying causal model allows one now to assess if the causal effect of interest can be identified from the probability distribution of the observed data. If that is not possible, then we state that the desired causal effect is not identifiable. If, on the other hand, our causal assumptions allow us to write the causal effect as a particular feature of the probability distribution of the observed data, then we have identified a target parameter of the probability distribution of the observed data that can be interpreted as a causal effect.

Let's assume that the causal effect is identifiable from the observed data. Our parameter of interest, here the causal effect of a toxin on death from cancer within 5 years, is now a parameter of our true probability distribution of the observed data. This definition as a parameter of the probability distribution of the observed data does not rely on the causal assumptions coded by the underlying causal model describing the ideal experiment for generating the desired full data, and the link between the observed data and the full data. Thus, if we ultimately do not believe these causal assumptions, the parameter is still an interesting statistical parameter. Our next goal becomes estimating this parameter of interest.

The open problem addressed in this book is the estimation of interesting parameters of the probability distribution of the data. This need not only be (causal) effect measures. Another problem researchers are frequently faced with is the generation of functions for the prediction of outcomes. For these problems, we do not make causal assumptions, but still define our realistic nonparametric or semiparametric statistical model based on actual knowledge. We view effect and prediction parameters of interest as features of the probability distribution of our data, well defined for each probability distribution in the nonparametric or semiparametric model. Statistical learning from data is concerned with efficient and unbiased estimation of these features and with an assessment of uncertainty of the estimator. Traditional approaches to estimation differ from this philosophy.

1.2 Traditional Approach to Estimation

We can sometimes implement one element of the ideal experiment: assigning a value for treatment or exposure in a controlled experiment. Controlled experiments are exactly what they sound like: they allow the investigator to control certain variables in the study. Randomized controlled trials (RCTs) are one type of controlled experiment where subjects are randomized to receive a specific level of treatment. For example, if each subject was assigned to one of two levels of treatment based on the flip of a fair coin, the differences between the two groups would be solely due to treatment as all other factors would be balanced, up to random error. However, most studies are so-called observational studies where exposure or treatment is not assigned. In many cases it may not be ethical to set the exposure of interest in an RCT, or an RCT is cost prohibitive.

1.2.1 Experimental Studies

The randomization in RCTs suggests that we can estimate the causal effect of the treatment. For example, the difference of means between the treatment and control groups equals an additive causal effect. Indeed, this randomization of treatment in RCTs allows us to go from the observed data to the causal effect of interest. The difference in means can be estimated using a saturated regression of the outcome on treatment in a parametric statistical model where covariates are ignored. Since the regression is saturated (i.e., there is a parameter for each of the two observed values of treatment), this parametric statistical model is not making any unreasonable assumptions, and is thus actually nonparametric. Therefore, this parametric statistical model is not wrong, although the resulting estimator of the causal effect of the treatment is not the most efficient estimator. This so-called unadjusted estimator of the treatment effect is a nonparametric maximum likelihood estimator based on the reduced observations that only consist of the outcome and the treatment.

Suppose randomization did not occur perfectly due to chance (as is common), and there is a single covariate that is predictive of the outcome. We now have more subjects in the treatment or control group with a covariate that is predictive of the outcome, and this saturated regression ignoring the covariate will potentially contain a lot of residual error due to the exclusion of the covariate. Now, one might propose conditioning on the covariate and taking the difference in means for each stratum of the covariate. This results in a treatment effect within each stratum of the covariate. One might now estimate the causal effect of treatment as the average over all strata of these strata-specific treatment effects. This adjusted estimator of the treatment effect is a nonparametric maximum likelihood estimator based on the reduced observations that consist of the outcome, treatment, and this single covariate. This approach is generally still not efficient, since it only uses one of the measured covariates, but it is more efficient than the unadjusted treatment effect estimator. However, this strategy is not practical with multiple covariates, or even one continuous covariate, and starts to suffer in practical performance due to strata with a very small number of subjects.

So why not run regressions in parametric statistical models (incorporating all covariates) for RCTs? The short answer is simple: the Food and Drug Administration (FDA) does not allow it. We will explain why this is so in a few sections. For now it is sufficient to know that the FDA requires researchers to specify a priori the method of estimation, and it must rely on a statistical model that reflects true knowledge.

1.2.2 Observational Studies

Recall that observational studies do not involve randomization to treatment or exposure. In most observational studies, standard practice for effect estimation involves assuming a parametric statistical model and using maximum likelihood estimation to estimate the parameters in that statistical model. Let us be very clear again about what a statistical model is: the statistical model represents the set of possible probability distributions of the data.

In traditional practice, one assumes the actual data as observed in practice can be represented as observations of n i.i.d. random variables, and that the goal of the traditional modeling approach is to learn the true underlying probability distribution that generated the data. (This is different than the goal of causal effect estimation.) Maximum likelihood estimation uses the likelihood function to estimate the unknown parameter(s) in the statistical model. Solutions are often found by differentiating the log-likelihood with respect to these parameters, setting the resulting equation equal to zero, and solving. If the score equation has multiple solutions, the solution with the largest likelihood is selected.

This procedure is detailed in most introductory statistics books, although the pervasiveness of statistical software allows the user to implement maximum likelihood estimation without the need to understand these concepts. This also means the assumptions that come with the use of parametric statistical models are frequently not well understood or ignored.

We already acknowledged in Sect. 1.1 that we usually know very little about how our data were generated; thus the use of parametric statistical models is troublesome. We typically know that our data can be represented as a number (representing the sample size) of i.i.d. observations, which is an assumption in parametric statistical models, but we do not know the underlying probability distribution that generated the data. Parametric statistical models assume the underlying probability distribution that generated the data is known up to a finite number of parameters. It is an accepted fact within the statistical community that nonsaturated *parametric statistical models are wrong*. Thus, making an assumption known to be untrue is not the best approach. When this assumption is violated and the statistical model is misspecified, the estimate of the probability distribution can be extremely biased, and it is not even clear what the parameter estimates are even estimating. The bias resulting from statistical model misspecification cannot be overcome with a large sample size.

This brings us to another problem that arises when using misspecified parametric statistical models. The target parameter is not defined as a parameter of the true probability distribution for any possible probability distribution. The target parameter, when defined as a coefficient in a (misspecified) parametric statistical model, is only defined within that parametric statistical model, as if the statistical model were true. There is only correct inference if the parametric statistical model is correct, but we know it is wrong.

Lastly, the traditional approach does not make any explicit (untestable) causal assumptions linking the observed data to a system that generated the data. Thus, there is no framework to make causal inference. There are also other assumptions that are part of the statistical model that are typically not addressed, such as positivity (discussed in Chaps. 2 and 10). When this (testable) assumption is violated, you may see groups of individuals where there is no experimentation in the treatment. For example, all the highly educated women received HRT, or all the wealthy women received mammograms. Since there are strata of certain covariates (e.g., level of education, socioeconomic status) where all subjects are treated, the regression will extrapolate what would have happened to these subjects had they not been treated, and this extrapolation is not based on any observed information.

To summarize, the use of parametric statistical models in observational studies is troublesome for several main reasons.

1. The statistical models are always misspecified in practice since we do not know the underlying data-generating distribution and we handle complex problems with many covariates.
2. The target parameter is not defined as a parameter of the true probability distribution that generated the data.
3. The traditional approach does not typically make causal assumptions allowing us to define the desired causal effect, and often neglects other key assumptions, such as the positivity assumption, that are part of the statistical model.

1.2.3 Regression in (Misspecified) Parametric Statistical Models

In this section we discuss briefly the traditional approach to effect estimation. Let us introduce our random variable O, which has probability distribution P_0. This is written $O \sim P_0$. Recall that a probability distribution P_0 assigns a probability to any possible event or set of possible outcomes for O. In particular, $P_0(O = o)$ for a particular value o of O can be defined as a probability if O is a discrete random variable, or we can use the concept of probability density if O is continuous. For simplicity and sake of presentation, we will often treat O as discrete so that we can refer to $P_0(O = o)$ as a probability.

We observe our random variable O n times, by repeating the same experiment n times. For a simple example, suppose our data structure is $O = (W, A, Y) \sim P_0$. We have a covariate or vector of covariates W, an exposure or treatment A, and a continuous outcome Y. These variables comprise the random variable O, which we observe repeatedly, and O has probability distribution P_0. Thus, for each possible value (w, a, y), $P_0(w, a, y)$ denotes the probability that (W, A, Y) equals (w, a, y). For example, the random variables $O_1, \ldots, O_n$ might be the result of randomly sampling n subjects from a population of patients, collecting baseline characteristics

W, assigning treatment or exposure A, and following the patients and measuring continuous outcome Y.

Suppose one poses a particular regression in a parametric statistical model, a so-called linear regression for the conditional mean of Y given A or Y given A and W. However, we leave the distributions of A and W unspecified. Linear regression in a parametric statistical model has varying levels of complexity, and what variables one includes impacts this complexity. The saturated regression for RCTs discussed in Sect. 1.2.1 includes only a treatment variable A. (This is sometimes called a crude regression.) For example, with a continuous outcome Y and a binary treatment A the regression of the conditional mean of Y given A is

$$E_0(Y \mid A) = \alpha_0 + \alpha_1 A.$$

The parameter $E_0(Y \mid A)$ is the conditional mean of Y given A, and (α_0, α_1) are the unknown regression parameters in the parametric statistical model for the conditional mean. We are estimating the regression $E_0(Y \mid A)$ based on the data $(A_1, Y_1), \ldots, (A_n, Y_n)$, ignoring the covariates W_i for subject i. Fitting this regression to the data will result in an estimate of the effect of treatment given by $\alpha_1 = E_0(Y \mid A = 1) - E_0(Y \mid A = 0)$.

In the analysis of observational studies, it is commonplace to include covariates associated with both A and Y in the regression, in an attempt to eliminate the contribution of these variables and isolate the effect of A on Y. With one covariate W, an example of such a regression in a parametric statistical model is

$$E_0(Y \mid A, W) = \alpha_0 + \alpha_1 A + \alpha_2 W.$$

The effect of A is again given by α_1, but α_1 now represents an effect of A adjusting for W, and is thus a different parameter of interest than the effect of A above. If effect modification is suspected, an interaction term between the effect modifier and A might be included:

$$E_0(Y \mid A, W) = \alpha_0 + \alpha_1 A + \alpha_2 W + \alpha_3 A \times W. \tag{1.1}$$

Effect modification between A and W occurs when the effect of A differs within strata of W. The consequence of including an interaction term in the regression is that there is now not one summary measure of the effect of A. For every level of W there is a different effect measure of A. For example, in the simple case where W is binary, such as smoking status, there will be two effect measures for A. If $W = 1$ indicates current smoker, the effect of A among current smokers is $\alpha_1 + \alpha_3$. When $W = 0$, α_3 is equal to zero thus the effect of A among current nonsmokers is α_1. As we add covariates and interaction terms to our regression, α_1 does not estimate a marginal population-level effect. In fact, each time we add a covariate or interaction the interpretation of the coefficients in the parametric statistical model changes.

In the situation where we only have one binary covariate, the regression specified in Eq. (1.1) is a saturated parametric statistical model. Let us also suppose the collection of the single covariate represents the truth, and there are no other covariates that should have been measured. This parametric statistical model is therefore suitable in that it is *not misspecified*. However, we still want a marginal effect estimate of treatment. This marginal-effect could be defined as $\alpha_1 + \alpha_3 E_0(W)$, where $E_0(W)$ denotes the true marginal mean of W. A simple nonparametric maximum likelihood estimator will accomplish this for the simple case posed here. But what happens when you have a continuous covariate? Or we have an increasing number of covariates? This approach to fitting a saturated linear regression quickly becomes problematic since the number of coefficients will grow exponentially with the number of covariates.

High-dimensional data have become increasingly common, and researchers often have dozens, hundreds, or even thousands of potential covariates to include in their parametric statistical model. Not only does this provide an impossible challenge to correctly specify the parametric statistical model for the conditional mean, but the complexity of the parametric statistical model may also increase to the point that there are more unknown parameters than observations. A fully saturated parametric statistical model will usually result in a gross overfit of the data. In addition, the true functional, $(A, W) \to E_0(Y \mid A, W)$, mapping the treatment and covariates into the conditional mean, might be described by a complex function not easily approximated by main terms or simple two-way interactions.

1.2.4 The Complications of Human Art in Statistics

We now highlight further the innate challenges of parametric statistical models and the problematic human art component of data analysis. Returning to our toxin and cancer study from Sect. 1.1, where an indicator of death is the outcome, let's say that the principal investigator (PI) asserts smoking status is the only relevant covariate that we must control for in our analysis. The PI also says to use the following logistic linear regression in a parametric statistical model for the probability of death, where the α_is are the unknown regression parameters in the statistical model:

$$P_0(Y = 1 \mid A, W) = \text{expit}(\alpha_0 + \alpha_1 A + \alpha_2 W).$$

Another subject matter expert on the project enters the conversation and says that one must also control for age and gender. Smoking is now denoted W_1, with age as W_2 and gender W_3. The covariates can be represented as a vector $W = \{W_1, W_2, W_3\}$ and the logistic linear regression given by

$$P_0(Y = 1 \mid A, W) = \text{expit}(\alpha_0 + \alpha_1 A + \alpha_2 W_1 + \alpha_3 W_2 + \alpha_4 W_3).$$

A data analyst enters the picture and explains that all covariates measured at baseline, listed in Table 1.1, should be thrown into a logistic linear regression. Using the results of this regression fit, all W_is with coefficients that do not have a p-value smaller than 0.05 should be removed from the list. The regression should then be fit again in a new (different) parametric statistical model with the variables remaining

Table 1.1 Baseline covariates from a study examining the effect of a toxin on death from cancer

W_i	Covariate
W_1	Smoking status
W_2	Age
W_3	Gender
W_4	Health status
W_5	Cardiac event
W_6	Chronic illness

in the list. This continues until all coefficients in front of the W_is in the regression have a p-value of less than 0.05. The regression coefficient α_1 in front of A changes with each new regression. It is highly dependent on which variables are included.

One can quickly see, even in this simplified example, the impossible challenge involved in selecting which variables to include in the parametric statistical model, and thereby assigning the underlying probability distribution of Y, conditional on the treatment and covariates, that generated the data up to a finite number of unknown parameters. The problem that we stress again here is that we do not know the true probability distribution of the data up to a finite number of unknown parameters.

The inference made using parametric statistical models assumes that the parametric statistical model is correct and was a priori selected. If the parametric statistical model is wrong, our estimates will approximate a noninterpretable parameter, and thereby be biased for the true hypothesized target parameter one had in mind under the assumption that the parametric statistical model was true. If we run several models with the full data, the statistical inference (e.g., the p-values) is meaningless, and this statistical model should be selected before looking at the data to avoid bias.

In addition, if the parametric statistical model was not a priori specified but data-adaptively selected as the data analyst suggests, then the statistical inference is misleading, claiming a certainty that does not exist. The final parametric statistical model is reported as if it were the only one considered and evaluated. The data analyst has performed a procedure that began the moment the data were used. In other words, once you start using the data, your estimation method has also started. Therefore, our data analyst has selected an approach that, while very common, blatantly leaves us with faulty inference.

Even without the approach defined by the data analyst, the PI and the subject matter expert might run both of their regressions and then decide between them based on the results. It should not be overlooked that the process of looking at the data, examining coefficient p-values, and trying multiple statistical models is not only incredibly prevalent but is taught to students learning statistics.

This is the human art component we eluded to in Sect. 1.2. The moment we use post-hoc arbitrary criteria and human judgment to select the parametric statistical model after looking at the data, the analysis becomes prone to additional bias. This bias manifests in both the effect estimate and the assessment of uncertainty for that estimator (i.e., standard errors). One cannot even define the procedure that was used

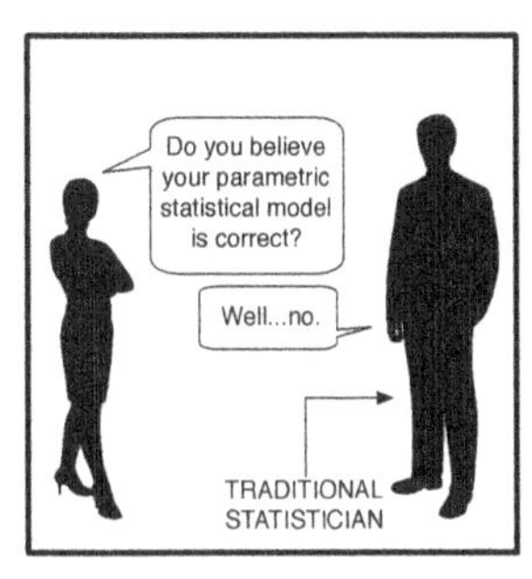

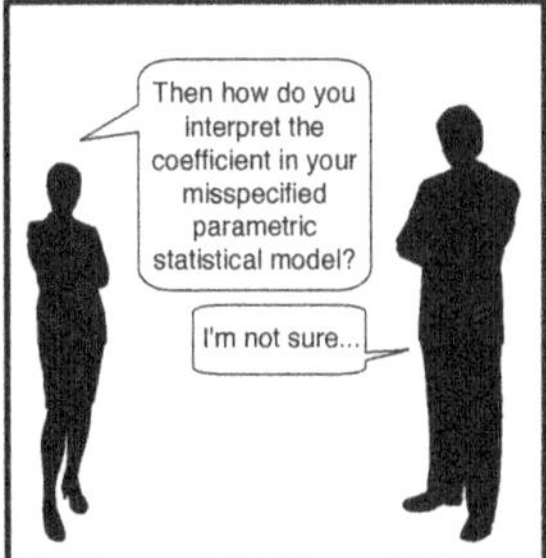

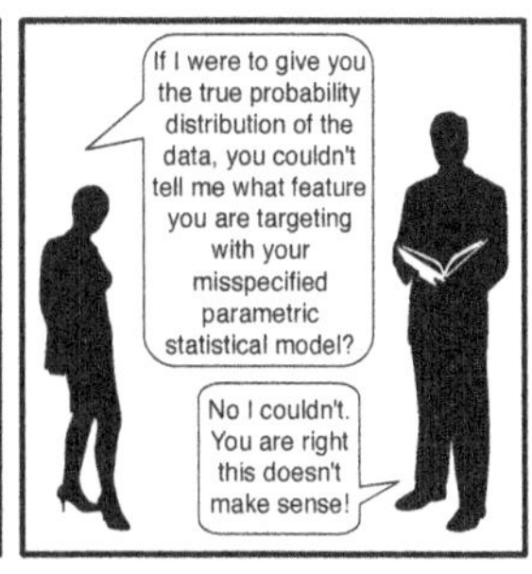

as a function of the data so that more appropriate standard errors can be calculated (e.g., by use of bootstrapping). Statistics is not an art, it is a science.

Standard practice focuses on estimating $E_0(Y \mid A, W)$ with an assumed parametric statistical model. One then extracts the coefficient in front of A as the effect estimate, ignoring that we know that most *parametric statistical models are wrong.* This criticism extends in general to estimation procedures (e.g., prediction) using misspecified parametric regression models. There is a more natural way to think about our parameter of interest, which we introduced abstractly in Sect. 1.1. The definitions of the data, model, and parameter will allow us to target parameters that are frequently of interest, such as causal effects. These concepts will be developed more concretely in the next section, and additionally in Chap. 2, as we set aside the traditional approach to effect estimation.

1.3 Data, Model, and Target Parameter

Our discussion of the data, model, and target parameter has been relatively abstract up to this point. We formalize these concepts in this section using notation. We define O as the random variable with P_0 as the corresponding probability distribution of interest. We write $O \sim P_0$ to mean that the probability distribution of O is P_0. Our random variable, which we observe n times, could be defined in a simple case as $O = (W, A, Y) \sim P_0$ if we are without common issues such as missingness and censoring. W, A, and Y are as defined in Sect. 1.2.3.

Complex data structures. While the data structure $O = (W, A, Y) \sim P_0$ makes for effective examples, data structures found in practice are frequently more complicated. Suppose we have a right-censored data structure. Right censoring means that we do not observe a particular variable or variables to the end of the study or time period. For example, if we are following subjects for 5 years, some subjects may drop out of the study for various reasons (e.g., relocation, death, voluntarily ending participation). If we are planning to measure an outcome Y, such as developing liver cancer, within 5 years of baseline, those subjects that drop out before 5 years (i.e., are censored) will not have measurements across the whole time period. All subjects will be censored at year 5 if they have not already been censored, but subjects that are observed for the full 5 years provide us with the desired full-data structure and are thereby referred to as uncensored.

Censoring is always defined with respect to a desired full-data structure. This type of censoring of a desired full-data structure is referred to as right censoring since timelines are frequently numbered from left to right, and it is some portion of the right side that is censored. Now, for each subject we will observe their time of censoring, and we may observe their time to event. For example, subject 1 may develop liver cancer at year 3. Another subject may be censored at year 2 due to dropout, and we never observe whether they develop liver cancer within the 5 years. Thus our data structure now has added complexity. We have T representing time to event Y, C a censoring time, $\tilde{T} = \min(T, C)$ which represents the T or C that was observed first, and $\Delta = I(T \leq \tilde{T}) = I(C \geq T)$ an indicator that T was observed at or before C. We then define $O = (W, A, \tilde{T}, \Delta) \sim P_0$. This is another example of a possible data structure.

1.3.1 The Model

We are considering the general case that one observed n i.i.d. copies of a random variable O with probability distribution P_0. The data-generating distribution P_0 is also known to be an element of a statistical model $\mathcal{M}$, which we write $P_0 \in \mathcal{M}$. Formally, a statistical model $\mathcal{M}$ is the set of possible probability distributions for P_0; it is a collection of probability distributions. What if all we know is that we have n i.i.d. copies of O? Well, then we've stated what we know, thus this can be our statistical model, which we call a nonparametric statistical model. We don't need to assign a parametric form to the distribution of our data; it is simply known to be an element of a nonparametric statistical model $\mathcal{M}$.

We might also consider a semiparametric statistical model if we have additional information about the way our data were generated that puts restrictions on the data-generating distribution P_0. For example, we may know that the effect of exposure A on the mean outcome is linear. Note, though, that semiparametric statistical models can be wrong by not containing the true P_0 if our "knowledge" is faulty. While we might have additional knowledge, we do not have enough knowledge to parameterize P_0 by a finite-dimensional parameter. These nonparametric and semiparametric statistical models should represent true knowledge about the underlying mechanism generating the data, that is, they are supposed to contain the true probability distribution P_0 of the experimental data.

We will frequently use *semiparametric* to include both nonparametric and semiparametric, such as the phrase "semiparametric estimation" referring to estimation in a nonparametric or semiparametric statistical model. When semiparametric excludes nonparametric and we make additional assumptions, this will be explicit.

Statistical model vs. model. A statistical model can be augmented with additional (causal) assumptions providing a parameterization so that $\mathcal{M} = \{P_\theta : \theta \in \Theta\}$, where the space of θ-values, Θ, is itself infinite dimensional. Even though such a parameterization does not change the statistical model, thereby providing nontestable causal assumptions, it does allow one to enrich the interpretation of $\Psi(P_0)$ in terms of a statement of an underlying truth θ_0. We refer to the statistical model augmented with a parameterization as a model. We will return to the issue of modeling, thereby making (causal) assumptions that go beyond specifying a statistical model $\mathcal{M}$, in Chap. 2. The important take-home message for now is that the statistical model is the only relevant information for the estimation problem, while the additional (causal) assumptions will provide enriched (or misleading, if wrong) interpretations of the target parameter.

1.3.2 The Target Parameter

What are we trying to learn from our data? Often the question of interest is related to quantifying some difference in the probability distribution of an outcome of interest between the treated and untreated or the exposed and unexposed groups. We want to understand the effect of treatment or exposure on the probability distribution of the outcome of interest. This difference could be measured on an additive scale or multiplicative scale, such as a relative risk or odds ratio.

Either way, once an agreement is reached concerning what one wants to learn, we can explicitly define the target parameter of the probability distribution P_0 as some function of P_0: $\Psi(P_0)$ for some function Ψ that maps the probability distribution P_0 into the target feature. That is, we are interested in estimating a parameter $\Psi(P_0)$ of the probability distribution $P_0 \in \mathcal{M}$, which is known to be an element of a nonparamteric or semiparametric statistical model $\mathcal{M}$. The parameter $\Psi(P_0)$ is a function of the unknown probability distribution P_0. We are not interested in estimating an effect defined by a coefficient of a (misspecified) parametric statistical model. Rather, we define a parameter as a feature of the true probability distribution P_0 of the data using true knowledge we have about P_0 as embodied by the statistical model $\mathcal{M}$. Thus, we are explicitly confronted with the fact that we need to know how to define our target parameter as a feature of P_0: it does not suffice to grab a parametric statistical model and just target the coefficients in that model.

First, one needs to define the parameter of interest as a function of the data-generating distribution varying over the nonparametric or semiparametric statistical model. Many practitioners are used to thinking of their parameter in terms of a regression coefficient, but that is often not possible in realistic nonparametric and semiparametric statistical models. Instead, one has to carefully think about what feature of the distribution of the data one wishes to target. With an experimental unit-specific data structure $O = (W, A, Y) \sim P_0$, the risk difference is the following function of the distribution P_0 of O:

$$\Psi(P_0) = E_{W,0}[E_0(Y \mid A = 1, W) - E_0(Y \mid A = 0, W)],$$

where $E_0(Y \mid A = a, W)$ is the conditional mean of Y given $A = a$ and W. Here A is binary and therefore a takes on two values, 1 and 0. E_W indicates that we take the average over the observed distribution of our covariate(s) W. Uppercase letters represent random variables and lowercase letters are a specific value for that variable. For example, if all variables are discrete, $P_0(W = w, A = a, Y = y)$ assigns a probability to any possible outcome (w, a, y) for $O = (W, A, Y)$. P_0 is like a calculator: we input (w, a, y) and it returns a probability. $\Psi(P_0)$ for the risk difference can then also be written:

$$\Psi(P_0) = \sum_w \Big[\sum_y y P_0(Y = y \mid A = 1, W = w) - \sum_y y P_0(Y = y \mid A = 0, W = w) \Big] P_0(W = w),$$

where
$$P_0(Y = y \mid A = a, W = w) = \frac{P_0(W = w, A = a, Y = y)}{\sum_y P_0(W = w, A = a, Y = y)}.$$

After obtaining an estimate of $\Psi(P_0)$ and a confidence interval, we can provide two interpretations, one as a purely statistical parameter of P_0, and one as a causal parameter under additional causal assumptions representing a causal model that goes beyond the specification of the statistical model $\mathcal{M}$. We discuss these causal assumptions in detail in Chap. 2.

1.3.3 Summary of Concepts

1. **Data.** Our data are comprised of n i.i.d. copies of a random variable $O \sim P_0$. P_0 is the true probability distribution for O.
2. **Model.** Our statistical model $\mathcal{M}$ is nonparametric or semiparametric and represents only what we know about our data-generating distribution P_0. $\mathcal{M}$ is the set of possible probability distributions for P_0. Our model includes possible additional causal assumptions, allowing an enriched interpretation of the parameter of interest.
3. **Target parameter.** Our parameter $\Psi(P_0)$ is a particular feature of the unknown probability distribution P_0. The explicit definition of this mapping Ψ on the statistical model requires that one defines $\Psi(P)$ at each P in the statistical model. The parameter typically has two interpretations, one as a parameter $\Psi(P_0)$ of a probability distribution P_0 and one as a causal parameter under additional (causal) assumptions to be discussed in Chap. 2.

1.4 The Need for Targeted Estimators

Let us step back for a moment. Suppose you were handed ten textbooks and told you would be asked one question in 12 h. The question might require understanding portions of several of these books. However, you are not told what the question is going to be. How would you prepare for such a test? You do not have time to read all ten textbooks, let alone master the material contained within them. You might read the chapter abstracts from each book in order to learn basic summary information.

Now, suppose you were handed the same ten textbooks, but instead you were told the question you would be asked 12 h later. Would this change your approach to studying? Yes! Since you know what question will be asked, you can more carefully discard books that will be completely unnecessary, keeping only those books with relevant chapters. You are able to spend 12 h working through the pertinent chapters and then give a thoughtful precise answer on the one question test.

This theoretical situation has a direct parallel to nontargeted learning vs. targeted learning. Maximum likelihood estimation in misspecified parametric statistical models is nontargeted learning; one estimates all the parameters (coefficients) in a parametric statistical model. One uses an empirical criterion that is only concerned with the overall fit of the entire probability distribution of the data instead of only the parameter of interest; we are trying to master all the books, spreading error uniformly across all content, when we only care about very specific portions of each book. The overall fit of the probability distribution based on the data set is then used to evaluate the target parameter of the probability distribution, i.e., the question is answered with the nontargeted fit of the distribution of the data. For a small *true* parametric statistical model, containing the true probability distribution, one with few terms or few unknown coefficients, the performance of the maximum likelihood estimator of the target parameter with regard to mean squared error may be satisfactory. However, the bigger the statistical model, the more problematic nontargeted learning becomes. We have no problem with maximum likelihood estimation for relatively low-dimensional parametric statistical models if they are correct, but this is not the case in practice, and we wish for our statistical models to represent true knowledge. Indeed, in semiparametric statistical models, maximum likelihood estimation breaks down completely. With targeted learning, we focus on our known question of interest; we focus on the relevant information in the books, and rank the information by its relevance for the question of interest.

1.5 Road Map for Targeted Learning

The first six chapters of this textbook are meant to provide the reader with a firm grasp of the targeted learning road map and the solution to prediction and causal inference estimation problems: super learning and targeted maximum likelihood estimation (TMLE). For the sake of presentation, in these introductory chapters we will focus on the data structure $(W, A, Y) \sim P_0$, the nonparametric statistical

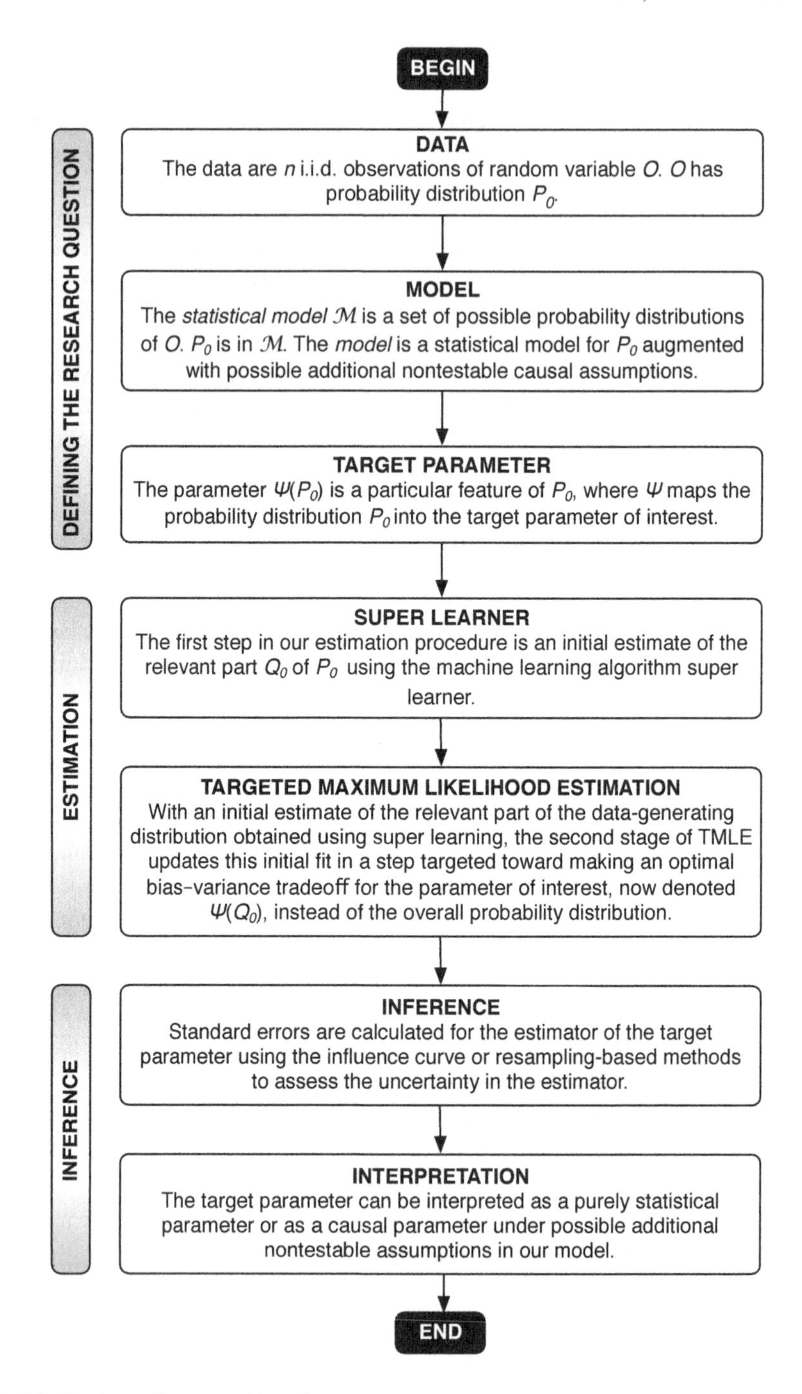

Fig. 1.2 Road map for targeted learning

model $\mathcal{M}$, and the additive causal effect target parameter $\Psi(P_0) = E_{W,0}[E_0(Y \mid A = 1, W) - E_0(Y \mid A = 0, W)]$. Our estimator of the treatment effect will be obtained by plugging in a (targeted) estimator of (or the relevant part of) P_0 into the parameter mapping Ψ. Such an estimator is called a plug-in or substitution estimator. Substitution estimators have the advantage of fully respecting the constraints implied by the statistical model $\mathcal{M}$ and respecting that the target parameter is a very specific function of P_0. As a consequence, substitution estimators are generally robust, even in small samples.

This first chapter was intended to motivate the need for improved estimation methods, highlight the troublesome nature of the traditional approach to estimation, and introduce important concepts such as the data, model, and target parameter. We develop the following concepts, as part of the road map for targeted learning, in the remaining five introductory chapters.

Defining the model and target parameter. By defining a structural causal model (SCM), we specify a model for underlying counterfactual outcome data, representing the data one would be able to generate in an ideal experiment. This is a translation of our knowledge about the data-generating process into causal assumptions. We can define our target parameter in our SCM, i.e., as a so-called causal effect of an intervention on a variable A on an outcome Y. The SCM also generates the observed data O, and one needs to determine if the target parameter can be identified from the distribution P_0 of O alone. In particular, one needs to determine what additional assumptions are needed in order to obtain such identifiability of the causal effect from the observed data.

Super learning for prediction. The first step in our estimation procedure is an initial estimate for the part of the data-generating distribution P_0 required to evaluate the target parameter. This estimator needs to recognize that P_0 is only known to be an element of a semiparametric statistical model. That is, we need estimators that are able to truly learn from data, allowing for flexible fits with increased amounts of information. We introduce cross-validation and machine learning as essential tools and then present the method of super learning for prediction with its theoretical grounding, demonstrating that super learning provides an optimal approach to estimation of P_0 (or infinite-dimensional parameters thereof) in semiparametric statistical models. Since prediction can be a research question of interest in itself, super learning for prediction is useful as a standalone tool as well.

TMLE. With an initial estimate of the relevant part of the data-generating distribution obtained using super learning, we are prepared to present the remainder of the TMLE procedure. The second stage of TMLE updates this initial fit in a step targeted towards making an optimal bias–variance tradeoff for the parameter of interest, instead of the overall probability distribution P_0. This results in a targeted estimator of the relevant part of P_0, and thereby in a corresponding substitution estimator of $\Psi(P_0)$.

Many of the topics we have presented in this road map may be new to you. They will be explained in detail in the coming chapters. This brief road map is introduced for the reader to see where we are going, how the pieces fit together, and why we will present material in this order.

1.6 Notes and Further Reading

We motivated this chapter with two real-world debates: HRT and screening guidelines for breast cancer. In a *New York Times* piece, Taubes (2007) discussed the merits of epidemiology using the HRT studies as an example. For those interested in reading more about this topic, it is an excellent comprehensive starting point with thorough references. For the statistician and researcher, it also raises one of the questions we seek to answer with this text. Can we estimate causal effects from observational studies? Two starting points for the mammography debate include U.S. Preventive Services Task Force (2009) for the official recommendation statement on breast cancer screenings, as well as Freedman et al. (2004) for a qualitative review of breast cancer mammography studies.

For additional background on study designs and covariate adjustment we direct readers to Rothman and Greenland (1998) and Jewell (2004). For a readable introductory statistics text on traditional regression techniques and key statistics concepts such as the central limit theorem (CLT) we refer readers to Freedman (2005).

A popular article drawing attention to false research findings, due in part to current statistical practice, is Ioannidis (2006). Ioannidis was also interviewed in journalist David H. Freedman's new book, *Wrong: Why Experts Keep Failing Us—And How to Know When to Trust Them*. This text focuses on problems in research fields, including the way data are analyzed and presented to the public (Freedman 2010).

George Box famously discussed that (parametric) statistical models are wrong, but may be useful (Box and Draper 1987). As presented in this chapter, misspecified parametric statistical models may not perform terribly for low-dimensional data structures and small sample sizes. Over 20 years after Box's statements, data sets have become increasingly high dimensional, and large studies are very common. We are also still left with the issue that the coefficients in misspecified parametric statistical models do not represent the target parameter of interest. Therefore, the usefulness of misspecified parametric statistical models is extremely limited. Note, however, that maximum likelihood estimators according to candidate parametric working statistical models can be included in the library of the super learner, discussed in Chap. 3, and can play a useful role in that manner.

The use of data-adaptive tools can be beneficial, although we discuss in this chapter (Sect. 1.2.4) a commonly used data-adaptive procedure in parametric statistical models that provides faulty inference. Data-adaptive methods, when guided by a priori benchmarks in a nonparametric or semiparametric statistical model, are advantageous for prediction and discussed in detail in Chap. 3. We use the terms *data-adaptive* and *machine learning* interchangeably in this text. Targeted estimators will be discussed in Chaps. 4–6.

Chapter 2
Defining the Model and Parameter

Sherri Rose, Mark J. van der Laan

Targeted statistical learning from data is often concerned with the estimation of causal effects and an assessment of uncertainty for the estimator. In Chap. 1, we identified the road map we will follow to solve this estimation problem. Now, we formalize the concepts of the model and target parameter. We will introduce additional topics that may seem abstract. While we attempt to elucidate these abstractions with tangible examples, depending on your background, the material may be quite dense compared to other textbooks you have read. Do not get discouraged. Sometimes a second reading and careful notes are helpful and sufficient to illuminate these concepts. Researchers and students at UC Berkeley have also had great success discussing these topics in groups. If this is your assigned text for a course or workshop, meet outside of class with your fellow classmates. We guarantee you that the effort is worth it so you can move on to the next step in the targeted learning road map. Once you have a firm understanding of the core material in Chap. 2, you can begin the estimation steps.

This chapter is based on methods pioneered by Judea Pearl, and we consider his text *Causality*, recently published in a second edition (Pearl 2009), a companion book to our book. Causal inference requires both a causal model to define the causal effect as a target parameter of the distribution of the data *and* robust semiparametric efficient estimation, with his book covering the former and ours the latter. We start by succinctly summarizing the open problem:

The statistical estimation problem begins by defining a statistical model $\mathcal{M}$ for P_0. The statistical model $\mathcal{M}$ is a collection of possible probability distributions P of O. P_0 is the true distribution of O. The estimation problem requires the description of a target parameter of P_0 one wishes to learn from the data. This definition of a target parameter requires specification of a mapping Ψ one can then apply to P_0. Clearly, this mapping Ψ needs to be defined on any possible probability distribution in the statistical model $\mathcal{M}$. Thus Ψ maps any $P \in \mathcal{M}$ into a vector of numbers $\Psi(P)$. We write the mapping as $\Psi : \mathcal{M} \rightarrow \mathbb{R}^d$ for a

d-dimensional parameter. We introduce ψ_0 as the evaluation of $\Psi(P_0)$, i.e., the true value of our parameter. The statistical estimation problem is now to map the observed data $O_1, \ldots, O_n$ into an estimator of $\Psi(P_0)$ that incorporates the knowledge that $P_0 \in \mathcal{M}$, accompanied by an assessment of the uncertainty in the estimator.

In the following sections, we will define a model that goes beyond a statistical model by incorporating nontestable assumptions, define a parameter of interest in that model that can be interpreted as a causal effect, determine the assumptions to establish the identifiability of the causal parameter from the distribution of the observed data, and, finally, based on this modeling and identifiability exercise, commit to a statistical model (i.e., $\mathcal{M}$) and target parameter (i.e., Ψ).

Recall that the data $O_1, \ldots, O_n$ consist of n i.i.d. copies of a random variable O with probability distribution P_0. For a data structure, such as $O = (W, A, Y)$ with covariates W, exposure A, and outcome Y discrete, which we use as a simple example in this chapter, uppercase letters represent random variables and lowercase letters are a specific value for that variable. For example, if all variables are discrete, $P_0(W = w, A = a, Y = y)$ assigns a probability to any possible outcome (w, a, y) for $O = (W, A, Y)$.

2.1 Defining the Structural Causal Model

We first specify a set of endogenous variables $X = (X_j : j)$. Endogenous variables are those variables for which the structural causal model (SCM) will state that it is a (typically unknown) deterministic function of some of the other endogenous variables and an exogenous error. Typically, the endogenous variables X include the observables O, but might also include some nonobservables that are meaningful and important to the scientific question of interest. Perhaps there was a variable you did not measure, but would have liked to, and it plays a crucial role in defining the scientific question of interest. This variable would then be an unobserved endogenous variable. For example, if you are studying the effect of hepatitis B on liver cancer, you might also want to measure hepatitis C and aflatoxin exposure. However, suppose you know the role aflatoxin plays in the relationships between hepatitis B and liver cancer, but you were unable to measure it. Aflatoxin exposure is, therefore, an unobserved endogenous variable. Liver cancer, hepatitis B, and hepatitis C are observed endogenous variables.

In a very simple example, we might have $j = 1, \ldots, J$, where $J = 3$. Thus, $X = (X_1, X_2, X_3)$. We can rewrite X as $X = (W, A, Y)$ if we say $X_1 = W$, $X_2 = A$, and $X_3 = Y$. Let W represent the set of baseline covariates for a subject, A the treatment or exposure, and Y the outcome. All the variables in X are observed. Suppose we are interested in estimating the effect of leisure-time physical activity (LTPA) on mortality in an elderly population. A study is conducted to estimate this effect where we sample individuals from the population of interest. The hypothesis is that LTPA at or above current recommended levels decreases mortality risk. Let us say that LTPA is a binary variable $A \in \{0, 1\}$ defined by the recommended level of energy expenditure. For all subjects meeting this level, $A = 1$ and all those below have $A = 0$. The mortality outcome is also binary $Y \in \{0, 1\}$ and defined as death within 5 years of the beginning of the study, with $Y = 1$ indicating death. W includes variables such as age, sex, and health history.

For each endogenous variable X_j one specifies the parents of X_j among X, denoted $Pa(X_j)$. In our mortality study example above, the parent of A is the set of baseline covariates W. Thus, $Pa(A) = W$. The specification of the parents might be known by the time ordering in which the X_j were collected over time: the parents of a variable collected at time t could be defined as the observed past at time t. This is true for our study of LTPA; $W = \{\text{age, sex, health history}\}$ all occur before the single measurement of LTPA. Likewise, LTPA was generated after the baseline covariates and before death but depends on the baseline covariates. Death was generated last and depends on both LTPA and the baseline covariates. We can see the time ordering involved in this process: the baseline covariates occurred before the exposure LTPA, which occurred before the outcome of death: $W \rightarrow A \rightarrow Y$.

We denote a collection of exogenous variables by $U = (U_{X_j} : j)$. These variables in U are never observed and are not affected by the endogenous variables in the model, but instead they affect the endogenous variables. They may also be referred to as background or error variables. One assumes that X_j is some function of $Pa(X_j)$ and an exogenous U_{X_j}:

$$X_j = f_{X_j}(Pa(X_j), U_{X_j}), \; j = 1 \ldots, J.$$

The collection of functions f_{X_j} indexed by all the endogenous variables is represented by $f = (f_{X_j} : j)$. Together with the joint distribution of U, these functions f_{X_j}, specify the data-generating distribution of (U, X) as they describe a deterministic system of structural equations (one for each endogenous variable X_j) that deterministically maps a realization of U into a realization of X. In an SCM one also refers to some of the endogenous variables as intervention variables. The SCM assumes that intervening on one of the intervention variables by setting their value, thereby making the function for that variable obsolete, does not change the form of the other functions. The functions f_{X_j} are often unspecified, but in some cases it might be reasonable to assume that these functions have to fall in a certain more restrictive class of functions. Similarly, there might be some knowledge about the joint distribution of U. The set of possible data-generating distributions of (U, X) can be obtained by varying the structural equations f over all allowed forms, and the distribution of the errors U over all possible error distributions defines the SCM for the full-data (U, X), i.e., the SCM is a statistical model for the random variable (U, X). An example of a fully parametric SCM would be obtained by assuming that all the functions f_{X_j} are known up to a finite number of parameters and that the error distribution is a multivariate normal distribution with mean zero and unknown covariance matrix. Such parametric structural equation models are not recommended, for the same reasons as outlined in Chap. 1.

The corresponding SCM for the observed data O also includes specifying the relation between the random variable (U, X) and the observed data O, so that the SCM for the full data implies a parameterization of the probability distribution of O in terms of f and the distribution P_U of U. This SCM for the observed data also implies a statistical model for the probability distribution of O.

Let's translate these concepts into our mortality study example. We have the functions $f = (f_W, f_A, f_Y)$ and the exogenous variables $U = (U_W, U_A, U_Y)$. The values of W, A, and Y are deterministically assigned by U corresponding to the functions f. We specify our structural equation models, based on investigator knowledge, as

$$\begin{aligned} W &= f_W(U_W), \\ A &= f_A(W, U_A), \\ Y &= f_Y(W, A, U_Y), \end{aligned} \tag{2.1}$$

where no assumptions are made about the true shape of f_W, f_A, and f_Y. These functions f are nonparametric as we have not put a priori restrictions on their functional form. We may assume that U_A is independent of U_Y, given W, which corresponds with believing that there are no unmeasured factors that predict both A and the outcome Y: this is often called the no unmeasured confounders assumption. This SCM represents a semiparametric statistical model for the probability distribution of the errors U and endogenous variables $X = (W, A, Y)$. We assume that the observed data structure $O = (W, A, Y)$ is actually a realization of the endogenous variables (W, A, Y) generated by this system of structural equations. This now defines the SCM for the observed data O. It is easily seen that any probability distribution of O can be obtained by selecting a particular data-generating distribution of (U, X) in this SCM. Thus, the statistical model for P_0 implied by this SCM is a nonparametric model. As a consequence, one cannot determine from observing O if the assumptions in the SCM contradict the data. One states that the SCM represents a set of nontestable causal assumptions we have made about how the data were generated in nature.

Specifically, with the SCM represented in (2.1), we have assumed that the underlying data were generated by the following actions:

1. Drawing unobservable U from some probability distribution P_U ensuring that U_A is independent of U_Y, given W,
2. Generating W as a deterministic function of U_W,
3. Generating A as a deterministic function of W and U_A,
4. Generating Y as a deterministic function of W, A, and U_Y.

What if, instead, our SCM had been specified as follows:

$$\begin{aligned} W &= f_W(U_W), \\ A &= f_A(U_A), \\ Y &= f_Y(W, A, U_Y). \end{aligned} \tag{2.2}$$

What different assumption are we making here? If you compare (2.1) and (2.2), you see that the only difference between the two is the structural equation for f_A. In (2.2), A is evaluated as a deterministic function of U_A only. The baseline variables W play no role in the generation of variable A. We say that (2.2) is a more restrictive SCM than (2.1) because of this additional assumption about data generation. When might a researcher make such an assumption? In Chap. 1, we discussed RCTs. RCTs are studies where the subjects are randomized to treatment in the study. If our study of LTPA had been an RCT, it would make sense to assume the SCM specified in (2.2) given our knowledge of the study design. However, since it would be unethical to randomize subjects to levels of exercise, given the known health benefits, our study of LTPA on mortality is observational and we assume the less restrictive (2.1).

Causal assumptions made by the SCM for the full data:

- For each endogenous X_j, $X_j = f_j(Pa(X_j), U_{X_j})$ only depends on the other endogenous variables through its parents $Pa(X_j)$.
- The exogenous variables have a particular joint distribution P_U.

The SCM for the observed data includes the following additional assumption:

- The probability distribution of observed data structure O is implied by the probability distribution of (U, X).

After having specified the parent sets $Pa(X_j)$ for each endogenous variable X_j, one might make an assumption about the joint distribution of U, denoted P_U, representing knowledge about the underlying random variable (U, X) as accurately as possible. This kind of assumption would typically not put any restrictions on the probability distribution of O. The underlying data (U, X) are comprised of the exogenous variables U and the endogenous variables X, which is why we use the notation (U, X). In a typical SCM, the endogenous variables are the variables for which we have some understanding, mostly or fully observed, often collected according to a time ordering, and are very meaningful to the investigator. On the other hand, typically much of the distribution of U is poorly understood. In particular, one would often define U_{X_j} as some surrogate of potential unmeasured confounders, collapsing different poorly understood phenomena in the real world in one variable. The latter is reflected by the fact that we do not even measure these confounders, or know how to measure them. However, in some applications something about the joint distribution of U might be understood, and some components of U might be measured. For example, it might be known that treatment was randomized as in an RCT, implying that the error U_A for that treatment variable is independent of all other errors. On the other hand, in an observational study, one might feel uncomfortable making the assumption that U_A is independent of U_Y, given W, since one might know that some of the true confounders were not measured and are thereby captured by U_A.

Relationship of X and O. Our observed random variable O is related to X, and has a probability distribution that is implied by the distribution of (U, X). Specification of this relation is an important assumption of the SCM for the observed data O. A typical example is that $O = \Phi(X)$ for some Φ, i.e., O is a function of X. This includes the special case that $O \subset X$, i.e., with O being a simple subset of X. Because of this relationship $O = \Phi(X)$, the marginal probability distribution of X,

$$P_X(x) = \sum_u P_f(X = x \mid U = u) P_U(U = u),$$

also identifies the probability distribution of O through the functions $f = (f_{X_j} : j)$ and the distribution of the exogenous errors U. [Note that the conditional probability distribution $P_f(X = x \mid U = u)$ of X, given a realization $U = u$, is indeed completely determined by the functions f, which explains our notation P_f.] For example, if $X = O$, then:

$$P(o) = \sum_u P_f(X = o \mid U = u) P_U(U = u).$$

In order to make explicit that the probability distribution P of O is implied by the probability distribution of (U, X), we use the notation $P = P(P_{U,X})$. The true probability distribution $P_{U,X,0}$ of (U, X) implies the true probability distribution P_0 of O through this relation: $P_0 = P(P_{U,X,0})$. Since the assumed SCM often does not put any restrictions on the functions f_{X_j}, and the selection of the parent sets $Pa(X_j)$ might be purely based on time ordering (thereby not implying conditional independencies among the X_js), for many types of restrictions one would put on P_U, the resulting SCM for (U, X) would still not provide any restriction on the distribution of O. In that case, these causal assumptions provide no restriction on the distribution of O itself and thus imply a nonparametric *statistical* model $\mathcal{M}$ for the distribution P_0 of O. This statistical model $\mathcal{M}$ implied by the SCM for the observed data is given by $\mathcal{M} = \{P(P_{U,X}) : P_{U,X}\}$, where $P_{U,X}$ varies over all possible probability distributions of (U, X) in the SCM.

Each possible probability distribution $P_{U,X}$ of (U, X) in the SCM for the full data, indexed by a choice of error distribution P_U and a set of deterministic functions $(f_{X_j} : j)$, implies a probability distribution $P(P_{U,X})$ of O. In this manner the SCM for the full data implies a parameterization of the true probability distribution of O in terms of a true probability distribution of (U, X), so that the statistical model $\mathcal{M}$ for the probability distribution P_0 of O can be represented as $\mathcal{M} = \{P(P_{U,X}) : P_{U,X}\}$, where $P_{U,X}$ varies over all allowed probability distributions of (U, X) in the SCM. If this statistical model $\mathcal{M}$ implied by the SCM is nonparametric, then it follows that none of the causal assumptions encoded by the SCM are testable from the observed data.

2.2 Causal Graphs

SCMs provide a system for assigning values to a set of variables from random input. They are also an effective and straightforward means for explicitly specifying causal assumptions and the identifiability of the causal parameter of interest based on the observed data. We can draw a causal graph from our SCM, which is a visual way to describe some of the assumptions made by the model and the restrictions placed on the joint distribution of the data (U, X). However, in this text we do not place heavy emphasis on causal graphs as their utility is limited in many situations (e.g., complicated longitudinal data structures), and simpler visual displays of time ordering may provide more insight. Causal graphs also cannot encode every assumption we make in our SCM, and, in particular, the identifiability assumptions derived from causal graphs alone are not specific for the causal parameter of interest. Identifiability assumptions derived from a causal graph will thus typically be stronger than required. In addition, the link between the observed data and the full-data model represented by the causal graph is often different than simply stating that O corresponds with observing a subset of all the nodes in the causal graph. In this case, the causal graph itself cannot be used to assess the identifiability of a desired causal parameter from the observed data distribution.

2.2.1 Terminology

Figure 2.1 displays a possible causal graph for (2.1). The graph is drawn based on the relationships defined in f. The parents $Pa(X_j)$ of each X_j are connected to each X_j with an arrow directed toward X_j. Each X_j also has a directed arrow connecting its U_{X_j}. For example, the parents of Y, those variables in X on the right-hand side of the equation f_Y, are A and W. In Fig. 2.1, A and W are connected to Y, the child, with directed arrows, as is the exogenous U_Y. The baseline covariates W are represented with one variable. All the variables X and U in the graph are called nodes, and the lines that connect nodes are edges. All ancestors of a node occur before that node and all descendants occur after that node. This is a directed graph, meaning that each edge has only one arrow.

A path is any sequence of edges in a graph connecting two nodes. An example of a directed path in Fig. 2.1 is $W \rightarrow A \rightarrow Y$. This path connects each node with arrows that point in the direction of the path. In this figure there are several backdoor paths, which are paths that start with a node that has a directed arrow pointing into that node. The path can then be followed without respect to the direction of the arrows. For example, the path from Y to A through W is a backdoor path. Likewise, the path from Y to W through A is a backdoor path. These graphs are also acyclic; you cannot start at a node in a directed path and then return back to the same node through a closed loop. A collider is a node in a path where both arrows are directed toward the node. There are no colliders in Fig. 2.1. A blocked path is any path with at least one collider. A direct effect is illustrated by a directed arrow between two nodes, with

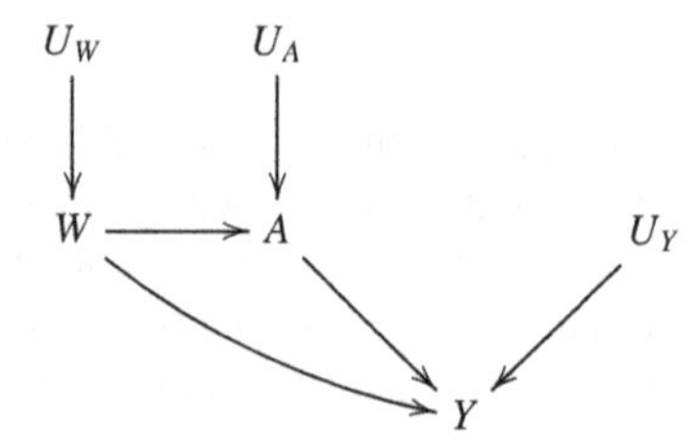

Fig. 2.1 A possible causal graph for (2.1).

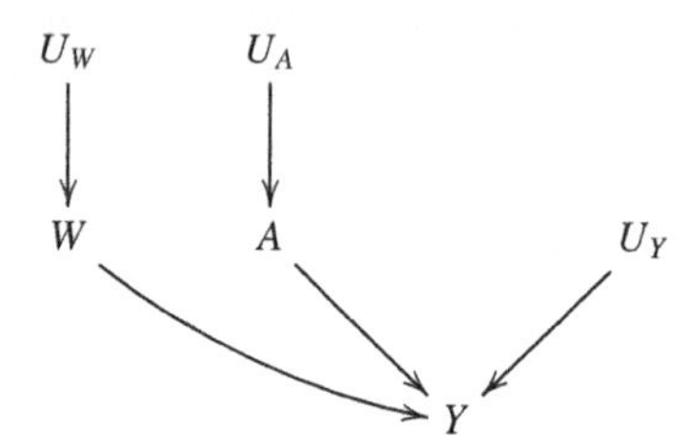

Fig. 2.2 A possible causal graph for (2.2)

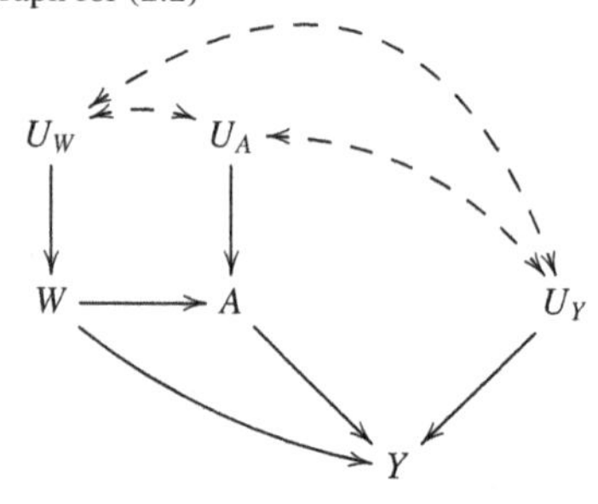

Fig. 2.3 A causal graph for (2.1) with no assumptions on the distribution of P_U

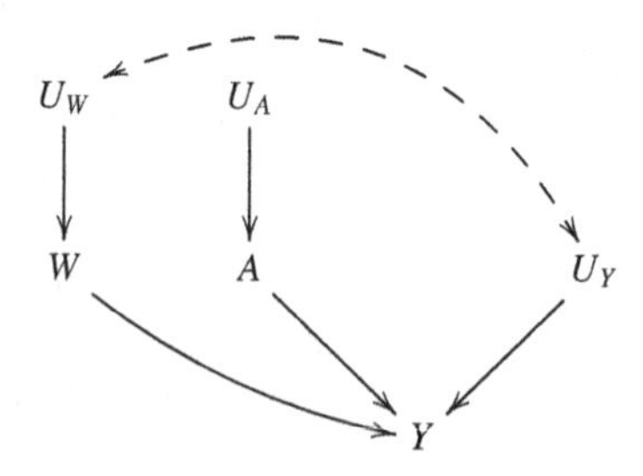

Fig. 2.4 A causal graph for (2.2) with no assumptions on the relationship between U_W and U_Y

no nodes mediating the path. Any unblocked path from A to Y other than the direct effect connecting A and Y represents an indirect effect of A on Y. One must block all unblocked backdoor paths from A to Y in order to isolate the causal effect of A on Y.

2.2.2 Assumptions

In Sect. 2.1, we discussed the typically nontestable causal assumptions made by an SCM. We make the first assumption by defining the parents $Pa(X_j)$ for each endogenous X_j. The second is any set of assumptions about the joint distribution P_U of the exogenous variables.

The assumptions made based on actual knowledge concerning the relationships between variables [i.e., defining the parents $Pa(X_j)$ for each endogenous X_j] are displayed in our causal graph through the presence and absence of directed arrows. The explicit absence of an arrow indicates a known lack of a direct effect. In many cases all arrows are included as it is not possible to exclude a direct effect based on a priori knowledge. In Fig. 2.1, the direction of the arrows is defined by the assignment of the parents to each node, including the time ordering assumed during the specification of (2.1). There is no explicit absence of any arrows; no direct effects are excluded. However, if we were to draw a graph for (2.2), it could look like Fig. 2.2. The direct effect between W and A is excluded because A is evaluated as a deterministic function of U_A only.

The assumptions on the distribution P_U are reflected in causal graphs through dashed double-headed arrows between the variables U. In Figs. 2.1 and 2.2, there are no arrows between the $U = (U_W, U_A, U_Y)$. Therefore, (2.1) and (2.2) included the assumption of joint independence of the endogenous variables U, which is graphically displayed by the lack of arrows. This is not an assumption one is usually able to make based on actual knowledge. More likely, we are able to make few or no assumptions about the distribution of P_U.

For (2.1), with no assumptions about the distribution of P_U, our causal graph would appear as in Fig. 2.3. For (2.2), our causal graph based on actual knowledge may look like Fig. 2.4. Since A is randomized, this implies that U_A is independent of U_Y and U_W, and we remove the arrows connecting U_A to U_Y and U_A to U_W. However, we have no knowledge to indicate the independence of U_Y and U_W, thus we cannot remove the arrows between these two variables.

The causal graph encodes some of the information and assumptions described by the SCM. It is an additional tool to visually describe assumptions encoded by the SCM. In more complex longitudinal data structures, it may be simpler to work with the SCM over the causal graph, as the intricacies of the causal relationships and abundance of arrows can limit the utility of the graphic.

2.3 Defining the Causal Target Parameter

Now that we have a way of modeling the data-generating mechanism with an SCM, we can focus on what we are trying to learn from the observed data. That is, we can define a causal target parameter of interest as a parameter of the distribution of the full-data (U, X) in the SCM. Formally, we denote the SCM for the full-data (U, X) by $\mathcal{M}^F$, a collection of possible $P_{U,X}$ as described by the SCM. In other words, $\mathcal{M}^F$, a model for the full data, is a collection of possible distributions for the underlying data (U, X). Ψ^F is a mapping applied to a $P_{U,X}$ giving $\Psi^F(P_{U,X})$ as the target parameter of $P_{U,X}$. This mapping needs to be defined for each $P_{U,X}$ that is a possible distribution of (U, X), given our assumptions coded by the posed SCM. In this way, we state $\Psi^F : \mathcal{M}^F \to \mathbb{R}^d$, where $\mathbb{R}^d$ indicates that our parameter is a vector of d real numbers. The SCM $\mathcal{M}^F$ consists of the distributions indexed by the deterministic function $f = (f_{X_j} : j)$ and distribution P_U of U, where f and this joint distribution P_U are identifiable from the distribution of the full-data (U, X). Thus the target parameter can also be represented as a function of f and the joint distribution of U.

Recall our mortality example with data structure $O = (W, A, Y)$ and SCM given in (2.1) with no assumptions about the distribution P_U. We can define $Y_a = f_Y(W, a, U_Y)$ as a random variable corresponding with intervention $A = a$ in the SCM. The marginal probability distribution of Y_a is thus given by

$$P_{U,X}(Y_a = y) = P_{U,X}(f_Y(W, a, U_Y) = y).$$

The causal effect of interest for a binary A (suppose it is the causal risk difference) could then be defined as a parameter of the distribution of (U, X) given by

$$\Psi^F(P_{U,X}) = E_{U,X}Y_1 - E_{U,X}Y_0.$$

In other words, $\Psi^F(P_{U,X})$ is the difference of marginal means of counterfactuals Y_1 and Y_0. We discuss this in more detail in the next subsection.

2.3.1 Interventions

We will define our causal target parameter as a parameter of the distribution of the data (U, X) under an intervention on one or more of the structural equations in f. The intervention defines a random variable that is a function of (U, X), so that the target parameter is $\Psi^F(P_{U,X})$. In Chap. 1, we discussed the "ideal experiment" which we cannot conduct in practice, where we observe each subject's outcome at all levels of A under identical conditions. Intervening on the system defined by our SCM describes the data that would be generated from the system at the different levels of our intervention variable (or variables). For example, in our study of LTPA on mortality, we can intervene on the exposure LTPA in order to observe the results of this intervention on the system. By assumption, intervening and changing the functions f_{X_j} of the intervention variables does not change the other functions in f. With the SCM given in (2.1) we can intervene on f_A and set $a = 1$:

$$\begin{aligned} W &= f_W(U_W), \\ a &= 1, \\ Y_1 &= f_Y(W, 1, U_Y). \end{aligned}$$

We can also intervene and set $a = 0$:

$$\begin{aligned} W &= f_W(U_W), \\ a &= 0, \\ Y_0 &= f_Y(W, 0, U_Y). \end{aligned}$$

The intervention defines a random variable that is a function of (U, X), namely, $Y_a = Y_a(U)$ for $a = 1$ and $a = 0$. The notation $Y_a(U)$ makes explicit that Y_a is random only through U. The probability distribution of the (X, U) under an intervention is called the postintervention distribution. Our target parameter is a parameter of the postintervention distribution of Y_0 and Y_1, i.e., it is a function of these two postintervention distributions, namely, some difference. Thus, the SCM for the full data allows us to define the random variable $Y_a = f_Y(W, a, U_Y)$ for each a, where Y_a represents the outcome that would have been observed under this system for a particular subject under exposure a. Thus, with the SCM we can carry out the "ideal experiment" and define parameters of the distribution of the data generated in this perfect experiment, even though our observed data are only the random variables $O_1, \ldots, O_n$.

Formally, and more generally, the definition of the target parameter involves first specifying a subset of the endogenous nodes X_j playing the role of intervention nodes. Let A_s denote the intervention nodes, $s = 0, \ldots, S$, so that $A = (A_s : s = 1, \ldots, S)$, which, in shorthand notation, we also denote by $A = (A_s : s)$. We will denote the other endogenous nodes in X by $L = (L_r : r)$. Thus, $X = ((A_s : s), (L_r : r))$. Static interventions on the A-nodes correspond with setting A to a fixed value a, while dynamic interventions deterministically set A_s according to a fixed rule applied to the parents of A_s. Static interventions are a subset of the dynamic interventions. We will denote such a rule for assigning d to the intervention nodes, but it should be observed that d defines a rule for each A_s. Thus $d = (d_s : s = 1, \ldots, S)$ is a set of S rules. Such rules d are also called dynamic treatment regimens.

For a particular intervention d on the A nodes, and for a given realization u, the SCM generates deterministically a corresponding value for L, obtained by erasing the f_{A_s} functions, and carrying out the intervention d on A in the parent sets of the remaining equations. We denote the resulting realization by $L_d(u)$ and note that $L_d(u)$ is implied by f and u. The actual random variable $L_d(U)$ is called a postintervention random variable corresponding with the intervention that assigns the intervention nodes according to rule d. The probability distribution of $L_d(U)$ can be described as

$$P(L_d(U) = l) = \sum_u P_f(L_d(u) = l \mid U = u)P_U(u) = \sum_u I(L_d(u) = l)P_U(u).$$

In other words, it is the probability that U falls in the set of u-realizations under which the SCM system deterministically sets $L_d(u) = l$. Indicator $I(L_d(u) = l)$ is uniquely determined by the function specifications f_{X_j} for the X_j nodes that comprise L. This shows explicitly that the distribution of $L_d(U)$ is a parameter of f and the distribution of U, and thus a well-defined parameter on the full-data SCM $\mathcal{M}^F$ for the distribution of (U, X). We now define our target parameter $\Psi^F(P_{U,X})$ as some function of $(P_{L_d} : d)$ for a set of interventions d. Typically, we define our target parameter as a so-called causal contrast that involves a difference between two of such d-specific postintervention probability distributions. This target parameter is referred to as a causal parameter since it is a parameter of the postintervention distribution of L as a function of an intervention choice on $A = (A_s : s)$ across one or more interventions.

2.3.2 *Counterfactuals*

We would ideally like to see each individual's outcome at all possible levels of exposure A. The study is only capable of collecting Y under one exposure, the exposure the subject experiences. We discussed interventions on our SCM in Sect. 2.3.1 and we intervened on A to set $a = 1$ and $a = 0$ in order to generate the outcome for each subject under $A = a$ in our mortality study. Recall that Y_a represents the outcome that would have been observed under this system for a particular subject under exposure a. For our binary exposure LTPA , we have $(Y_a : a)$, with $a \in \mathcal{A}$, and where $\mathcal{A}$ is the set of possible values for our exposure LTPA. Here, this set is simply $\{0, 1\}$, but in other examples it could be continuous or otherwise more complex. Thus, in our example, for each realization u, which might correspond with an individual randomly drawn from some target population, by intervening on (2.1), we can generate so-called counterfactual outcomes $Y_1(u)$ and $Y_0(u)$. These counterfactual outcomes are implied by our SCM; they are consequences of it. That is, $Y_0(u) = f_Y(W, 0, u_Y)$, and $Y_1(u) = f_Y(W, 1, u_Y)$, where $W = f_W(u_W)$ is also implied by u. The random counterfactuals $Y_0 = Y_0(U)$ and $Y_1 = Y_1(U)$ are random through the probability distribution of U. Now we have the expected outcome had everyone in the target population met or exceeded recommended levels of LTPA, and the expected outcome had everyone had levels of LTPA below health recommendations. For example, the expected outcome of Y_1 is the mean of $Y_1(u)$ with respect to the probability distribution of U. Our target parameter is a function of the probability distributions of these counterfactuals: $E_0Y_1 - E_0Y_0$.

2.3.3 Establishing Identifiability

Are the assumptions we have already made enough to express the causal parameter of interest as a parameter of the probability distribution P_0 of the observed data? We want to be able to write $\Psi^F(P_{U,X,0})$ as $\Psi(P_0)$ for some parameter mapping Ψ, where we remind the reader that the SCM also specifies how the distribution P_0 of the observed data structure O is implied by the true distribution $P_{U,X,0}$ of (U, X). Since the true probability distribution of (U, X) can be any element in the SCM $\mathcal{M}^F$, and each such choice $P_{U,X}$ implies a probability distribution $P(P_{U,X})$ of O, this requires that we show that $\Psi^F(P_{U,X}) = \Psi(P(P_{U,X}))$ for all $P_{U,X} \in \mathcal{M}^F$.

This step involves establishing possible additional assumptions on the distribution of U, or sometimes also on the deterministic functions f, so that we can identify the target parameter from the observed data distribution. Thus, for each probability distribution of the underlying data (U, X) satisfying the SCM with these possible additional assumptions on P_U, we have $\Psi^F(P_{U,X}) = \Psi(P(P_{U,X}))$ for some Ψ. O is implied by the distribution of (U, X), such as $O = X$ or $O \subset X$, and $P = P(P_{X,U})$, where $P(P_{U,X})$ is a distribution of O implied by $P_{U,X}$.

Let us denote the resulting full-data SCM by $\mathcal{M}^{F*} \subset \mathcal{M}^F$ to make clear that possible additional assumptions were made that were driven purely by the identifiability problem, not necessarily reflecting reality. To be explicit, $\mathcal{M}^F$ is the full-data SCM under the assumptions based on real knowledge, and $\mathcal{M}^{F*}$ is the full-data SCM under possible additional causal assumptions required for the identifiability of our target parameter. We now have that for each $P_{U,X} \in \mathcal{M}^{F*}$, $\Psi^F(P_{U,X}) = \Psi(P)$, with $P = P(P_{U,X})$ the distribution of O implied by $P_{U,X}$ (whereas P_0 is the true distribution of O implied by the true distribution $P_{U,X,0}$).

Theorems exist that are helpful to establish such a desired identifiability result. For example, if $O = X$, and the distribution of U is such that, for each s, A_s is independent of L_d, given $Pa(A_s)$, then the well-known g-formula expresses the distribution of L_d in terms of the distribution of O:

$$P(L_d = l) = \prod_{r=1}^{R} P(L_r = l_r \mid Pa_d(L_r)) = Pa_d(l_r)),$$

where $Pa_d(L_r)$ are the parents of L_r with the intervention nodes among these parent nodes deterministically set by intervention d.

This so-called sequential randomization assumption can be established for a particular independence structure of U by verifying the backdoor path criterion on the corresponding causal graph implied by the SCM and this independence structure on U. The backdoor path criterion states that for each A_s, each backdoor path from A_s to an L_r node that is realized after A_s is blocked by one of the other L_r nodes.

In this manner, one might be able to generate a number of independence structures on the distribution of U that provide the desired identifiability result. That is, the resulting model for U that provides the desired identifiability might be represented as a union of models for U that assume a specific independence structure.

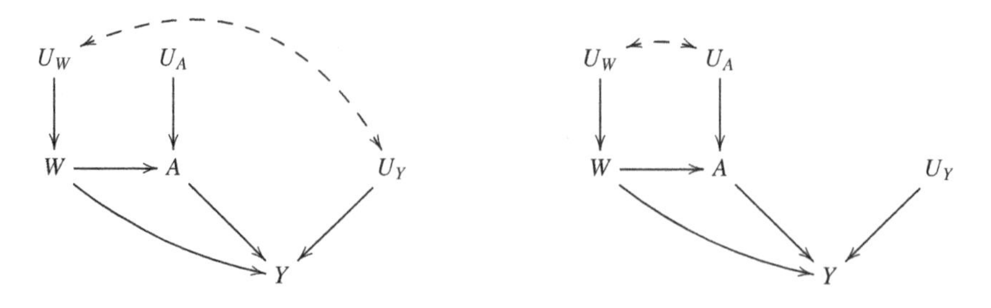

Fig. 2.5 Causal graphs for (2.1) with various assumptions about the distribution of P_U

If there is only one intervention node, i.e., $S = 1$, so that $O = (W, A, Y)$, the sequential randomization assumption reduces to the randomization assumption. The randomization assumption states that treatment node A is independent of counterfactual Y_a, conditional on W: $Y_a \perp A \mid Pa(A) = W$. You may be familiar with the (sequential) randomization assumption by another name, the no unmeasured confounders assumption. For our purposes, confounders are those variables in X one needs to observe in O in order to establish the identifiability of the target parameter of interest. We note that different such subsets of X may provide a desired identifiability result.

If we return to our mortality example and the structural equation models found in (2.1), the union of several independence structures allows for the identifiability of our causal target parameter $E_0Y_1 - E_0Y_0$ by meeting the backdoor path criterion. The independence structure in Fig. 2.3 does not meet the backdoor path criterion, but the two in Fig. 2.5 do. Thus in these two graphs the randomization assumption holds: A and Y_a are conditionally independent given W, which is implied by U_A being independent of U_Y, given W. It should be noted that Fig. 2.1 is a special case of the first graph in Fig. 2.5, so the union model for the distribution of U only represents two conditional independence models.

2.3.4 Commit to a Statistical Model and Target Parameter

The identifiability result provides us with a purely statistical target parameter $\Psi(P_0)$ on the distribution P_0 of O. The full-data model $\mathcal{M}^{F*}$ implies a statistical observed data model $\mathcal{M} = \{P(P_{X,U}) : P_{X,U} \in \mathcal{M}^{F*}\}$ for the distribution $P_0 = P(P_{U,X,0})$ of O. This now defines a target parameter $\Psi : \mathcal{M} \rightarrow \mathbb{R}^d$. The statistical observed data model for the distribution of O might be the same for $\mathcal{M}^F$ and $\mathcal{M}^{F*}$. If not, then one might consider extending the Ψ to the larger statistical observed data model implied by $\mathcal{M}^F$, such as possibly a fully nonparametric model allowing for all probability distributions. In this way, if the more restricted SCM holds, our target parameter would still estimate the target parameter, but one now also allows the data to contradict the more restricted SCM based on additional doubtful assumptions.

We can return to our example of the effect of LTPA on mortality and define our parameter, the causal risk difference, in terms of the corresponding statistical parameter $\Psi(P_0)$:

$$\Psi^F(P_{U,X,0}) = E_0 Y_1 - E_0 Y_0 = E_0[E_0(Y \mid A = 1, W) - E_0(Y \mid A = 0, W)] \equiv \Psi(P_0),$$

where the outer expectation in the definition of $\Psi(P_0)$ is the mean across the strata for W. This identifiability result for the additive causal effect as a parameter of the distribution P_0 of O required making the randomization assumption stating that A is independent of the counterfactuals (Y_0, Y_1) within strata of W. This assumption might have been included in the original SCM $\mathcal{M}^F$, but, if one knows there are unmeasured confounders, then the model $\mathcal{M}^{F*}$ would be more restrictive by enforcing this "known to be wrong" randomization assumption.

Another required assumption is that $P_0(A = 1, W = w) > 0$ and $P_0(A = 0, W = w) > 0$ are positive for each possible realization w of W. Without this assumption, the conditional expectations of Y in $\Psi(P_0)$ are not well defined. This positivity assumption is often called the experimental treatment assignment (ETA) assumption. Here we are assuming that the conditional treatment assignment probabilities are positive for each possible w: $P_0(A = 1 \mid W = w) > 0$ and $P_0(A = 0 \mid W = w) > 0$ for each possible w. However, the positivity assumption is a more general name for the condition that is necessary for the target parameter $\Psi(P_0)$ to be well defined, and it often requires the censoring or treatment mechanism to have certain support.

So, to be very explicit about how this parameter corresponds with mapping P_0 into a number, as presented in Chap. 1:

$$\Psi(P_0) = \sum_w \Big[\sum_y y P_0(Y = y \mid A = 1, W = w) - \sum_y y P_0(Y = y \mid A = 0, W = w) \Big] P_0(W = w),$$

where

$$P_0(Y = y \mid A = a, W = w) = \frac{P_0(W = w, A = a, Y = y)}{\sum_y P_0(W = w, A = a, Y = y)}$$

is the conditional probability distribution of $Y = y$, given $A = a$, $W = w$, and

$$P_0(W = w) = \sum_{y,a} P_0(Y = y, A = a, W = w)$$

is the marginal probability distribution of $W = w$. This statistical parameter Ψ is defined on all probability distributions of (W, A, Y). The statistical model $\mathcal{M}$ is nonparametric and $\Psi : \mathcal{M} \rightarrow \mathbb{R}$.

We note again that we use the term statistical model for the collection of possible probability distributions, while we use the word model for the statistical model augmented with the nontestable causal assumptions coded by the underlying SCM and its relation to the observed data distribution of O. In our LTPA example, the model is the nonparametric statistical model augmented with the nontestable SCM. If this model includes the randomization assumption, and the experimental treatment assignment assumption, then this model allows the identifiability of the additive causal effect $E_0 Y_1 - E_0 Y_0$ through the statistical target parameter $\Psi(P_0) = E_0(E_0(Y \mid A = 1, W) - E_0(Y \mid A = 0, W))$.

2.3.5 Interpretation of Target Parameter

The observed data parameter $\Psi(P_0)$ can be interpreted in two possibly distinct ways:

1. $\Psi(P_0)$ with $P_0 \in \mathcal{M}$ augmented with the truly reliable additional nonstatistical assumptions that are known to hold (e.g., $\mathcal{M}^F$). This may involve bounding the deviation of $\Psi(P_0)$ from the desired target causal effect $\Psi^F(P_{U,X,0})$ under a realistic causal model $\mathcal{M}^F$ that is not sufficient for the identifiability of this causal effect.
2. The truly causal parameter $\Psi^F(P_{U,X}) = \Psi(P_0)$ under the more restricted SCM $\mathcal{M}^{F*}$, thereby now including all causal assumptions that are needed to make the desired causal effect identifiable from the probability distribution P_0 of O.

The purely statistical (noncausal) parameter given by interpretation 1 is often of interest, such as $E_W[E_0(Y \mid A = 1, W) - E_0(Y \mid A = 0, W)]$, which can be interpreted as the average of the difference in means across the strata for W. With this parameter we can assume nothing, beyond the experimental treatment assignment assumption, except perhaps time ordering $W \to A \to Y$, to have a meaningful interpretation of the difference in means. Since we do not assume an underlying system, the SCM for (U, X) and thereby Y_a, or the randomization assumption, the parameter is a statistical parameter only. This type of parameter is sometimes referred to as a variable importance measure.

For example, if A = age, the investigator may not be willing to assume an SCM defining interventions on age (a variable one cannot intervene on and set in practice). Thus, if one does not assume $\mathcal{M}^F$, the statistical parameter $\Psi(P_0)$ under interpretation 1 can still be very much of interest. In some cases, however, these two interpretations coincide. What is known about the generation of data and distribution

P_U may imply the assumptions necessary to interpret $\Psi(P_0)$ as the causal parameter $\Psi^F(P_{U,X})$: for example, in an RCT, by design, assuming full compliance and no missingness or censoring, the causal assumptions required will hold.

2.4 Revisiting the Mortality Example

For the sake of presentation, we intentionally assumed that the exposure LTPA was binary and worked with an SCM that generated a binary exposure A. In the actual mortality study A is continuous valued. Consider the more realistic SCM $W = f_W(U_W)$, $A = f_A(W, U_A)$, $Y = f_Y(W, A, U_Y)$, where A is now continuous valued. Let $Y_a(u)$ be the counterfactual obtained by setting $A = a$ and $U = u$, so that Y_a is the random variable representing survival at 5 years under LTPA at level a. Suppose one wishes to consider a cut-off value δ for LTPA level so that one can recommend that the population at least exercise at this level δ. A causal quantity of interest is now

$$\psi_0^F = \sum_a w_1(a) E_0 Y_a - \sum_a w_0(a) E_0 Y_a,$$

where $w_1(a)$ is a probability distribution on excercise levels larger than δ, and $w_0(a)$ is a probability distribution on exercise levels smaller than or equal to δ. This corresponds to $E_0 Y_1 - E_0 Y_0$, where Y_1 is defined by the random intervention on the SCM in which one randomly draws A from w_1, and similarly Y_0 is defined by randomly drawing A from w_0. This causal effect $E_0 Y_1 - E_0 Y_0$ can be identified from the probability distribution P_0 of $O = (W, A, Y)$ as follows:

$$\psi_0^F = \sum_a (w_1 - w_0)(a) E_0 E_0(Y \mid A = a, W) \equiv \psi_0.$$

2.5 Road Map for Targeted Learning

In Chap. 1, we introduced the road map for targeted learning. In this chapter we have discussed defining the research question, which involved describing the data and committing to a statistical model and target parameter. The estimation problem we wish to solve is now fully defined. The next stage of the road map addresses estimation of the target parameter, which will be covered in the next three chapters.

The statistical estimation problem. We observe n i.i.d. copies $O_1, .., O_n$ from a probability distribution P_0 known to be in a statistical model $\mathcal{M}$, and we wish to infer statistically about the target parameter $\Psi(P_0)$. Often, this target parameter only depends on P_0 through a relevant (infinite-dimensional) parameter $Q_0 = Q_0(P_0)$ of P_0, so that we can also write $\Psi(Q_0)$.

Targeted substitution estimator. We construct a substitution estimator $\Psi(Q_n^*)$ obtained by plugging in an estimator Q_n^* of Q_0. This involves super learning and

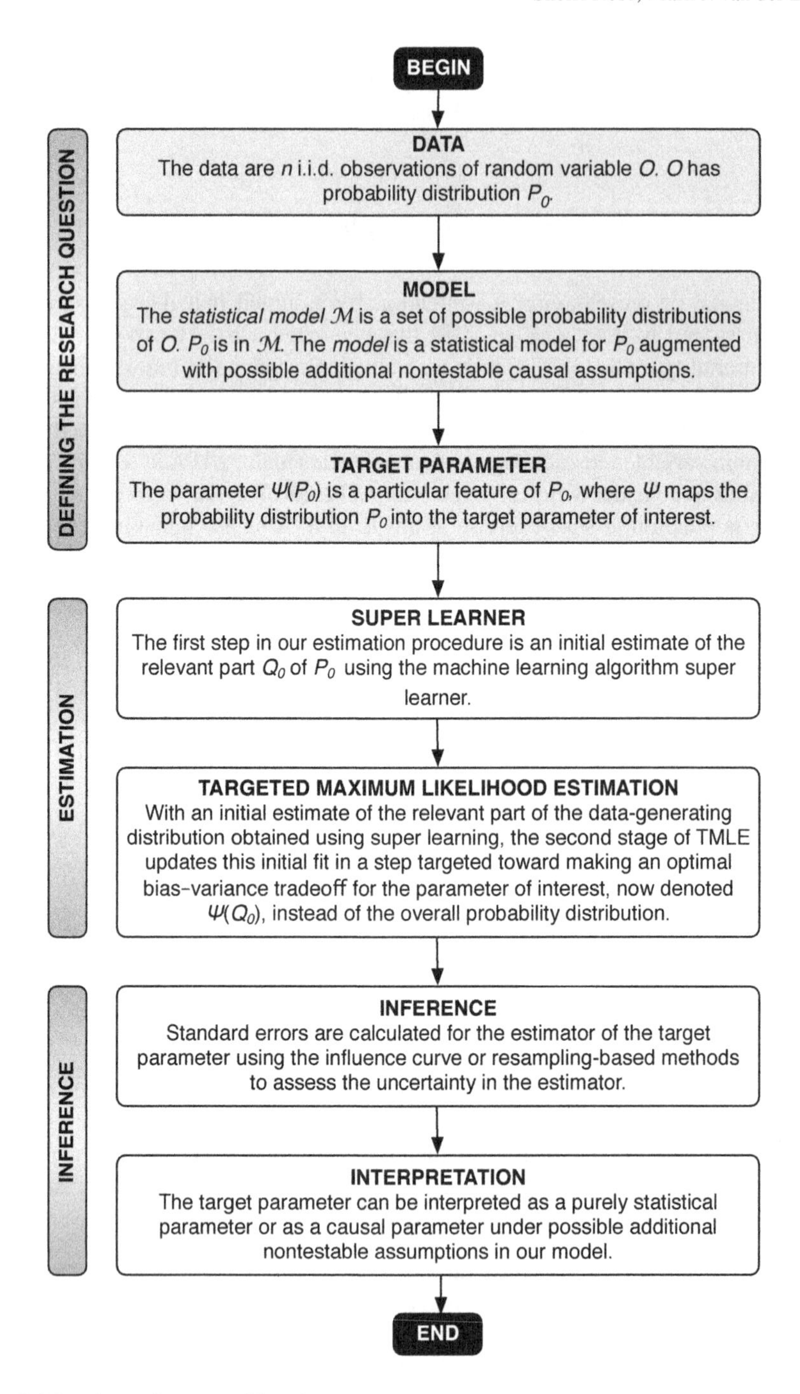

Fig. 2.6 Road map for targeted learning

TMLE, so that we obtain, under regularity conditions, an asymptotically linear, double robust, and efficient normally distributed estimator of $\psi_0 = \Psi(Q_0)$, and, in general, put in the maximal effort to minimize the mean squared error with respect to the true value ψ_0. In addition, we provide statistical inference about ψ_0 based on the estimation of the normal limit distribution of $\sqrt{n}(\Psi(Q_n^*) - \psi_0)$.

2.6 Conceptual Framework

This section provides a rigorous conceptual framework for the topics covered in this chapter. If you find it too abstract on your initial reading, we advise you to come back as you become more familiar with the material. It is meant for more advanced readers.

Data are meaningless without knowledge about the experiment that generated the data. That is, data are realizations of a random variable with a certain probability distribution on a set of possible outcomes, and statistical learning is concerned with learning something about the probability distribution of the data. Typically, we are willing to view our data as a realization of n independent identical replications of the experiment, and we accept this as our first modeling assumption. If we denote the random variable representing the data generated by the experiment by O, having a probability distribution P_0, then the data set corresponds with drawing a realization of n i.i.d. copies $O_1, \ldots, O_n$ with some common probability distribution P_0.

A statistical estimation problem corresponds with defining a statistical model $\mathcal{M}$ for P_0, where the statistical model $\mathcal{M}$ is a collection of possible probability distributions of O. The estimation problem also requires a mapping Ψ on this statistical model $\mathcal{M}$, where Ψ maps any $P \in \mathcal{M}$ into a vector of numbers $\Psi(P)$. We write $\Psi : \mathcal{M} \rightarrow \mathbb{R}^d$ for a d-dimensional parameter. We introduce ψ_0, and the interpretation of ψ_0 as $\Psi(P_0)$, i.e., a well-defined feature of P_0, is called the pure statistical interpretation of the parameter value ψ_0. The statistical estimation problem is now to map the data set $O_1, \ldots, O_n$ into an estimator of $\Psi(P_0)$ that incorporates the knowledge that $P_0 \in \mathcal{M}$, accompanied by an assessment of the uncertainty in the estimator of ψ_0.

When thinking purely about the construction of an estimator, the only concern is to construct an estimator of ψ_0 that has small mean squared error (MSE), or some other measure of dissimilarity between the estimator and the true ψ_0. This does not require any additional knowledge (or nontestable causal assumptions). As a consequence, for the construction of a targeted maximum likelihood estimator, which we introduce in Chaps. 4 and 5, the only input is the statistical model $\mathcal{M}$ and the mapping Ψ representing the target parameter.

Making assumptions about P_0 that do not change the statistical model, so-called nontestable assumptions, will not change the statistical estimation problem. However, such assumptions allows one to interpret a particular parameter $\Psi(P_0)$ in a new way. If such nontestable assumptions are known to be true, it enriches the interpretation of the number ψ_0. If they are wrong, then it results in misinterpretation of ψ_0.

This is called causal modeling when it involves nontestable assumptions that allow $\Psi(P_0)$ to be interpreted as a causal effect, and, in general, it is modeling with nontestable assumptions with the goal of providing an enriched interpretation of this parameter $\Psi(P_0)$.

It works as follows. One proposes a parameterization $\theta \rightarrow P_\theta$ for θ varying over a set Θ so that the statistical model $\mathcal{M}$ can be represented as $\mathcal{M} = \{P_\theta : \theta \in \Theta\}$, where θ represents $P_{U,X}$ in our SCM framework, but it can represent any underlying structure (not necessarily causal). That is, we provide a parameterization for the statistical model $\mathcal{M}$. In addition, since $P_0 \in \mathcal{M}$, there exists a θ_0 such that $P_0 = P_{\theta_0}$. Assume that this θ_0 is actually uniquely identified by P_0. θ_0 has its own interpretation, such as the probability distribution of counterfactual random variables in the SCM. Suddenly, the P_0 allows us to infer $\theta_0 = \Theta(P_0)$ for a mapping Θ. As a consequence, with this "magic trick" of parameterizing P_0 we succeeded in providing a new interpretation of P_0 and, in particular, of any parameter $\Psi(P_0) = \Psi(P_{\theta_0})$ as a function of θ_0.

As one can imagine, there are millions of possible magic tricks one can carry out, each one creating a new interpretation of P_0 by having it mapped into an interpretation of a θ_0 implied by a particular parameterization. The data cannot tell you if one magic trick will provide a more accurate description of reality than another magic trick, since data can only provide information about P_0 itself. As a consequence, which magic trick is applied, or if any trick is applied at all, should be driven by true knowledge about the underlying mechanism that resulted in the generation of O. In that case, the selection of the parameterization is not a magic trick but represents the incorporation of true knowledge allowing us to interpret the parameter ψ_0 for what it is. Note that this modeling could easily correspond with a nonparametric statistical model $\mathcal{M}$ for P_0.

Two important mistakes can occur in statistical practice, before the selection of an estimator, given that one has specified a statistical model $\mathcal{M}$ and parameter $\Psi : \mathcal{M} \rightarrow \mathbb{R}^d$. The first mistake is that one specifies the statistical model $\mathcal{M}$ incorrectly so that $P_0 \notin \mathcal{M}$, resulting in misinterpretation of $\Psi(P_0)$, even as a purely statistical parameter, i.e., as a mapping Ψ applied to P_0. The second mistake is that one misspecifies additional nontestable assumptions as coded by the selected parameterization for $\mathcal{M}$ that were used to provide an enriched interpretation of $\Psi(P_0)$, again resulting in misinterpretation of $\Psi(P_0)$. These two mistakes can be collapsed into one, namely, misspecification of the model for P_0. By the model we now mean the statistical model for P_0 augmented with the additional nontestable structural assumptions, even though these do not change the statistical model.

So a model now includes the additional parameterization, such that two identical statistical models that are based on different parameterizations are classified as different models. Thus, a model is defined by a mapping $P_\cdot : \Theta \rightarrow \mathcal{M}, \theta \rightarrow P_\theta$, and the statistical model implied by this model is given by the range $\mathcal{M} = \{P_\theta : \theta\}$ of this mapping. Regarding statistical vocabulary, we will use the word model for the parameterization mapping $P_\cdot : \Theta \rightarrow \mathcal{M}$, and statistical model for the set of possible probability distributions, i.e., the range of this mapping. Note, that if the parameterization is simply the identity mapping defined on $\mathcal{M}$, then the model equals the statistical model.

Even though it is healthy to be cynical about modeling and extremely aware of its dangers and its potential to lie with data, it is of fundamental importance to statistical learning that we can incorporate structural knowledge about the data-generating process and utilize that in our interpretation. In addition, even if these structural assumptions implied by the model/parameterization are uncertain, it is worthwhile to know that, *if* these were true, then our parameter would allow its corresponding interpretation. One could then report both the statistical interpretation, or the reliable statistical model interpretation, as well as the *if also, then* interpretation to our target ψ_0.

In addition, this structural modeling allows one to create truly interesting parameters in an underlying world and one can then establish under what assumptions one can identify these truly interesting parameters from the observed data. This itself teaches us how to generate new data so that these parameters will be identifiable. The identifiability results for these truly interesting parameters provide us with statistical parameters $\Psi(P_0)$ that might be interesting as statistical parameters anyway, without these additional structural assumptions, and have the additional flavor of having a particularly powerful interpretation if these additional structural assumptions happen to be true. In particular, one may be able to interpret $\Psi(P_0)$ as the best possible approximation of the wished causal quantity of interest based on the available data. Overall, this provides us with more than enough motivation to include (causal) modeling as an important component in the road map of targeted learning from data.

2.7 Notes and Further Reading

As noted in the introduction, a thorough presentation of SCMs, causal graphs, and related identifiability theory can be found in Pearl (2009). We also direct the interested reader to Judea Pearl's Web site (http://bayes.cs.ucla.edu/jp_home.html) for easily organized references and presentations on these topics. The g-formula for identifying the distribution of counterfactuals from the observed data distribution, under the sequential randomization assumption, was originally published in Robins (1986). The simplified data example we introduce in this chapter, a mortality study examining the effect of LTPA, is based on data presented in Tager et al. (1998). We carry this example through the next three chapters, and in Chap. 4, we analyze this data using super learning and targeted maximum likelihood estimation.

In our road map we utilize causal models, such as SCMs and the Neyman–Rubin model, to generate statistical effect parameters $\psi_0 = \Psi(P_0)$ of interest. The interpretation of the estimand ψ_0, beyond its pure statistical interpretation, depends on the required causal assumptions necessary for identifiability of the desired causal quantity ψ_0^F (defined as target quantity in causal model for full data or counterfactuals) from the observed data distribution. Such an interpretation might be further enriched if one could define an actual experiment that would reproduce this causal quantity. Either way, our road map poses these causal models as working models to derive these statistical target parameters that can be interpreted as causal effects under explicitly stated causal assumptions. The latter assumptions are fully exposed and for anybody to criticize.

We wish to stress that the learning of these estimands with their pure statistical interpretation already represents progress in science. In addition, the required causal assumptions that would allow a richer interpretation of the estimand teach us how to improve our design of the observational or RCT.

Somehow, we think that a statistical target parameter that has a desired causal interpretation under possibly unrealistic assumptions is a "best" approximation of the ideal causal quantity, given the limitations set by the available data. For example, $E_0(E_0(Y \mid A = 1, W) - E_0(Y \mid A = 0, W))$ is an effect of treatment, controlling for the measured covariates, with a clear statistical interpretation, and, if people feel comfortable talking about $E_0 Y_1 - E_0 Y_0$, then we think that this statistical estimand represents a "best" effort to target this additive causal effect under the constraints set by the available data.

Instead of making a hard decision regarding the causal assumptions necessary for making the estimand equal to the causal quantity, one may wish to investigate the potential distance between the estimand and the causal quantity. In this manner, one still allows for a causal interpretation of the estimand (such as that the asymptotic bias of the estimand with respect to the desired causal quantity is bounded from above by a certain number), even if the causal assumptions required for making the estimand equal to the causal quantity are violated. Such an approach relies on the ability to bound this distance by incorporation of realistic causal knowledge. Such a sensitivity analysis will require input from subject matter people such as a determination of an upper bound of the effect of unmeasured confounders beyond the measured time-dependent confounders. Even a highly trained statistician will have an extremely hard time getting his/her head around such a question, making such sensitivity analyses potentially unreliable and extremely hard to communicate. Still, this is an important research area since it allows for a continuous range from pure statistical interpretation of the estimand to a pure causal effect interpretation.

Either way, we should not forget that using poor methods for estimation with the actual observed data, while investing enormous effort in such a sensitivity analysis. makes no sense. By the same token, estimation of the estimand is a separate problem from determining the distance between the estimand and the causal quantity of interest and is obviously as important as carefully defining and interpreting the estimand: the careful definition and interpretation of an estimand has little value if one decides to use a misspecified parametric model to fit it!

Chapter 3
Super Learning

Eric C. Polley, Sherri Rose, Mark J. van der Laan

This is the first chapter in our text focused on estimation within the road map for targeted learning. Now that we've defined the research question, including our data, the model, and the target parameter, we are ready to begin. For the estimation of a target parameter of the probability distribution of the data, such as target parameters that can be interpreted as causal effects, we implement TMLE. The first step in this estimation procedure is an initial estimate of the data-generating distribution P_0, or the relevant part Q_0 of P_0 that is needed to evaluate the target parameter. This is the step presented in Chap. 3, and TMLE will be presented in Chaps. 4 and 5.

We introduce these concepts using our mortality study example from Chap. 2 examining the effect of LTPA. Our outcome Y is binary, indicating death within 5 years of baseline, and A is also binary, indicating whether the subject meets recommended levels of physical activity. The data structure in this example is $O = (W, A, Y) \sim P_0$. Our target parameter is $\Psi(P_0) = E_{W,0}[E_0(Y \mid A = 1, W) - E_0(Y \mid A = 0, W)]$, which represents the causal risk difference under causal assumptions. Since this target parameter only depends on P_0 through the conditional mean $\bar{Q}_0(A, W) = E_0(Y \mid A, W)$, and the marginal distribution $Q_{W,0}$ of W, we can also write $\Psi(Q_0)$, where $Q_0 = (\bar{Q}_0, Q_{W,0})$. We estimate the expectation over W with the empirical mean over W_i, $i = 1, \ldots, n$. With this target parameter, $\bar{Q}_0(A, W) = E_0(Y \mid A, W)$ is the only object we will still need to estimate. Therefore, the first step of the TMLE of the risk difference $\Psi(P_0)$ is to estimate this conditional mean function $\bar{Q}_0(A, W)$. Our substitution TMLE will be of the type

$$\psi_n = \Psi(Q_n) = \frac{1}{n}\sum_{i=1}^{n}\{\bar{Q}_n(1, W_i) - \bar{Q}_n(0, W_i)\},$$

where this estimate is obtained by plugging $Q_n = (\bar{Q}_n, Q_{W,n})$ into the parameter mapping Ψ.

We could estimate the entire conditional probability distribution of Y, instead of estimating the conditional mean of Y, but then (except when Y is binary) we are estimating portions of the density we do not need. Targeted estimation of only the relevant portion of the probability distribution of O in this first step of the TMLE procedure provides us with maximally efficient and unbiased estimators. This will be further discussed in Chaps. 4 and 5.

3.1 Background

Let's start our discussion with studies where Y is binary, such as in our mortality study example. When Y is binary, there is no difference between the conditional mean or conditional probability distribution, so this distinction plays no role. Now, what do we know about our probability distribution P_0 of O? We know that the data are n i.i.d. observations (realizations) on n i.i.d. copies $O_1, \ldots, O_n$ of $O \sim P_0$. These realizations are denoted $o_1, \ldots, o_n$. In our mortality study example, we have no knowledge about P_0. Thus we have a nonparametric statistical model for P_0. In scenarios where we have some knowledge about data generation, we can include this knowledge in a semiparametric statistical model. Our parameter of interest is this chapter is $\bar{Q}_0(A, W) = P_0(Y = 1 \mid A, W)$.

How are we to estimate $P_0(Y = 1 \mid A, W)$ if we assume only a nonparametric (or, in general, a large semiparametric) statistical model? We do not know anything about the shape of $\bar{Q}_0(A, W)$ as a function of exposure and covariates. Standard practice would assume a parametric statistical model, making assumptions we know are wrong, and proceeding to estimate $P_0(Y = 1 \mid A, W)$ under the assumptions of the parametric statistical model, thereby forcing the shape of this function of (A, W) to follow an incorrect user-supplied structure. Since the parametric statistical model is wrong, the estimate of $P_0(Y = 1 \mid A, W)$ will be biased, and increasing the sample size will not make it any better. What we want is an automated algorithm to nonparametrically (or semiparametrically) estimate $P_0(Y = 1 \mid A, W)$, i.e., we want an estimator that is able to learn from the data using the true knowledge represented by the actual statistical model for P_0.

In the computer science literature, this is called machine learning. In statistics, these methods are often referred to as nonparametric or semiparametric estimators, or data-adaptive estimators. We will use the terms *data-adaptive* and *machine learning* interchangeably in this text. The essential point is that there are nonparametric methods that also aim to "smooth" the data and estimate this regression function flexibly, adapting it to the data given a priori guidelines, without overfitting the data.

For example, one could use local averaging of the outcome Y within covariate "neighborhoods." Here, neighborhoods are bins for covariate observations that are close in value, where these bins are defined by partitioning the covariate space. The number of bins will determine the smoothness of our fitted regression function. Such a regression estimator is also called a histogram regression estimator. How do you choose the size of these neighborhoods or bins? This becomes a bias–variance trade-off question. If we have many small neighborhoods, the estimate will not be smooth and will have high variance since some neighborhoods will be empty or contain only a small number of observations. The result is a sample mean of the outcome over the observations in the neighborhood that is imprecise. On the other hand, if we have very few large neighborhoods, the estimate is much smoother, but it will be biased since the neighborhoods fail to capture the complexity of the data. Suppose we choose the number of neighborhoods in a smart way. With n large enough, this will result in a good estimator in our nonparametric statistical model. Formally, we say such a histogram regression estimator is asymptotically consistent in the sense that it approximates the true regression function as sample size increases.

However, if the true data-generating distribution is very smooth, a logistic regression in a misspecified parametric statistical model might beat the nonparametric estimator. This is frustrating! We want to create a smart nonparametric estimator that is consistent, but in some cases it may "lose" to a misspecified parametric model because it is more variable. There are other ways of approaching the truth that will be smoother than local averaging. One method, locally weighted regression and scatterplot smoothing (loess), is a weighted polynomial regression method that fits the data locally, iteratively within neighborhoods. Spline functions, another method, are similar to polynomial functions, as splines are piecewise polynomial functions. Smoothing splines use penalties to adjust for a lack of smoothness, and regression splines use linear combinations of basis functions. There are many other potential algorithms we could implement to estimate $P_0(Y = 1 \mid A, W)$. However, how are we to know priori which one to use? We cannot bet on a logistic regression in a misspecified parametric statistical model, but we have the problem that one particular algorithm is going to do better than the other candidate estimators for the particular data-generating distribution P_0, and we do not know which one is the best.

To be very explicit, an algorithm is an estimator of $\bar{Q}_0$ that maps a data set of n observations (W_i, A_i, Y_i), $i = 1, \ldots, n$, into a prediction function that can be used to map input (A, W) into a predicted value for Y. The algorithms may differ in the subset of the covariates used, the basis functions, the loss functions, the searching algorithm, and the range of tuning parameters, among others. We use *algorithm* in a general sense to mean any mapping from data into a predictor, so that the word *algorithm* is equivalent to the word *estimator*. As long as the algorithm takes the observed data and outputs a fitted prediction function, we consider it a prediction algorithm. For example, a collection of algorithms could include least squares regression estimators, algorithms indexed by set values of the fine-tuning parameters for a collection of values, algorithms using internal cross-validation to set fine-tuning parameters, algorithms coupled with screening procedures to reduce the dimension of the covariate vector, and so on.

Effect Estimation vs. Prediction

Both causal effect and prediction research questions are inherently *estimation* questions. In the first, we are interested in estimating the causal effect of A on Y adjusted for covariates W. For prediction, we are interested in generating a function to input the variables (A, W) and predict a value for Y. These are separate and distinct research questions. However, many (causal) effect estimators, such as TMLE, involve prediction steps within the procedure. Thus, understanding prediction is a core concept even when one has an effect estimation research question. Effect parameters where no causal assumptions are made are often referred to as variable importance measures (VIMs).

3.2 Defining the Estimation Problem

Our data structure is $O = (W, A, Y) \sim P_0$, and we observe n i.i.d. observations on $O_1, \ldots, O_n$. An estimator maps these observations into a value for the parameter it targets. We can view estimators as mappings from the empirical distribution P_n of the data set, where P_n places probability $1/n$ on each observed O_i, $i = 1, \ldots, n$. In our mortality study example, we need an estimator of $\bar{Q}_0(A, W) = P_0(Y = 1 \mid A, W)$.

Before we can choose a "best" algorithm to estimate the function $\bar{Q}_0 : (A, W) \rightarrow \bar{Q}_0(A, W)$, we must have a way to define what "best" means. We do this in terms of a loss function, which assigns a measure of performance to a candidate function $\bar{Q}$ when applied to an observation O. That is, a loss function is a function L given by

$$L : (O, \bar{Q}) \rightarrow L(O, \bar{Q}) \in \mathbb{R}.$$

It is a function of the random variable O and parameter value $\bar{Q}$. Examples of loss functions include the L_1 absolute error loss function

$$L(O, \bar{Q}) = |Y - \bar{Q}(A, W)|,$$

the L_2 squared error (or quadratic) loss function

$$L(O, \bar{Q}) = (Y - \bar{Q}(A, W))^2,$$

and the negative log loss function for a binary Y

$$L(O, \bar{Q}) = -\log(\bar{Q}(A, W)^Y (1 - \bar{Q}(A, W))^{1-Y}).$$

A loss function defines a function $\bar{Q}_0$ that has the optimal expected performance with respect to that loss function among all candidate functions $\bar{Q}$. For example, the function $\bar{Q}_0$ that minimizes the expected absolute error, $\bar{Q} \rightarrow E_0|Y - \bar{Q}(A, W)|$, is the conditional median of Y, as a function of (A, W). On the other hand, the function that minimizes the expected squared error is the conditional mean of Y, while the function that minimizes the expected negative log loss function for a binary Y is the conditional probability distribution of Y, as a function of (A, W). For binary Y, both the L_2 loss and negative log loss target the same function $\bar{Q}_0(A, W) = P_0(Y = 1 \mid A, W)$.

We can now define our parameter of interest, $\bar{Q}_0(A, W) = E_0(Y \mid A, W)$, as the minimizer of the expected squared error loss:

$$\bar{Q}_0 = \arg\min_{\bar{Q}} E_0 L(O, \bar{Q}),$$

where $L(O, \bar{Q}) = (Y - \bar{Q}(A, W))^2$. $E_0 L(O, \bar{Q})$, which we want to be small, evaluates the candidate $\bar{Q}$, and it is minimized at the optimal choice of $\bar{Q}_0$. We refer to expected loss as the risk. Thus we have a way to define the "best" algorithm. We want the estimator of the regression function $\bar{Q}_0$ whose realized value minimizes the expectation of the squared error loss function. If we have two estimates $\bar{Q}_n^a$ and $\bar{Q}_n^b$, then we prefer the estimator for which $\sum_o P_0(O = o) L(o, \bar{Q}_n)$ is smallest.

This makes sense intuitively. We want an estimator that is close to the true $\bar{Q}_0$ and the difference between the risk at a candidate $\bar{Q}$ and the risk at the true $\bar{Q}_0$ corresponds with an expected squared error between $\bar{Q}$ and $\bar{Q}_0$ across all values of (A, W):

$$E_0 L(O, \bar{Q}) - E_0 L(O, \bar{Q}_0) = E_0(\bar{Q} - \bar{Q}_0)^2(A, W).$$

Minimizing the expected loss will bring the chosen candidate closer to the true $\bar{Q}_0$ with respect to the dissimilarity measure implied by the loss function, namely, the difference of the risk at $\bar{Q}$ and the optimal risk at $\bar{Q}_0$. How do we find out which algorithm among a library of algorithms yields the smallest expected loss, or, equivalently, which one has the best performance with respect to the dissimilarity implied by the loss function?

3.3 Super (Machine) Learning

Let us return to our simplified mortality study example. The outcome Y is binary, indicating death within 5 years of baseline, and A is also binary, indicating whether the subject meets recommended levels of physical activity. The data structure is $O = (W, A, Y) \sim P_0$. For now let us consider only the covariates $W = \{W_1, W_2, W_3\}$. Age (W_1) is a continuous measure, gender (W_2) is binary, and chronic health history (W_3) is a binary measure indicating whether the subject has a chronic health condition at baseline. While we are ultimately interested in the effect of LTPA on death demonstrated in the next chapter, if we were strictly interested in a *prediction* research question, we could also include LTPA as a covariate in vector W.

Suppose there are three subject matter experts, and they each have a different proposal about the specification of a logistic regression in a parametric statistical model, incorporating their subject matter knowledge. The first believes a main terms statistical model is sufficient for the estimation of the prediction target parameter:

$$\bar{Q}_n^a(A, W) = P_n^a(Y = 1 \mid A, W) = \text{expit}\,(\alpha_{0,n} + \alpha_{1,n} A + \alpha_{2,n} W_1 + \alpha_{3,n} W_2 + \alpha_{4,n} W_3).$$

The second expert proposes including all covariates W and exposure A, as well as an interaction term between age and gender:

$$\bar{Q}_n^b(A, W) = \text{expit}\,(\alpha_{0,n} + \alpha_{1,n}A + \alpha_{2,n}W_1 + \alpha_{3,n}W_2 + \alpha_{4,n}W_3 + \alpha_{5,n}(W_1 \times W_2)).$$

The third expert wants to use a statistical model with main terms and age^2:

$$\bar{Q}_n^c(A, W) = \text{expit}\,(\alpha_{0,n} + \alpha_{1,n}A + \alpha_{2,n}W_1 + \alpha_{3,n}W_2 + \alpha_{4,n}W_3 + \alpha_{5,n}W_1^2).$$

The investigators would ideally like to run all three of these statistical models. Now that we've defined a criterion for the best estimator of $\bar{Q}_0$, how can we responsibly select the optimal estimator from a collection of algorithms, such as the collection of estimators $\bar{Q}_n^a$, $\bar{Q}_n^b$, and $\bar{Q}_n^c$?

3.3.1 Discrete Super Learner

We start by introducing discrete super learning, which will give us an estimate of the cross-validated risk for each algorithm. The entire data set (learning set) is divided into V groups of size $\sim n/V$. These groups are mutually exclusive and exhaustive sets. Our mortality data set has $n = 2066$ subjects. If we want to perform V-fold cross-validation in our discrete super learning procedure, using 10 folds, we will divide our data set into groups of size $\sim 2066/10$. (This gives us four groups with 206 subjects and six groups with 207 subjects.) We label each group from 1 to 10.

Let us focus first on understanding the procedure with just one of the regressions in the collection of algorithms. The observations in group 1 are set aside, and the first regression is fit on the remaining nine groups (called the training set). Then we take the observations in group 1 (called the validation set) and obtain predicted probabilities of death for these 206 or 207 observations using the regression fit on the training set. It is important to note that the observations in group 1 *were not included in the fitting process* and will only be used to evaluate the performance of the predictor that was obtained on the training sample. In this way, we have succeeded in obtaining predicted probabilities of death for approx. 10% of our data, where the prediction function used to obtain these predicted probabilities was fit based on the remaining 90% of data. At this stage, we calculate the estimated risk within the validation set using their predicted probabilities. This procedure is performed for all of the algorithms in the collection of algorithms, so that we have, at the end of the first fold, predicted probabilities for each of the three regressions. We also have an estimate of risk within the validation set (group 1) for each of the three regressions, calculated using their corresponding predicted probabilities.

We need to perform this procedure nine more times, so that each group has the opportunity to take on the role of the validation set and obtain predicted probabilities for each algorithm fit on the corresponding training set. Thus, the procedure continues until we have predicted probabilities of death for all 2066 subjects for each algorithm, and also estimated risk within each validation set for each algorithm. We then have 10 estimated risks for each of the three algorithms, and these risks are averaged across validation sets resulting in one estimated cross-validated risk for each algorithm. The discrete super learner algorithm selects the algorithm with the smallest cross-validated risk. The algorithm with the smallest cross-validated risk is the "best" estimator according to our criterion: minimizing the estimated expected squared error loss function. See Fig. 3.1 for a diagram of this procedure.

We have now described a new algorithm that took as input the three algorithms. This new estimator is what we call the discrete super learner, and it is indexed by this collection of three algorithms.

By incorporating a rich collection of algorithms that vary in bias and degree of data-fitting, the cross-validation within the discrete super learner prevents overfitting and it also prevents selecting a fit that is too biased. There are many forms of cross-validation, and here we discussed V-fold cross-validation due to its low computational burden while still providing the desirable finite sample and asymptotic optimality properties, which will be discussed later. The collection of algorithms can be large and includes other algorithms besides parametric statistical models, for example, the collection of algorithms may include random forest algorithms and support vector machines.

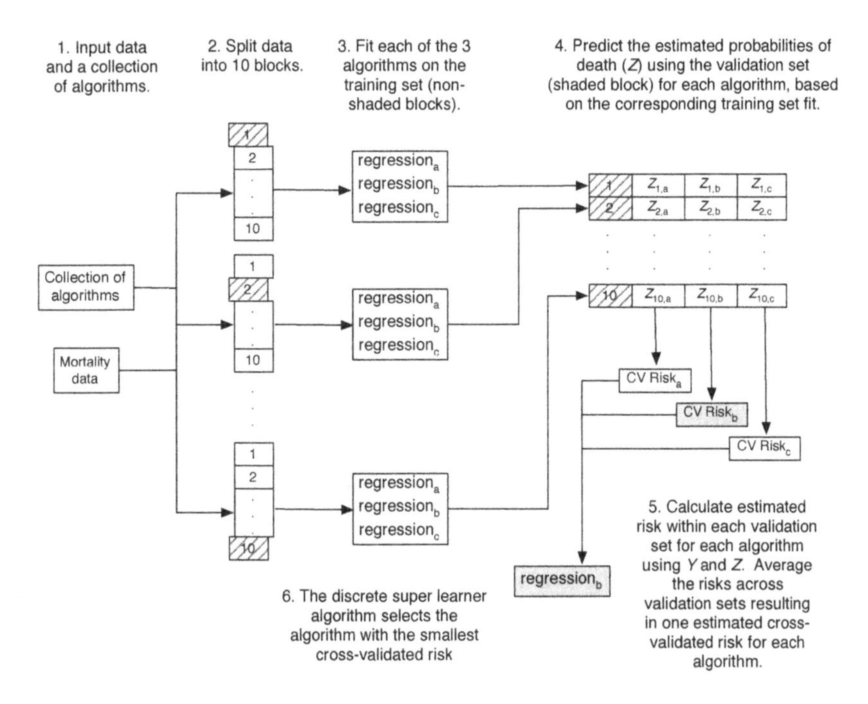

Fig. 3.1 Discrete super learner algorithm for the mortality study example where $\bar{Q}_n^b(A, W)$ is the algorithm with the smallest cross-validated risk

When the loss function is bounded, it has been shown that this discrete super learner will, for large sample sizes, perform as well as the algorithm that is the minimizer of the expected loss function. The latter impossible choice is called the oracle selector, which corresponds with simply selecting the estimator that is closest to the true $\bar{Q}_0$. In addition, cross-validation selection is tailored for small sample sizes, thus one should not be misled that cross-validation requires large sample sizes.

3.3.2 Super Learner

Can we improve upon the discrete super learner? Yes! We can use our three regressions to build a library of algorithms consisting of all weighted averages of these regressions. It is reasonable to expect that one of these weighted averages might perform better than one of the three regressions alone. This simple principle allows us to map a collection of candidate algorithms (in this case, our three regressions) into a library of weighted averages of these algorithms. Each weighted average is a unique candidate algorithm in this augmented library. We can then apply the same cross-validation selector to this augmented set of candidate algorithms, resulting in the super learner. It might seem that the implementation of such an estimator is problematic, since it requires minimizing the cross-validated risk over an infinite set of candidate algorithms (the weighted averages). The contrary is true. The super learner is not more computer intensive than the discrete super learner. If the discrete super learner has been implemented, then all the work has been done! Only the relatively trivial calculation of the optimal weight vector needs to be completed.

Consider that the discrete super learner has already been completed as described in Sect. 3.3.1. We then propose a family of weighted combinations of the three regression algorithms, which we index by the weight vector α. We want to determine which combination minimizes the cross-validated risk over the family of weighted combinations. The (cross-validated) probabilities of death (Z) for each algorithm are used as inputs in a working (statistical) model to predict the outcome Y. Therefore, we have a working model with three $\alpha = \{\alpha_a, \alpha_b, \alpha_c\}$ coefficients that need to be estimated, one for each of the three algorithms. Selecting the weights that minimize the cross-validated risk is a simple minimization problem, formulated as a regression of the outcomes Y on the predicted values of the algorithms (Z) according to the user-supplied parametric family of weighted combinations. The weighted combination with the smallest cross-validated risk is the "best" estimator according to our criterion: minimizing the estimated expected squared error loss function.

The selected weighted combination is a new estimator we can now use to input data (e.g., our complete mortality data set) to estimate predicted probabilities. Thus, we fit each of the three algorithms on our complete data (learning set). Combining these algorithm fits with our new estimator generates the super learner prediction function. This prediction function is the weighted combination of the candidate algorithms applied to the whole data set. See Fig. 3.2 for a full diagram of the super learner algorithm. In order to calculate an honest risk for the super learner, the super

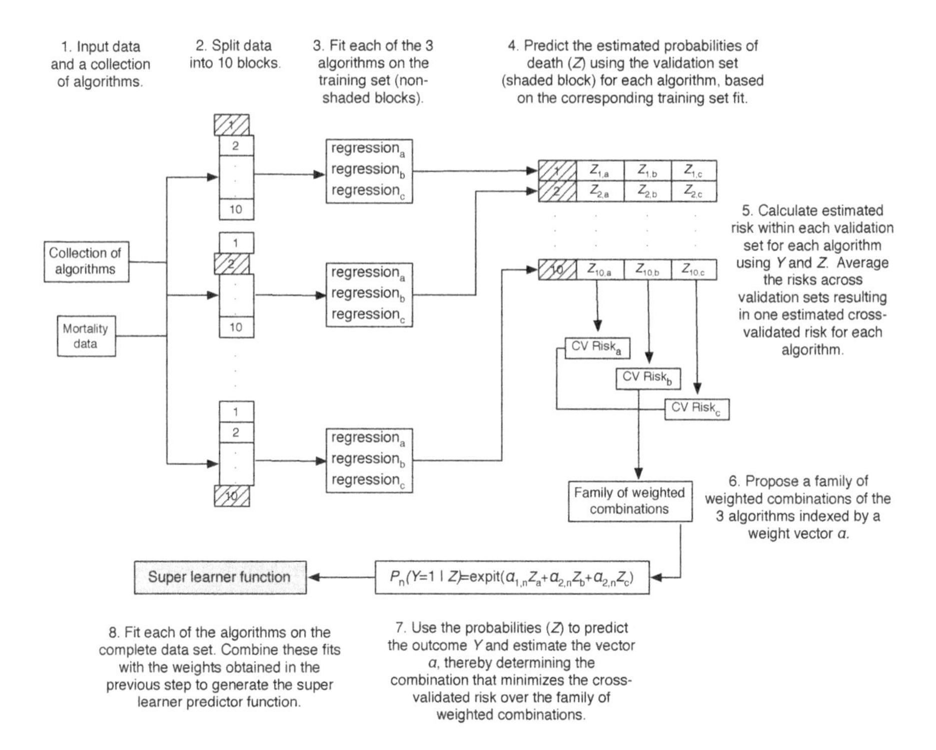

Fig. 3.2 Super learner algorithm for the mortality study example

learner itself must be externally cross-validated after the procedure described above has been implemented.

The family of weighted combinations includes only those α-vectors that have a sum equal to one, and where each weight is positive or zero. Theory does not dictate any restrictions on the family of weighted combinations used for assembling the algorithms; however, the restriction of the parameter space for α to be the convex combination of the algorithms provides greater stability for the final super learner prediction. The convex combination is not only empirically motivated, but also supported by theory. The oracle results for the super learner require a bounded loss function. Restricting oneself to a convex combination of algorithms implies that if each algorithm in the library is bounded, the convex combination will also be bounded.

The super learner improves asymptotically on the discrete super learner by working with a larger library. We reiterate that asymptotic results prove that in realistic scenarios (where none of the algorithms are a correctly specified parametric model), the cross-validated selector performs asymptotically as well as the oracle, which we define as the best estimator given the algorithms in the collection of algorithms. Consequently, the super learner performs asymptotically as well as the best choice among the family of weighted combinations of estimators. Thus, by adding more competitors, we only improve the performance of the super learner. The asymptotic equivalence remains true if the number of algorithms in the library grows very quickly with sample size. Even when the collection of algorithms contains a correctly specified parametric statistical model, the super learner will approximate the truth as fast as the parametric statistical model, although it will be more variable.

The super learner algorithm provides a system to combine multiple estimators into an improved estimator, and returns a function we can also use for prediction in new data sets.

3.3.3 Finite Sample Performance and Applications

To examine the finite sample performance of the super learner we present a series of simulations and data applications. (For those readers unfamiliar with simulation, simulated data are ideal for methodology validation, as the true underlying distribution of the data is known.) We then demonstrate the super learner on a collection of real data sets and a microarray cancer data set.

Four different simulations are presented in this section. All four simulations involve a univariate X drawn from a uniform distribution in $[-4, 4]$. The outcomes follow the functions described below:

$$\begin{aligned}
\textbf{Simulation 1: } Y &= -2 \times \mathrm{I}(X < -3) + 2.55 \times \mathrm{I}(X > -2) - 2 \times \mathrm{I}(X > 0) \\
&\quad + 4 \times \mathrm{I}(X > 2) - 1 \times \mathrm{I}(X > 3) + U; \\
\textbf{Simulation 2: } Y &= 6 + 0.4X - 0.36X^2 + 0.005X^3 + U; \\
\textbf{Simulation 3: } Y &= 2.83 \times \sin\left(\frac{\pi}{2} \times X\right) + U; \\
\textbf{Simulation 4: } Y &= 4 \times \sin(3\pi \times X) \times \mathrm{I}(X > 0) + U,
\end{aligned}$$

where $\mathrm{I}(\cdot)$ is the usual indicator function and U, our exogenous background error, is drawn from an independent standard normal distribution in all simulations. A sample of size 100 was drawn for each scenario. Figure 3.3 contains a scatterplot with a sample from each of the four simulations. The true curve for each simulation is represented by the solid line. These four simulations were chosen because they represent a diverse set of true regression functions, but all four have the same optimal $R^2 = 0.80$. The empirical R^2 is computed as $R^2 = 1 - (\sum(Y_i - Y_{i,n})^2 / \sum(Y_i - \bar{Y})^2)$, where $\bar{Y} = 1/n \sum_{i=1}^{n} Y_i$ and $Y_{i,n}$ is the predicted value of Y_i reported by the algorithm when applied to the whole data set. The optimal R^2 is the value attained when the true regression function (i.e., true conditional mean) is used and an infinite test sample is used to evaluate the mean squared errors in the numerator and denominator. Knowledge of the true regression function and using an infinite test sample implies $\sum(Y_i - Y_{i,n})^2 = \mathrm{var}(U) \times n = 1 \times n$. Hence the optimal R^2 in all four simulations

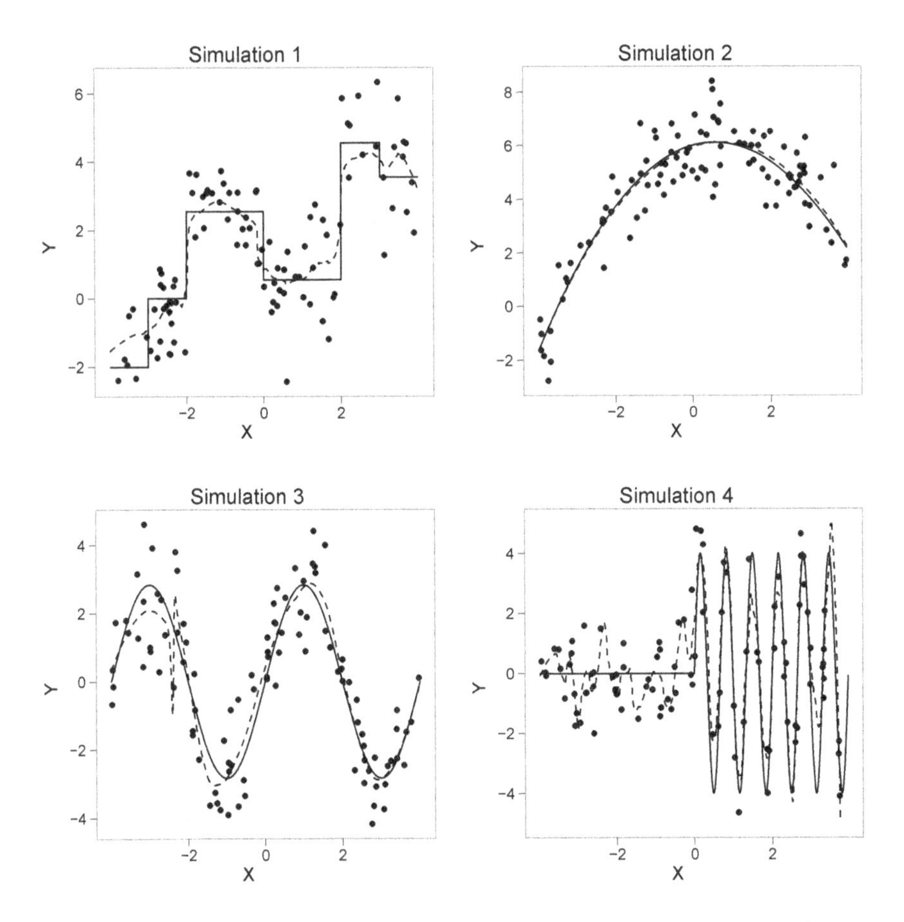

Fig. 3.3 Scatterplots of the four simulations. The *solid line* is the true relationship. The *points* represent one of the simulated data sets of size $n = 100$. The *dashed line* is the super learner fit for the shown data set

is $R^2_{opt} = 1 - (1/\text{var}(Y))$. The variance of Y is set such that $R^2_{opt} = 0.80$ in each simulation.

The collection of algorithms should ideally be a diverse set. One common aspect of many prediction algorithms is the need to specify values for tuning parameters. For example, generalized additive models require a degrees-of-freedom value for the spline functions and the neural network requires a size value. The tuning parameters could be selected using cross-validation or bootstrapping, but the different values of the tuning parameters could also be considered different prediction algorithms. A collection of algorithms could contain three generalized additive models with degrees of freedom equal to 2, 3, and 4. When one considers different values of tuning parameters as unique prediction algorithms in the collection, it is easy to see how the number of algorithms in the collection can become large.

Table 3.1 Collection of prediction algorithms for the simulations and citations

R Algorithm	Description	Source
glm	Linear model	R Development Core Team (2010)
interaction	Polynomial linear model	R Development Core Team (2010)
randomForest	Random forest	Liaw and Wiener (2002) Breiman (2001b)
bagging	Bootstrap aggregation of trees	Peters and Hothorn (2009) Breiman (1996d)
gam	Generalized additive models	Hastie (1992) Hastie and Tibshirani (1990)
gbm	Gradient boosting	Ridgeway (2007) Friedman (2001)
nnet	Neural network	Venables and Ripley (2002)
polymars	Polynomial spline regression	Kooperberg (2009) Friedman (1991)
bart	Bayesian additive regression trees	Chipman and McCulloch (2009) Chipman et al. (2010)
loess	Local polynomial regression	Cleveland et al. (1992)

In all four simulations, we started with the same collection of 21 prediction algorithms. Table 3.1 contains a list of the algorithms in the library. A linear model and a linear model with a quadratic term were considered. The default random forest algorithm, along with a collection of bagging regression trees with values of the complexity parameter (cp) equal to 0.10, 0.01, and 0.00 and a bagging algorithm adjusting the minimum split parameter to be 5, with default cp of 0.01, was also within the collection of algorithms. Generalized additive models with degrees of freedom equal to 2, 3, and 4 were added along with the default gradient boosting model. Neural networks with sizes 2 through 5, the polymars algorithm, and the Bayesian additive regression trees were added. Finally, we considered the loess curve with spans equal to 0.75, 0.50, 0.25, and 0.10.

Figure 3.3 contains the super learner fit on a single simulated data set for each scenario. With the given collection of algorithms, the super learner is able to adapt to the underlying structure of the data-generating function. For each algorithm we evaluated the true R^2 on a test set of size 10,000. The optimal R^2 is the value attained with knowledge of the true regression function. This value gives us an upper bound on the possible R^2 for each algorithm.

To assess the performance of the super learner in comparison to each algorithm, we simulated 100 samples of size 100 and computed the R^2 for each fit of the true regression function. The results are presented in Table 3.2. Negative R^2 values indicate that the mean is a better predictor of Y than the algorithm. In the first simulation, the regression-tree-based methods perform the best. Bagging complete regression trees (cp = 0) has the largest R^2. In the second simulation, the best algorithm is the quadratic linear regression (SL.interaction). In both of these cases, the super learner is able to adapt to the underlying structure and has an average R^2 close to the best algorithm. The same trend is exhibited in simulations 3 and 4; the super learner method of combining algorithms does nearly as well as the individual best

Table 3.2 Results for four simulations. Average R^2 based on 100 simulations and the corresponding standard errors

Algorithm	Sim 1		Sim 2		Sim 3		Sim 4	
	R^2	SE(R^2)	R^2	SE(R^2)	R^2	SE(R^2)	R^2	SE(R^2)
Super learner	0.741	0.032	0.754	0.025	0.760	0.025	0.496	0.122
Discrete SL	0.729	0.079	0.758	0.029	0.757	0.055	0.509	0.132
SL.glm	0.422	0.012	0.189	0.016	0.107	0.016	−0.018	0.021
SL.interaction	0.428	0.016	0.769	0.011	0.100	0.020	−0.018	0.029
SL.randomForest	0.715	0.021	0.702	0.027	0.724	0.018	0.460	0.109
SL.bagging(0.01)	0.751	0.022	0.722	0.036	0.723	0.018	0.091	0.054
SL.bagging(0.1)	0.635	0.120	0.455	0.195	0.661	0.029	0.020	0.025
SL.bagging(0.0)	0.752	0.021	0.722	0.034	0.727	0.017	0.102	0.060
SL.bagging(ms5)	0.747	0.020	0.727	0.030	0.741	0.016	0.369	0.104
SL.gam(2)	0.489	0.013	0.649	0.026	0.213	0.029	−0.014	0.023
SL.gam(3)	0.535	0.033	0.748	0.024	0.412	0.037	−0.017	0.029
SL.gam(4)	0.586	0.027	0.759	0.020	0.555	0.022	−0.020	0.034
SL.gbm	0.717	0.035	0.694	0.038	0.679	0.022	0.063	0.040
SL.nnet(2)	0.476	0.235	0.591	0.245	0.283	0.285	−0.008	0.030
SL.nnet(3)	0.700	0.096	0.700	0.136	0.652	0.218	0.009	0.035
SL.nnet(4)	0.719	0.077	0.730	0.062	0.738	0.102	0.032	0.052
SL.nnet(5)	0.705	0.079	0.716	0.070	0.731	0.077	0.042	0.060
SL.polymars	0.704	0.033	0.733	0.032	0.745	0.034	0.003	0.040
SL.bart	0.740	0.015	0.737	0.027	0.764	0.014	0.077	0.034
SL.loess(0.75)	0.599	0.023	0.761	0.019	0.487	0.028	−0.023	0.033
SL.loess(0.50)	0.695	0.018	0.754	0.022	0.744	0.029	−0.033	0.038
SL.loess(0.25)	0.729	0.016	0.738	0.025	0.772	0.015	−0.076	0.068
SL.loess(0.1)	0.690	0.044	0.680	0.064	0.699	0.039	0.544	0.118

algorithm. Since the individual best algorithm is not known a priori, if a researcher selected a single algorithm, they may do well in some data sets, but the overall performance will be worse than that of the super learner. For example, an individual who always uses bagging complete trees (SL.bagging(0.0)) will do well on the first three simulations, but will perform poorly on the fourth simulation compared to the average performance of the super learner.

In the first three simulations the super learner approaches the optimal R^2 value because algorithms in the collection approximate the truth well. However, in the fourth simulation, the collection is not rich enough to contain a combination of algorithms that approaches the optimal value. The super learner does as well as the best algorithms in the library but does not attain the optimal R^2. Upon supplementation of the collection of algorithms, the super learner achieves an average $R^2 = 0.76$, which is close to the optimal R^2 (results not shown; see Polley and van der Laan 2010).

To study the super learner in real data examples, we collected a number of publicly available data sets. Table 3.3 contains descriptions of the data sets, which can be found either in public repositories or in textbooks, with the corresponding citation listed in the table. Sample sizes ranged from 200 to 654 observations, and the number of covariates ranged from 3 to 18. All 13 data sets have a continuous outcome and no missing values. The collection of prediction algorithms included

Table 3.3 Description of data sets, where n is the sample size and p is the number of covariates

Name	n	p	Source
ais	202	10	Cook and Weisberg (1994)
diamond	308	17	Chu (2001)
cps78	550	18	Berndt (1991)
cps85	534	17	Berndt (1991)
cpu	209	6	Kibler et al. (1989)
FEV	654	4	Rosner (1999)
Pima	392	7	Newman et al. (1998)
laheart	200	10	Afifi and Azen (1979)
mussels	201	3	Cook (1998)
enroll	258	6	Liu and Stengos (1999)
fat	252	14	Penrose et al. (1985)
diabetes	366	15	Harrell (2001)
house	506	13	Newman et al. (1998)

the applicable algorithms from the univariate simulations along with the algorithms listed in Table 3.4. These algorithms represent a diverse set and should allow the super learner to work well in most practical settings. For comparison across data sets, we kept the collection of algorithms fixed for all data analyses.

In order to compare the performance of the K prediction algorithms across diverse data sets with outcomes on different scales, we used the relative mean squared error, which we denote RE for relative efficiency. The denominator is the mean squared error of a linear model:

$$\mathrm{RE}(k) = \frac{\mathrm{MSE}(k)}{\mathrm{MSE}(lm)}, \quad k = 1, \ldots, K.$$

The results for the super learner, the discrete super learner, and each individual algorithm can be found in Fig. 3.4. Each point represents the 10-fold cross-validated relative mean squared error for a data set, and the plus sign is the geometric mean of the algorithm across all 13 data sets. The super learner outperformed the discrete super learner, and both outperformed any individual algorithm. With real data, it is unlikely that one single algorithm would contain the true relationship, and the benefit of the combination of the algorithms vs. the selection of a single algorithm is demonstrated. The additional estimation of the combination parameters (α) does not cause an overfit in terms of the risk assessment. Among the individual algorithms, the Bayesian additive regression trees perform the best, but they overfit one of the data sets with a relative mean squared error of almost 3.0.

A common application of prediction is in microarray data. Super learning is well suited for this setting. Microarray data are often high dimensional, i.e., the number of covariates is larger than the sample size. We demonstrate the super learner in microarray data using a publicly available breast cancer data set published in van't Veer et al. (2002). This study was conducted to develop a gene-expression-based predictor for 5-year distant metastases. The outcome is a binary indicator that a

Table 3.4 Additional prediction algorithms in the collection of algorithms for the real data examples to be combined with the algorithms from Table 3.1

R Algorithm	Description	Source
bayesglm	Bayesian linear model	Gelman et al. (2010)
		Gelman et al. (2009)
glmnet	Elastic net	Friedman et al. (2010a)
		Friedman et al. (2010b)
DSA	DSA algorithm	Neugebauer and Bullard (2009)
		Sinisi and van der Laan (2004)
step	Stepwise regression	Venables and Ripley (2002)
ridge	Ridge regression	Venables and Ripley (2002)
svm	Support vector machine	Dimitriadou et al. (2009)
		Chang and Lin (2001)

Fig. 3.4 Tenfold cross-validated relative mean squared error compared to glm across 13 real data sets. Sorted by geometric mean, denoted by the plus (+) sign

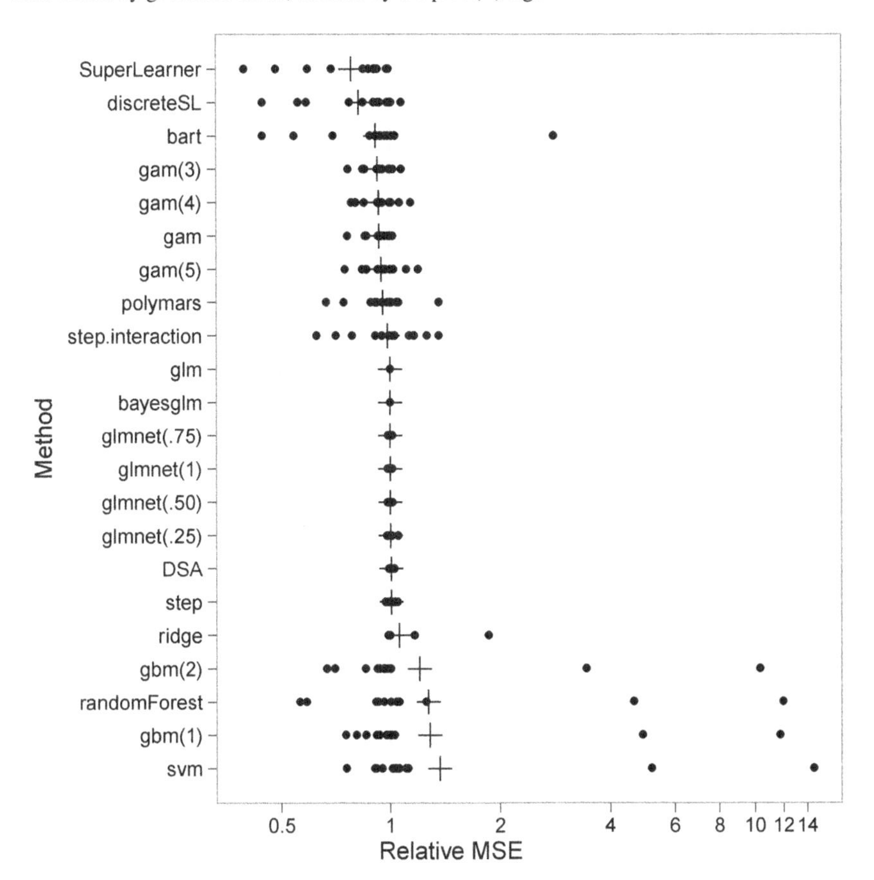

Table 3.5 Twentyfold cross-validated mean squared error for each algorithm and the standard error in the breast cancer study

Algorithm	Subset	Risk	SE
Super learner	–	0.194	0.0168
Discrete SL	–	0.238	0.0239
SL.knn(10)	All	0.249	0.0196
SL.knn(10)	Clinical	0.239	0.0188
SL.knn(10)	cor($p < 0.1$)	0.262	0.0232
SL.knn(10)	cor($p < 0.01$)	0.224	0.0205
SL.knn(10)	glmnet	0.219	0.0277
SL.knn(20)	All	0.242	0.0129
SL.knn(20)	Clinical	0.236	0.0123
SL.knn(20)	cor($p < 0.1$)	0.233	0.0168
SL.knn(20)	cor($p < 0.01$)	0.206	0.0176
SL.knn(20)	glmnet	0.217	0.0257
SL.knn(30)	All	0.239	0.0128
SL.knn(30)	Clinical	0.236	0.0119
SL.knn(30)	cor($p < 0.1$)	0.232	0.0139
SL.knn(30)	cor($p < 0.01$)	0.215	0.0165
SL.knn(30)	glmnet	0.210	0.0231
SL.knn(40)	All	0.240	0.0111
SL.knn(40)	Clinical	0.238	0.0105
SL.knn(40)	cor($p < 0.1$)	0.236	0.0118
SL.knn(40)	cor($p < 0.01$)	0.219	0.0151
SL.knn(40)	glmnet	0.211	0.0208
SL.glmnet(1.0)	cor(Rank = 50)	0.229	0.0285
SL.glmnet(1.0)	cor(Rank = 20)	0.208	0.0260
SL.glmnet(0.75)	cor(Rank = 50)	0.221	0.0269
SL.glmnet(0.75)	cor(Rank = 20)	0.209	0.0258
SL.glmnet(0.50)	cor(Rank = 50)	0.226	0.0269
SL.glmnet(0.50)	cor(Rank = 20)	0.211	0.0256
SL.glmnet(0.25)	cor(Rank = 50)	0.230	0.0266
SL.glmnet(0.25)	cor(Rank = 20)	0.216	0.0252
SL.randomForest	Clinical	0.198	0.0186
SL.randomForest	cor($p < 0.01$)	0.204	0.0179
SL.randomForest	glmnet	0.220	0.0245
SL.bagging	Clinical	0.207	0.0160
SL.bagging	cor($p < 0.01$)	0.205	0.0184
SL.bagging	glmnet	0.206	0.0219
SL.bart	Clinical	0.202	0.0183
SL.bart	cor($p < 0.01$)	0.210	0.0207
SL.bart	glmnet	0.220	0.0275
SL.mean	All	0.224	0.1016

patient had a distant metastasis within 5 years of initial therapy. In addition to the expression data, six clinical variables were attained. The clinical information was age, tumor grade, tumor size, estrogen receptor status, progesterone receptor status, and angioinvasion. The array data contained 4348 genes after the unsupervised screening steps outlined in the original article. We used the entire sample of 97 individuals (combining the training and validation samples from the original article) to fit the super learner.

In high-dimensional data, it is often beneficial to screen the variables before running prediction algorithms. Screening is part of the algorithm and should thus also be included when calculating the cross-validated risk of an algorithm in the super learner. Screening algorithms can be coupled with prediction algorithms to create new algorithms in the library. For example, we may consider k-nearest neighbors using all features and k-nearest neighbors on the subset of only clinical variables. These two algorithms are considered unique algorithms. Another screening algorithm involves testing the pairwise correlations of each variable with the outcome and ranking the variables by the corresponding p-value. With the ranked list of variables, we consider the screening cutoffs as follows: variables with a p-value less than 0.1, variables with a p-value less than 0.01, variables in the bottom 20, and variables in the bottom 50. An additional screening algorithm involves running the glmnet algorithm and selecting the variables with nonzero coefficients.

The results for the breast cancer data can be found in Table 3.5. The algorithms in the collection are k-nearest neighbors with $k = \{10, 20, 30, 40\}$, elastic net with $\alpha = \{1.0, 0.75, 0.50, 0.25\}$, random forests, bagging, bart, and an algorithm that uses the mean value of the outcome as the predicted probability. We coupled these algorithms with the screening algorithms to produce the full list of 38 algorithms. Within this collection of algorithms, the best algorithm in terms of minimum risk estimate is the random forest algorithm using only the clinical variables (MSE = 0.198). As we observed in the previous examples, the super learner was able to attain a risk comparable to the best algorithm (MSE = 0.194).

3.4 Road Maps

In previous chapters, we introduced our road map for targeted learning (Fig. 3.5), the first steps of which involved defining our data, model, and target parameter. This chapter dealt with obtaining the best initial estimator of the relevant portion Q_0 of the distribution P_0 of O. The next stage of the road map addresses estimation of the target parameter using TMLE, taking this initial estimator as input.

We also present a separate road map for prediction estimation questions in Fig. 3.6. We note that inference for prediction is not covered in detail in this text and we refer readers in Sect. 3.7 to literature using the permutation distribution for obtaining exact tests of the null hypothesis of independence of the covariates and the outcome, allowing the incorporation of machine learning.

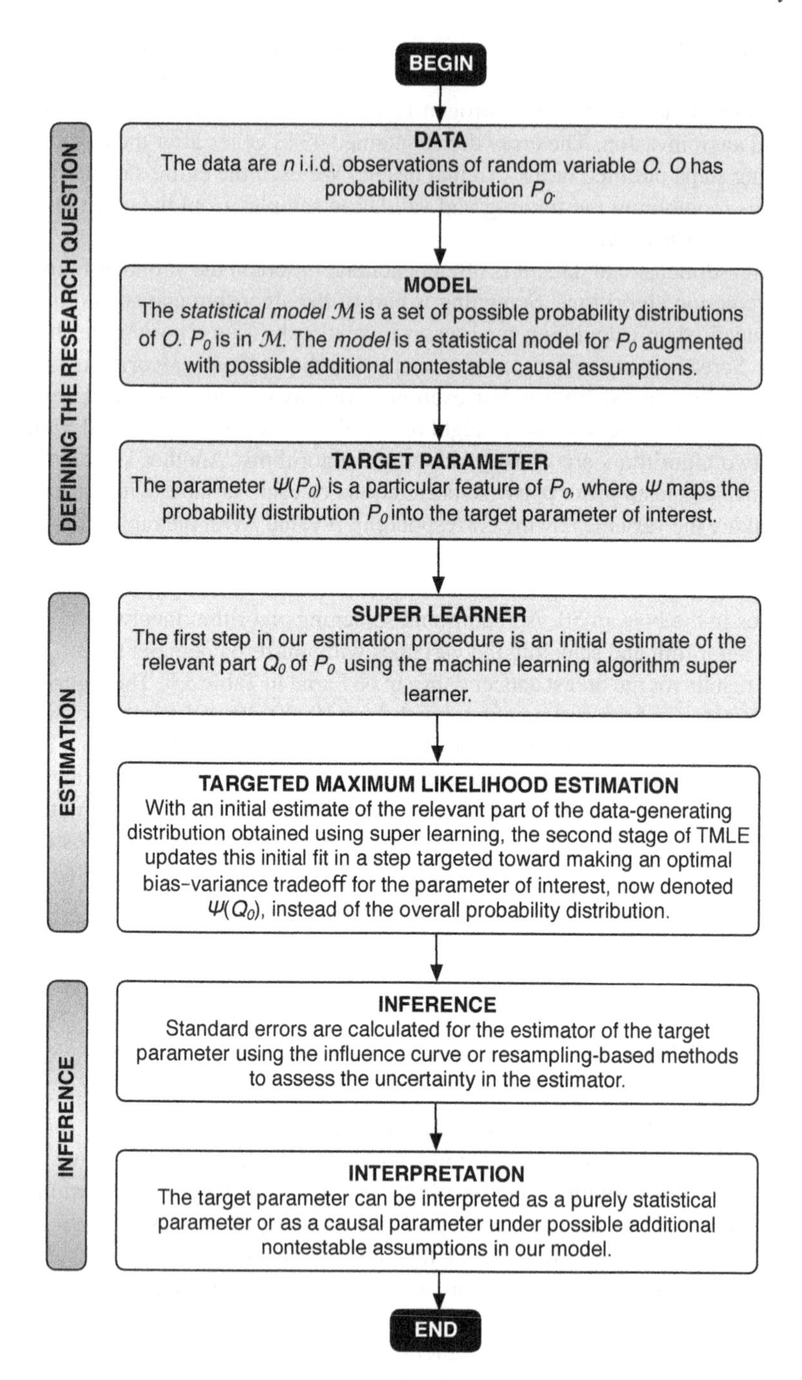

Fig. 3.5 Road map for targeted learning

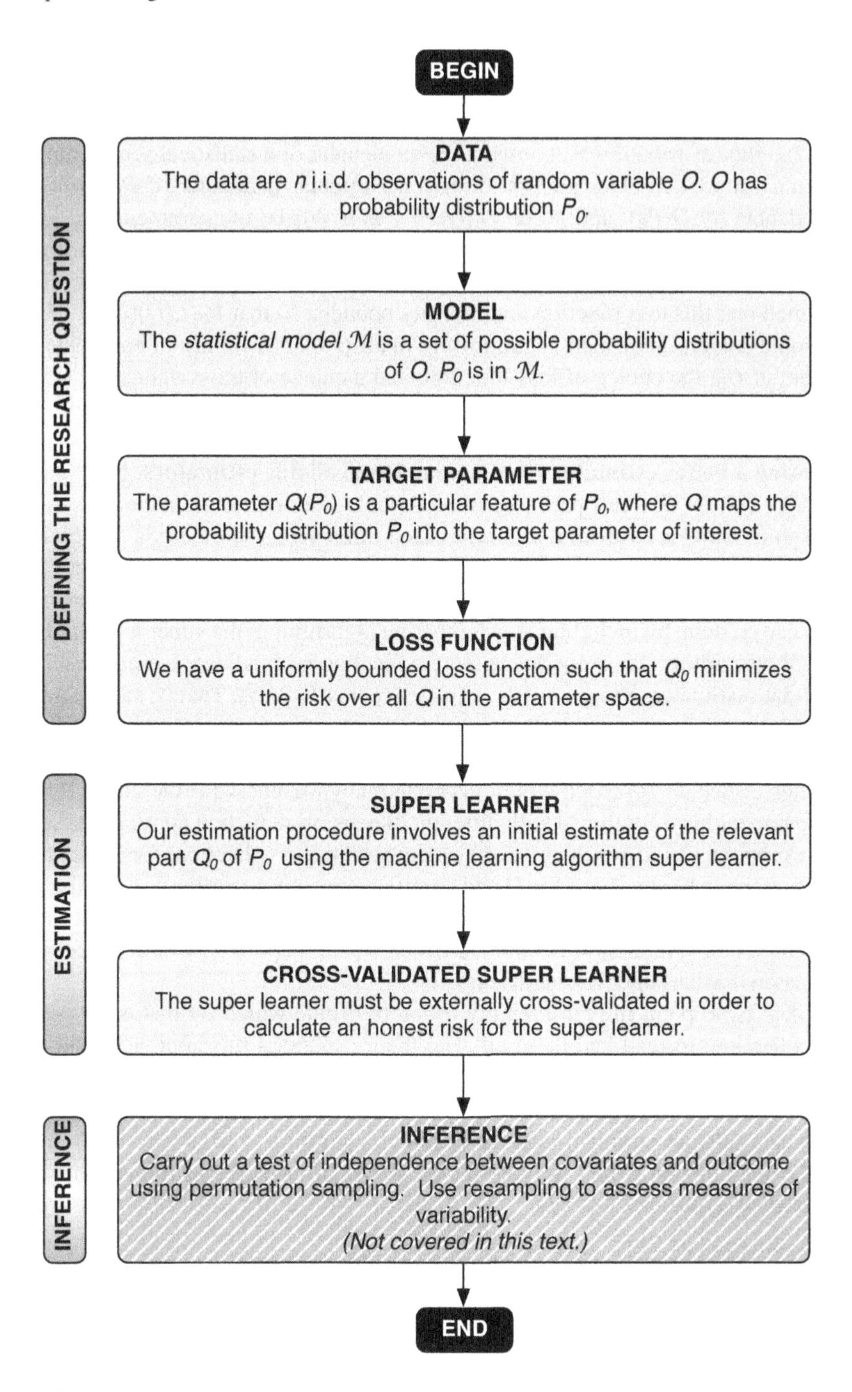

Fig. 3.6 Road map for prediction

3.5 Conceptual Framework of Loss-Based Super Learning

Suppose we observe n i.i.d. observations $O_1, \ldots, O_n$ on a random variable O from a probability distribution P_0 known to be an element of a statistical semiparametric statistical model $\mathcal{M}$. Our goal is to learn a particular parameter of P_0, which we will denote by $Q(P_0)$, and let $\mathcal{Q} = \{Q(P) : P \in \mathcal{M}\}$ be the parameter space. We assume that we have available a loss function $L(Q)(O)$ such that Q_0 minimizes the risk $P_0 L(Q) \equiv E_0 L(Q)(O)$ of Q over all Q in the parameter space $\mathcal{Q}$. In addition, it is assumed that this loss function is uniformly bounded so that $P_0(L(Q)(O) < M) = 1$ for some universal constant M, uniformly in all $Q \in \mathcal{Q}$. A library of candidate estimators of Q_0, the choice of loss function, and a choice of cross-validation scheme now define the super learner of Q_0.

Creating a better estimator from among the available estimators. If the parameter $Q : \mathcal{M} \to \mathcal{Q}$ is not pathwise differentiable (i.e., not identifiable and smooth enough to allow central-limit-theorem-based inference), then there is no efficiency theory. That is, even asymptotically, there is no best estimator of Q_0. As a consequence, the best one can do is to make sure that one is better than any competitor. This can be done by including any competing algorithm in the super learner collection of algorithms. Thus one has a large collection of candidate estimators. These candidate estimators should use the knowledge that $P_0 \in \mathcal{M}$. That is, each estimator should at a minimum map the data into functions in the parameter space $\mathcal{Q}$.

One particular approach might require a choice of a number of fine-tuning parameters. Such an approach would generate many members for the collection. An estimator could be combined with different dimension-reduction approaches, so that one estimator would result in several members in the collection. One might also partition the outcome space for O and stratify estimators accordingly, and also consider applying different estimators to different strata. In this manner, one estimation procedure and several stratification variables would map into a whole collection of estimators for the super learner library.

There is no point in painstakingly trying to decide which estimators to enter in the collection; instead add them all. The theory supports this approach, and finite sample simulations and data analyses only confirm that it is very hard to overfit the super learner by augmenting the collection, but benefits are obtained. Indeed, for large data sets, we simply do not have enough algorithms available to build the desired collection that would fully utilize the power of the super learning principle as established by the oracle result.

The free lunch: fully robust application-specific modeling. This is not enough. In a particular application, there are always many experts with creative ideas. Put them in a room and let them generate ideas about effective dimension reductions, propose parametric statistical models they find interesting, and let them propose strategies for approximating this unknown true target-function Q_0. Translate these into new candidate algorithms for the collection of algorithms. For example, one professor might think that certain specific summary measures of the history of the unit at baseline should be particularly effective in predicting the outcome of interest. This then translates into estimators that only use these summaries and algorithms that add these summary measures to the existing set of (nontransformed) variables. If there are competing theories about how the truth is best approximated, translate them all into candidate estimators for the super learning library. The super learner will not select an estimator that performs poorly, but even mediocre algorithms can still improve the super learner. That is, there is no risk in adding candidate estimators that are heavily model-based to the super learner; there is only benefit.

Concerned about overfitting the super learner? Indeed, let the data speak to answer this question. That is why one should evaluate the performance of the super learner itself by determining its cross-validated risk. It can then be determined if the super learner does as well or better than any of the candidate algorithms in the collection. In particular, one might diagnose that one has reached a point at which adding more algorithms harms the super learner performance, but our experience has not reached that point by any meaningful standard. If anything, it appears to flatten out, but not deteriorate. However, it is important that one use quite high-fold cross-validation when evaluating the super learner itself (say 20-fold), especially when the sample size gets small. Above all, it is crucial that the family of combinations respects a universal bound on the loss functions across all combinations.

Computational challenge. The super learning system of learning is perfectly tailored for parallel programming. The different candidate estimators can do their job separately, and the applications of the candidate estimators to the different training sets can be separated as well.

Generality of super learning. Super learning can be applied to estimate an immense class of parameters across different data structures O and different statistical models $\mathcal{M}$. One can use it to estimate marginal densities, conditional densities, conditional hazards, conditional means, conditional medians, conditional quantiles, conditional survival functions, and so on, under biased sampling, missingness, and censoring.

It is a matter of defining Q_0 as a parameter of P_0 and determining an appropriate loss function. For example, the minus log loss function can be used for conditional densities and hazards. However, one might come up with loss functions that are indexed by unknown parameters: $L_h(Q)$ for some unknown h. Many such examples are now provided in the literature, such as the double robust augmented inverse probability of treatment-weighted loss function for the treatment-specific mean outcome as a function of effect modifiers. In this case h includes a conditional distribution of treatment as a function of the covariates. This nuisance parameter would be known in an RCT, but it will need to be estimated in an observational study. We discuss the statistical property of double robustness in Chap. 6.

In these situations one will need to estimate h from the data and then employ this estimated loss function as before. The basic messsage is that one needs the estimation of h to be easier than the estimation of Q_0 in order to get the full benefit of super learner, as if h was known from the start. It should also be remarked that h could represent an index that does not affect the validity of the loss function in the sense that for each choice of h, Q_0 minimizes the risk of $L_h(Q)$ over all Q. In these cases, the choice of h only affects the dissimilarity measure for which the performance of the super learner is optimized. For example, h might represent a weight function in a squared-error loss function, or it might represent a covariance matrix for the generalized squared-error loss function for a conditional mean $E(\mathbf{Y} \mid W)$ of a multivariate outcome:

$$L_h(Q)(W, \mathbf{Y}) = (\mathbf{Y} - Q(W))^\top h(W)(\mathbf{Y} - Q(W)).$$

Choice of loss function. If several choices are available, the loss function that maps into the desired dissimilarity measure $d_L(Q, Q_0) = E_0 L(Q) - E_0 L(Q_0)$ should be selected. It should be kept in mind that the super learner optimizes the approximation of Q_0 with respect to this dissimilarity d_L implied by the loss function. For example, suppose one wishes to estimate a conditional survival function at a time point t_0, $Q_0 = P(T > t_0 \mid W)$. Then one could still use the minus log loss function for the conditional density of T, given W, which, by substitution, also implies a valid loss function for Q_0, since Q_0 is determined by this conditional density. However, this loss function is trying to determine an entire conditional density, and is thus not very targeted towards its goal. Instead, we can use

$$L(Q)(W, T) = [I(T > t_0) - Q(W)]^2 .$$

This loss function is minimized over all functions Q of W by $Q_0 = P(T > t_0 \mid W)$, and thereby targets exactly our parameter of interest. Indeed, the super learner will now be aiming to minimize the dissimilarity:

$$d_L(Q, Q_0) = E_0[Q(W) - Q_0(W)]^2,$$

i.e., the expected squared error between the candidate survival function at t_0 and the true survival function at t_0.

Formal oracle result for cross-validation selector. Consider a loss function that satisfies

$$\sup_Q \frac{\mathrm{var}_{P_0}\{L(Q) - L(Q_0)\}}{P_0\{L(Q) - L(Q_0)\}} \leq M_2 \qquad (3.1)$$

and that is uniformly bounded:

$$\sup_{O,Q} \mid L(Q) - L(Q_0) \mid (O) < M_1 < \infty,$$

where the supremum is over the support of P_0 and over all possible candidate estimators of Q_0 that will ever be considered. We used the notation $P_0 f = \int f(o) dP_0(o)$ for the expectation of $f(O)$ under P_0. The first property (3.1) applies to the log-likelihood loss function and any weighted squared residual loss function, among others. Property (3.1) is essentially equivalent to the assumption that the loss-function-based dissimilarity $d(Q, Q_0) = P_0\{L(Q) - L(Q_0)\}$ is quadratic in a distance between Q and Q_0. Property (3.1) has been proven for log-likelihood loss functions and weighted L^2-loss functions and is in essence equivalent to stating that the loss function implies a quadratic dissimilarity $d(Q, Q_0)$ (van der Laan and Dudoit 2003). If this property does not hold for the loss function, the rates $1/n$ for second-order terms in the below stated oracle inequality reduce to the rate $1/\sqrt{n}$.

Let $B_n \in \{0, 1\}^n$ be a random variable that splits the learning sample in a training sample $\{i : B_n(i) = 0\}$ and validation sample $\{i : B_n(i) = 1\}$, and let P^0_{n,B_n} and P^1_{n,B_n} denote the empirical distribution of the training and validation sample, respectively. Given candidate estimators $P_n \to \hat{Q}_k(P_n)$, the loss-function-based cross-validation selector is now defined by

$$k_n = \hat{K}(P_n) = \arg\min_k E_{B_n} P^1_{n,B_n} L(\hat{Q}_k(P^0_{n,B_n})).$$

The resulting estimator, the discrete super learner, is given by $\hat{Q}(P_n) = \hat{Q}_{\hat{K}(P_n)}(P_n)$.

For quadratic loss functions, the cross-validation selector satisfies the following (so-called) oracle inequality: for any $\delta > 0$

$$E_{B_n}\{P_0 L(\hat{Q}_{k_n}(P^0_{n,B_n}) - L(Q_0)\} \leq (1 + 2\delta) E_{B_n} \min_k P_0\{L(\hat{Q}_k(P^0_{n,B_n})) - L(Q_0)\}$$
$$+ 2C(M_1, M_2, \delta)\frac{1 + \log K(n)}{np},$$

where the constant $C(M_1, M_2, \delta) = 2(1+\delta)^2(M_1/3+M_2/3)$ (van der Laan and Dudoit 2003, p. 25). This result proves [see van der Laan and Dudoit (2003) for the precise statement of these implications] that if the number of candidates $K(n)$ is polynomial in sample size, then the cross-validation selector is either asymptotically equivalent to the oracle selector (based on a sample of training sample sizes, as defined on the right-hand side of the above inequality), or it achieves the parametric rate $\log n/n$ for convergence with respect to $d(Q, Q_0) \equiv P_0\{L(Q) - L(Q_0)\}$.

So in most realistic scenarios, in which none of the candidate estimators achieves the rate of convergence one would have with an a priori correctly specified parametric statistical model, the cross-validated estimator selector performs asymptotically exactly as well (not only in rate, but also up to the constant!) as the oracle-selected estimator. These oracle results are generalized for estimated loss functions $L_n(Q)$ that approximate a fixed loss function $L(Q)$. If $\arg\min_Q P_0 L_n(Q) \neq Q_0$, then the oracle inequality also presents second-order terms due to the estimation of the loss function (van der Laan and Dudoit 2003).

3.6 Notes and Further Reading

We've discussed in this chapter the notion of estimator selection. We use this terminology over "model selection," since the formal meaning of a (statistical) model in the field of statistics is the set of possible probability distributions, and most algorithms are not indexed by a statistical model choice. The general loss-based super learner was initially presented in van der Laan et al. (2007b). Super learner is a generalization of the stacking algorithm introduced in the neural networks context by Wolpert (1992) and adapted to the regression context by Breiman (1996c), and its name was introduced due to the theoretical oracle property and its consequences as presented in van der Laan and Dudoit (2003). The stacking algorithm is examined in LeBlanc and Tibshirani (1996) and the relationship to the model-mix algorithm of Stone (1974) and the predictive sample-reuse method of Geisser (1975) is discussed. Recent literature on aggregation and ensemble learners includes Tsybakov (2003), Juditsky et al. (2005), Bunea et al. (2006, 2007a,b), and Dalalyan and Tsybakov (2007, 2008). As noted previously, inference for prediction, such as permutation resampling, is not covered in this text. We refer the interested reader to Lehmann (1986), Hastie et al. (2001), Ruczinski et al. (2002), Birkner et al. (2005), and Chaffee et al. (2010). The simulations and data analyses contained in this chapter were previously published as a technical report (Polley and van der Laan 2010).

Chapter 15 uses super learning to estimate the risk score of mortality in a Kaiser Permanente database. Additionally, Chap. 16 discusses the use of super learning in right-censored data. We refer readers to Polley and van der Laan (2009) for a chapter in the book *Design and Analysis of Clinical Trials with Time-to-Event Endpoints* that discusses the use of super learning to assess effect modification in clinical trials.

Theory for loss-function-based cross-validation is presented in van der Laan and Dudoit (2003), including the finite sample oracle inequality, the asymptotic equivalence of the cross-validation selector, and the oracle selector. See also van der Laan et al. (2006), van der Vaart et al. (2006), van der Laan et al. (2004), Dudoit and van der Laan (2005), Keleş et al. (2002), and Sinisi and van der Laan (2004). A finite sample result for the single-split cross-validation selector for the squared error loss function was established in Györfi et al. (2002) and then generalized in van der Laan and Dudoit (2003) and Dudoit and van der Laan (2005) for both general cross-validation schemes and a general class of loss functions.

Other types of cross-validation beyond V-fold cross-validation include bootstrap cross-validation, Monte Carlo cross-validation, and leave-one-out cross-validation (Stone 1974, 1977; Breiman et al. 1984; Breiman and Spector 1992; Efron and Tibshirani 1993; Breiman 1996a,b; Ripley 1996; Breiman 1998; Hastie et al. 2001; Ambroise and McLachlan 2002; Györfi et al. 2002). Simulation studies (Pavlic and van der Laan 2003) show that likelihood-based cross-validation performs well when compared to common validity-functionals-based approaches, such as Akaike's information criterion (Akaike 1973; Bozdogan 2000), Bayesian Information criterion (Schwartz 1978), minimum description length (Rissanen 1978), and informational complexity (Bozdogan 1993).

Hastie et al. (2001) covers a variety of machine learning algorithms and related topics. Areas include stepwise selection procedures, ridge regression, LASSO, principal component regression, least angle regression, nearest neighbor methods, random forests, support vector machines, neural networks, classification methods, kernel smoothing methods, and ensemble learning.

Chapter 4
Introduction to TMLE

Sherri Rose, Mark J. van der Laan

This is the second chapter in our text to deal with estimation. We started by defining the research question. This included our data, model for the probability distribution that generated the data, and the target parameter of the probability distribution of the data. We then presented the estimation of prediction functions using super learning. This leads us to the estimation of causal effects using the TMLE. This chapter introduces TMLE, and a deeper understanding of this methodology is provided in Chap. 5. Note that we use the abbreviation *TMLE* for *targeted maximum likelihood estimation* and the *targeted maximum likelihood estimator*. Later in this text, we discuss *targeted minimum loss-based estimation*, which can also be abbreviated *TMLE*.

For the sake of demonstration, we have considered the data structure $O = (W, A, Y) \sim P_0$. Our statistical model for the probability distribution P_0 is nonparametric. The target parameter for this example is $E_{W,0}[E_0(Y \mid A = 1, W) - E_0(Y \mid A = 0, W)]$, which can be interpreted as a causal effect under nontestable assumptions formalized by an SCM, including the randomization assumption and the positivity assumption. In Chap. 3, we estimated $E_0(Y \mid A, W)$ using super learning. With super learning we are able to respect that the statistical model does not allow us to assume a particular parametric form for the prediction function $E_0(Y \mid A, W)$. We could have estimated the entire conditional density of the outcome Y, but then we would be estimating portions of the density we do not need. In particular, this would mean that our initial estimator, such as a super learner of this conditional density of Y, would be targeted toward the complete conditional density, even though it is better to target it toward the conditional mean of Y. Estimating only the relevant portion of the density of O in this first step of the TMLE procedure provides us with a maximally efficient (precise) and unbiased procedure: the practical and asymptotic performance of the TMLE of ψ_0 only cares about how well $\bar{Q}_0$ is estimated.

The super learner fit can be plugged into the target parameter mapping to obtain a corresponding estimator of the target parameter. In other words, for each subject in the sample, one would evaluate the difference between the predicted value of Y under treatment ($A = 1$) and control ($A = 0$) and average these differences across all subjects in the sample.

However, this super learner maximum likelihood (ML)-based substitution estimator is not targeted toward the parameter of interest. The super learner prediction function was tailored to optimally fit the overall prediction function $E_0(Y \mid A, W)$, spreading its errors uniformly to (successfully) optimize average squared prediction errors, and thereby suffers from a nonoptimal bias–variance tradeoff for the causal effect of interest. Specifically, this ML-based super learner of the causal effect will be biased.

Our TMLE procedure improves on the ML-based substitution estimator by reducing bias for the target parameter of interest. The initial super learner fit for $E_0(Y \mid A, W)$ is the first step in the TMLE procedure. The second stage of the TMLE procedure is a step targeted toward modifying the initial estimator of $E_0(Y \mid A, W)$ in order to make it less biased for the target parameter. That is, the second stage of TMLE is tailored to get the best estimate of our target parameter of interest, with respect to bias and variance, instead of a best estimate of the overall prediction function $E_0(Y \mid A, W)$. We cover the entire TMLE procedure in this chapter, assuming the reader has knowledge based on the material presented in Chap. 3.

We explain the TMLE procedure in multiple ways in these two chapters, with the goal of reinforcing the method and targeting different levels of understanding (conceptual, applied, theoretical). Thus, the applied researcher may only be interested in a thorough understanding of the conceptual and applied sections, whereas the more theoretically inclined mathematician may wish to also read the technical derivations and Appendix A.

TMLE Methodology Summary

TMLE is a two-step procedure where one first obtains an estimate of the data-generating distribution P_0, or the relevant portion Q_0 of P_0. The second stage updates this initial fit in a step targeted toward making an optimal bias–variance tradeoff for the parameter of interest $\Psi(Q_0)$, instead of the overall density P_0. The procedure is double robust and can incorporate data-adaptive likelihood-based estimation procedures to estimate Q_0 and the treatment mechanism. The double robustness of TMLE has important implications in both randomized controlled trials and observational studies, with potential reductions in bias and gains in efficiency.

We use our mortality study example to present an application of TMLE. As a reminder, in this study we are interested in the effect of LTPA on death. We have binary Y, death within 5 years of baseline, and binary A indicating whether the subject meets recommended levels of physical activity. The data structure in this example is $O = (W, A, Y) \sim P_0$. While we use this basic data structure and a particular target parameter to illustrate the procedure, TMLE is a very flexible general method for estimating any particular target parameter of a true probability distribution that is known to be an element of any particular statistical model. We will demonstrate its implementation with a variety of specific data structures throughout this text. In Appendix A, we also present a general TMLE of causal effects of multiple time point interventions for complex longitudinal data structures. However, we find introducing TMLE in the context of a simple data structure is helpful for many people. Starting with Appendix A is often overwhelming, and that appendix is geared toward those who desire a comprehensive and rigorous statistical understanding or wish to develop TMLE for unique applications encountered in practice, corresponding with a choice of data structure, statistical model, and target parameter, not previously addressed.

TMLE has many attractive properties that make it preferable to other existing estimators of a target parameter of the probability distribution of the data. We fully detail these properties in Chaps. 5 and 6, after introducing them in this chapter, and compare other estimators to TMLE based on these properties. Of note, TMLE removes all the asymptotic residual bias of the initial estimator for the target parameter, if it uses a consistent estimator of the treatment mechanism. If the initial estimator was already consistent for the target parameter, the slight additional fitting of the data in the targeted step will potentially remove some finite sample bias, and certainly preserve this consistency property of the initial estimator.

As a consequence, the TMLE is a so-called double robust estimator. In addition, if the initial estimator and the estimator of the treatment mechanism are both consistent, then it is also asymptotically efficient according to semiparametric statistical model efficiency theory. It allows the incorporation of machine learning (i.e., super learning) methods for the estimation of both $\bar{Q}_0$ and g_0 so that we do not make assumptions about the probability distribution P_0 we do not believe. In this manner, every effort is made to achieve minimal bias and the asymptotic semiparametric efficiency bound for the variance.

TMLE is also a substitution estimator. Substitution estimators are plug-in estimators, taking an estimator of the relevant part of the data-generating distribution and plugging it into the mapping $\Psi()$. Substitution estimators respect the statistical model space (i.e., the global constraints of the statistical model) and respect that the target parameter ψ_0 is a number obtained by applying the target parameter mapping Ψ to a particular probability distribution in the statistical model. Substitution estimators are therefore more robust to outliers and sparsity than nonsubstitution estimators.

4.1 Motivation

Let us step back for a moment and discuss why we are here. We want to estimate a parameter $\Psi(P_0)$ under a semiparametric statistical model that represents actual knowledge. Thus we don't want to use a misspecified parametric statistical model that makes assumptions we know to be false. We also know that an ML-based substitution estimator is not targeted to the parameter we care about. While we like this approach as it is flexible, it is still not a targeted approach. TMLE is a *targeted* substitution estimator that incorporates super learning to get the best estimate of our

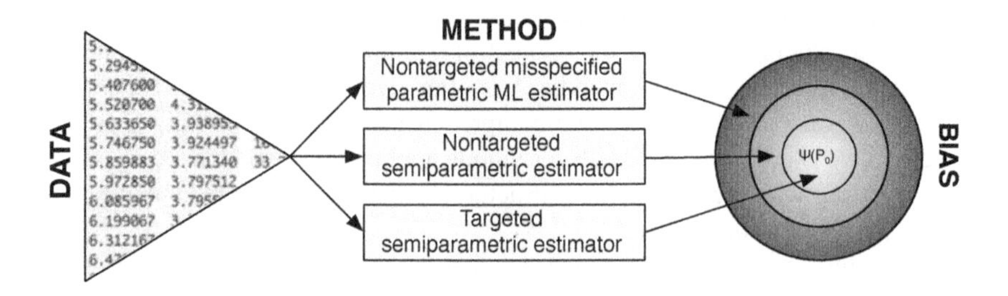

Fig. 4.1 Illustration of bias for different methods

target parameter; it is tailored to be a minimally biased method while also being tailored to fully utilize all the information in the data.

We illustrate this in Fig. 4.1. The outermost ring is furthest from the truth, and that represents the estimate we achieve using a misspecified parametric statistical model. The middle ring in our target improves on the misspecified parametric statistical model, but it still does not contain the truth. This ring is our nontargeted semiparametric statistical model approach (super learning). The innermost circle contains the true $\Psi(P_0)$, and this is what we have the potential to achieve with super learning *and* TMLE combined. We refer to the combined two-stage approach as TMLE, even though it is understood that the initial estimator and estimator of the treatment mechanism should be based on super learning respecting the actual knowledge about P_0.

4.2 TMLE in Action: Mortality Study Example

In Chap. 3, we discussed the implementation of super learning for our simplified mortality study example. In this section we analyze the actual data, updating the super learner estimate of $\bar{Q}_0$ with a targeting step. This section serves as an introduction to the implementation of TMLE in a concrete example: the data structure is $O = (W, A, Y) \sim P_0$, the nonparametric statistical model is augmented with causal assumptions, and the targeted parameter is $\Psi(P_0) = E_{W,0}[E_0(Y \mid A = 1, W) - E_0(Y \mid A = 0, W)]$, which represents the causal risk difference under these causal assumptions. The mean over the covariate vector W in $\Psi(P_0)$ is simply estimated with the empirical mean, so that our substitution TMLE will be of the type

$$\psi_n = \Psi(Q_n) = \frac{1}{n} \sum_{i=1}^{n} \{\bar{Q}_n(1, W_i) - \bar{Q}_n(0, W_i)\},$$

where $Q_n = (\bar{Q}_n, Q_{W,n})$ and $Q_{W,n}$ is the empirical distribution for the marginal distribution of W. The second step in the TMLE will update our initial estimate of $\bar{Q}_0$. We will use the superscript 0 to denote this initial estimate, in conjunction with the

Table 4.1 SPPARCS variables

Variable	Description
Y	Death occurring within 5 years of baseline
A	LTPA score $\geq$ 22.5 METs at baseline‡
W_1	Health self-rated as "excellent"
W_2	Health self-rated as "fair"
W_3	Health self-rated as "poor"
W_4	Current smoker
W_5	Former smoker
W_6	Cardiac event prior to baseline
W_7	Chronic health condition at baseline
W_8	$x \leq 60$ years old
W_9	$60 < x \leq 70$ years old
W_{10}	$80 < x \leq 90$ years old
W_{11}	$x > 90$ years old
W_{12}	Female

‡ LTPA is calculated from answers to a detailed questionnaire where prior performed vigorous physical activities are assigned standardized intensity values in metabolic equivalents (METs). The recommended level of energy expenditure for the elderly is 22.5 METs.

subscript n thus we have $\bar{Q}_n^0$ as our initial estimate of $\bar{Q}_0$. Information from the treatment mechanism (or exposure mechanism; we use these terms interchangeably) is used to update $\bar{Q}_n^0$ and target it toward the parameter of interest. In this example, our treatment mechanism is $g_0 = P_0(A \mid W)$. Our updated estimate of $\bar{Q}_0$ is denoted $\bar{Q}_n^1$.

Data. The National Institute of Aging-funded Study of Physical Performance and Age-Related Changes in Sonomans (SPPARCS) is a population-based, census-sampled, study of the epidemiology of aging and health. Participants of this longitudinal cohort were recruited if they were aged 54 years and over and were residents of Sonoma, CA or surrounding areas. Study recruitment of 2092 persons occurred between May 1993 and December 1994 and follow-up continued for approx. 10 years. The data structure is $O = (W, A, Y)$, where $Y = I(T \leq 5 \text{ years})$, T is time to the event death, A is a binary categorization of LTPA, and W are potential confounders. These variables are further defined in Table 4.1. Of note is the lack of any right censoring in this cohort. The outcome (death within or at 5 years after baseline interview) and date of death was recorded for each subject. Our parameter of interest is the causal risk difference, the average treatment effect of LTPA on mortality 5 years after baseline interview. The cohort was reduced to a size of $n = 2066$, as 26 subjects were missing LTPA values or self-rated health score (1.2% missing data).

4.2.1 Estimator

Estimating $\bar{Q}_0$. In Chap. 3, we generated a super learner prediction function. This is the first step in our TMLE procedure. Thus, we take as inputs our super learner

Table 4.2 Collection of algorithms

Algorithm	Description
glm	Linear model
bayesglm	Bayesian linear model
polymars	Polynomial spline regression
randomForest	Random forest
glmnet,$\alpha = 0.25$	Elastic net
glmnet,$\alpha = 0.50$	
glmnet,$\alpha = 0.75$	
glmnet,$\alpha = 1.00$	
gam, degree = 2	Generalized additive models
gam, degree = 3	
gam, degree = 4	
gam, degree = 5	
nnet,size = 2	Neural network
nnet, size = 4	
gbm, interaction depth=1	Gradient boosting
gbm, interaction depth=2	

prediction function, the initial estimate $\bar{Q}_n^0$, and our data matrix. The data matrix includes columns for each of the covariates W found in Table 4.1, exposure LTPA (A), and outcome Y indicating death within 5 years of baseline. This is step 1 as described in Fig. 4.2. We implemented super learner in the R programming language (R Development Core Team 2010), using the 16 algorithms listed in Table 4.2, recalling that algorithms of the same class with different tuning parameters are considered individual algorithms. Then we calculated predicted values for each of the 2066 observations in our data set, using their observed value of A, and added this as an n-dimensional column labeled $\bar{Q}_n^0(A_i, W_i)$ in our data matrix. Then we calculated a predicted value for each observation where we set $a = 1$, and also $a = 0$, forming two additional columns $\bar{Q}_n^0(1, W_i)$ and $\bar{Q}_n^0(0, W_i)$. Note that for those observations with an observed value of $A_i = 1$, the value in column $\bar{Q}_n^0(A_i, W_i)$ will be equal to the value in column $\bar{Q}_n^0(1, W_i)$. For those with observed $A_i = 0$, the value in column $\bar{Q}_n^0(A_i, W_i)$ will be equal to the value in column in $\bar{Q}_n^0(0, W_i)$. This is depicted in step 2 of Fig. 4.2. At this stage we could plug our estimates $\bar{Q}_n^0(1, W_i)$ and $\bar{Q}_n^0(0, W_i)$ for each subject into our substitution estimator of the risk difference:

$$\psi_{MLE,n} = \Psi(Q_n) = \frac{1}{n}\sum_{i=1}^{n}\{\bar{Q}_n^0(1, W_i) - \bar{Q}_n^0(0, W_i)\}.$$

This is the super learner ML-based substitution estimator discussed previously, plugging in the empirical distribution $Q_{W,n}^0$ for the marginal distribution of W, and the super learner $\bar{Q}_n^0$ for the true regression $\bar{Q}_0$. We know that this estimator is not targeted towards the parameter of interest, so we continue on to a targeting step.

Estimating g_0. Our targeting step required an estimate of the conditional distribution of LTPA given covariates W. This estimate of $P_0(A \mid W) \equiv g_0$ is denoted g_n and was obtained using super learning and the same algorithms listed in Table 4.2. We estimated predicted values using this new super learner prediction function, adding two more columns to our data matrix: $g_n(1 \mid W_i)$ and $g_n(0 \mid W_i)$. This can be seen in Fig. 4.2 as step 3.

Determining a parametric working model to fluctuate the initial estimator. The targeting step used the estimate g_n in a clever covariate to define a parametric working model coding fluctuations of the initial estimator. This clever covariate $H_n^*(A, W)$ is given by

$$H_n^*(A, W) \equiv \left(\frac{I(A = 1)}{g_n(1 \mid W)} - \frac{I(A = 0)}{g_n(0 \mid W)} \right).$$

Thus, for each subject with $A_i = 1$ in the observed data, we calculated the clever covariate as $H_n^*(1, W_i) = 1/g_n(1 \mid W_i)$. Similarly, for each subject with $A_i = 0$ in the observed data, we calculated the clever covariate as $H_n^*(0, W_i) = -1/g_n(0 \mid W_i)$. We combined these values to form a single column $H_n^*(A_i, W_i)$ in the data matrix. We also added two columns $H_n^*(1, W_i)$ and $H_n^*(0, W_i)$. The values for these columns were generated by setting $a = 0$ and $a = 1$. This is step 4 in Fig. 4.2.

Updating $\bar{Q}_n^0$. We then ran a logistic regression of our outcome Y on the clever covariate using as intercept the offset $\text{logit}\bar{Q}_n^0(A, W)$ to obtain the estimate ϵ_n, where ϵ_n is the resulting coefficient in front of the clever covariate $H_n^*(A, W)$. We next wanted to update the estimate $\bar{Q}_n^0$ into a new estimate $\bar{Q}_n^1$ of the true regression function $\bar{Q}_0$:

$$\text{logit}\,\bar{Q}_n^1(A, W) = \text{logit}\,\bar{Q}_n^0(A, W) + \epsilon_n H_n^*(A, W).$$

This parametric working model incorporated information from g_n, through $H_n^*(A, W)$, into an updated regression. One can now repeat this updating step by running a logisitic regression of outcome Y on the clever covariate $H_n^*(A, W)$ using as intercept the offset $\text{logit}\,\bar{Q}_n^1(A, W)$ to obtain the next update $\bar{Q}_n^2$. However, it follows that this time the coefficient in front of the clever covariate will be equal to zero, so that subsequent steps do not result in further updates. Convergence of the TMLE algorithm was achieved in one step. The TMLE of Q_0 was given by $Q_n^* = (\bar{Q}_n^1, Q_{W,n}^0)$. With ϵ_n, we were ready to update our prediction function at $a = 1$ and $a = 0$ according to the logistic regression working model. We calculated

$$\text{logit}\,\bar{Q}_n^1(1, W) = \text{logit}\bar{Q}_n^0(1, W) + \epsilon_n H_n^*(1, W),$$

for all subjects, and then

$$\text{logit}\,\bar{Q}_n^1(0, W) = \text{logit}\bar{Q}_n^0(0, W) + \epsilon_n H_n^*(0, W)$$

for all subjects and added a column for $\bar{Q}_n^1(1, W_i)$ and $\bar{Q}_n^1(0, W_i)$ to the data matrix. Updating $\bar{Q}_n^0$ is also illustrated in step 5 of Fig. 4.2.

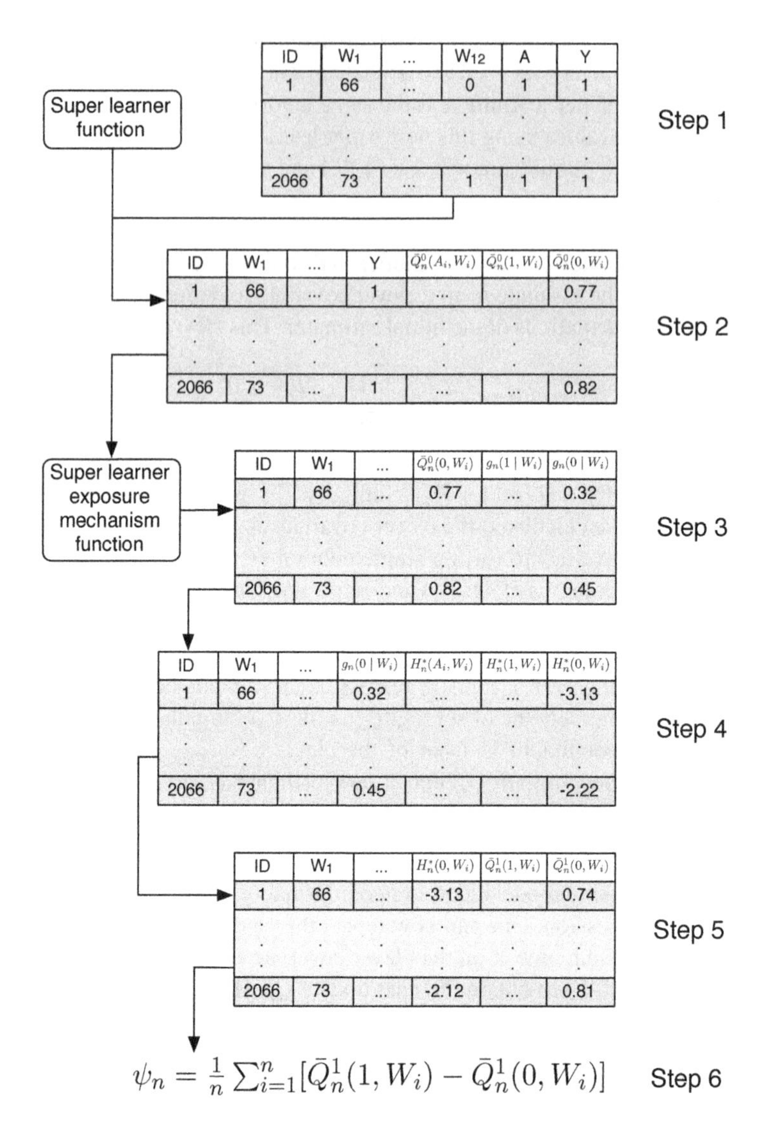

Fig. 4.2 Flow diagram for TMLE of the risk difference in the mortality study example

Targeted substitution estimator of the target parameter. We are at the last step! We computed the plug-in targeted maximum likelihood substitution estimator using the updated estimates $\bar{Q}_n^1(1, W)$ and $\bar{Q}_n^1(0, W)$ and the empirical distribution of W, as seen in step 6 of Fig. 4.2. Our formula from the first step becomes

$$\psi_{TMLE,n} = \Psi(Q_n^*) = \frac{1}{n}\sum_{i=1}^{n}\{\bar{Q}_n^1(1, W_i) - \bar{Q}_n^1(0, W_i)\}.$$

This mapping was accomplished by evaluating $\bar{Q}_n^1(1, W_i)$ and $\bar{Q}_n^1(0, W_i)$ for each observation i, and plugging these values into the above equation. Our estimate of the causal risk difference for the mortality study was $\psi_{TMLE,n} = -0.055$.

4.2.2 Inference

Standard errors. We then needed to calculate the influence curve for our estimator in order to obtain standard errors:

$$IC_n(O_i) = \left(\frac{I(A_i = 1)}{g_n(1 \mid W_i)} - \frac{I(A_i = 0)}{g_n(0 \mid W_i)} \right) (Y - \bar{Q}_n^1(A_i, W_i)) \\ + \bar{Q}_n^1(1, W_i) - \bar{Q}_n^1(0, W_i) - \psi_{TMLE,n},$$

where I is an indicator function: it equals 1 when the logical statement it evaluates, e.g., $A_i = 1$, is true. Note that this influence curve is evaluated for each of the n observations O_i. The beauty of the influence curve of an estimator is that one can now proceed with statistical inference as if the estimator minus its estimand equals the empirical mean of the influence curve. Next, we calculated the sample mean of these estimated influence curve values: $\bar{IC}_n = \frac{1}{n} \sum_{i=1}^n IC_n(o_i)$, where we use o_i to stress that this mean is calculated with our observed realizations of the random variable O_i. For the TMLE we have $\bar{IC}_n = 0$. Using this mean, we calculated the sample variance of the estimated influence curve values:

$$S^2(IC_n) = \frac{1}{n} \sum_{i=1}^n \left(IC_n(o_i) - \bar{IC}_n \right)^2 .$$

Lastly, we used our sample variance to estimate the standard error of our estimator:

$$\sigma_n = \sqrt{\frac{S^2(IC_n)}{n}}.$$

This estimate of the standard error in the mortality study was $\sigma_n = 0.012$.

Confidence intervals and p-values. With the standard errors, we can now calculate confidence intervals and p-values in the same manner you may have learned in other statistics texts. A 95% Wald-type confidence interval can be constructed as:

$$\psi_{TMLE,n} \pm z_{0.975} \frac{\sigma_n}{\sqrt{n}},$$

where z_α denotes the α-quantile of the standard normal density $N(0, 1)$. A p-value for $\psi_{TMLE,n}$ can be calculated as:

$$2 \left[1 - \Phi \left(\left| \frac{\psi_{TMLE,n}}{\sigma_n / \sqrt{n}} \right| \right) \right],$$

where Φ denotes the standard normal cumulative distribution function. The p-value was < 0.001 and the confidence interval was $[-0.078, -0.033]$.

Interpretation

The interpretation of our estimate $\psi_{TMLE,n} = -0.055$, under causal assumptions, is that meeting or exceeding recommended levels of LTPA decreases 5-year mortality in an elderly population by 5.5%. This result was significant, with a p-value of < 0.001 and a confidence interval of $[-0.078, -0.033]$.

4.3 Practical Implications

The double robustness and semiparametric efficiency of the TMLE for estimating a target parameter of the true probability distribution of the data has important implications for both the analysis of RCTs and observational studies.

4.3.1 Randomized Controlled Trials

In 2010, a panel of the National Academy of Sciences made a recommendation to the FDA regarding the use of statistical methods for dealing with missing data in RCTs. The panel represented the split in the literature, namely, those supporting maximum-likelihood-based estimation, and specifically the use of multiple imputation (MI) methods, and the supporters of (augmented) inverse probability of censoring weighted (A-IPCW) estimators based on solving estimating equations. As a consequence, the committee's report ended up recommending both methods: a split decision.

Both camps at the table have been right in their criticism. The MI camp has been stating that the IPCW methods are too unstable and cannot be trusted in finite samples as demonstrated in various simulation studies, even though these methods can be made double robust. The A-IPCW camp has expressed that one cannot use methods that rely on parametric models that may cause severe bias in the resulting estimators of the treatment effect.

TMLE provides the solution to this problem of having to choose between two methods that have complementary properties: TMLE is a maximum-likelihood-based method and thus inherits all the attractive properties of maximum-likelihood-based substitution estimators, while it is still double robust and asymptotically efficient. TMLE has all the good properties of both the MI and the A-IPCW estimators, but it does not have the bad properties such as reliance on misspecified parametric models of the maximum-likelihood-based estimation the instability of the IPCW estimators due to not being substitution estimator. The FDA has also repeatedly expressed a desire for methods that can be communicated to medical researchers. As with maximum-likelihood-based estimation, the TMLE is easier to communicate: it is hard to communicate estimators that are defined as a solution of an estimating equation instead of a maximizer of a well-defined criterion.

TMLE can also be completely aligned with the highly populated maximum-likelihood-based estimation camp: TMLE can use maximum-likelihood-based estimation as the initial estimator, but it will carry out the additional targeting step. Of course, we recommend using the super learner (i.e., machine learning) as the initial estimator, but in an RCT in which one assumes that missingness is noninformative, the use of the parametric maximum likelihood estimation as initial estimator will not obstruct unbiased estimation of the causal effect of interest.

Consider an RCT in which we observe on each unit $(W, A, \Delta, \Delta Y)$, where Δ is an indicator of the clinical outcome being observed. Suppose we wish to estimate the additive causal effect $E_0 Y_1 - E_0 Y_0$, which is identified by the estimand $E_0[\bar{Q}_0(0, W) - \bar{Q}_0(1, W)]$, where $\bar{Q}_0(A, W) = E_0(Y \mid A, W, \Delta = 1)$ under causal assumptions, including that no unmeasured predictors of Y predict the missingness indicator. The TMLE of this additive causal effect only involves a minor modification of the TMLE presented above, and is derived in Appendix A. That is, the clever covariate is modified by multiplying it by $1/P_0(\Delta = 1 \mid A, W)$, and all outcome regressions are based on the complete observations only.

In an RCT the treatment assignment process, $g_0(1 \mid W) = P_0(A = 1 \mid W)$, is known (e.g., 0.5), and it is often assumed that missingness of outcomes is noninformative, also called missing completely at random. When this assumption holds, the g_n, comprising both the treatment assignment and the censoring or missingness mechanism, is always correctly estimated. Specifically, one can consistently estimate the missingness mechanism $P_0(\Delta = 1 \mid A, W)$ with the empirical proportions for the different treatment groups, thus ignoring the value of W. The TMLE will provide valid type I error control and confidence intervals for the causal effect of the investigated treatment, even if the initial regression estimator $\bar{Q}_n^0$ is completely misspecified.

The use of TMLE also often results in efficiency and bias gains with respect to the unadjusted or other ad hoc estimators commonly employed in the analysis of RCT data. For example, consider the additive causal effect example discussed in this chapter. The unadjusted estimator is restricted to considering only complete cases, ignoring observations where the outcome is missing, and ignoring any covariate information. In this particular example, the efficiency and bias gain is already apparent from the fact that the targeted maximum likelihood approach averages an estimate of an individual effect $\bar{Q}_0(1, W) - \bar{Q}_0(0, W)$ over all observations in the sample, including the observations that had a missing outcome.

TMLE can exploit information in measured baseline and time-dependent covariates, even when there is no missingness or right censoring. This allows for bias reduction due to empirical confounding, i.e., it will adjust for empirical imbalances in the treatment and control arm, and thereby improve finite sample precision (efficiency). To get an insight into the potential gains of TMLE relative to the current standard, we note that the relative efficiency of the TMLE relative to the unadjusted estimator of the causal additive risk in a standard RCT with two arms and randomization probability equal to 0.5, and no missingness or censoring, is given by 1 minus the R squared of the regression of the clinical outcome Y on the baseline covariates W implied by the targeted maximum likelihood fit of the regression of Y on the binary treatment and baseline covariates. That is, if the baseline covariates are predictive, one will gain efficiency, and one can predict the amount of improvement from the actual regression fit.

Perhaps more importantly, the TMLE naturally adjusts for dropout (missingness) as well and can also be used to assess the effect of treatment under noncompliance, i.e., it is unbiased when standard methods are biased. Unlike an unadjusted estimator that ignores covariate information, TMLE does not rely on an assumption of noninformative missingness or dropout, but allows that missingness and dropout depend on the observed covariates, including time-dependent covariates.

In RCTs, including sequentially randomized controlled trials, one can still fully respect the likelihood of the data and obtain fully efficient and unbiased estimators, without taking the risk of bias due to statistical model misspecification (which has been the sole reason for the application of inefficient unadjusted estimators). On the contrary, the better one fits the true functions Q_0 and g_0, as can be evaluated with the cross-validated log-likelihood, the more bias reduction and efficiency gain will have been achieved.

Prespecification of the TMLE in the statistical analysis plan allows for appropriate adjustment with measured confounders while avoiding the possible introduction of bias should that decision be based on human intervention. Therefore, TMLEs can be used for both the efficacy as well as the safety analysis in Phase II, III, and IV clinical trials. In addition, just like for unadjusted estimators, permutation distributions can be used to obtain finite sample inference and more robust inference.

4.3.2 Observational Studies

At many levels of society one builds large electronic databases that keep track of large patient populations. One wishes to use these dynamic databases to assess safety signals of drugs, evaluate the effectiveness of different interventions, and so on. Comparative effectiveness research concerns the research involved to make such comparisons. These comparisons often involve observational studies, so that one cannot assume that the treatment was randomly assigned. In such studies, standard off-the-shelf methods are biased due to confounding as well as informative missingness, censoring, and possibly biased sampling.

In observational studies, the utilization of efficient and maximally unbiased estimators is thus extremely important. One cannot analyze the effect of high dose of a drug on heart attack in a postmarket safety analysis using logistic regression in a parametric statistical model or Cox proportional hazards models, and put much trust in a p-value. It is already a priori known that these statistical models are misspecified and that the effect estimate will be biased, so under the null hypothesis of no treatment effect, the resulting test statistic will reject the null hypothesis incorrectly with probability tending to 1 as sample size increases. For example, if the high dose is preferentially assigned to sicker people, then the unadjusted estimator is biased high, a maximum likelihood estimator according to a misspecified parametric model will still be biased high by its inability to let the data speak and thereby adjust for the measured confounders.

As a consequence, the only alternative is to use semiparametric statistical models that acknowledge what is known and what is not known, and use robust and efficient substitution estimators. Given such infinite-dimensional semiparametric statistical models, we need to employ machine learning, and, in fact, as theory suggests, we should not be married to one particular machine learning algorithm but let the data speak by using super learning. That is, one cannot foresee what kind of algorithm should be used, but one should build a rich library of approaches, and use cross-validation to combine these estimators into an improved estimator that adapts the choice to the truth. In addition, and again as theory teaches us, we have to target the fit toward the parameter of interest, to remove bias for the target parameter, and to improve the statistical inference based on the central limit theorem. TMLE combined with super learning provides such a robust and semiparametric efficient substitution estimator, while we maintain the log-likelihood or other appropriate loss function as the principal criterion.

4.4 Summary

TMLE is a general algorithm where we start with an initial estimator of P_0, or a relevant parameter Q_0 of P_0. We then create a parametric statistical model with parameter ϵ through this given initial estimator whose score at $\epsilon = 0$ spans the efficient influence curve of the parameter of interest at the given initial estimator. It estimates ϵ with maximum likelihood estimation in this parametric statistical model and finally updates the new estimator as the corresponding fluctuation of the given initial estimator. The algorithm can be iterated until convergence, although in many common cases it converges in one step.

4.5 Road Map for Targeted Learning

We have now completed the road map for targeted learning depicted in Fig. 4.3. This chapter covered effect estimation using super learner and TMLE, as well as inference. In many cases, we may be interested in a ranked list of effect measures, often referred to as variable importance measures (VIMs). We provided an additional road map (Fig. 4.4) for research questions involving VIMs, which are common in medicine, genomics, and many other fields. We address questions of variable importance in Chaps. 22 and 23.

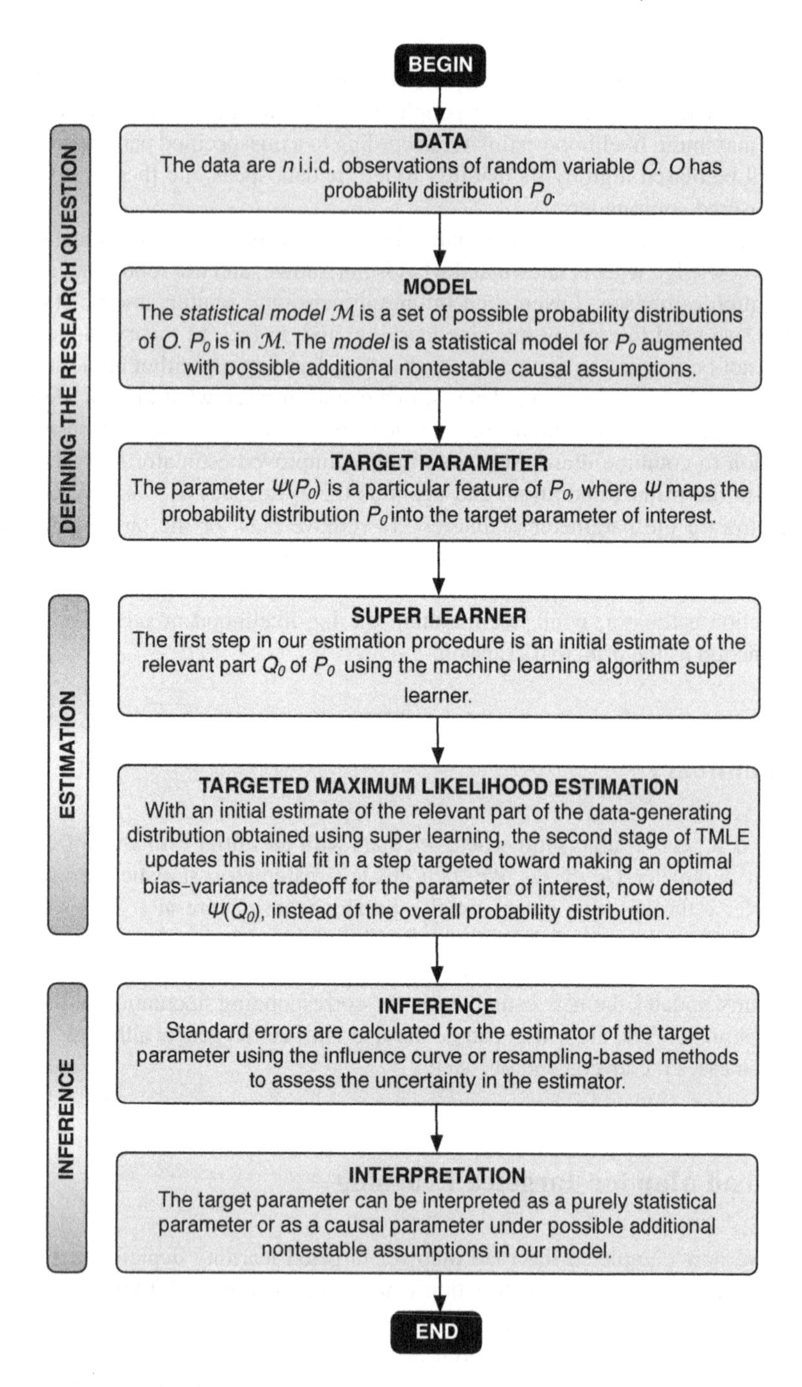

Fig. 4.3 Road map for targeted learning

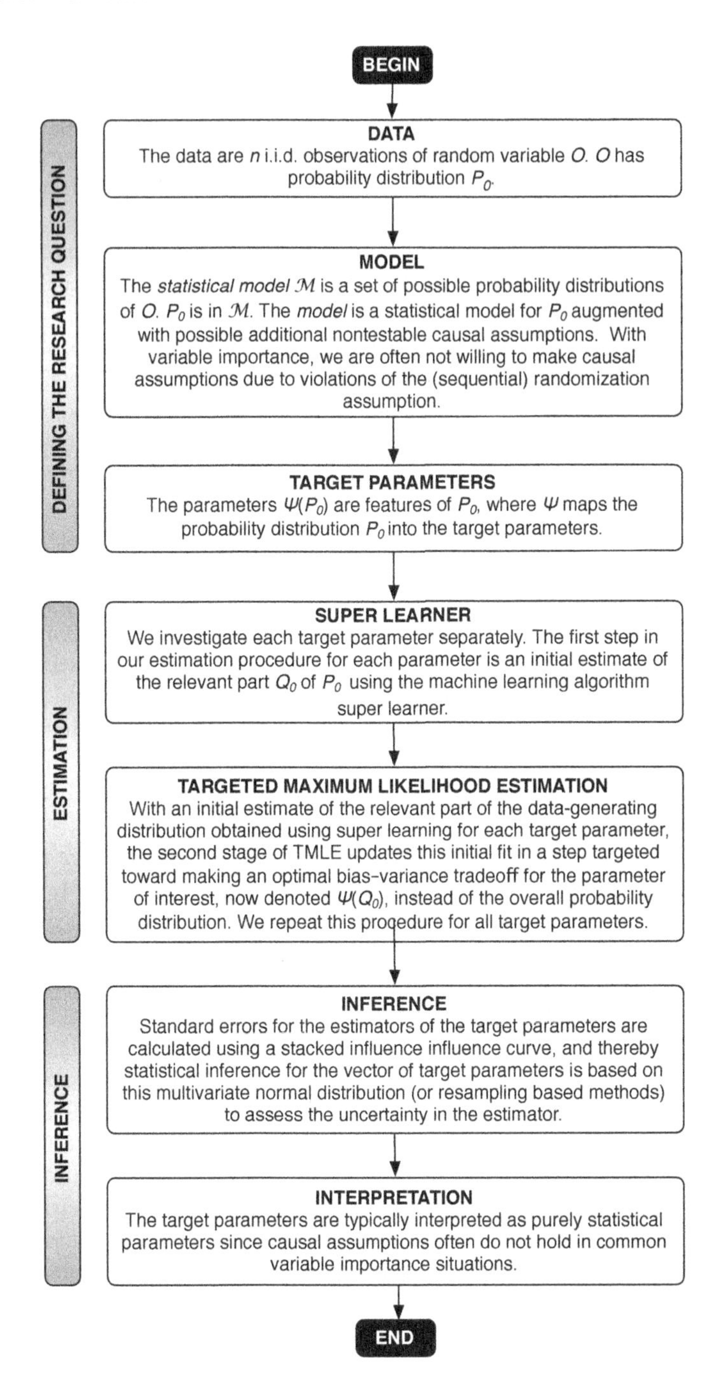

Fig. 4.4 Road map for targeted learning of variable importance measures

4.6 Notes and Further Reading

MLE has been referred to elsewhere as g-formula and g-computation. It is a maximum-likelihood-based substitution estimator of the g-formula parameter. The g-formula for identifying the distribution of counterfactuals from the observed data distribution, under the sequential randomization assumption, was originally published in Robins (1986). We also refer readers to an introductory implementation of a maximum-likelihood-based substitution estimator of the g-formula (Snowden et al. 2011; Rose et al. 2011).

Estimating equation methodology, including IPTW (Robins 1999b; Hernan et al. 2000) and A-IPTW (Robins et al. 2000b; Robins 2000; Robins and Rotnitzky 2001), is discussed in detail in van der Laan and Robins (2003). Detailed references and a bibliographic history on locally efficient A-IPTW estimators, double robustness, and estimating equation methodology can be found in Chap. 1 of that text. A key seminal paper in this literature is Robins and Rotnitzky (1992). A-IPTW was previously referred to as the double robust estimator in some publications. Didactic presentations of IPTW can be found in Robins et al. (2000a), Mortimer et al. (2005), and Cole and Hernan (2008).

For the original paper on TMLE we refer readers to van der Laan and Rubin (2006). Subsequent papers on TMLE in observational and experimental studies include Bembom and van der Laan (2007a), van der Laan (2008a), Rose and van der Laan (2008, 2009, 2011), Moore and van der Laan (2009a,b,c), Bembom et al. (2009), Polley and van der Laan (2009), Rosenblum et al. (2009), van der Laan and Gruber (2010), Gruber and van der Laan (2010a), Rosenblum and van der Laan (2010a), and Wang et al. (2010).

A detailed discussion of multiple hypothesis testing and inference for variable importance measures is presented in Dudoit and van der Laan (2008). We also refer readers to Chaps. 22 and 23. The mortality study analyzed in this chapter with TMLE is based on data discussed in Tager et al. (1998).

Previous work related to estimators in RCTs (and in general in observational studies with known probabilities of treatment) that are robust to model misspecification include, for example, Robins (1994), Robins et al. (1995), Scharfstein et al. (1999), van der Laan and Robins (2003), Leon et al. (2003), Tan (2006), Tsiatis (2006), Moore and van der Laan (2009b), Zhang et al. (2008), Rubin and van der Laan (2008), Freedman (2008a,b), and Rosenblum and van der Laan (2009a).

We refer readers to Bickel et al. (1997) for a text on semiparametric estimation and asymptotic theory. Tsiatis (2006) is a text applying semiparametric theory to missing data, including chapters on Hilbert spaces and influence curves. We also refer to Hampel et al. (1986) for a text on robust statistics, including presentation of influence curves. Van der Vaart (1998) provides a thorough introduction to asymptotic statistics, and van der Vaart and Wellner (1996) discuss stochastic convergence, empirical process theory, and weak convergence theory.

Chapter 5
Understanding TMLE

Sherri Rose, Mark J. van der Laan

This chapter focuses on understanding TMLE. We go into more detail than the previous chapter to demonstrate how this estimator is derived. Recall that TMLE is a two-step procedure where one first obtains an estimate of the data-generating distribution P_0 or the relevant portion Q_0 of P_0. The second stage updates this initial fit in a step targeted toward making an optimal bias–variance tradeoff for the parameter of interest $\Psi(Q_0)$, instead of the overall density P_0. The procedure is double robust and can incorporate data-adaptive-likelihood-based estimation procedures to estimate Q_0 and the treatment mechanism.

5.1 Conceptual Framework

We begin the discussion of TMLE at a conceptual level to give an overall picture of what the method achieves. In Fig. 5.1 we depict a flow chart for TMLE, and in this section, we walk the reader through the illustration and provide a conceptual foundation for TMLE. We start with our observed data and some (possibly) real valued function $\Psi()$, the target parameter mapping. These two objects are our inputs. We have an initial estimator of the probability distribution of the data (or something smaller than that – the relevant portion). This is P_n^0 and is estimated semiparametrically using super learning. This initial estimator is typically already somewhat informed about the target parameter of interest by, for example, only focusing on fitting the relevant part Q_0 of P_0. P_n^0 falls within the statistical model, which is the set of all possible probability distributions of the data. P_0, the true probability distribution, also falls within the statistical model, since it is assumed that the statistical model is selected to represent true knowledge. In many applications the statistical model is necessarily nonparametric. We update P_n^0 in a particular way, in a targeted way by incorporating the target parameter mapping Ψ, and now denote this targeted update as P_n^*. If we map P_n^* using our function $\Psi()$, we get our estimator $\Psi(P_n^*)$ and thereby a value on the real line. The updating step is tailored to result in values

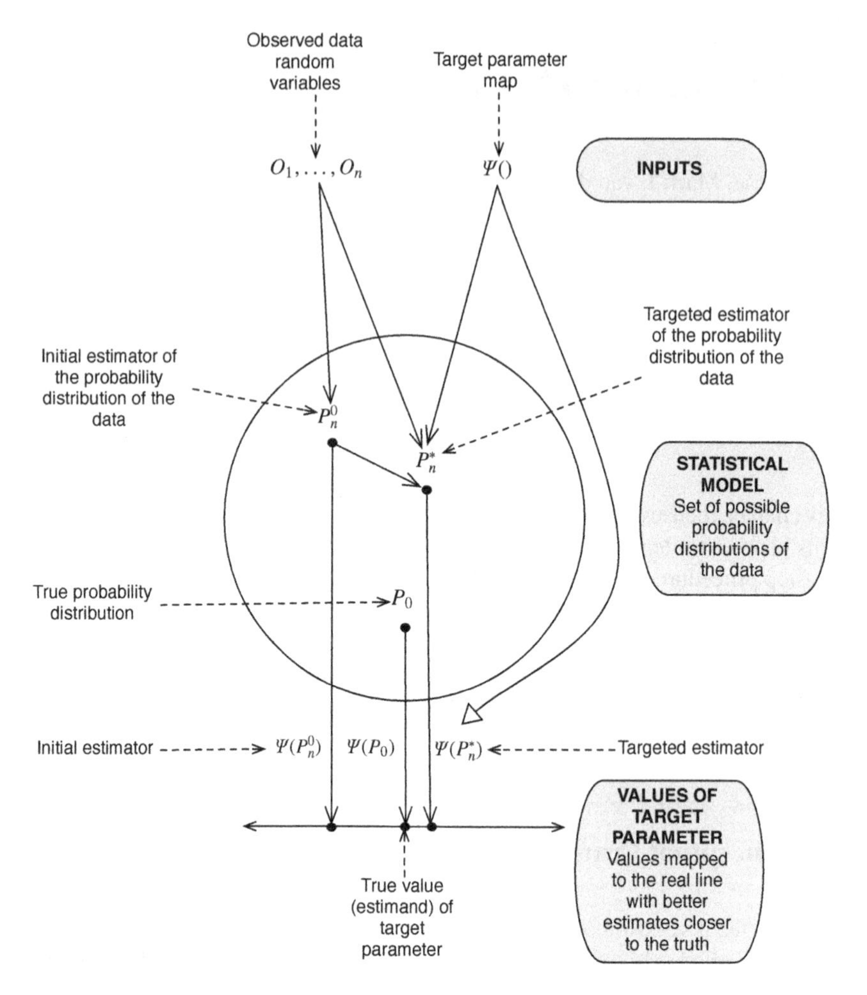

Fig. 5.1 TMLE flow chart.

$\Psi(P_n^*)$ that are closer to the truth than the value generated using the initial estimate P_n^0: specifically, $\Psi(P_n^*)$ is less biased than $\Psi(P_n^0)$.

TMLE provides a concrete methodology for mapping the initial estimator P_n^0 into a targeted estimator P_n^*, which is described below in terms of an arbitrary statistical model $\mathcal{M}$ and target parameter mapping $\Psi()$ defined on this statistical model. In order to make this more accessible to the reader, we then demonstrate this general template for TMLE with a nonparametric statistical model for a univariate random variable and a survival probability target parameter. Specifically, TMLE involves the following steps:

- Consider the target parameter $\Psi : \mathcal{M} \rightarrow \mathbb{R}$. Compute its pathwise derivative at P and its corresponding canonical gradient $D^*(P)$, which is also called the efficient influence curve. This object $D^*(P)$, a function of O with mean zero under P, is now available for each possible probability distribution P.

- Define a loss function $L()$ so that $P \to E_0 L(P)$ is minimized at the true probability distribution P_0. One could select the log-likelihood loss function $L(P) = -\log P$. However, typically, this loss function is chosen so that it only depends on P through a relevant part $Q(P)$ and $Q \to L(Q)$ is minimized at $Q_0 = Q(P_0)$. This loss function could also be used to construct a super-learner-based initial estimator of Q_0.
- For a P in our model $\mathcal{M}$, define a parametric working model $\{P(\epsilon) : \epsilon\}$ with finite-dimensional parameter ϵ so that $P(\epsilon = 0) = P$, and a "score" $\frac{d}{d\epsilon} L(P(\epsilon))$ at $\epsilon = 0$ for which a linear combination of the components of this "score" equals the efficient influence curve $D^*(P)$ at P. Typically, we simply choose the parametric working model so that this score equals the efficient influence curve $D^*(P)$. If the loss function $L()$ only depends on P through a relevant part $Q = Q(P)$, then this translates into a parametric working model $\{Q(\epsilon) : \epsilon\}$ chosen so that a linear combination of the components of the "score" $\frac{d}{d\epsilon} L(Q(\epsilon))$ at $\epsilon = 0$ equals the efficient influence curve $D^*(P)$ at P.
- Given an initial estimator P_n^0 of P_0, we compute $\epsilon_n^0 = \arg\min_\epsilon \sum_{i=1}^n L(P_n^0(\epsilon))(O_i)$. This yields the first step TMLE $P_n^1 = P_n^0(\epsilon_n^0)$. This process is iterated: start with $k = 1$, compute $\epsilon_n^k = \arg\min_\epsilon \sum_{i=1}^n L(P_n^k(\epsilon))(O_i)$ and $P_n^{k+1} = P_n^k(\epsilon_n^k)$, increase k to $k+1$, and repeat these updating steps until $\epsilon_n^k = 0$. The final update P_n^K at the final step K is denoted by P_n^* and is the TMLE of P_0. The same algorithm can be directly applied to Q_n^0 of $Q_0 = Q(P_0)$ for the case that the loss function only depends on P through $Q(P)$.
- The TMLE of ψ_0 is now the substitution estimator obtained by plugging P_n^* into the target parameter mapping: $\psi_n^* = \Psi(P_n^*)$. Similarly, if $\psi_0 = \Psi(Q_0)$ and the above loss function $L()$ is a loss function for Q_0, then we plug the TMLE Q_n^* into the target parameter mapping: $\psi_n^* = \Psi(Q_n^*)$.
- The TMLE P_n^* solves the efficient influence curve equation $0 = \sum_{i=1}^n D^*(P_n^*)(O_i)$, which provides a basis for establishing the asymptotic linearity and efficiency of the TMLE $\Psi(P_n^*)$.

For further presentation of TMLE at this general level we refer the interested reader to Appendix A.

Demonstration of TMLE template. In this section we demonstrate the TMLE template for estimation of survival probability. Suppose we observe n i.i.d. univariate random variables $O_1, \ldots, O_n$ with probability distribution P_0, where O_i represents a time to failure such as death. Suppose that we have no knowledge about this probability distribution, so that we select as statistical model the nonparametric model $\mathcal{M}$. Let $\Psi(P) = P(O > 5)$ be the target parameter that maps any probability distribution in its survival probability at 5 years, and let $\psi_0 = P_0(O > 5)$ be our target parameter of the true data-generating distribution.

The pathwise derivative $\Psi(P(\epsilon))$ at $\epsilon = 0$ for a parametric submodel (i.e., path) $\{P_S(\epsilon) = (1 + \epsilon S(P))P : \epsilon\}$ with univariate parameter ϵ is given by

$$\frac{d}{d\epsilon}\Psi(P_S(\epsilon))\bigg|_{\epsilon=0} = E_P\{I(O > 5) - \Psi(P)\}S(P)(O).$$

Note that indeed, for any function S of O that has mean zero under P and is uniformly bounded, it follows that $P_S(\epsilon)$ is a probability distribution for a small enough choice of ϵ, so that the family of paths indexed by such functions S represents a valid family of submodels through P in the nonparametric model. By definition, it follows that the canonical gradient of this pathwise derivative at P (relative to this family of parametric submodels) is given by $D^*(P)(O) = I(O > 5) - \Psi(P)$. The canonical gradient is also called the efficient influence curve at P.

We could select the log-likelihood loss function $L(P) = -\log P(O)$ as loss function. A parametric working model through P is given by $P(\epsilon) = (1 + \epsilon D^*(P))P$, where ϵ is the univariate fluctuation parameter. Note that this parametric submodel includes P at $\epsilon = 0$ and has a score at $\epsilon = 0$ given by $D^*(P)$, as required for the TMLE algorithm. We are now ready to define the TMLE.

Let P_n^0 be an initial density estimator of the density P_0. Let

$$\epsilon_n^0 = \arg\max_{\epsilon} \sum_{i=1}^{n} \log P_n^0(\epsilon)(O_i),$$

and let $P_n^1 = P_n^0(\epsilon_n^0)$ be the corresponding first-step TMLE of P_0. It can be shown that the next iteration yields $\epsilon_n^1 = 0$, so that convergence of the iterative TMLE algorithm occurs in one step (van der Laan and Rubin 2006). The TMLE is thus given by $P_n^* = P_n^1$, and the TMLE of ψ_0 is given by the plug-in estimator $\psi_n^* = \Psi(P_n^*) = P_n^*(O > 5)$. Since P_n^* solves the efficient influence curve equation, it follows that $\psi_n^* = \frac{1}{n}\sum_{i=1}^n I(O_i > 5)$ is the empirical proportion of subjects that has a survival time larger than 5. This estimator is asymptotically linear with influence curve $D^*(P_0)$ since $\psi_n^* - \psi_0 = \frac{1}{n}\sum_{i=1}^n D^*(P_0)(O_i)$, which proves that the TMLE of ψ_0 is efficient for every choice of initial estimator: apparently, all bias of the initial estimator is removed by this TMLE update step.

Consider a kernel density estimator with an optimally selected bandwidth (e.g., based on likelihood-based cross-validation). Since this optimally selected bandwidth trades off bias and variance for the kernel density estimator as an estimate of the true density P_0, it will, under some smoothness conditions, select a bandwidth that converges to zero in sample size at a rate $n^{-1/5}$. The bias of such a kernel density estimator converges to zero at the rate $n^{-2/5}$. As a consequence, the substitution estimator of the survival function at t for this kernel density estimator has a bias that converges to zero at a slower rate than $1/\sqrt{n}$ in the sample size n. We can conclude that the substitution estimator of a survival function at 5 years based on this optimal kernel density estimator will have an asymptotic relative efficiency of zero (!) relative to the empirical survival function at 5 years. This simple example demonstrates that a regularized maximum likelihood estimator of P_0 is not targeted toward the target parameter of interest and, by the same token, that current Bayesian inference is not targeted toward the target parameter. However, if we apply the TMLE step to the kernel density estimator, then the resulting TMLE of the survival function is unbiased and asymptotically efficient, and it even remains unbiased and asymptotically efficient if the kernel density estimator is replaced by an incorrect guess of the true density.

The point is: the best estimator of a density is not a good enough estimator of a particular feature of the density, but the TMLE step takes care of this.

5.2 Definition of TMLE in Context of the Mortality Example

This section presents the definition of TMLE in the context of our mortality example, thereby allowing the reader to derive the TMLE presented in the previous chapter. The reader may recognize the general recipe for TMLE as presented in Sect. 5.1 that can be applied in any semiparametric model with any target parameter. After having read this section, the reader might consider revisiting this general TMLE presentation. Our causal effect of interest is the causal risk difference, and the estimand is the corresponding statistical W-adjusted risk difference, which can be interpreted as the causal risk difference under causal assumptions. The data structure in the illustrative example is $O = (W, A, Y) \sim P_0$. TMLE follows the basic steps enumerated below, which we then illustrate in more detail.

TMLE for the Risk Difference

1. Estimate $\bar{Q}_0$ using super learner to generate our prediction function $\bar{Q}_n^0$. Let $Q_n^0 = (\bar{Q}_n^0, Q_{W,n})$ be the estimate of $Q_0 = (\bar{Q}_0, Q_{W,0})$, where $Q_{W,n}$ is the empirical probability distribution of $W_1, \ldots, W_n$.
2. Estimate the treatment mechanism using super learning. The estimate of g_0 is g_n.
3. Determine a parametric family of fluctuations $\{Q_n^0(\epsilon) : \epsilon\}$ of the initial estimator Q_n^0 with fluctuation parameter ϵ, and a loss function $L(Q)$ so that a linear combination of the components of the derivative of $L(Q_n^0(\epsilon))$ at $\epsilon = 0$ equals the efficient influence curve $D^*(Q_n^0, g_n)$ at any initial estimator $Q_n^0 = (\bar{Q}_n^0, Q_{W,n}^0)$ and g_n. Since the initial estimate $Q_{W,n}^0$ of the marginal distribution of W is the empirical distribution (i.e., nonparametric maximum likelihood estimator), the TMLE using a separate ϵ for fluctuating $Q_{W,n}^0$ and $\bar{Q}_n^0$ will only fluctuate $\bar{Q}_n^0$. The parametric family of fluctuations of $\bar{Q}_n^0$ is defined by parametric regression including a clever covariate chosen so that the above derivative condition holds with ϵ playing the role of the coefficient in front of the clever covariate. This "clever covariate" $H_n^*(A, W)$ depends on (Q_n^0, g_n) only through g_n, and in the TMLE procedure it needs to be evaluated for each observation (A_i, W_i), and at $(0, W_i)$, $(1, W_i)$.

4. Update the initial fit $\bar{Q}_n^0(A, W)$ from step 1. This is achieved by holding $\bar{Q}_n^0(A, W)$ fixed (i.e., as intercept) while estimating the coefficient ϵ for $H_n^*(A, W)$ in the parametric working model using maximum likelihood estimation. Let ϵ_n be this parametric maximum likelihood estimator. The updated regression is given by $\bar{Q}_n^1 = \bar{Q}_n^0(\epsilon_n)$. For the risk difference, no iteration is necessary, since the next iteration will not result in any change: that is, the next ϵ_n will be equal to zero. The TMLE of Q_0 is now $Q_n^* = (\bar{Q}_n^1, Q_{W,n}^0)$, where only the conditional mean estimator $\bar{Q}_n^0$ was updated.
5. Obtain the substitution estimator of the causal risk difference by application of the target parameter mapping to Q_n^*:

$$\psi_n = \Psi(Q_n^*) = \frac{1}{n} \sum_{i=1}^{n} \{\bar{Q}_n^1(1, W_i) - \bar{Q}_n^1(0, W_i)\}.$$

6. Calculate standard errors based on the influence curve of the TMLE ψ_n, and then calculate p-values and confidence intervals.

There are several concepts in this enumerated step-by-step list that may be somewhat opaque for the reader: the parametric working model coding the fluctuations of the initial estimator, the corresponding clever covariate, the efficient influence curve, and the influence curve. We expand upon the list, including these topics, below. For the nontechnical reader, we provide gray boxes so that you can read these to understand the essential topics relevant to each step. The white boxes outlined in black contain additional technical information for the more theoretical reader.

5.2.1 Estimating $\bar{Q}_0$

The first step in TMLE is obtaining an estimate $\bar{Q}_n^0$ for $\bar{Q}_0$. This initial fit is achieved using super learning, avoiding assuming a misspecified parametric statistical model.

5.2.2 Estimating g_0

The TMLE procedure uses the estimate of $\bar{Q}_0$ obtained above in conjunction with an estimate of g_0. We estimate g_0 with g_n, again using super learning.

5.2.3 Determining the Efficient Influence Curve $D^*(P)$

To obtain such a parametric working model to fluctuate the initial estimator Q_n^0 we need to know the efficient influence curve of the target parameter mapping at a particular P in the statistical model. This is a mathematical exercise that takes as input the definition of the statistical model $\mathcal{M}$ (i.e, the nonparametric model) and the target parameter mapping from this statistical model to the real line (i.e., $\Psi : \mathcal{M} \to \mathbb{R}$). We refer to Appendix A for required background material. It follows that the efficient influence curve at P_0 only depends on (Q_0, g_0) and is given by

$$D^*(Q_0, g_0)(W, A, Y) = \left(\frac{I(A=1)}{g_0(1 \mid W)} - \frac{I(A=0)}{g_0(0 \mid W)}\right)(Y - \bar{Q}_0(A, W)) \\ + \bar{Q}_0(1, W) - \bar{Q}_0(0, W) - \Psi(Q_0).$$

More on the efficient influence curve. Calculation of the efficient influence curve, and of components of the efficient influence curve, requires calculations of projections of an element onto a subspace within a Hilbert space. These projections are defined in the Hilbert space $L_0^2(P)$ of functions of O that have mean zero under P endowed with an inner product $\langle S_1, S_2 \rangle_P = E_P S_1(O) S_2(O)$, being the covariance of two functions of O. Two elements in an Hilbert space are orthogonal if the inner product equals zero: so two functions of O are defined as orthogonal if their correlation or covariance equals zero. Recall that a projection of a function S onto a subspace of $L_0^2(P)$ is defined as follows: (1) the projection is an element of the subspace and (2) the difference of S minus the projection is orthogonal to the subspace. The subspaces on which one projects are so-called tangent spaces and subtangent spaces. The tangent space at P is defined as the closure of the linear span of all scores of submodels through P. The tangent space is a subspace of $L_0^2(P)$. The tangent space of a particular variation-independent parameter of P is defined as the closure of the linear span of all scores of submodels through P that only vary this particular factor. We can denote the tangent spaces by $T(P)$ and a projection of a function S onto a $T(P)$ by $\Pi(S \mid T(P))$.

5.2.4 Determining the Fluctuation Working Model

Now, can we slightly modify the initial estimator $\bar{Q}_n^0$ to reduce bias for the additive causal effect? Let $Q_{W,n}^0$ be the empirical probability distribution of $W_1, \ldots, W_n$. We refer to the combined conditional probability distribution of Y and the marginal probability distribution of W as Q_0. $Q_n^0 = (\bar{Q}_n^0, Q_{W,n}^0)$ denotes the initial estimator of this Q_0. We also remind the reader that the target parameter ψ_0 only depends on

P_0 through $\bar{Q}_0$ and $Q_{W,0}$. Since the empirical distribution $Q^0_{W,n}$ is already a nonparametric maximum likelihood estimator of the true marginal probability distribution of W, for the sake of bias reduction for the target parameter, we can focus on only updating $\bar{Q}^0_n$, as explained below.

We want to reduce the bias of our initial estimator, where the initial estimator is a random variable that has bias and variance. We only need to update $\bar{Q}^0_n$ since the empirical distribution $Q^0_{W,n}$ is a nonparametric maximum likelihood estimator (and can thus not generate bias for our target parameter).

Our parametric working model is denoted as $\{\bar{Q}^0_n(\epsilon) : \epsilon\}$, which is a small parametric statistical model, a one-dimensional submodel that goes through the initial estimate $\bar{Q}^0_n(A, W)$ at $\epsilon = 0$. If we use the log-likelihood loss function

$$L(\bar{Q})(O) = -\log \bar{Q}(A, W)^Y (1 - \bar{Q}(A, W))^{1-Y},$$

then the parametric working model for fluctuating the conditional probability distribution of Y, given (A, W), needs to have the property

$$\frac{d}{d\epsilon} \log \bar{Q}^0_n(\epsilon)(A, W)^Y (1 - \bar{Q}^0_n(A, W))^{1-Y}|_{\epsilon=0} = D^*_Y(Q^0_n, g_n)(W, A, Y), \qquad (5.1)$$

where $D^*_Y(Q^0_n, g_n)$ is the appropriate component of the efficient influence curve $D^*(Q^0_n, g_n)$ of the target parameter mapping at (Q^0_n, g_n). Formally, the appropriate component D^*_Y is the component of the efficient influence curve that equals a score of a fluctuation of a conditional distribution of Y, given (A, W). These components of the efficient influence curve that correspond with scores of fluctuations that only vary certain parts of factors of the probability distribution can be computed with Hilbert space projections. We provide the required background and tools in Appendix A and various subsequent chapters.

More on fluctuating the initial estimator. If the target parameter ψ_0 depends on different variation-independent parts $(Q_{W,0}, \bar{Q}_0)$ of the probability distribution P_0, then one can decide to fluctuate the initial estimators $(Q^0_{W,n}, \bar{Q}_n)$ with separate submodels and separate loss functions $L(Q_W) = -\log Q_W$ and $L(\bar{Q})$, respectively. The submodels $\{Q^0_{W,n}(\epsilon) : \epsilon\}$, $\{\bar{Q}_n(\epsilon) : \epsilon\}$ and their corresponding loss functions $L(Q_W)$ and $L(\bar{Q})$ need to be chosen such that a linear combination of the components of the derivative $\frac{d}{d\epsilon} L(Q^0_n(\epsilon))\big|_{\epsilon=0}$ equals $D^*(Q^0_n, g_n)$ for the sum-loss function $L(Q) = L(Q_W) + L(\bar{Q})$. This corresponds with requiring that each of the two loss functions generates a "score" so that the sum of these two "scores" equals the efficient influence curve. If the initial estimator $Q^0_{W,n}$ is a nonparametric maximum likelihood estimator, the TMLE using a separate ϵ_1 and ϵ_2 for the two submodels will not update $Q^0_{W,n}$.

Following the protocol of TMLE, we also need to fluctuate the marginal distribution of W. For that purpose we select as loss function of $Q_{W,0}$ the log-likelihood loss function $-\log Q_W$. Then we would select a parametric working model coding fluctuations $Q^0_{W,n}(\epsilon)$ of $Q^0_{W,n}$ so that

$$\frac{d}{d\epsilon} \log Q^0_{W,n}(\epsilon)\Big|_{\epsilon=0} = D^*_W(Q^0_n, g_n),$$

where D^*_W is the component of the efficient influence curve that is a score of a fluctuation of the marginal distribution of W.

Tangent spaces. Since Q_W and $\bar{Q}$ represent parameters of different factors P_W and $P_{Y|A,W}$ in a factorization of $P = P_W P_{A|W} P_{Y|A,W}$, these components $D^*_W(P)$ and $D^*_Y(P)$ can be defined as the projection of the efficient influence curve $D^*(P)$ onto the tangent space of P_W at P and $P_{Y|A,W}$ at P, respectively. The tangent space T_W of P_W is given by all functions of W with mean zero. The tangent space T_Y of $P_{Y|A,W}$ is given by all functions of W, A, Y for which the conditional mean, given A, W, equals zero. The tangent space T_A of $P_{A|W}$ is given by all functions of A, W, with conditional mean zero, given W. These three tangent spaces are orthogonal, as a general consequence of the factorization of P into the three factors. The projection of a function S onto these three tangent spaces is given by $\Pi(S \mid T_W) = E_P(S(O) \mid W)$, $\Pi(S \mid T_Y)) = S(O) - E_P(S(O) \mid A, W)$, and $\Pi(S \mid T_A) = E_P(S(O) \mid A, W) - E_P(S \mid W)$, respectively. From these projection formulas and setting $S = D^*(P)$, the explicit forms of $D^*_W(P) = \Pi(D^*(P) \mid T_W)$ and $D^*_Y(P) = \Pi(D^*(P) \mid T_Y)$ can be calculated as provided below, and for each choice of P. It also follows that the projection of $D^*(P)$ onto the tangent space of $P_{A|W}$ equals zero: $\Pi(D^*(P) \mid T_A) = 0$. The latter formally explains that the TMLE does not require fluctuating the initial estimator of g_0. It follows that the efficient influence curve $D^*(P)$ at P can be decomposed as:

$$D^*(P) = D^*_Y(P) + D^*_W(P).$$

Our loss function for Q is now $L(Q) = L(\bar{Q}) + L(Q_W)$, and with this parametric working model coding fluctuations $Q^0_n(\epsilon) = (Q^0_{W,n}(\epsilon), \bar{Q}^0_n(\epsilon))$ of Q^0_n, we have that the derivative of $\epsilon \to L(Q^0_n(\epsilon))$ at $\epsilon = 0$ equals the efficient influence curve at (Q^0_n, g_n). If we use different ϵ for each component of Q^0_n, then the two derivatives span the efficient influence curve, since the efficient influence curve equals the sum of the two scores D^*_Y and D^*_W. Either way, the derivative condition is satisfied:

$$\langle \frac{d}{d\epsilon} L(Q^0_n(\epsilon))\Big|_{\epsilon=0} \rangle \supset D^*(Q^0_n, g_n), \tag{5.2}$$

where $D^*(Q_n^0, g_n) = D_Y^*(Q_n^0, g_n) + D_W^*(Q_n^0, g_n)$. Here we used the notation $\langle (h_1, \ldots, h_k) \rangle$ for the linear space consisting of all linear combinations of the functions $h_1, \ldots, h_k$. That is, the task of obtaining a loss function and parametric working model for fluctuating Q_n^0 so that the derivative condition holds has been completed.

Due to this property (5.2) of the parametric working model, the TMLE has the important feature that it solves the efficient influence curve equation $0 = \sum_i D^*(Q_n^*, g_n)(O_i)$ (also called the efficient score equation). Why is this true? Because at the next iteration of TMLE, the parametric maximum likelihood estimator $\epsilon_n = 0$, and a parametric maximum likelihood estimator solves its score equation, which exactly yields this efficient score equation. This is a strong feature of the procedure as it implies that TMLE is double robust and (locally) efficient under regularity conditions. In other words, TMLE is consistent and asymptotically linear if either Q_n or g_n is a consistent estimator, and if both estimators are asymptotically consistent, then TMLE is asymptotically efficient.

However, if one uses a separate ϵ_W and ϵ for the two parametric working models through $Q_{W,n}^0$ and $\bar{Q}_n^0$, respectively, then the maximum likelihood estimator of ϵ_W equals zero, showing that TMLE will only update $\bar{Q}_n^0$. Therefore, it was never necessary to update the part of Q_n^0 that was already nonparametrically estimated.

If the initial estimator of $Q_{W,0}$ is a nonparametric maximum likelihood estimator, then the TMLE does not update this part of the initial estimator Q_n^0.

Of course, we have not been explicit yet about how to construct this submodel $\bar{Q}_n^0(\epsilon)$ through $\bar{Q}_n^0$. For that purpose, we now note that $D_Y^*(Q_n^0, g_n)$ equals a function $H_n^*(A, W)$ times the residual $(Y - \bar{Q}_n^0(A, W))$, where

$$H_n^*(A, W) \equiv \left(\frac{I(A = 1)}{g_n(A = 1 \mid W)} - \frac{I(A = 0)}{g_n(A = 0 \mid W)} \right).$$

Here $I(A = 1)$ is an indicator variable that takes the value 1 when $A = 1$. One can see that for $A = 1$ the second term disappears, and for $A = 0$ the first term disappears.

It can be shown (and it is a classical result for parametric logistic main term regression in a parametric statistical model) that the score of a coefficient in front of a covariate in a logistic linear regression in a parametric statistical model for a conditional distribution of a binary Y equals the covariate times the residual. Therefore, we can select the following parametric working model for fluctuating the initial estimate of the conditional probability distribution of Y, given (A, W), or, equivalently, for the estimate of the probability of $Y = 1$, given (A, W):

$$\bar{Q}_n^0(\epsilon)(Y = 1 \mid A, W) = \frac{1}{1 + \exp\left(-\log \frac{\bar{Q}_n^0}{(1 - \bar{Q}_n^0)}(A, W) - \epsilon H_n^*(A, W)\right)}.$$

By this classical result, it follows that indeed the score of ϵ of this univariate logistic regression submodel at $\epsilon = 0$ equals $D^*_Y(Q^0_n, g_n)$. That is, we now have really fully succeeded in finding a parametric submodel through the initial estimator Q^0_n that satisfies the required derivative condition. Since $H^*_n(A, W)$ now just plays the role of a covariate in a logistic regression, using an offset, this explains why we call the covariate $H^*_n(A, W)$ a clever covariate.

More on constructing the submodel. If one needs a submodel through an initial estimator of a conditional distribution of a binary variable Y, given a set of parent variables $Pa(Y)$, and it needs to have a particular score D^*_Y, then one can define this submodel as a univariate logistic regression model, using the initial estimator as offset, with univariate clever covariate defined as $H^*(Pa(Y)) = E(D^*_Y \mid Y = 1, Pa(Y)) - E(D^*_Y \mid Y = 0, Pa(Y))$. Application of this general result to the above setting yields the clever covariate $H^*(A, W)$ presented above.

If our goal was to target $P_0(Y_1 = 1)$ or $P_0(Y_0 = 1)$, then going through the same protocol for the TMLE shows that one would use as clever covariate

$$H^*_{0,n}(A, W) \equiv \left(\frac{I(A = 0)}{g_n(A = 0 \mid W)}\right) \text{ or } H^*_{1,n}(A, W) \equiv \left(\frac{I(A = 1)}{g_n(A = 1 \mid W)}\right).$$

By targeting these two parameters simultaneously, using a two-dimensional clever covariate with coefficients ϵ_1, ϵ_2, one automatically obtains a valid TMLE for parameters that are functions of these two marginal counterfactual probabilities, such as a causal relative risk and causal odds ratio.

By computing the TMLE that targets a multidimensional target parameter, one also obtains a valid TMLE for any (say) univariate summary measure of the multidimensional target parameter. By valid we mean that this TMLE will still satisfy the same asymptotic properties, such as efficiency and double robustness, as the TMLE that directly targets the particular summary measure. The TMLE that targets the univariate summary measure of the multidimensional parameter may have a better finite sample performance than the TMLE that targets the whole multidimensional target parameter, in particular, if the dimension of the multidimensional parameter is large.

5.2.5 Updating $\bar{Q}^0_n$

We first perform a logistic linear regression of Y on $H^*_n(A, W)$ where $\bar{Q}^0_n(A, W)$ is held fixed (i.e., used as an offset), and an additional intercept is suppressed in order to estimate the coefficient in front of $H^*_n(A, W)$, denoted ϵ. The TMLE procedure is then able to incorporate information from g_n, through $H_n^*(A, W)$, into an updated regression. It does this by extracting ϵ_n, the maximum likelihood estimator of ϵ, from the fit described above, and updating the estimate $\bar{Q}_n^0$ according to the logistic regression working model. This updated regression is then given by $\bar{Q}_n^1$:

$$\text{logit } \bar{Q}_n^1(A, W) = \text{logit } \bar{Q}_n^0(A, W) + \epsilon_n H_n^*(A, W).$$

One iterates this updating process until the next $\epsilon_n = 0$ or has converged to zero, but, in this example, convergence is achieved in one step. The TMLE of Q_0 is now $Q_n^* = (Q_{W,n}^0, \bar{Q}_n^1)$. Note that this step is equivalent to $(\epsilon_{1n}, \epsilon_{2n}) = \arg\min_{\epsilon_1,\epsilon_2} \sum_i L(Q_n^0(\epsilon_1, \epsilon_2))(O_i)$, and setting $Q_n^1 = Q_n^0(\epsilon_{1n}, \epsilon_{2n})$, where, as noted above, $\epsilon_{1n} = 0$, so that only $\bar{Q}_n^0$ is updated.

Given a parametric working model $Q_n^0(\epsilon)$ with fluctuation parameter ϵ, and a loss function $L(Q)$ satisfying (5.2), the first-step TMLE is defined by determining the minimum ϵ_n^0 of $\sum_{i=1}^n L(Q_n^0(\epsilon))(O_i)$ and setting $Q_n^1 = Q_n^0(\epsilon_n^0)$. This updating process is iterated until convergence of $\epsilon_n^k = \arg\min_\epsilon \sum_{i=1}^n L(Q_n^k(\epsilon))$ to zero, and the final update Q_n^* is referred to as the TMLE of Q_0. In this case, the next $\epsilon_n^1 = 0$, so that convergence is achieved in one step and $Q_n^* = Q_n^1$.

5.2.6 Estimating the Target Parameter

The estimate $\bar{Q}_n^* = \bar{Q}_n^1$ obtained in the previous step is now plugged into our target parameter mapping, together with the empirical distribution of W, resulting in the targeted substitution estimator given by

$$\psi_n = \Psi(Q_n^*) = \frac{1}{n}\sum_{i=1}^n \{\bar{Q}_n^1(1, W_i) - \bar{Q}_n^1(0, W_i)\}.$$

This mapping is accomplished by evaluating $\bar{Q}_n^1(1, W_i)$ and $\bar{Q}_n^1(0, W_i)$ for each observation i and plugging these values into the above equation.

5.2.7 Calculating Standard Errors

The calculation of standard errors for TMLE can be based on the central limit theorem, relying on δ-method conditions. (See Appendix A for an advanced introduction to these topics.) Under such regularity conditions, the asymptotic behavior of the estimator, that is, its asymptotic normal limit distribution, is completely characterized by the so-called influence curve of the estimator in question. In our example, we need to know the influence curve of the TMLE of its estimand.

Note that, in order to recognize that an estimator is a random variable, an estimator should be represented as a mapping from the data into the parameter space, where the data $O_1, \ldots, O_n$ can be represented by the empirical probability distribution function P_n. Therefore, let $\hat{\Psi}(P_n)$ be the TMLE described above. Since the TMLE is a substitution estimator, we have $\hat{\Psi}(P_n) = \Psi(P_n^*)$ for a targeted estimator P_n^* of P_0. An estimator $\hat{\Psi}(P_n)$ of ψ_0 is asymptotically linear with influence curve $IC(O)$ if it satisfies:

$$\sqrt{n}(\hat{\Psi}(P_n) - \psi_0) = \frac{1}{\sqrt{n}} \sum_{i=1}^{n} IC(O_i) + o_{P_0}(1).$$

Here the remainder term, denoted by $o_{P_0}(1)$, is a random variable that converges to zero in probability when the sample size converges to infinity. The influence curve $IC(O)$ is a random variable with mean zero under P_0.

More on estimators and the influence curve. An estimator $\hat{\Psi}(P_n)$ is a function $\hat{\Psi}$ of the empirical probability distribution function P_n. Specifically, one can express the estimator as a function $\hat{\Psi}$ of a large family of empirical means $1/n \sum_{i=1}^n f(O_i)$ of functions f of O varying over a class of functions $\mathcal{F}$. We say the estimator is a function of $P_n = (P_n f : f \in \mathcal{F})$, where we use the notation $P_n f \equiv 1/n \sum_{i=1}^n f(O_i)$. By proving that the estimator is a differentiable function $\hat{\Psi}$ of $P_n = (P_n f : f \in \mathcal{F})$ at $P_0 = (P_0 f : f \in \mathcal{F})$, and that a uniform central limit theorem applies to P_n based on empirical process theory, it follows that the estimator minus its estimand $\psi_0 = \hat{\Psi}(P_0)$ behaves in first order as an empirical mean of $IC(O_i)$: we write $\hat{\Psi}(P_n) - \psi_0 = (P_n - P_0)IC + o_P(1/\sqrt{n})$. This function $IC(O)$ is called the influence curve of the estimator, and it is uniquely determined by the derivative of $\hat{\Psi}$. Specifically, $IC(O) = \sum_{f \in \mathcal{F}} \frac{d}{dP_0 f} \hat{\Psi}((P_0 f : f)(f(O) - P_0 f)$, where, formally, the $\sum$ becomes an integral when $\mathcal{F}$ is not finite.

Asymptotic linearity is a desirable property as it indicates that the estimator behaves like an empirical mean, and, as a consequence, its bias converges to zero in sample size at a rate faster than $1/\sqrt{n}$, and, for n large enough, it is approximately normally distributed. The influence curve of an estimator evaluated as a function in O measures how robust the estimator is toward extreme values. The influence curve $IC(O)$ has mean zero under sampling from the true probability distribution P_0, and its (finite) variance is the asymptotic variance of the standardized estimator $\sqrt{n}(\hat{\Psi}(P_n) - \psi_0)$.

In other words, the variance of $\hat{\Psi}(P_n)$ is well approximated by the variance of the influence curve, divided by sample size n. If ψ_0 is multivariate, then the covariance matrix of $\hat{\Psi}(P_n)$ is well approximated by the covariance matrix of the multivariate influence curve divided by sample size n. More importantly, the probability distribution of $\hat{\Psi}(P_n)$ is well approximated by a normal distribution with mean ψ_0 and the covariance matrix of the influence curve, divided by sample size.

An estimator is asymptotically efficient if its influence curve is equal to the efficient influence curve, $IC(O) = D^*(O)$. The influence curve of the TMLE indeed equals D^* if Q_n^* is a consistent estimator of Q_0, and g_n is a consistent estimator of g_0. A complete technical understanding of influence curve derivation is not necessary to implement the TMLE procedure. However, we provide Appendix A for a detailed methodology for deriving the influence curve of an estimator.

More on asymptotic linearity and efficiency. The TMLE is a consistent estimator of ψ_0 if either $\bar{Q}_n$ is consistent for $\bar{Q}_0$ or g_n is consistent for g_0. The TMLE is asymptotically linear under additional conditions. For a detailed theorem establishing asymptotic linearity and efficiency of the TMLE, we refer the reader to Chap. 27. In particular, if for some $\delta > 0$, $\delta < g_0(1 \mid W) < 1 - \delta$, and the product of the L^2-norm of $\bar{Q}_n - \bar{Q}_0$ and the L^2-norm of $g_n - g_0$ converges to zero at faster rate than $1/\sqrt{n}$, then the TMLE is asymptotically efficient. If g_n is a consistent estimator of g_0, then the influence curve of the TMLE $\hat{\Psi}(P_n)$ equals $IC = D^*(Q^*, g_0) - \Pi(D^*(Q^*, g_0) \mid T_g)$, the efficient influence curve at the possibly misspecified limit of Q_n^* minus its projection on the tangent space of the model for the treatment mechanism g_0. The projection term makes $D^*(Q^*, g_0)$ a conservative working influence curve, and the projection term equals zero if either $Q^* = Q_0$ or g_0 was known and $g_n = g_0$.

From these formal asymptotic linearity results for the TMLE it follows that if g_n is a consistent estimator of g_0, then the TMLE $\hat{\Psi}(P_n)$ is asymptotically linear with an influence curve that can be conservatively approximated by $D^*(Q^*, g_0)$, where Q^* denotes the possibly misspecified estimand of Q_n^*. If g_0 was known, as in a randomized controlled trial, and g_n was not estimated, then the influence curve of the TMLE equals $D^*(Q^*, g_0)$. If, on the other hand, g_n was estimated under a correctly specified model for g_0, then the influence curve of the TMLE has a smaller variance than the variance of $D^*(Q^*, g_0)$, except if $Q^* = Q_0$, in which case the influence curve of the TMLE equals the efficient influence curve $D^*(Q_0, g_0)$. As a consequence, we can use as a working estimated influence curve for the TMLE

$$IC_n(O) = \left(\frac{I(A=1)}{g_n(1 \mid W)} - \frac{I(A=0)}{g_n(0 \mid W)}\right)(Y - \bar{Q}_n^1(A, W)) + \bar{Q}_n^1(1, W) - \bar{Q}_n^1(0, W) - \psi_n.$$

Even if $\bar{Q}_n^1$ is inconsistent, but g_n is consistent, this influence curve can be used to obtain an asymptotically *conservative* estimator of the variance of the TMLE

$\hat{\Psi}(P_n)$. This is very convenient since the TMLE requires calculation of $D^*(Q_n^*, g_n)$, and apparently we can use the latter as influence curve to estimate the normal limit distribution of the TMLE.

If one assumes that g_n is a consistent maximum-likelihood-based estimator of g_0, then one can (asymptotically) conservatively estimate the variance of the TMLE with the sample variance of the estimated efficient influence curve $D^*(Q_n^*, g_n)$.

An estimate of the asymptotic variance of the standardized TMLE, $\sqrt{n}(\hat{\Psi}(P_n)-\psi_0)$, viewed as a random variable, using the estimate of the influence curve $IC_n(O)$ is thereby given by

$$\sigma_n^2 = \frac{1}{n}\sum_{i=1}^{n} IC_n^2(o_i).$$

5.3 Foundation and Philosophy of TMLE

TMLE in semiparametric statistical models for P_0 is the extension of maximum likelihood estimation in parametric statistical models. Three key ingredients are needed for this extension. Firstly, one needs to define the parameter of interest semiparametrically as a function of the data-generating distribution varying over the (large) semiparametric statistical model. Many practitioners are used to thinking of their parameter in terms of a regression coefficient, but that luxury is not available in semi- or nonparametric statistical models. Instead, one has to carefully think of what feature of the distribution of the data one wishes to target.

Secondly, one needs to estimate the true distribution P_0, or at least its relevant factor or portion as needed to evaluate the target parameter, and this estimate should respect the actual semiparametric statistical model. As a consequence, nonparametric maximum likelihood estimation is often ill defined or results in a complete overfit, and thereby results in estimators of the target parameter that are too variable. We discussed this issue in Chap. 3. The theoretical results obtained for the cross-validation selector (discrete super learner) inspired the general super learning methodology for estimation of probability distributions of the data, or factors of other high-dimensional parameters of the probability distributions of the data. In the sequel, a reference to a true probability distribution of the data is meant to refer to this relevant part of the true probability distribution of the data. This super learning methodology takes as input a collection of candidate estimators of the distribution of the data and then uses cross-validation to determine the best weighted combination of these estimators. It is assumed or arranged that the loss function is uniformly bounded so that oracle results for the cross-validation selector apply. The super learning methodology results now in an estimator of the distribution of the data that will be used as an initial estimator in the TMLE procedure. The oracle results for this super learner teach us that the initial estimator is optimized with respect to a global loss function such as the log-likelihood loss function and is thereby not targeted toward the target parameter, $\Psi(P_0)$. That is, it will be too biased for $\Psi(P_0)$ due to a bias–variance tradeoff with respect to the more ambitious full P_0 (or relevant portion thereof) instead of having used a bias–variance tradeoff with respect to $\Psi(P_0)$. The targeted maximum likelihood step is tailored to remove bias due to the nontargeting of the initial estimator.

The targeted maximum likelihood step involves now updating this initial (super-learning-based) estimator P_n^0 of P_0 to tailor its fit to estimation of the target ψ_0, the value of the parameter $\Psi(P_0)$. This is carried out by determining a cleverly chosen parametric working model modeling fluctuations $P_n^0(\epsilon)$ of the initial estimator P_n^0 with a (say) univariate fluctuation parameter ϵ. The value $\epsilon = 0$ corresponds with no fluctuation so that $P_n^0(0) = P_n^0$. One now estimates ϵ with maximum likelihood estimation, treating the initial estimator as a fixed offset, and updates the initial estimator accordingly. If needed, this updating step is iterated to convergence, and the final update P_n^* is called the TMLE of P_0, while the resulting substitution estimator $\hat{\Psi}(P_n^*)$ of $\Psi(P_0)$ is the TMLE of ψ_0. This targeted maximum likelihood step thus uses a parametric maximum likelihood estimator, accordingly to a cleverly chosen parametric working model that includes the initial estimator, to obtain a bias reduction for the target $\Psi(P_0)$.

This is not just any parametric working model. That is, we wish to select a parametric working model such that the parametric maximum likelihood estimator is maximally effective in removing bias for the target parameter, at minimal increase in variance. So if ϵ_n is the parametric maximum likelihood estimator of ϵ, then we want the mean squared error of $\Psi(P_n^0(\epsilon_n)) - \psi_0$ to be as small as possible. We want this parametric working model to really listen to the information in the data that is relevant for the target parameter. In fact, we would like the parametric maximum likelihood estimator to be as responsive to the information in the data that is relevant for the target parameter as an estimator that is asymptotically efficient in the semiparametric model.

To get insight into what kind of choice of parametric working model may be as adaptive to such target-parameter-specific features in the data as a semiparametric efficient estimator, we make the following observations. Suppose one is interested in determining the parametric working model coding fluctuations $P_0(\epsilon)$ of P_0 so that the maximum likelihood estimator of $\psi_0 = \Psi(P_0(\epsilon = 0))$ according to this parametric working model is asymptotically equivalent to an efficient estimator in the large semiparametric model. Note that this parametric working model is not told that the true value of ϵ equals zero. It happens to be the case that from an asymptotic efficiency perspective this can be achieved as follows. Among all possible parametric working models that code fluctuations $P_0(\epsilon)$ of the true P_0 we chose the one for which the Cramer–Rao lower bound for the target parameter $\Psi(P_0(\epsilon))$ at $\epsilon = 0$ is equivalent to the semiparametric information bound for the target parameter at P_0. The Cramer–Rao lower bound for a parametric working model $P_0(\epsilon)$ is given by

$$\frac{\left\{\frac{d}{d\epsilon}\Psi(P_0(\epsilon))\Big|_{\epsilon=0}\right\}^2}{I(0)},$$

where $I(0)$ denotes the variance of the score of the parametric working model at $\epsilon = 0$. In parametric model theory $I(0)$ is called the information at parameter value 0. The semiparametric information bound for the target parameter at P_0 is defined as the supremum over all these possible Cramer–Rao lower bounds for the parametric working models. That is, the semiparametric information bound is defined as the Cramer–Rao lower bound for the hardest parametric working model. Thus, the parametric working model for which the parametric maximum likelihood estimator is as responsive to the data with respect to the target parameter as a semiparametric efficient estimator is actually given by this hardest parametric working model. Indeed, the TMLE selects this hardest parametric working model, but through P_n^0.

Note also that this hardest working parametric model can also be interpreted as the one that maximizes the change of the target parameter relative to a change $P_0(\epsilon) - P_0$ under small amounts of fluctuations. Thus this hardest working parametric model through an initial estimator P_n^0 will maximize the change of the target parameter relative to the initial value $\Psi(P_n^0)$ for small values of ϵ.

Beyond the practical appeal of this TMLE update that uses the parametric likelihood to fit the target parameter of interest, an important feature of the TMLE is that it solves the efficient influence curve equation, also called the efficient score equation, of the target parameter. We refer the reader to Sect. 5.2 and Appendix A for relevant material on the efficient influence curve. For now, it suffices to know that an estimator is semiparametric efficient if the estimator minus the true target parameter behaves as an empirical mean of $D^*(P_0)(O_i)$, $i = 1, \ldots, n$, showing the incredible importance of this transformation $D^*(P_0)$ of O, which somehow captures all the relevant information of O for the sake of learning the statistical parameter $\Psi(P_0)$. If $D^*(P)(O)$ is the efficient influence curve at P, a possible probability distribution for O in the statistical model, and P_n^* is the TMLE of P_0, then, $0 = \sum_{i=1}^n D^*(P_n^*)(O_i)$.

Just as a parametric maximum likelihood estimator solves a score equation by virtue of its maximizing the likelihood over the unknown parameters, a TMLE solves the target-parameter-specific score equation for the target parameter by virtue of maximizing the likelihood in a targeted direction. This can then be used to establish that the TMLE is asymptotically efficient if the initial estimator is consistent and remarkably robust in the sense that for many data structures and semiparametric statistical models, the TMLE of ψ_0 remains consistent even if the initial estimator is inconsistent. By using submodels that have a multivariate fluctuation parameter ϵ, the TMLE will solve the score equation implied by each component of ϵ. In this manner, one can obtain TMLEs that solve not only the efficient influence curve/efficient score equation for the target parameter, but also an equation that characterizes other interesting properties, such as being an imputation estimator (Gruber and van der Laan 2010a).

In particular, in semiparametric models used to define causal effect parameters, the TMLE is a double robust estimator. In such semiparametric models the probability distribution function P_0 can be factorized as $P_0(O) = Q_0(O)g_0(O)$, where g_0

is the treatment mechanism and Q_0 is the relevant factor that defines the g-formula for the counterfactual distributions. The TMLE $\Psi(Q_n^*)$ of $\psi_0 = \Psi(Q_0)$ is consistent if either Q_n^* or g_n is consistent. In our example, g_n is the estimator of the treatment mechanism $g_0(A \mid W) = P_0(A \mid W)$, and Q_n^* is the TMLE of Q_0.

5.4 Summary

TMLE of a parameter $\Psi(Q_0)$ distinguishes from nonparametric or regularized maximum likelihood estimation by fully utilizing the power of cross-validation (super learning) to fine-tune the bias–variance tradeoff with respect to the part Q_0 of the data-generating distribution, thereby increasing adaptivity to the true Q_0, and by targeting the fit to remove bias with respect to ψ_0. The loss-based super learner of Q_0 already outperforms with respect to bias and variance a regularized maximum likelihood estimator for the semiparametric statistical model with respect to estimation of Q_0 itself by its asymptotic equivalence to the oracle selector: one could include the regularized maximum likelihood estimator in the collection of algorithms for the super learner. Just due to using the loss-based super learner it already achieves higher rates of convergence for Q_0 itself, thereby improving both in bias and variance for Q_0 as well as $\Psi(Q_0)$. In addition, due to the targeting step, which again utilizes super learning for estimation of the required g_0 in the fluctuation function, it is less biased for ψ_0 than the initial loss-function-based super learner estimator, and, as a bonus, the statistical inference based on the central limit theorem is also heavily improved relative to just using a nontargeted regularized maximum likelihood estimator.

Overall it comes down to the following: the TMLE is a semiparametric efficient substitution estimator. This means it fully utilizes all the information in the data (super learning and asymptotic efficiency), in addition to fully using knowledge about global constraints implied by the statistical semiparametric statistical model $\mathcal{M}$ and the target parameter mapping (by being a substitution estimator), thereby making it robust under sparsity with respect to the target parameter. It fully incorporates the power of super learning for the benefit of getting closer to the truth in finite samples.

Chapter 6
Why TMLE?

Sherri Rose, Mark J. van der Laan

In the previous five chapters, we covered the targeted learning road map. This included presentation of the tools necessary to estimate causal effect parameters of a data-generating distribution. We illustrated these methods with a simple data structure: $O = (W, A, Y) \sim P_0$. Our target parameter for this example was $\Psi(P_0) = E_{W,0}[E_0(Y \mid A = 1, W) - E_0(Y \mid A = 0, W)]$, which represents the causal risk difference under causal assumptions.

Throughout these chapters, the case for TMLE using super learning is compelling, but many of its properties have not been fully discussed, especially in comparison to other estimators. This chapter makes a comprehensive case for TMLE based on statistical properties and compares TMLE to maximum-likelihood-based substitution estimators of the g-formula (MLE) and estimating-equation-based methodology. We continue to refer to the simple data structure $O = (W, A, Y) \sim P_0$ and causal risk difference as the target parameter in some comparisons, but also discuss the performance of TMLE and other estimators globally, considering many target parameters and data structures.

As we introduced in Chaps. 4 and 5, TMLE has many attractive properties that make it preferable to other existing procedures for estimation of a target parameter of a data-generating distribution for arbitrary semiparametric statistical models. TMLE removes all the asymptotic residual bias of the initial estimator for the target parameter if it uses a consistent estimator of the treatment mechanism. If the initial estimator is already consistent for the target parameter, the minimal additional fitting of the data in the targeting step may potentially remove some finite sample bias and certainly preserve this consistency property of the initial estimator. As a consequence, TMLE is a so-called double robust estimator.

In addition, if the initial estimator and the estimator of the treatment mechanism are both consistent, then it is also asymptotically efficient according to semiparametric statistical model efficiency theory. That is, under this condition, other competing estimators will underperform in comparison for large enough sample sizes with respect to variance, assuming that the competitors are required to have a bias for the target parameter smaller than $1/\sqrt{n}$ across a neighborhood of distributions of the true P_0 that shrinks to P_0 at this same rate $1/\sqrt{n}$. It allows the incorporation of machine learning (i.e., super learning) methods for the estimation of both the relevant part of P_0 and the nuisance parameter g_0 required for the targeting step, so that we do not make assumptions about the probability distribution P_0 we do not believe. In this manner, every effort is made to achieve minimal bias and the asymptotic semiparametric efficiency bound for the variance. We further explain these issues in the pages that follow.

Portions of this chapter are technical, but a general understanding of the essential concepts can be gleaned from reading the introduction to each of the sections and the tables at the end of each section. For example, Sect. 6.1 explains that there are two general types of estimators and provides a list of various estimators that may be familiar to the reader. Similarly, Sects. 6.2–6.6 discuss properties of TMLE: it is a loss-based, well-defined, unbiased, efficient substitution estimator of target parameters of a data-generating distribution. The introductions explain these concepts and the closing tables summarize these properties among competing estimators and TMLE. Therefore, a strong math background is not required to understand the basic concepts, and some readers may find it useful to skim or skip certain subsections.

6.1 Landscape

In order to effectively establish the benefits of TMLE, we must enumerate competing estimators. For example, what are our competitors for the estimation of causal effect parameters, such as $E_0Y_1 - E_0Y_0$, as well as other target parameters? We group these estimators into two broad classes: MLE and estimating equation methodology. For each specific estimation problem, one can come up with a number of variations of an estimator in such a class. In Chaps. 7 and 21, among others, we provide a finite sample comparison of TMLE with a number of estimators, including estimators specifically tailored for this simple data structure. Recall that the conditional expectation of Y given (A, W) is denoted $E_0(Y \mid A, W) \equiv \bar{Q}_0(A, W)$. Additionally, we let $Q_n = (\bar{Q}_n, Q_{W,n})$ be the estimate of the conditional mean and the empirical distribution for the marginal distribution of W, representing the estimator of the true $Q_0 = (\bar{Q}_0, Q_W)$.

6.1.1 MLE

A maximum likelihood estimator for a parametric statistical model $\{p_\theta : \theta\}$ is defined as a maximizer over all densities in the parametric statistical model of the empirical mean of the log density:

$$\theta_n = \arg\max_\theta \sum_{i=1}^{n} \log p_\theta(O_i).$$

The $L(p)(O) = -\log p(O)$ is called a loss function at candidate density p for the true density p_0 since its expectation is minimized across all densities p by the true density $p = p_0$. This minimization property of the log-likelihood loss function is the principle behind maximum likelihood estimation providing the basis for establishing that maximum likelihood estimators for correctly specified statistical models approximate the true distribution P_0 for large sample size.

An estimator that is based on maximizing the log-likelihood over the whole statistical model or submodels of the statistical model or utilizes algorithms that involve maximization of the log-likelihood will be called a maximum-likelihood-based estimator. We use the abbreviation MLE to refer specifically to maximum-likelihood-based substitution estimators of the g-formula.

This chapter can be equally applied to the case where $L(p)(O)$ is replaced by any other loss function $L(Q)$ for a relevant part Q_0 of p_0, satisfying that $E_0 L(Q_0)(O) \leq E_0 L(Q)(O)$ for each possible Q. In that case, we might call this estimator a minimum-loss-based estimator. TMLE incorporates this case as well, in which it could be called targeted minimum-loss-based estimation (still abbreviated as TMLE). In this chapter we focus our comparison on the log-likelihood loss function and will thereby refer to MLE, including ML-based super learning.

The g-formula was previously discussed in Chaps. 1–4. Recall that uppercase letters represent random variables and lowercase letters are a specific value for that variable. $\Psi(P_0)$ for the causal risk difference can be written as the g-formula:

$$\Psi(P_0) = \sum_w \Big[\sum_y y P_0(Y = y \mid A = 1, W = w) - \sum_y y P_0(Y = y \mid A = 0, W = w) \Big] P_0(W = w), \tag{6.1}$$

where

$$P_0(Y = y \mid A = a, W = w) = \frac{P_0(W = w, A = a, Y = y)}{\sum_y P_0(W = w, A = a, Y = y)}$$

is the conditional probability distribution of $Y = y$, given $A = a$, $W = w$, and

$$P_0(W = w) = \sum_{y,a} P_0(W = w, A = a, Y = y).$$

Recall that our target parameter only depends on P_0 through the conditional mean $\bar{Q}_0(A, W) = E_0(Y \mid A, W)$ and the marginal distribution Q_W of W; thus we can also write $\Psi(Q_0)$.

Maximum-likelihood-based substitution estimators of the g-formula are obtained by substitution of a maximum-likelihood-based estimator of Q_0 into the parameter mapping $\Psi(Q_0)$. The marginal distribution of W can be estimated with the nonparametric maximum likelihood estimator, which happens to be the empirical distribution that puts mass $1/n$ on each W_i, $i = 1, \ldots, n$. In other words, we estimate the expectation over W with the empirical mean over W_i, $i = 1, \ldots, n$. Maximum-likelihood-based estimation of $\bar{Q}_0$ can range from the use of stratification to super learning. We introduced nonparametric estimation of $\bar{Q}_0$ in Chap. 3. Maximum-likelihood-based substitution estimators will be of the type

$$\psi_n = \Psi(Q_n) = \frac{1}{n} \sum_{i=1}^{n} \{\bar{Q}_n(1, W_i) - \bar{Q}_n(0, W_i)\}, \tag{6.2}$$

where this estimate is obtained by plugging in $Q_n = (\bar{Q}_n, Q_{W,n})$ into the mapping Ψ.

MLE using stratification. The simplest maximum likelihood estimator of $\bar{Q}_0$ stratifies by categories or possible values for (A, W). One then simply averages across the many categories (also called bins or treatment/covariate combinations). In most data sets, there will be a large number of categories with few or zero observations. One might refer to this as the curse of dimensionality, making the MLE for nonparametric statistical models typically ill defined, and an overfit to the data resulting in poor finite sample performance. One can refer to this estimator as the nonparametric MLE (NPMLE).

MLE after dimension reduction: propensity score methods. To deal with the curse of dimensionality, one might propose a dimension reduction W^r of W and apply the simple MLE to the reduced-data structure (W^r, A, Y). However, such a dimension reduction could easily result in a biased estimator of $\Psi(Q_0)$ by excluding confounders. One can show that a sufficient confounder is given by the propensity score $g_0(1 \mid W) = P_0(A = 1 \mid W)$, allowing one to reduce the dimension of W to only a single covariate, without inducing bias. A maximum likelihood estimator of $E_0(Y \mid A, W^r)$ can then be applied, where $W^r = g_0(1 \mid W)$, using stratification. For example, one creates five categories for the propensity score, thereby creating a total of ten categories for (A, W^r), and estimates $E_0(Y \mid A, W^r)$ with the empirical average of the outcomes within each category. Of course, this propensity score is typically unknown and will thus first need to be estimated from the data.

MLE using regression in a parametric working model. $\bar{Q}_0(A, W)$ is estimated using regression in a parametric working (statistical) model and plugged into the formula given in (6.2).

ML-based super learning. We estimate $\bar{Q}_0$ with the super learner, in which the collection of estimators may include stratified maximum likelihood estimators, maximum likelihood estimators based on dimension reductions implied by the propensity score, and maximum likelihood estimators based on parametric working models, beyond many other machine learning algorithms for estimation of $\bar{Q}_0$. Super learning requires a choice of loss function. If the loss function is a log-likelihood loss, $L(P_0)(O) = -\log p_0(O)$, then we would call this maximum-likelihood-based super learning. However, one might use a loss function for the relevant part $\bar{Q}_0$ that is not necessarily a log-likelihood loss, in which case we should call it minimum-loss-based super learning. For example, if Y is a continuous random variable with outcomes in $[0, 1]$, then one can select as loss function for $\bar{Q}_0$ the following function:

$$L(\bar{Q}_0)(O) = -Y \log \bar{Q}_0(A, W) + (1 - Y) \log(1 - \bar{Q}_0(A, W)),$$

which indeed satisfies that the expectation $E_0 L(\bar{Q})(O)$ is minimized by $\bar{Q} = \bar{Q}_0$. This loss function is an example of a loss function that is not a log-likelihood loss function. In this chapter we will not stress this additional important gain in generality of loss-based super learning relative to maximum-likelihood-based estimation, allowing us to proceed directly after the relevant parts of the distribution of P_0 required for evaluation of our target parameter $\Psi(P_0)$.

6.1.2 Estimating Equation Methods

Estimating-equation-based methodology for estimation of our target parameter $\Psi(P_0)$ includes inverse probability of treatment-weighted (IPTW) estimators and augmented IPTW (A-IPTW) estimators. These methods aim to solve an estimating equation in candidate ψ-values. An estimating function is a function of the data O and the parameter of interest. If $D(\psi)(O)$ is an estimating function, then we can define a corresponding estimating equation:

$$0 = \sum_{i=1}^{n} D(\psi)(O_i),$$

and solution ψ_n satisfying $\sum_{i=1}^{n} D(\psi_n)(O_i) = 0$. Most estimating functions for ψ will also depend on an unknown "nuisance" parameter of P_0. So we might define the estimating function as $D(\psi, \eta)$, where η is a candidate for the nuisance parameter. Given an estimator η_n of the required true nuisance parameter η_0 of P_0, we would define the estimating equation as

$$0 = \sum_{i=1}^{n} D(\psi, \eta_n)(O_i),$$

with solution ψ_n satisfying $\sum_{i=1}^{n} D(\psi_n, \eta_n)(O_i) = 0$. The theory of estimating functions teaches us that for each semiparametric statistical model and each target parameter, a class of estimating functions can be mathematically derived in terms of the gradients of the pathwise derivative of the target parameter, and the optimal estimating function that may yield an estimator with minimal asymptotic variance needs to be defined by the efficient influence curve (also called canonical gradient of the pathwise derivative) of the target parameter.

When the notation $D^*(\psi_0, \eta_0)$ is used for the estimating function $D(\psi_0, \eta_0)$, $D^*(\psi_0, \eta_0)$ is an estimating function implied by the efficient influence curve. An efficient influence curve is $D^*(P_0)(O)$, i.e., a function of O, but determined by P_0, and may be abbreviated $D^*(P_0)$ or $D^*(O)$. An optimal estimating function is one such that $D(\psi_0, \eta_0) = D^*(P_0)$.

For estimation of the causal risk difference, the following are two popular examples of estimating-equation-based methods, where the A-IPTW estimator is based on the estimating function implied by the efficient influence curve.

IPTW. One estimates our target parameter, the causal risk difference $\Psi(P_0)$, with

$$\psi_n = \frac{1}{n}\sum_{i=1}^{n}\{I(A_i = 1) - I(A_i = 0)\}\frac{Y_i}{g_n(A_i, W_i)}.$$

This estimator is a solution of an IPTW estimating equation that relies on an estimate of the treatment mechanism, playing the role of a nuisance parameter of the IPTW estimating function.

A-IPTW. One estimates $\Psi(P_0)$ with

$$\psi_n = \frac{1}{n}\sum_{i=1}^{n}\frac{\{I(A_i = 1) - I(A_i = 0)\}}{g_n(A_i, W_i)}(Y_i - \bar{Q}_n(A_i, W_i))$$
$$+ \frac{1}{n}\sum_{i=1}^{n}\{\bar{Q}_n(1, W_i) - \bar{Q}_n(0, W_i)\}.$$

This estimator is a solution of the A-IPTW estimating equation that relies on an estimate of the treatment mechanism g_0 and the conditional mean $\bar{Q}_0$. Thus $(g_0, \bar{Q}_0)$ plays the role of the nuisance parameter of the A-IPTW estimating function. The A-IPTW estimating function evaluated at the true $(g_0, \bar{Q}_0)$ and true ψ_0 actually equals the efficient influence curve at the true data-generating distribution P_0, making it an optimal estimating function.

6.2 TMLE is Based on (Targeted) Loss-Based Learning

Suppose one is given a loss function $L()$ for a parameter $Q_0 = Q(P_0)$ while the estimand ψ_0 of interest is determined by Q_0. Thus, $Q_0 = \arg\min_Q E_0 L(Q)(O)$, where the minimum is taken over all possible parameter values of Q. One can proceed by defining a collection of candidate estimators $\hat{Q}_k$ that map the data P_n into an estimate of Q_0, where such estimators can be based on aiming to minimize the expected loss $Q \rightarrow E_0 L(Q)(O)$. This family of estimators can be used as a library of the loss-based super learner, which will use cross-validation to determine the best weighted combination of all these candidate estimators. The resulting super learner estimate Q_n can now be mapped into the estimate $\Psi(Q_n)$ of the estimand ψ_0.

Such estimators have the following properties. Firstly, these estimators are generally well defined by being based on minimizing empirical risk and cross-validated risk with respect to the loss function $L()$ over the statistical model. Secondly, by definition, these substitution estimators fully respect the global constraints implied by the statistical model and the target parameter mapping Ψ. Thirdly, such estimators can incorporate the state of the art in machine learning. Fourthly, the loss function

$L(Q)$ can be selected to result in good estimators of the estimand ψ_0: in particular, the TMLE chooses a loss function and a cleverly chosen parametric working model to construct a targeted loss function whose empirical risk represents the fit of the TMLE. Finally, such estimators can be constrained to also solve a particular estimating equation that might be considered to yield advantageous statistical properties of the substitution estimator of $\Psi(Q_n)$: The TMLE enforces such a constraint by iteratively minimizing the empirical risk over the parametric working model through the current initial estimate.

6.2.1 Competitors

MLE is a loss-based learning methodology based on the log-likelihood loss function $L(P_0) = -\log P_0$. This explains many of the popular properties of maximum-likelihood-based estimation. Since the log-likelihood loss function measures the performance of a candidate probability distribution as a whole, it does not represent a targeted loss function when the parameter of interest is a small feature of P_0. The lack of targeting of the MLE is particularly apparent when the data structure O is high dimensional and the statistical model is large.

An estimating equation method (e.g., A-IPTW) is not a loss-based learning method. It takes as input not a particular loss function but an estimating function, and the estimator is defined as a solution of the corresponding estimating equation. The estimating function is derived from local derivatives of the target parameter mapping and thereby ignores the global constraints implied by the statistical model and by the target parameter mapping. These global constraints are important to put a natural brake on estimators, so that it is no surprise that estimating equation methods are often notoriously unstable under sparsity.

6.2.2 TMLE

TMLE (targeted minimum-loss-based estimation) is a targeted-loss-based learning methodology. It is targeted by its choice of loss function $L()$ and by the targeted minimization over cleverly chosen parametric working models through an initial estimate. The TMLE is driven by the *global* choices of the loss function and parametric working model, and not defined by its consequence that it solves the efficient influence curve estimating equation, as implied by the *local* derivative condition. For example, consider the data structure $O = (W, A, Y)$, with Y continuous and bounded between 0 and 1.

Suppose that the statistical model is nonparametric and that the estimand is the additive treatment effect $E_{W,0}[E_0(Y \mid A = 1, W) - E_0(Y \mid A = 0, W)]$, as in our mortality example. To define a TMLE we could select the squared error loss function $L(\bar{Q})(O) = (Y - \bar{Q}_0(A, W))^2$ for the conditional mean $\bar{Q}_0$, and the linear parametric working model $\bar{Q}(\epsilon) = \bar{Q} + \epsilon H^*$. Alternatively, we could define a TMLE implied by the "quasi"-log-likelihood loss function $-Y \log \bar{Q}_0(A, W) - (1-Y)\log(1-\bar{Q}_0(A, W))$, and the logistic linear parametric working model $\text{logit}\bar{Q}(\epsilon) = \text{logit}\bar{Q} + \epsilon H^*$.

Both TMLEs solve the efficient influence curve estimating equation, but they have very different properties regarding utilization of the global constraints of the statistical model. The TMLE with the squared error loss does not respect that it is known that $P_0(0 < Y < 1) = 1$, and, as a consequence, the TMLE $\bar{Q}_n^*$ can easily predict far outside $[0, 1]$, making it an unstable estimator under sparsity. In fact, this TMLE violates the very principle of TMLE in that TMLE should use a parametric *submodel* through the initial estimator, and the linear fluctuations of an initial estimator $\bar{Q}_n^0$ do *not* respect that $0 < \bar{Q}_0 < 1$, and are thus not a *submodel* of the statistical model. On the other hand, the other *valid* TMLE uses a logistic fluctuation of the initial estimator that fully respects this constraint, and is therefore a sensible substitution estimator fully respecting the global constraints of the statistical model. We refer to Chap. 7 for a full presentation of the latter TMLE for continuous and bounded Y.

Table 6.1 Summary of loss-based estimators for a general $\Psi(P_0)$

	MLE					Estimating equations	
	TMLE	Stratification	Propensity score	Parametric regression	ML-based super learning	IPTW	A-IPTW
Loss-based estimator of $\Psi(P_0)$	×	×	×	×	×		

6.3 TMLE Is Well Defined

An estimator that is well defined is desirable. Well-defined estimators have one solution in the space of possible solutions. It is easy to see why a well-defined estimator would be preferable to one that is not well defined. We seek the best estimate of $\Psi(P_0)$, and if our estimator gives multiple or no solutions, that presents a problem.

6.3.1 Competitors

MLEs aim to maximize a log-likelihood over candidate parameter values. Thus, MLE is often well defined, since, even if there are local maxima, the empirical log-likelihood or cross-validated log-likelihood can be used to select among such local maxima. Estimating equation methods are not well defined in general since the only criterion is that it solves the equation. A maximum likelihood estimator in a parametric statistical model often cannot be uniquely defined as a solution of the score equation since each local maximum will solve the score equation. The estimating equation methods are well defined for our target parameter with the simple data structure $O = (W, A, Y)$ and nonparametric statistical model for P_0, as is obvious from the definition of the IPTW and A-IPTW estimators given above. This is due to the fact that the estimating functions happen to be linear in ψ, allowing for a simple closed-form solution to their corresponding estimating equations.

When defining an estimator as a solution of the optimal efficient score/influence curve estimating equation, one may easily end up having to solve nonlinear equations that can have multiple solutions. The estimating equation itself provides no information about how to select among these candidate estimates of the target parameter. Also, one cannot use the likelihood since these estimators cannot be represented as $\hat{\Psi}(P_n)$ for some candidate P_n, i.e., these solutions ψ_n of the estimating equation are not substitution estimators (Sect. 6.6). This goes back to the basic fact that estimating functions (such as those defined by the efficient score/efficient influence curve) might not asymptotically identify the target parameter, and, even if they did, the corresponding estimating equation might not uniquely identify an estimator for a given finite sample.

In addition, for many estimation problems, the efficient influence curve $D^*(P_0)$ of the target parameter cannot be represented as an estimating function $D^*(\psi_0, \eta_0)$, so that the estimating equation methodology is not directly applicable. This means that the estimating equation methodology can only be applied if the efficient influence curve allows a representation as an estimating function. This is not a natural requirement, since the efficient influence curve $D^*(P_0)$ is defined as a gradient of the pathwise derivative of the target parameter along paths through P_0, and thereby only defines it as a function of P_0. There is no natural reason why the dependence of $D^*(P_0)$ on P_0 can be expressed in a dependence on two variation-independent parameters (ψ_0, η_0). Indeed, in some of our chapters we encounter target parameters where the efficient influence curve does not allow a representation as an estimating function.

6.3.2 TMLE

Unlike estimating function methodology (e.g., A-IPTW), TMLE does not aim to solve an estimating equation but instead uses the log-likelihood as a criterion. The super learner, representing the initial estimator in the TMLE, uses the (cross-validated) log-likelihood, or other loss function, to select among many candidate estimators. Even in the unlikely event that more than one global maximum exists, both would provide valid estimators so that a simple choice could make the super learner well defined. The targeting step involves computing a maximum likelihood estimator in a parametric working model of the same dimension as the target parameter, fluctuating the initial estimator, and is therefore as well defined as a parametric maximum likelihood estimator; again, the log-likelihood can be used to select among different local maxima. See Table 6.2 for a summary of well-defined estimators of $\Psi(P_0)$.

Table 6.2 Summary of well-defined estimators for a general $\Psi(P_0)$

	MLE					Estimating equations	
	TMLE	Stratification	Propensity score	Parametric regression	ML-based super learning	IPTW	A-IPTW
Well-defined estimator of $\Psi(P_0)$	×	×	×	×	×		

6.4 TMLE Is Unbiased

An estimator is asymptotically unbiased if it is unbiased as the sample size approaches infinity. Bias is defined as follows: bias$(\psi_n) = E_0(\psi_n) - \psi_0$, where $E_0(\psi_n)$ denotes the expectation of the estimator ψ_n viewed as a function of the n i.i.d. copies $O_1, \ldots, O_n$ drawn from P_0. An estimator is unbiased if bias$(\psi_n) = 0$. It is rare that an estimator is exactly unbiased. If we restricted ourselves to using only unbiased estimators, then in most estimation problems we would have no estimators available. Therefore, one wants to focus on estimators where bias is negligible for the purpose of obtaining confidence intervals for ψ_0 and tests of null hypotheses about ψ_0. This can be achieved by requiring that the bias converge to zero when sample size n increases, at a rate smaller than $1/\sqrt{n}$, such as $1/n$. Indeed, most correctly specified parametric maximum likelihood estimators have a bias of the order $1/n$.

Why do we care about bias? In the real world, biased estimators can lead to false positives in multimillion-dollar studies. That is, the true causal risk difference might be equal to zero, but if the estimator is biased, then a test that ignores this bias will interpret the bias as a deviation from the null hypothesis. This deviation from the null hypothesis would be declared statistically significant if sample size was large enough. In addition, bias against the null hypothesis (for example, one wishes to test for a positive treatment effect, but the effect estimate is biased low) results in less power to reject the null hypothesis. Overall, bias causes incorrect statistical inference.

One might wonder why one would not aim to estimate the bias of an estimator. The problem is that estimation of bias is typically an impossible goal, inducing more error than the bias: often the best one can do is to diagnose the presence of unusual bias, and that is indeed a task that should be incorporated in a data analysis (Chap. 10). Again, our goal is the best estimator of the true effect, and an asymptotically biased estimator is an estimator that cannot even learn the truth. We also want the bias to be asymptotically negligible so that statistical assessment of uncertainty based on an estimator of the variance of the estimator is reasonably valid.

6.4.1 Competitors

MLEs using stratification, super learning, or parametric regression are asymptotically unbiased if $\bar{Q}_0$ is consistently estimated. In order for propensity score methods that fit a nonparametric regression on treatment A and the propensity score to be asymptotically unbiased, the estimator of g_0 must be consistent. MLEs using stratification can easily suffer from large finite sample bias in sparse data. In other words, using a nonparametric MLE with a limited data set provides no recipe for an unbiased estimator of the target parameter $\Psi(P_0)$. IPTW is asymptotically unbiased for $\Psi(P_0)$ if the estimator of g_0 is consistent, and A-IPTW is asymptotically unbiased for $\Psi(P_0)$ if either $\bar{Q}_0$ or g_0 is consistently estimated. The asymptotic bias of the A-IPTW is characterized by the same expression provided in the next paragraph for TMLE. The finite sample bias is very much a function of how g_0 is estimated, in particular with respect to what covariates are included in the treatment mechanism and how well it approximates the true distribution. Since g_n is by necessity estimated based on the log-likelihood for the treatment mechanism, its fit is not affected by data on Y. As a consequence, covariates that have no effect on Y but a strong effect on A will be included, only harming the bias reduction effort.

6.4.2 TMLE

Using super learning within TMLE makes our estimator of the outcome regression $\bar{Q}_0$ and estimator of the treatment mechanism g_0 maximally asymptotically unbiased. In our flexible nonparametric statistical model, we can show that the asymptotic bias in our procedure involves a product of the bias of $\bar{Q}_n^*$ and g_n relative to the true $\bar{Q}_0$ and g_0, respectively. For example, with data structure $O = (W, A, Y)$ in an observational study (where g_0 is unknown), our asymptotic bias of the TMLE $\Psi(Q_n^*)$ given by

$$\text{bias}(\psi_n) = P_0\left\{\frac{g_0(1 \mid W) - g(1 \mid W)}{g(1 \mid W)}(\bar{Q}_0 - \bar{Q}^*)(1, W) - \frac{g_0(0 \mid W) - g(0 \mid W)}{g(0 \mid W)}(\bar{Q}_0 - \bar{Q}^*)(0, W)\right\},$$

where $\bar{Q}^*$ and g denote the limits of $\bar{Q}_n^*$ and g_n. This teaches us that the asymptotic bias behaves as a second-order difference involving the product of approximation errors for g_0 and $\bar{Q}_0$. The empirical counterpart of this term plays the role of second-order term for the TMLE approximation of the true ψ_0, and thereby also drives the finite sample bias. For reliable confidence intervals one wants $\sqrt{n}$ times the empirical counterpart of this bias term to converge to zero in probability as sample size converges to infinity. If one wants to make this second-order term and the resulting bias as small as possible, then theory teaches us that we should use super learning for both $\bar{Q}_0$ and g_0. As we point out in the next subsection, to minimize the variance of the first-order mean zero linear approximation of the TMLE approximation of the true ψ_0, one needs to estimate $\bar{Q}_0$ consistently. In other words, the use of super learning is essential for both maximizing efficiency as well as minimizing bias. For a formal theorem formalizing these statements we refer the interested reader to Chap. 27.

From this bias term one concludes that if the estimator of g_0 is correct, our estimator will have no asymptotic bias. This is an important scenario: consider again $O = (W, A, Y)$, and suppose we know the treatment mechanism, such as an RCT. In this instance, TMLE is always unbiased. Additionally, finite sample bias can be removed in RCTs by estimating g_0. If $\bar{Q}_n^*$ is already close to $\bar{Q}_0$, then the targeting step will further reduce the bias if g_n is also consistent. Finally, since running an additional univariate regression of the clever covariate on the outcome using the initial estimator as offset is a robust operation (assuming the clever covariate is bounded), even if g_n is misspecified, the targeting step will not cause harm to the bias.

In fact, one can show that if one replaces $g_0(A \mid W)$ by a true (sufficient) conditional distribution g_0^s of A, given a subset W^s of all covariates W, and W^s is chosen such that $Q^* - Q_0$ only depends on W through W^s, then the TMLE using this g_0 is also an unbiased estimator of the estimand ψ_0. Here Q^* represents the possibly misspecified estimand of the TMLE $\bar{Q}_n^*$. That is, the TMLE already achieves its full bias reduction by only incorporating the covariates in the treatment mechanism that explain the residual bias of $\bar{Q}_n^*$ with respect to $\bar{Q}_0$. We say that the TMLE is collaborative double robust to stress that consistency of the TMLE of ψ_0 is already achieved if g_n appropriately adapts to the residual bias of $\bar{Q}_n^*$: the TMLE is collaborative double robust, which is a stronger type of robustness with respect to misspecification of the nuisance parameters $\bar{Q}_0$ and g_0 than double robustness. In particular, an estimator g_n of g_0 used by the TMLE does not need to include covariates that are not predictive of Y, and are thus not confounders, even if the true treatment mechanism used these covariates. Apparently, the selection of covariates to be included in the estimator of the treatment mechanism should not be based on how well it fits g_0, but on the gain in fit of $\bar{Q}_0$ obtained by fitting the parametric working model (that uses this estimate of g_0) through the initial estimator $\bar{Q}_n^0$, relative to the fit of the initial estimator.

That is, TMLE naturally allows for the fine-tuning of the choice of g_n based on the fit of the corresponding TMLE of $\bar{Q}_0$, and can thereby data-adaptively select covariates into the treatment mechanism that actually matter and yield effective bias reduction in the TMLE step. For example, consider two possible estimators g_n^1 and g_n^2. These two choices combined with the initial estimator $\bar{Q}_n^0$ yield two different TMLEs, $\bar{Q}_{n1}^*$ and $\bar{Q}_{n2}^*$. These results suggest that one should select the estimator of g_0 for which the TMLE has the best fit of $\bar{Q}_0$. Note that this is equivalent to selecting covariates for the treatment mechanism based on how well the resulting estimate of the treatment mechanism improves the predictiveness of the corresponding clever covariate in predicting the outcome Y beyond the initial regression. This insight that the choice of g_n should be based on an evaluation of the resulting TMLE of $\bar{Q}_0$ is formalized by collaborative TMLE (C-TMLE), which is presented in Chaps. 19–21 and 23. See Table 6.3 for a summary of conditions for unbiased estimation among the estimators for a general $\Psi(P_0)$. Table 6.4 summarizes targeted estimation of the treatment mechanism for a general $\Psi(P_0)$.

Table 6.3 Summary of conditions for unbiased estimation for a general $\Psi(P_0)$

	MLE					Estimating equations	
	TMLE	Stratification	Propensity score	Parametric regression	ML-based super learning	IPTW	A-IPTW
Consistent estimation of $\bar{Q}_0$		×		×	×		
Consistent estimation of g_0			×			×	
Consistent estimation of $\bar{Q}_0$ or g_0	×						×
Problems in finite samples		×					

Table 6.4 Summary of targeted estimation of the treatment mechanism for a general $\Psi(P_0)$

	MLE					Estimating equations	
	(C-)TMLE	Stratification	Propensity score	Parametric regression	ML-based super learning	IPTW	A-IPTW
Targeted estimation of treatment mechanism	×						

6.5 TMLE Is Efficient

Efficiency is another measure of the desirability of an estimator. Finite sample efficiency for an estimator ψ_n can be defined as

$$\text{efficiency}(\psi_n) = \frac{\left(\frac{1}{I(\Psi(P_0))}\right)}{n\text{var}(\psi_n)},$$

where $I(\Psi(P_0))$ is the Fisher information, defined as 1 over the variance of the efficient influence curve. The variance of the efficient influence curve is also called the generalized Cramer–Rao lower bound for the variance of locally (approximately) unbiased estimators. Thus, efficiency(ψ_n) is the ratio of the minimum possible asymptotic variance for an approximately unbiased estimator over its actual finite sample variance. The asymptotic efficiency is defined as the limit of efficiency(ψ_n) for n converging to infinity. If the estimator of $\Psi(P_0)$ is unbiased and the asymptotic efficiency(ψ_n) = 1, the estimator is asymptotically efficient. Asymptotically efficient estimators achieve the Cramer–Rao bound (i.e., the variance of an unbiased estimator is, at a minimum, the inverse of the Fisher information) for large n. What we really care about, though, is performance in finite samples. So we would like to see that the finite sample efficiency efficiency(ψ_n) is close to 1. Minimally, we want an asymptotically efficient estimator, but we also want our estimator to perform well in realistic finite sample sizes.

Efficiency theory is concerned with an admission criterion: it is restricted to only those estimators that have negligible bias (i.e., small bias in finite samples) along small fluctuations of the true data-generating distribution, and among such estimators it defines a best estimator as the estimator that has the smallest asymptotic variance. This best estimator will be asymptotically linear with influence curve the efficient influence curve $D^*(O)$. An estimator $\hat{\Psi}(P_n)$ of ψ_0 is asymptotically linear with influence curve $IC(O)$ if it satisfies

$$\sqrt{n}(\psi_n - \psi_0) = \frac{1}{\sqrt{n}} \sum_{i=1}^{n} IC(O_i) + o_{P_0}(1).$$

Here the remainder term, denoted by $o_{P_0}(1)$, is a random variable that converges to zero in probability when the sample size converges to infinity. Asymptotic linearity is a desirable property as it indicates that the estimator behaves like an empirical mean, and, as a consequence, its bias converges to zero in sample size at a rate faster than $1/\sqrt{n}$, and, for n large enough, it is approximately normally distributed. The influence curve of an estimator evaluated as a function in O measures how robust the estimator is toward extreme values. The influence curve $IC(O)$ has a mean of zero under sampling from the true probability distribution P_0, and its (finite) variance is the asymptotic variance of the standardized estimator $\sqrt{n}(\psi_n - \psi_0)$. In other words, the variance of $\hat{\Psi}(P_n)$ is well approximated by the variance of the influence curve, divided by sample size n. An estimator is asymptotically efficient if and only if its influence curve is equal to the efficient influence curve, $IC(O) = D^*(O)$.

If we already agree that we want unbiased estimators, why do we care about efficiency? Given two unbiased estimators why should we choose the one that is also efficient? An unbiased estimator that has a large spread (i.e., huge confidence intervals) may be uninformative. A practical real-world result of this, aside from improved interpretation, is huge potential cost savings. If we can extract more information out of the our data with an efficient estimator, we can reduce the sample size required for an inefficient estimator. This savings may be nontrivial. For example, in a large multicenter RCT with a projected budget of \$100 million, reducing sample size by 30% results in close to \$30 million saved.

6.5.1 Competitors

If the covariate W is discrete, MLE using stratification is efficient asymptotically, but falls apart in finite samples if the number of categories is large. Suppose we have 30 discrete covariates, each with 3 levels. This gives us 3^{30} different covariate combinations, over 200 trillion! It is clear it becomes hopeless to wish for efficiency in finite sample sizes.

If W also includes continuous components, and some form of smoothing is used in the maximum likelihood estimation of $\bar{Q}_0$, then the maximum likelihood estimator will have approximation errors of the form $\sum_w E(\bar{Q}_n(1,w) - \bar{Q}_0(1,w))P_0(W = w)$ (minus the same term with $A = 0$). That is, the bias of $\bar{Q}_n$ will translate directly into a bias for the substitution estimator, and this bias will typically not be $o_P(1/\sqrt{n})$. The bias will also be larger than it would have been using super learning. In these cases, the bias causes the MLE to not be asymptotically linear and thereby also not achieve asymptotic efficiency. As discussed above, TMLE reduces the bias into a second-order term, so that it can still be asymptotically linear and thus efficient when the MLE will not (e.g., if g_0 can be well estimated).

Estimating equation methodology using the optimal estimating function (implied by the efficient influence curve) is asymptotically efficient if both $\bar{Q}_n$ and g_n are estimated consistently and if these estimators approximate the truth fast enough so that the estimator of ψ_0 succeeds in being asymptotically linear. This would require using super learning to estimate the nuisance parameters of the optimal estimating function. Due to the fact that estimating-equation-based estimators are not substitution estimators (Sect. 6.6), these estimators ignore global constraints, which harms the finite sample efficiency, in particular in the context of sparsity.

6.5.2 TMLE

Like the optimal estimating equation based estimator (i.e., A-IPTW), TMLE is double robust and (locally) efficient under regularity conditions. In other words, if the second-order term discussed above is asymptotically negligible, then the TMLE is consistent and asymptotically linear if either $\bar{Q}_n$ or g_n is a consistent estimator, and if both estimators are asymptotically consistent, then the TMLE is asymptotically efficient. TMLE also has excellent finite sample performance because it is driven by a log-likelihood (or other loss function) criterion, and a substitution estimator respecting all global constraints. The finite sample efficiency is further enhanced by the natural potential to fine-tune the estimator of the treatment mechanism through the predictiveness of the corresponding clever covariate, so that the treatment mechanism can be fitted in a way that is beneficial to its purpose in the targeting step. As previously noted, this is formalized by C-TMLE considered in later chapters. See Table 6.5 for a summary of efficiency among estimators for a general $\Psi(P_0)$.

Table 6.5 Summary of efficiency among estimators for a general $\Psi(P_0)$

	MLE					Estimating equations	
	TMLE	Stratification	Propensity score	Parametric regression	ML-based super learning	IPTW	A-IPTW
Efficient estimator of $\Psi(P_0)$	×	×					×
Problems in finite samples		×	×			×	×

6.6 TMLE Is a Substitution Estimator

Substitution estimators can be written as a mapping, taking an estimator of the relevant part of the data-generating distribution (e.g., P_n, P_n^*, Q_n, Q_n^*) and plugging it into the mapping $\Psi()$. The substitution estimator respects the statistical model space (i.e., the global constraints of the statistical model). Knowing and using information about the global constraints of the statistical model is helpful for precision (efficiency), particularly in the context of sparsity. For example, a substitution estimator of the risk difference ψ_0 respects knowledge that the mean outcome regression $\bar{Q}_0$ is bounded between [0, 1], or that ψ_0 is a difference of two probabilities.

To understand why respecting global constraints in a statistical model is important in the context of sparsity (i.e., the data carry little information for target parameter), suppose one wishes to estimate the mean of an outcome Y based on observing n i.i.d. copies $Y_1, \ldots, Y_n$. Suppose it is also known that $E_0 Y$ is larger than 0 and smaller than 0.1. This knowledge is not needed if the sample size is large enough such that the standard error of the estimator is much smaller than 0.1, but for small sample sizes, it cannot be ignored.

6.6.1 Competitors

MLEs using stratification, super learning, propensity scores, and parametric regression are substitution estimators. An estimator of ψ_0 that is obtained as a solution of an estimating equation is often *not* a substitution estimator, i.e., it cannot be written as $\Psi(P_n)$ for a specified estimator P_n of P_0 in the statistical model. Indeed, IPTW and A-IPTW are not substitution estimators. To be specific, suppose one wishes to estimate the treatment-specific mean $E_0Y_1 = E_0[E_0(Y \mid A = 1, W)]$ based on n i.i.d. copies of (W, A, Y), Y being binary. In this case, the A-IPTW estimator ψ_n, which solves the efficient influence curve estimating equation, can fall outside the range $[0, 1]$, due to inverse probability of treatments being close to zero. This proves that it is not a substitution estimator, which results in a loss of finite sample efficiency.

6.6.2 TMLE

The TMLE of ψ_0 is obtained by substitution of an estimator P_n^* into the mapping $\Psi()$. For the risk difference, this mapping is given in (6.1). As a consequence, it respects the knowledge of the statistical model. TMLE for the treatment-specific mean, discussed above, would result in E_0Y_1 between $[0, 1]$. See Table 6.6 for a summary of substitution estimators for a general $\Psi(P_0)$.

Table 6.6 Substitution estimators for a general $\Psi(P_0)$

	MLE					Estimating equations	
	TMLE	Stratification	Propensity score	Parametric regression	ML-based super learning	IPTW	A-IPTW
Substitution estimator of $\Psi(P_0)$	×	×	×	×	×		

6.7 Summary

The TMLE procedure produces a well-defined, unbiased, efficient substitution estimator of target parameters of a data-generating distribution. Competing estimators, falling into the broad classes of MLE and estimating equation methodology, do not have all of these properties and will underperform in many scenarios in comparison to TMLE. See Table 6.7 for a summary of statistical properties among estimators for a general $\Psi(P_0)$.

6.8 Notes and Further Reading

We refer readers to the references listed in Chap. 4. Appendix A covers further theoretical development of TMLE. A key reference for propensity score methods is Rosenbaum and Rubin (1983), and we also refer readers to Chap. 21.

Table 6.7 Summary of statistical properties among estimators for a general $\Psi(P_0)$

	MLE					**Estimating equations**	
	TMLE	Stratification	Propensity score	Parametric regression	ML-based super learning	IPTW	A-IPTW
Loss-based:							
Loss-based estimator of $\Psi(P_0)$	×	×	×	×	×		
Well-defined:							
Well-defined estimator of $\Psi(P_0)$	×	×	×	×	×		
Unbiased under:							
Consistent estimation of $\bar{Q}_0$		×		×	×		
Consistent estimation of g_0			×			×	
Consistent estimation of $\bar{Q}_0$ or g_0	×						×
Problems in finite samples		×					
Efficiency:							
Efficient estimator of $\Psi(P_0)$	×	×					×
Problems in finite samples		×	×			×	×
Substitution estimator:							
Substitution estimator of $\Psi(P_0)$	×	×	×	×	×		

Part II
Additional Core Topics

Chapter 7
Bounded Continuous Outcomes

Susan Gruber, Mark J. van der Laan

This chapter presents a TMLE of the additive treatment effect on a bounded continuous outcome. A TMLE is based on a choice of loss function and a corresponding parametric submodel through an initial estimator, chosen so that the loss-function-specific score of this parametric submodel at zero fluctuation equals or spans the efficient influence curve of the target parameter. Two such TMLEs are considered: one based on the squared error loss function with a linear regression model, and one based on a quasi-log-likelihood loss function with a logistic regression submodel. The problem with the first TMLE is highlighted: the linear regression model is not a submodel and thus does not respect global constraints implied by the statistical model. It is theoretically and practically demonstrated that the TMLE with the logistic regression submodel is more robust than a TMLE based on least squares linear regression. Some parts of this chapter assume familiarity with the core concepts, as presented in Chap. 5. The less theoretically trained reader should aim to navigate through these parts and focus on the practical implementation and importance of the presented TMLE procedure. This chapter is adapted from Gruber and van der Laan (2010b).

7.1 Introduction

TMLE of a target parameter of the data-generating distribution, known to be an element of a semiparametric model, involves selecting a loss function (e.g., log-likelihood) and constructing a parametric *submodel* through an initial density estimator with parameter ϵ, so that the loss-function-specific "score" at $\epsilon = 0$ equals or spans the efficient influence curve (canonical gradient) at the initial estimator. This ϵ represents an amount of fluctuation of the initial density estimator. The latter "score" constraint can be satisfied by many loss functions and parametric submodels, since it represents only a local constraint of the submodels' behavior at zero fluctuation.

However, it is very important that the fluctuations encoded by the parametric model stay within the semiparametric model for the observed data distribution (otherwise it is not a submodel!), even if the target parameter can be defined on fluctuations that fall outside the assumed observed data model.

In particular, in the context of sparse data, by which we mean situations where the generalized Cramer–Rao lower bound is high, a violation of this property can significantly affect the performance of the estimator. We demonstrate this in the context of estimation of a causal effect of a binary treatment on a continuous outcome that is bounded. It results in a TMLE that inherently respects known bounds and consequently is more robust in sparse data situations than a TMLE using a naive parametric fluctuation working model that is actually not a *submodel* of the assumed statistical model.

Sparsity is defined as low information in a data set for the purpose of learning the target parameter. Formally, the Fisher information I is defined as sample size n divided by the variance of the efficient influence curve: $I = n/\text{var}(D^*(O))$, where $D^*(O)$ is the efficient influence curve of the target parameter at the true data-generating distribution. The reciprocal of the variance of the efficient influence curve can be viewed as the information one observation contains for the purpose of learning the target parameter. Since the variance of the efficient influence curve divided by n is the asymptotic variance of an asymptotically efficient estimator, one can also think of the information I as the reciprocal of the variance of an efficient estimator of the target parameter. Thus, sparsity with respect to a particular target parameter corresponds with small sample size relative to the variance of the efficient influence curve for that target parameter.

The following section begins with background on the application of TMLE methodology in the context of sparsity and its power relative to other semiparametric efficient estimators since it is a substitution estimator respecting global constraints of the semiparametric model. Even though an estimator can be asymptotically efficient without utilizing global constraints, the global constraints are instrumental in the context of sparsity with respect to the target parameter, motivating the need for semiparametric efficient *substitution* estimators, and for a careful choice of fluctuation function for the targeting step that fully respects these global constraints. A rigorous demonstration of the proposed TMLE of the causal effect of a binary treatment on a bounded continuous outcome follows, and the TMLE using a linear fluctuation function (i.e., that does not represent a parametric submodel) is compared with the proposed TMLE using a logistic fluctuation function. In Sect. 7.3, we carry out simulation studies that compare the two TMLEs of the causal effect, with and without sparsity in the data. Results for other commonly applied estimators discussed in Chap. 6 (MLE according to a parametric statistical model, IPTW, and A-IPTW) are also presented.

7.2 TMLE for Causal Estimation on a Continuous Outcome

We first review general TMLE so that we can clarify the important role of the choice of parametric working model, and thereby the fluctuation function, that defines the targeting update step of the initial estimator. Subsequently, in order to be specific, we define TMLE of the additive causal effect of a binary treatment on a bounded continuous outcome, which fully respects the known global bounds. Finally, we discuss its robustness in finite samples in the context of sparsity.

7.2.1 A Substitution Estimator Respecting the Statistical Model

A TMLE is a semiparametric efficient substitution estimator of a target parameter $\Psi(P_0)$ of a true distribution $P_0 \in \mathcal{M}$, known to be an element of a statistical model $\mathcal{M}$, based on sampling n i.i.d. $O_1, \ldots, O_n$ from P_0. Firstly, one notes that $\Psi(P_0) = \Psi(Q_0)$ only depends on P_0 through a relevant part $Q_0 = Q(P_0)$ of P_0. Secondly, one proposes a loss function $L(Q)$ such that

$$Q_0 = \arg\min_{Q \in \mathcal{Q}} E_0 L(Q)(O),$$

where $\mathcal{Q} = \{Q(P) : P \in \mathcal{M}\}$ is the set of possible values for Q_0. Thirdly, one uses minimum-loss-based learning, such as super learning, fully utilizing the power and optimality results for loss-based cross-validation to select among candidate estimators, to obtain an initial estimator Q_n^0 of Q_0. Fourthly, one proposes a parametric fluctuation $Q_{g_n,n}^0(\epsilon)$, possibly indexed by the estimator g_n of nuisance parameter $g_0 = g(P_0)$, such that

$$\frac{d}{d\epsilon} L(Q_{g_n,n}^0(\epsilon))(O)\Big|_{\epsilon=0} = D^*(Q_n^0, g_n)(O), \tag{7.1}$$

where $D^*(P) = D^*(Q(P), g(P))$ is the efficient influence curve of the pathwise derivative of the statistical target parameter mapping $\Psi : \mathcal{M} \to \mathbb{R}$ at $P \in \mathcal{M}$. If a multivariate ϵ is used, then the derivatives with respect to each of their components ϵ_j must span the efficient influence curve $D^*(Q_n^0, g_n)$. Fifthly, one computes the amount of fluctuation with minimum-loss-based estimation:

$$\epsilon_n = \arg\min_{\epsilon} \sum_{i=1}^{n} L(Q_{g_n,n}^0(\epsilon))(O_i).$$

This yields an update $Q_n^1 = Q_{g_n,n}^0(\epsilon_n)$. This updating of an initial estimator Q_n^0 into a next Q_n^1 is iterated until convergence, resulting in a final update Q_n^*. Since at the last step the amount of fluctuation $\epsilon_n \approxeq 0$, this final Q_n^* will solve the efficient influence curve estimating equation:

$$0 = \frac{1}{n}\sum_{i=1}^{n} D^*(Q_n^*, g_n)(O_i),$$

representing a fundamental ingredient for establishing the asymptotic efficiency of $\Psi(Q_n^*)$. Recall that an estimator is efficient if and only if it is asymptotically linear with an influence curve equal to the efficient influence curve $D^*(Q_0, g_0)$. Finally, the TMLE of ψ_0 is the substitution estimator $\Psi(Q_n^*)$.

Thus we see that TMLE involves constructing a parametric submodel $\{Q_n^0(\epsilon) : \epsilon\}$, and thereby its corresponding fluctuation function $\epsilon \rightarrow Q_n^0(\epsilon)$, through the initial estimator Q_n^0 with parameter ϵ, where the score of this parametric submodel at $\epsilon = 0$ equals the efficient influence curve at the initial estimator. The latter constraint can be satisfied by many parametric submodels, since it represents only a local constraint of its behavior at zero fluctuation. However, it is very important that the fluctuations stay within the statistical model for the observed data distribution, even if the target parameter Ψ can be defined on fluctuations of densities that fall outside the assumed observed data model. In particular, in the context of sparse data (i.e., data that will not allow for precise estimation of the target parameter), a violation of this property can significantly affect the performance of the estimator.

One important strength of the semiparametric efficient TMLE relative to the alternative semiparametric efficient estimating equation methodology is that it respects the global constraints of the observed data model. This is due to the fact that it is a substitution estimator $\Psi(Q_n^*)$ with Q_n^*, an estimator of a relevant part Q_0 of the true distribution of the data in the observed data model. The estimating equation methodology does not result in substitution estimators and consequently often ignores important global constraints of the observed data model, which comes at a price in the context of sparsity. Indeed, simulations have confirmed this gain of TMLE relative to the efficient estimating equation method in the context of sparsity (see Chap. 20 and also Stitelman and van der Laan 2010), which is demonstrated in this chapter. However, if TMLE violates the principle of being a substitution estimator by allowing Q_n^* to fall outside the assumed observed data model, this advantage is compromised. Therefore, it is crucial that TMLE use a fluctuation function that is guaranteed to map the fluctuated initial estimator into the statistical model.

7.2.2 Procedure

To demonstrate the important consideration of selecting a fluctuation function in the construction of TMLE that corresponds with a parametric *sub*model, we consider the problem of estimating the additive causal effect of a binary treatment A on a continuous outcome Y, based on observing n i.i.d. copies of $O = (W, A, Y) \sim P_0$, where W is the set of confounders. Consider the following SCM: $W = f_W(U_W)$, $A = f_A(W, U_A)$, $Y = f_Y(W, A, U_Y)$ with the functions f_W, f_A, and f_Y unspecified, representing a set of assumptions about how O is generated. We assume that U_A is independent of U_Y such that the randomization assumption ($A \perp Y_a \mid W$) holds with respect to the counterfactuals $Y_a = f_Y(W, a, U_Y)$ as defined by this SCM. In this SCM for the data-generating distribution of the observed data O, the additive causal effect $E_0(Y_1 - Y_0)$ can be identified from the observed data distribution through the statistical parameter of P_0:

$$\Psi(P_0) = E_0[E_0(Y \mid A = 1, W) - E_0(Y \mid A = 0, W)].$$

Suppose that it is known that $Y \in [a, b]$ for some $a < b$. Alternatively, one might have truncated the original data to fall in such an interval and focus on the causal effect of treatment on this truncated outcome, motivated by the fact that estimating the conditional means of unbounded, or very heavy tailed, outcomes requires very large data sets. The SCM implies no assumptions about the statistical model $\mathcal{M}$ so that the statistical model is nonparametric. The target parameter mapping $\Psi : \mathcal{M} \rightarrow \mathbb{R}$ and the estimand $\psi_0 = \Psi(P_0)$ are now defined. The statistical estimation problem is to estimate ψ_0 based on observing n i.i.d. copies $O_1, \ldots, O_n$.

Let $Y^* = (Y - a)/(b - a)$ be the linearly transformed outcome within $[0, 1]$, and we define the statistical parameter

$$\Psi^*(P_0) = E_0[E_0(Y^* \mid A = 1, W) - E_0(Y^* \mid A = 0, W)],$$

which can be interpreted as the causal effect of treatment on the bounded outcome Y^* in the postulated SCM. We note the following relation between the causal effect on the original outcome Y and the causal effect on the transformed outcome Y^*:

$$\Psi(P_0) = (b - a)\Psi^*(P_0).$$

An estimate, normal limit distribution, and confidence interval for $\Psi^*(P_0)$ is now immediately mapped into an estimate, normal limit distribution, and confidence interval for $\Psi(P_0)$ by simple multiplication. Suppose $\sqrt{n}(\psi_n - \Psi^*(P_0)) \xrightarrow{d} N(0, \sigma^{2*})$, then $\sqrt{n}((b - a)\psi_n - \Psi(P_0)) \xrightarrow{d} N(0, \sigma^2)$, with $\sigma^2 = (b - a)^2\sigma^{2*}$. Upper and lower bounds on the confidence interval for $\Psi^*(P_0)$, given as (c^*_{lb}, c^*_{ub}), are multiplied by $(b - a)$ to obtain upper and lower bounds on $\Psi(P_0)$, $c_{lb} = (b - a)c^*_{lb}$, and $c_{ub} = (b - a)c^*_{ub}$. As a consequence, for notational convenience, without loss of generality, we can assume $a = 0$ and $b = 1$ so that $Y \in [0, 1]$.

To determine a loss function and corresponding fluctuation function, and thereby the definition of the TMLE, we need to know the efficient influence curve. The efficient influence curve of the statistical parameter $\Psi : \mathcal{M} \rightarrow \mathbb{R}$, defined on a nonparametric statistical model $\mathcal{M}$ for P_0 at the true distribution P_0, is given by

$$D^*(P_0) = \frac{2A - 1}{g_0(A \mid W)}(Y - \bar{Q}_0(A, W)) + \bar{Q}_0(1, W) - \bar{Q}_0(0, W) - \Psi(Q_0), \qquad (7.2)$$

where $\bar{Q}_0(A, W) = E_0(Y \mid A, W)$ and $Q_0 = (Q_{W,0}, \bar{Q}_0)$ denotes both this conditional mean $\bar{Q}_0$ and the marginal distribution $Q_{W,0}$ of W. Note that indeed $\Psi(P_0)$ only depends on P_0 through the conditional mean $\bar{Q}_0$ and the marginal distribution of W. We will use the notation $\Psi(P_0)$ and $\Psi(Q_0)$ interchangeably. Note also that the efficient influence curve only depends on P_0 through Q_0, g_0, so that we will also denote the efficient influence curve $D^*(P_0)$ with $D^*(Q_0, g_0)$. In order to stress that $D^*(P_0)$ can also be represented as an estimating function in ψ, we also now and then denote it by $D^*(Q_0, g_0, \psi_0)$.

We are ready to define a TMLE of $\Psi(Q_0)$, completely analogous to the TMLE presented in Chaps. 4 and 5 for a binary outcome. Let $\bar{Q}_n^0$ be an initial estimate of $\bar{Q}_0(A, W) = E_0(Y \mid A, W)$ with predicted values in (0, 1). This could be a loss-based super learner based on the squared error loss function or the quasi-log-likelihood loss function presented below. In addition, we estimate $Q_{W,0}$ with the empirical distribution of $W_1, \ldots, W_n$. Let Q_n^0 denote the resulting initial estimate of Q_0. The targeting step will also require an estimate g_n of $g_0 = P_{A|W}$. As we will see, only the estimate $\bar{Q}_n^0$ of the conditional mean $\bar{Q}_0$ will be modified by the TMLE procedure defined below: this makes sense since the empirical distribution of W is already a nonparametric maximum likelihood estimator so that no bias gain with respect to the target parameter will be obtained by modifying it.

We use as fluctuation function for the empirical distribution $Q_{W,n}$, $Q_{W,n}(\epsilon_1) = (1 + \epsilon_1 D_2^*(Q_n^0))Q_{W,n}$, where $D_2^*(Q_n^0) = \bar{Q}_n^0(1, W) - \bar{Q}_n^0(0, W) - \Psi(Q_n^0)$ is the second component of the efficient influence curve $D^*(Q_n^0, g_n)$. We use the log-likelihood loss function, $-\log Q_W$, as loss function for the marginal distribution of W. It follows that

$$\frac{d}{d\epsilon} \log Q_{W,n}(\epsilon_1)\bigg|_{\epsilon_1=0} = D_2^*(Q_n^0),$$

showing that this fluctuation function and log-likelihood loss function for the marginal distribution of W indeed generates the wished score at zero fluctuation.

We can represent the estimate $\bar{Q}_n^0$ as

$$\bar{Q}_n^0 = \frac{1}{1 + \exp(-f_n^0)},$$

with $f_n^0 = \log(\bar{Q}_n^0/(1 - \bar{Q}_n^0))$. Consider now the following fluctuation function:

$$\bar{Q}_n^0(\epsilon_2) = \frac{1}{1 + \exp(-\{f_n^0 + \epsilon_2 H_{g_n}^*\})},$$

which maps a fluctuation parameter value ϵ_2 into a modification $\bar{Q}_n^0(\epsilon_2)$ of the initial estimate. This fluctuation function is indexed by a function

$$H_{g_n}^*(A, W) = \frac{2A - 1}{g_n(A \mid W)}.$$

Equivalently, we can write this fluctuation function in terms of fluctuations of the logit of $\bar{Q}_n^0$: $\text{logit}\bar{Q}_n^0(\epsilon_2) = \text{logit}\bar{Q}_n^0 + \epsilon_2 H^*(g_n)$.

Consider now the following quasi-log-likelihood loss function for the conditional mean $\bar{Q}_0$:

$$-L(\bar{Q})(O) = Y \log \bar{Q}(A, W) + (1 - Y) \log(1 - \bar{Q}(A, W)).$$

Note that this is the log-likelihood of the conditional distribution of a binary outcome Y, but now extended to continuous outcomes in $[0, 1]$. It is thus known that this loss function is a valid loss function for the conditional distribution of a binary Y, but we need it to be a valid loss function for a conditional mean of a continuous $Y \in [0, 1]$. It is indeed a valid loss function for the conditional mean of a continuous outcome in $[0, 1]$, as has been previously noted. See Wedderburn (1974) and McCullagh (1983) for earlier uses of logistic regression for continuous outcomes in $[0, 1]$. We formally prove this result in Lemma 7.1 at the end of this chapter. The proposed fluctuation function $\bar{Q}_n^0(\epsilon_2)$ and the quasi-log-likelihood loss function satisfy

$$\frac{d}{d\epsilon_2} L(\bar{Q}_n^0(\epsilon_2))\Big|_{\epsilon_2=0} = H^*(A, W)(Y - \bar{Q}_n^0(A, W)),$$

giving us the desired first component $D_1^*(\bar{Q}_n^0, g_n)$ of the efficient influence curve $D^* = D_1^* + D_2^*$, where $D_2^*(Q_0) = \bar{Q}_0(1, W) - \bar{Q}_0(0, W) - \Psi(Q_0)$.

Our combined loss function is given by $L(Q) = -\log Q_W + L(\bar{Q})$, and, for $\epsilon = (\epsilon_1, \epsilon_2)$, our parametric fluctuation function for the combined Q is given by $Q(\epsilon) = (Q_W(\epsilon_1), \bar{Q}(\epsilon_2))$. With these choices of loss function $L(Q)$ for Q_0 and fluctuation function $Q(\epsilon)$ of Q, we indeed now have that

$$\frac{d}{d\epsilon_j} L(Q(\epsilon))\Big|_{\epsilon=0} = D_j^*(Q, g),\ j = 1, 2.$$

This shows that we succeeded in defining a loss function for $Q_0 = (Q_{W,0}, \bar{Q}_0)$ and fluctuation function such that the derivatives as defined in (7.1) span the efficient influence curve. The TMLE is now defined!

In this first targeting step, the maximum likelihood estimator of ϵ_1 equals zero, so that the update of $Q_{W,n}$ equals $Q_{W,n}$ itself. As a consequence of $\epsilon_{1,n}^0 = 0$ being the maximum likelihood estimator, the empirical mean of the component $D_2^*(Q_n^*) = \bar{Q}_n^*(1, W) - \bar{Q}_n^*(0, W) - \Psi(Q_n^*)$ of the efficient influence curve at the final TMLE equals zero: of course, this is trivially verified.

The maximum likelihood estimator of ϵ_2 for fluctuating $\bar{Q}_n^0$ is given by

$$\epsilon_{2n}^0 = \arg\min_{\epsilon_2} P_n L(\bar{Q}_n^0(\epsilon_2)),$$

where we used the notation $P_n f = 1/n \sum_i f(O_i)$. This "maximum likelihood" estimator of ϵ_2 can be computed with generalized linear regression using the binomial link, i.e., the logistic regression maximum likelihood estimation procedure, simply ignoring that the outcome is not binary, which also corresponds with iterative reweighted least squares estimation using iteratively updated estimated weights of the form $1/(\bar{Q}_n(1 - \bar{Q}_n))$.

This provides us with the targeted update $Q_n^1 = Q_n^0(\epsilon_n^0)$, where the empirical distribution of W was not updated, but $\bar{Q}_n^0$ did get updated to $\bar{Q}_n^0(\epsilon_n^0)$. Iterating this procedure now defines the TMLE Q_n^*, but, as in the binary outcome case, we have that $\bar{Q}_n^2 = \bar{Q}_n^1(\epsilon_n^1) = \bar{Q}_n^1$ since the next maximum likelihood estimator $\epsilon_n^1 = 0$, and, of course, the maximum likelihood estimator of ϵ_1 remains 0. Thus convergence occurs in one step, so that $Q_n^* = Q_n^1$. The TMLE of ψ_0 is thus given by $\Psi(Q_n^*) = \Psi(Q_n^1)$. As a consequence of the definition of the TMLE, we have that the TMLE Q_n^* solves the efficient influence curve estimating equation $P_n D^*(Q_n^*, g_n, \Psi(Q_n^*)) = 0$.

7.2.3 Robustness of TMLE in the Context of Sparsity

We note that, even if there is strong confounding causing some large values of $H^*_{g_n}$, the resulting TMLE $\bar{Q}_n^*$ remains bounded in (0, 1), so that the TMLE $\Psi(Q_n^*)$, which just averages values of $\bar{Q}_n^*$, fully respects the global constraints of the observed data model. An inspection of the efficient influence curve (7.2), $D^*(P_0)$, reveals that there are two potential sources of sparsity. Small values for $g_0(A \mid W)$ and large outlying values of Y inflate the variance. Enforcing (e.g., known) bounds on Y and g_0 in the estimation procedure provides a means for controlling these sources of variance. We note that, even if there is strong confounding causing some large values of $h_{g_n^0}$, the resulting TMLE $\bar{Q}_n^*$ remains bounded in (0, 1), so that the TMLE $\Psi(Q_n^*)$ fully respects the global constraints of the observed data model. On the other hand, the A-IPTW estimator obtained by solving the efficient influence curve estimating equation, $P_n D^*(Q_n^0, g_n, \psi) = 0$, in ψ yields the estimator

$$\psi_n = \frac{1}{n}\sum_{i=1}^{n} H^*_{g_n}(A_i, W_i)(Y_i - \bar{Q}_n^0(A_i, W_i)) + \bar{Q}_n^0(1, W) - \bar{Q}_n^0(0, W).$$

This estimator can easily fall outside [0, 1] if for some observations $g_n(1 \mid W_i)$ is close to 1 or 0. This represents the price of not being a substitution estimator.

It is also important to contrast this TMLE with the TMLE using the linear fluctuation function. The latter TMLE would use the $L(\bar{Q}) = (Y - \bar{Q}(A, W))^2$ loss function, and fluctuation function $\bar{Q}_n^0(\epsilon) = \bar{Q}_n^0 + \epsilon H^*(g_n)$, so that (7.1) is still satisfied. The TMLE is defined as above, and again converges in one step. One estimates the fluctuation ϵ with univariate least squares linear regression, using $\bar{Q}_n^0$ as offset. In this case, large values of $H^*(g_n)$ will result in predicted values of $\bar{Q}_n^0(\epsilon_n)$ that are outside the bounds $[a, b]$. Therefore, this version of TMLE does not repect the global constraints of the model, i.e., the knowledge that $Y \in [a, b]$. In the next section, an analysis of a simulated data set provides a comparison of TMLE using the logistic fluctuation function and TMLE using this linear fluctuation.

7.3 Simulations

Two simulation studies illustrate the effects of employing a logistic vs. linear fluctuation function in the definition of the TMLE. These two studies evaluate practical performance with and without sparsity in the data, where a high degree of sparsity corresponds to a target parameter that is borderline identifiable. As above, the parameter of interest is defined as the additive effect of a binary point treatment on the outcome, $\psi_0 = E_0[E_0(Y \mid A = 1, W) - E_0(Y \mid A = 0, W)]$. We also implement three additional estimators: MLE, IPTW, and A-IPTW.

7.3.1 Estimators

In the simulation setting, Y is not bounded, so that we do not have an a priori a and b bound on Y. Instead of truncating Y and redefining the target parameter as the causal effect on the truncated Y, we still aim to estimate the causal effect on the original Y. Therefore, in the TMLE using a logistic fluctuation function we set $a = \min(Y)$, $b = \max(Y)$, and $Y^* = (Y - a)/(b - a)$. In this TMLE, the initial estimate $\bar{Q}_n^{0,Y^*}$ of $E_0(Y^*|A, W)$ needs to be represented as a logistic function of its logit transformation. Note that logit(x) is not defined when $x = 0$ or 1. Therefore, in practice $\bar{Q}_n^{0,Y^*}$ needs to be bounded away from 0 and 1 by truncating at $(\alpha, (1 - \alpha))$ for some small $\alpha > 0$. In the reported simulations we used $\alpha = 0.005$. We also obtained results for $\alpha = 0.001$ or $\alpha = 0.01$, but no notable difference was observed.

In our simulations, we also included the A-IPTW estimator of ψ_0, defined as

$$\psi_n^{A-IPTW} = \frac{1}{n}\sum_{i=1}^{n}\left\{\frac{2A_i - 1}{g_n(A_i \mid W_i)}(Y_i - \bar{Q}_n^0(A_i, W_i)) + (\bar{Q}_n^0(1, W_i) - \bar{Q}_n^0(0, W_i))\right\}.$$

The two TMLEs and the A-IPTW estimator are double robust so that these estimators will be consistent for ψ_0 if either g_n or $\bar{Q}_n^0$ is consistent for g_0 and $\bar{Q}_0$, respectively. In addition, the two TMLEs and the A-IPTW estimator are asymptotically efficient if both g_n and $\bar{Q}_n^0$ consistently estimate the true g_0 and $\bar{Q}_0$, respectively.

In this simulation study we will use simple parametric maximum likelihood estimators as initial estimators $\bar{Q}_n^0$ and g_n, even though we recommend the use of super learning in practice. The goal of this simulation is to investigate the performance of the updating step under misspecified and correctly specified $\bar{Q}_n^0$, and for that purpose we can work with parametric maximum likelihood estimation fits.

We also report the MLE $\Psi(Q_n^0)$ of ψ_0 according to a parametric model for $\bar{Q}_0$, and an IPTW estimator of ψ_0 that uses g_n as estimator of g_0:

$$\psi_n^{MLE} = \frac{1}{n}\sum_{i-1}^{n}\left\{\bar{Q}_n^0(1, W_i) - \bar{Q}_n^0(0, W_i)\right\},$$

$$\psi_n^{IPTW} = \frac{1}{n}\sum_{i=1}^{n}(2A - 1)\frac{Y_i}{g_n(A_i, W_i)}.$$

The MLE of ψ_0 is included for the sake of evaluating the bias reduction step carried out by the TMLEs and the A-IPTW estimator.

7.3.2 Data-Generating Distributions

Covariates W_1, W_2, W_3 were generated as independent binary random variables: $W_1, W_2, W_3 \sim$ *Bernoulli*(0.5). Two treatment mechanisms were defined that differ only in the values of the coefficients for each covariate. They are of the form

$$g_0(1 \mid W) = \text{expit}(\beta W_1 + \delta W_2 + \gamma W_3).$$

We considered the following two settings for the treatment mechanism:

$$\beta_1 = 0.5, \delta_1 = 1.5, \gamma_1 = -1, \text{ and}$$
$$\beta_2 = 1.5, \delta_2 = 4.5, \gamma_2 = -3.$$

We refer to these two treatment mechanisms as $g_{0,1}$ and $g_{0,2}$, respectively. The observed outcome Y was generated as

$$Y = A + 2W_1 + 3W_2 - 4W_3 + e, \; e \sim N(0, 1).$$

For both simulations the true additive causal effect equals one: $\psi_0 = 1$. Treatment assignment probabilities based on mechanism $g_{0,1}$ range from 0.269 to 0.881, indicating no sparsity in the data for simulation 1. In contrast, treatment assignment probabilities based on mechanism $g_{0,2}$ range from (0.047 to 0.998). Simulation 2 poses a more challenging estimation problem in the context of sparse data.

Estimates were obtained for 1000 samples of size $n = 1000$ from each data-generating distribution. Treatment assignment probabilities were estimated using a correctly specified logistic regression model. In both simulations predicted values for $g_n(A \mid W)$ were bounded away from 0 and 1 by truncating at $(p, 1-p)$, with $p = 0.01$. In one set of results a correctly specified main terms regression model was used to compute the initial estimate $\bar{Q}_n^0$, while in the other set of results the initial estimate was defined as the least squares regression Y on A only.

7.3.3 Results

Table 7.1 reports the average estimate, bias, empirical variance, and MSE for each estimator, under different specifications of the initial estimator $\bar{Q}_n^0$. In simulation 1, when $\bar{Q}_0$ is correctly estimated, all estimators perform quite well, though as expected IPTW is the least efficient. However, when $\bar{Q}_0$ is incorrectly estimated, the MLE is biased and has high variance relative to the other estimators. Since $g_n(A \mid W)$ is correctly specified, IPTW and A-IPTW provide unbiased estimates, as do both TMLEs: the TMLE$_{Y^*}$ based on the logistic regression model is similar to the TMLE based on the linear regression model, as there is no sparsity in the data, and both are asymptotically efficient estimators.

Table 7.1 Estimator performance for simulations 1 and 2 when the initial estimator of $\bar{Q}_0$ is correctly specified and misspecified. Results are based on 1000 samples of size $n = 1000$, g_n is consistent,and bounded at (0.01,0.99)

	$\bar{Q}_0$ correctly specified				$\bar{Q}_0$ misspecified			
	ψ_n	Bias	Var	MSE	ψ_n	Bias	Var	MSE
Simulation 1								
MLE	1.003	0.003	0.005	0.005	3.075	2.075	0.030	4.336
IPTW	1.006	0.006	0.009	0.009	1.006	0.006	0.009	0.009
A-IPTW	1.003	0.003	0.005	0.005	1.005	0.005	0.010	0.010
TMLE_{Y^*}	0.993	−0.007	0.005	0.005	0.993	−0.007	0.006	0.006
TMLE	0.993	−0.007	0.005	0.005	0.993	−0.007	0.006	0.006
Simulation 2								
MLE	1.001	0.001	0.009	0.009	4.653	3.653	0.025	13.370
IPTW	1.554	0.554	0.179	0.485	1.554	0.554	0.179	0.485
A-IPTW	0.999	−0.001	0.023	0.023	1.708	0.708	0.298	0.798
TMLE_{Y^*}	0.989	−0.011	0.037	0.037	0.722	−0.278	0.214	0.291
TMLE	0.986	−0.014	0.042	0.042	−0.263	−1.263	2.581	4.173

In simulation 2, all estimators except IPTW are unbiased when $\bar{Q}_0$ is correctly estimated. In this case, both TMLEs have higher variance than A-IPTW, even though all three are asymptotically efficient. All three are more efficient than IPTW but less efficient than MLE. Though asymptotically the IPTW estimator is expected to be unbiased in this simulation, since g_n is a consistent estimator of $g_{0,2}$, these results demonstrate that in finite samples, heavily weighting a subset of observations not only increases variance but can also bias the estimate.

When the model for $\bar{Q}_0$ is misspecified in simulation 2, MLE is even more biased than it was in simulation 1. The efficiency of all three double robust efficient estimators suffers in comparison with simulation 1 as well. Nevertheless, TMLE_{Y^*}, using the logistic fluctuation, has the lowest MSE of all estimators. Its superiority over TMLE, using linear least squares regression, in terms of bias and variance is clear. TMLE_{Y^*} also outperforms A-IPTW with respect to both bias and variance and performs much better than IPTW or MLE.

7.4 Discussion

For the sake of demonstration, we considered estimation of the additive causal effect. However, the same TMLE, using the logistic fluctuation, can be used to estimate other point-treatment causal effects, including parameters of a marginal structural model. The proposed quasi-log-likelihood loss function can be used to define a super learner for prediction of a bounded continuous outcome. It will be of interest to evaluate such a super learner relative to a super learner that does not incorporate these known bounds. The quasi-log-likelihood loss function and the logistic fluctuation function can also be applied in a TMLE of the causal effect of a multiple time point intervention in which the final outcome is bounded and continuous. In this case, one uses the loss function and logistic fluctuation function to fluctuate the last factor of the likelihood of the longitudinal structure. Our simulations show that the proposed fluctuation function and loss function, and corresponding TMLEs, should also be used for continuous outcomes for which no a priori bounds are known. In this case, one simply uses the minimal and maximal observed outcome values. In this way, these choices naturally robustify the TMLEs by enforcing that the updated initial estimator will not predict outcomes outside the observed range. TMLE using the logistic fluctuation function can also be incorporated in C-TMLE (Chaps. 19–21 and 23) without modification.

Appendix

The following lemma proves that the quasi-log-likelihood loss function is indeed a valid loss function for the conditional mean $\bar{Q}_0$ of a continuous outcome in $[0, 1]$.

Lemma 7.1. *We have that*

$$\bar{Q}_0 = \underset{\bar{Q}}{\text{argmin}}\ E_0 L(\bar{Q}),$$

where the minimum is taken over all functions of (A, W) *that map into* $[0, 1]$. *In addition, given a function* H^*, *define the fluctuation function*

$$logit(\bar{Q}(\epsilon)) = logit(\bar{Q}) + \epsilon H^*.$$

For any function H^* *we have*

$$\frac{d}{d\epsilon} L(\bar{Q}(\epsilon))\bigg|_{\epsilon=0} = H^*(A, W)(Y - \bar{Q}(A, W)).$$

Proof. Let $\bar{Q}_1$ be a local minimum of $\bar{Q} \rightarrow E_0 L(\bar{Q})(O)$, and consider the fluctuation function $\epsilon \rightarrow \bar{Q}_1(\epsilon)$ defined above. Then the derivative of $\epsilon \rightarrow E_0 L(\bar{Q}_1(\epsilon))$ at $\epsilon = 0$ equals zero. However, we also have

$$-\frac{d}{d\epsilon} L(\bar{Q}_1(\epsilon))\bigg|_{\epsilon=0} = H^*(A, W)(Y - \bar{Q}_1(A, W)).$$

Thus, it follows that

$$E_0[H^*(A, W)(Y - \bar{Q}_1(A, W))] = E_0[H^*(A, W)(\bar{Q}_0 - \bar{Q}_1)(A, W)].$$

But this needs to hold for any function $H^*(A, W)$, which proves that $\bar{Q}_1 = \bar{Q}_0$ almost everywhere. The final statement follows as well. □

Chapter 8
Direct Effects and Effect Among the Treated

Alan E. Hubbard, Nicholas P. Jewell, Mark J. van der Laan

Researchers are frequently interested in assessing the direct effect of one variable on an outcome of interest, where this effect is not mediated through a set of intermediate variables. In this chapter, we will examine direct effects in a gender salary equity study example. Such studies provide one measure of the equity of procedures used to set salaries and of decisions in promoting and advancing faculty based on performance measures. The goal is to assess whether gender, as determined at birth, has a direct effect on the salary at which a faculty member is hired, not mediated through intermediate performance of the subject up until the time the subject gets hired. If such a direct effect exists, then that means the salary was set in response not only to merit but also to the gender of the person, indicating a gender inequality issue.

We will start by defining the SCM and a natural direct effect of gender on salary controlling for the intermediate variables. In addition, we present the identifiability assumptions under which this causal quantity can be identified from the distribution of the observed data. We commit to an estimand and nonparametric statistical model, even though we accept that the estimand cannot be interpreted as the desired causal direct effect in the gender inequality study. Nevertheless, it represents an effect of gender that controls for the *measured* intermediate variables, and thereby represents a "best" approximation of the desired causal direct effect, given the restrictions of the observed data. We present TMLE for this estimand in a nonparametric statistical model and apply it to our gender equity data set.

8.1 Defining the Causal Direct Effect

The observed data structure is $O = (W, A, Y) \sim P_0$. Here, Y represents the salary for a specific year, A refers to gender with $A = 1$ for females and $A = 0$ for males, and W is the set of intermediate predictive factors available. In our data these intermediate factors include (1) the nature of the highest degree received, (2) years since receipt of highest degree, and (3) years since appointment at the institution.

We define the full data modeled by an SCM as $(X, U) \sim P_{X,U,0}$, where $X = (A, W, H, Y)$ are the endogenous nodes and U denotes the exogenous factors drawn from some distribution $P_{U,0}$. That is, given $U = u$, $X = (A, W, H, Y)$ is deterministically generated by a collection of functions, $f_A(u_A)$,$f_W(A, u_W)$, $f_H(A, W, u_H)$, $f_Y(A, W, H, u_Y)$. This SCM implies a counterfactual random variable $Y(a, w, h) = Y(a, w, h)(U)$ corresponding with intervening on the SCM by setting $A = a, W = w, H = h$, while keeping U random. H is a binary variable indicating whether or not a person is hired.

Because we only observe subjects if they have been hired, the actual observed data O follows the conditional distribution of (A, W, Y), given $H = 1$. We can now define a definition of the "gender" effect as a weighted average of the w-specific controlled direct effects of gender, where the weights are with respect to the probability distribution of the intermediate variables, given one is female ($A = 1$) and hired ($H = 1$). We will refer to this causal quantity as a generalized natural direct effect (NDE) parameter:

$$\Psi^F_{NDE}(P_{X,U,0}) = \sum_w E_{X,U,0}[Y(1, w, H = 1) - Y(0, w, H = 1)]Q_{W,0}(w), \tag{8.1}$$

with $Q_{W,0}(w) \equiv P_0(W = w \mid A = 1, H = 1)$. As discussed in van der Laan and Petersen (2008), the so-called NDE of treatment A on outcome Y, controlling for intermediate variables W, can be presented as $E_0[\sum_w(Y(1, w) - Y(0, w))P_0(W = w \mid A = 0)]$. In our case the only difference is that we are averaging the counterfactual differences within strata w with weights $P_0(W = w \mid A = 1, H = 1)$, so that we should indeed use the same terminology.

Under the causal graph assumption of no unblocked backdoor path from (A, W, H) to Y through the Us, or, equivalently, that (A, W, H) is independent of the counterfactuals $Y(a, w, h) = f_Y(a, w, h, U_Y)$, we can identify this causal quantity $\Psi^F_{NDE}(P_{X,U,0})$ from the probability distribution of the observed data structure O. Specifically, one can write parameter (8.1) as the following parameter mapping applied to the true observed data distribution P_0:

$$\begin{aligned}\Psi_{NDE}(P_0) &= E_0[E_0(Y \mid A = 1, W, H = 1) - E_0(Y \mid A = 0, W, H = 1) \mid A = 1, H = 1] \\ &= E_0[Y - E_0(Y \mid A = 0, W, H = 1) \mid A = 1, H = 1]. \end{aligned} \tag{8.2}$$

Note that the estimand defines a statistical parameter mapping $\Psi_{NDE} : \mathcal{M} \to \mathbb{R}$, where $\mathcal{M}$ is the nonparametric statistical model. For notational convenience, henceforth we suppress the conditioning on $H = 1$ in all conditional distributions.

Standard practice for estimating the estimand in gender equity studies is to fit a standard parametric regression among the men for $E_0[Y \mid A = 0, W]$, use the resulting fit to predict the outcomes among the women, compute for each female the difference between the observed outcome and this predicted outcome, and average all these differences. This is indeed a particular method for estimation of estimand (8.2) obtained by substitution of a parametric regression fit for $E_0(Y \mid A = 0, W)$, and the empirical distribution for the conditional distribution of W, given $A = 1$. Since in truth we lack the knowledge that warrants a parametric model, we pose a nonparametric statistical model $\mathcal{M}$ for the probability distribution of $O = (W, A, Y)$. We now have to develop an estimator of the desired estimand in this nonparametric statistical model.

It is understood that the causal interpretation of the estimand as an actual natural direct causal effect is very questionable as relevant variables were not collected, such as merit, on the pathway from gender to the outcome. However, the causal model makes explicit the desired causal quantity of interest and provides a framework to understand what intermediate variables W need to be measured to make estimand (8.2) approach the causal direct effect one desires. For example, if one wishes to exclude certain intermediate variables due to other considerations, then the bias resulting from such steps could be studied analytically or through Monte Carlo simulations.

Conveniently, a causal effect among the treated defined in another SCM as $W = f_W(U_W)$, $A = f_A(W, U_A)$, $Y = f_Y(W, A, U_Y)$, under the randomization assumption that U_A is independent of U_Y, is identified by the same estimand (8.2) above (van der Laan 2010c). In that case, W are confounders of the treatment of interest, A, instead of being on the causal pathway.

As a consequence, the TMLE of the estimand for the effect among the treated in one SCM is identical to the TMLE of the estimand for the NDE in our SCM. Of course, the interpretation of the estimand is a function of the assumed SCM. So, though we present a TMLE of an average controlled direct effect among the treated in our causal model, we can also use this TMLE to estimate the causal effect among the treated for another causal model. This example nicely shows the distinct tasks of defining a causal parameter of interest in a causal model for the full data (that is, a function of the distribution of U, X) and developing estimators of the corresponding statistical estimand.

8.2 TMLE

We have defined a specific estimand $\Psi_{NDE}(P_0)$ as well as provided identifiability conditions under which one can interpret the parameter value as a type of weighted-average controlled direct effect. In this section we will now and then suppress the NDE in the notation of this estimand since no other estimands are considered. Suppressing the conditioning on hiring ($H = 1$), the estimand can be represented as

$$\Psi_{NDE}(P_0) = E_0[E_0(Y \mid A = 1, W) - E_0(Y \mid A = 0, W) \mid A = 1]. \qquad (8.3)$$

We factorize P_0 in terms of the marginal distribution $Q_{W,0}$ of W, the conditional distribution g_0 of A, given W, and the conditional distribution $Q_{Y,0}$ of Y, given A, W.

We note that $\psi_{NDE,0}$ depends on P_0 through $\bar{Q}_0(A,W) = E_0(Y \mid A,W)$, $Q_{W,0}$, and g_0. The TMLE presented below will yield a targeted estimator $\bar{Q}_n^*$ and g_n^* of $\bar{Q}_0$ and g_0, and the empirical distribution $Q_{W,n}$ of the marginal distribution $Q_{W,0}$ of W. Let $Q_0 = (Q_{W,0}, \bar{Q}_0)$, so that we can also present the estimand as $\Psi_{NDE}(Q_0, g_0)$. The TMLE of $\Psi_{NDE}(Q_0, g_0)$ is a substitution estimator $\Psi(Q_n^*, g_n^*)$ obtained by plugging in this estimator (Q_n^*, g_n^*). Due to the particular form of g_n^*, we show below that this substitution estimator corresponds with using the empirical distribution for the conditional distribution of W, given $A = 1$, so that the TMLE of the estimand $\psi_{NDE,0}$ can also be represented as

$$\Psi_{NDE}(Q_n^*, g_n^*) = \frac{1}{\sum_{i=1}^n I(A_i = 1)} \sum_{i=1}^n I(A_i = 1) * [\bar{Q}_n^*(1, W_i) - \bar{Q}_n^*(0, W_i)]. \tag{8.4}$$

To develop the TMLE we first need an initial estimator of the outcome regression $\bar{Q}_0$, and the treatment mechanism g_0, while estimating the marginal distribution of W with the empirical probability distribution of $W_1, \ldots, W_n$. We can estimate both $\bar{Q}_0$ and g_0 with loss-based super learning using the appropriate loss function for $\bar{Q}_0$ and log-likelihood loss function for g_0, respectively. If Y is binary, then we would use the log-likelihood loss function $L(\bar{Q})(O) = Y \log \bar{Q}(A,W) + (1 - Y)\log(1 - \bar{Q}(A,W))$ for $\bar{Q}_0$. This same loss function can also be used if $Y \in [0,1]$, as shown in Chap. 7. If Y is continuous and bounded between a and b so that $P_0(a < Y < b) = 1$, we can either use the squared error loss function or this quasi-log-likelihood loss function applied to a linearly transformed $Y^* = (Y - a)/(b - a)$. Let $\bar{Q}_n^0, g_n^0$ be the resulting super learner fits of $\bar{Q}_0$ and g_0, respectively. This provides us with our initial estimator (Q_n^0, g_n^0) of (Q_0, g_0).

To determine the parametric submodel through the initial estimator that can be used to encode the fluctuations in the TMLE algorithm, we need to know the efficient influence curve of the target parameter $\Psi_{NDE} : \mathcal{M} \to \mathbb{R}$. This statistical target parameter was studied in van der Laan (2010c) in the context of a causal model for the causal effect among the treated, and the efficient influence curve at a $P \in \mathcal{M}$ was derived as (see also Appendix A)

$$\begin{aligned} D^*(P) = &\left(\frac{I(A=1)}{P(A=1)} - \frac{I(A=0)g(1 \mid W)}{P(A=1)g(0 \mid W)} \right) [Y - \bar{Q}(A,W)] \\ &+ \frac{I(A=1)}{P(A=1)} [\bar{Q}(1,W) - \bar{Q}(0,W) - \Psi(P)], \end{aligned} \tag{8.5}$$

where $\bar{Q} = \bar{Q}(P)$ and $g = g(P)$ are the conditional mean and probability distribution, respecively, under P. The first component, $D_Y^*(P)$, is a score of the conditional distribution of Y, given A, W, and the second component is a score $D_{A,W}^*(P)$ of the joint distribution of (A, W). The latter component of the efficient influence curve $D^*(P)$ can be orthogonally decomposed as $D_{A,W}^*(P) = D_W^*(P) + D_A^*(P)$, where

$$D^*_W(P) = \frac{g(1 \mid W)}{P(A = 1)}(\bar{Q}(1, W) - \bar{Q}(0, W) - \Psi(P)) \text{ and}$$
$$D^*_A(P) = \frac{I(A = 1) - g(1 \mid W)}{P(A = 1)}(\bar{Q}(1, W) - \bar{Q}(0, W) - \Psi(P))$$

are scores for the marginal distribution of W and the conditional distribution of A, given W. One can represent (8.5) as a function of the parameter of interest, ψ, Q, and g, or $D^*(Q, g, \psi)$. The resulting estimating function is double robust, or, formally,

$$P_0 D^*(Q, g, \psi_0) = 0 \text{ if } Q = Q_0 \text{ or } g = g_0,$$

where $Pf \equiv \int f(o)dP(o)$. Since the TMLE Q^*_n, g^*_n solves the efficient influence curve equation, $P_n D^*(Q^*_n, g^*_n, \Psi(Q^*_n, g^*_n)) = 0$, this double robustness implies that the TMLE $\Psi(Q^*_n, g^*_n)$ is consistent for ψ_0 if either Q^*_n is consistent for Q_0 or g^*_n is consistent for g_0. Apparently, even though the estimand depends on both Q_0 and g_0, we still obtain a consistent estimator if either Q_0 or g_0 is consistently estimated!

The next step in defining the TMLE is to select loss functions $L_1(\bar{Q})$ and $L_2(g) = -\log g$ for $\bar{Q}_0$ and g_0, respectively, and construct parametric submodels $\{\bar{Q}^0_n(\epsilon_1) : \epsilon_1\}$ and $\{g^0_n(\epsilon_2) : \epsilon_2\}$ so that the two "scores"

$$\frac{d}{d\epsilon_1} L_1(\bar{Q}^0_n(\epsilon_1)) \text{ and}$$

$$\frac{d}{d\epsilon_2} L_2(g^0_n(\epsilon_2))$$

at $\epsilon_1 = \epsilon_2 = 0$ span the efficient influence curve $D^*(Q^0_n, g^0_n)$ at the initial estimator. If we use the squared error loss function $L_1(\bar{Q})(O) = (Y - \bar{Q}(A, W))^2$, then we select the linear fluctuation working model $\bar{Q}^0_n(\epsilon_1)(A, W) = \bar{Q}^0_n(A, W) + \epsilon_1 C_1(g^0_n)(A, W)$, where

$$C_1(g)(A, W) = I(A = 1) - \frac{I(A = 0)g(1 \mid W)}{g(0 \mid W)}.$$

If Y is binary or continuous in $[0, 1]$ and we select the quasi-log-likelihood loss function for $L_1(\bar{Q})$, then we select the logisitic fluctuation working model logit $\bar{Q}^0_n(\epsilon_1) =$ logit $\bar{Q}^0_n + \epsilon_1 C_1(g^0_n)$. In the context of theoretical or practical violations of the positivity assumption, $P_0(g_0(0 \mid W) > 0) = 1$, as required for a bounded variance of the efficient influence curve, and Y being continuous, we strongly recommend the quasi-log-likelihood loss function $L_1(\bar{Q})$ for $\bar{Q}_0$, since the resulting TMLE will then fully respect the global bounds $[a, b]$ of the statistical model. As parametric submodel through g^0_n, we select $\text{logit}(g^0_n(\epsilon_2)(1 \mid W)) = \text{logit}(g^0_n(1 \mid W)) + \epsilon_2 C_2(g^0_n, Q^0_n)(W)$, where

$$C_2(Q, g)(W) = \bar{Q}(1, W) - \bar{Q}(0, W) - \Psi(Q, g).$$

Finally, we select the log-likelihood loss function $L(Q_W) = -\log Q_W$ for the probability distribution $Q_{W,0}$, and, as a parametric submodel through $Q_{W,n}$, we select $\{Q_{W,n}(\epsilon_3) = (1 + \epsilon_3 D^*_W(Q^0_n, g^0_n))Q_{W,n} : \epsilon_3\}$, where

$$D_W^*(Q_n^0, g_n^0)(W) = g_n^0(1 \mid W)\left\{\bar{Q}_n^0(1, W) - \bar{Q}_n^0(0, W) - \Psi(Q_n^0)\right\}.$$

We note that the scores with respect to the loss functions $L_1(\bar{Q})$, $L_2(g)$ and $L(Q_W)$ generated by these three submodels are $D_Y^*(Q_n^0, g_n^0) \equiv C_1(g_n^0)(Y - \bar{Q}_n^0)$, $D_A^*(Q_n^0, g_n^0) \equiv C_2(g_n^0, Q_n^0)(A - g_n^0(1 \mid W))$, and $D_W^*(Q_n^0, g_n^0)$, respectively, and the sum of these three scores equals $D^*(Q_n^0, g_n^0)$ up till the scalar $P_0(A = 1)$. Thus, if we define the single loss function $L(Q_n^0, g_n^0) = L_1(\bar{Q}_n^0) + L(Q_{W,n}) + L_2(g_n^0)$, then

$$\frac{d}{d\epsilon} L(Q_n^0(\epsilon), g_n^0(\epsilon))$$

at $\epsilon = 0$ spans the efficient influence curve $D^*(Q_n^0, g_n^0)$. That is, we successfully carried out the second step in defining the TMLE involving the selection of a loss function and corresponding parametric submodel through the initial estimator whose score spans the efficient influence curve at the initial estimator. The TMLE algorithm is now defined.

The maximum likelihood estimator of $\epsilon_n = (\epsilon_{1,n}, \epsilon_{2,n}, \epsilon_{3,n})$, according to the working parametric submodel through (Q_n^0, g_n^0), defines an updated fit $(Q_n^1 = Q_n^0(\epsilon_{1,n}, \epsilon_{3,n}),\ g_n^1 = g_n^0(\epsilon_{2,n}))$. Since we selected $Q_{W,n}$ to be the nonparametric maximum likelihood estimator of $Q_{W,0}$, we have that $\epsilon_{3,n} = 0$, so that the empirical distribution of W is not updated. This TMLE updating of $\bar{Q}_n^0$ and g_n^0 is iterated until convergence, and we denote the final fit with $(Q_n^* = (\bar{Q}_n^*, Q_{W,n}), g_n^*)$. The TMLE of ψ_0 is the corresponding substitution estimator $\Psi(Q_n^*, g_n^*)$.

Due to the fact that $P_n D_{A,W}^*(Q_n^*, g_n^*) = 0$, it follows immediately that the TMLE equals the substitution estimator (8.4) obtained by plugging in $\bar{Q}_n^*$ for $\bar{Q}_0$, and plugging in the empirical probability distribution for the conditional distribution of W, given $A = 1$. Suppose that we replace in the TMLE algorithm the parametric submodel $\bar{Q}_n^0(\epsilon_1)$ with

$$\bar{Q}_n^0(\epsilon_{11}, \epsilon_{12}) = \bar{Q}_n^0 + \epsilon_{11} C_{11} + \epsilon_{12} C_{12}(g_n^0),$$

where $C_{11}(A, W) = I(A = 1)$, and $C_{12}(g)(A, W) = I(A = 0)g(1 \mid W)/g(0 \mid W)$, and thus fit $\epsilon_1 = (\epsilon_{11}, \epsilon_{12})$ accordingly. Then the TMLE $\bar{Q}_n^*$ also solves the equation $\sum_{i=1}^n I(A_i = 1)(Y_i - \bar{Q}_n^*(1, W_i))$, so that we obtain the following representation of the TMLE:

$$\Psi(Q_n^*, g_n^*) = \frac{1}{\sum_{i=1}^n I(A_i = 1)} \sum_{i=1}^n I(A_i = 1)\left\{Y_i - \bar{Q}_n^*(0, W_i)\right\}. \tag{8.6}$$

That is, the difference between this TMLE and the standard practice in assessing gender inequality is only in the choice of estimator of $\bar{Q}_0$: the TMLE uses a targeted data-adaptive estimator, while standard practice would use a maximum likelihood estimator according to a parametric model.

Regarding implementation of this TMLE, we make the following remark. Technically, in each TMLE update step for $\bar{Q}_0$ one treats the most recent updated estimate of $\bar{Q}_0$ as offset, and one computes the appropriate maximum likelihood estimate of

ϵ_1 according to the parametric working model $\bar{Q}_n^k(\epsilon_1) = \bar{Q}_n^{k-1} + \epsilon_1 C_1(g_n)$. So if it takes K iterations until convergence, then the final fit can be represented as

$$\bar{Q}_n^* = \bar{Q}_n^0 + \sum_{k=1}^{K} \epsilon_{1n}^k C_1(g_n^{k-1}),$$

where g_n^k represents the estimated g after the kth iteration of estimation (and convergence would imply that $\epsilon_{1n}^K \approx 0$). Similarly, this applies to the final fit g_n^*. From a programming standpoint, this means that all one needs to save from the estimation procedure is the sequence, $(\epsilon_{1n}^k, \epsilon_{2n}^k), k = 1, \ldots, K$, as well as the initial fits, $(\bar{Q}_n^0, g_n^0)$. Finally, statistical inference can be based on the sample variance of the estimated efficient influence curve $D^*(Q_0, g_0)$, or the bootstrap.

One may also wish to employ a C-TMLE (Chaps. 19–21 and 23) approach, which would choose among a sequence of candidate estimates of g_0 in a targeted fashion. Remarkably, the efficient influence curve also satisfies collaborative double robustness results so that the C-TMLE can indeed be utilized to build a targeted regression estimator of g_0.

8.3 Simulation

To demonstrate the double robustness of the TMLE, we perform a simple simulation. Specifically, we have a binary $A \in \{0, 1\}$ with $P_0(A = 1) = 0.5$, a simple binary W where $P_0(W = 1|A = 1) = 0.27$ and $P(W = 1|A = 0) = 0.12$, and Y is normally distributed with a conditional mean given by $50000 + 4000W - 1000A + 3000A \times W$, and constant variance 100. The NDE is given by $\Psi_{NDE}(Q_0, g_0) = -192$. We simulate from this same data-generating distribution for sample sizes of $10^i, i = 2, \ldots, 6$, and for each data set we use a correctly specified model for the conditional probability distribution g_0 of A, given W, but a misspecified parametric regression model $E_0(Y \mid A, W) = \beta_0 A + \beta_1 A$ for $\bar{Q}_0$. Thus, the MLE of the estimand will be substantially biased, but the TMLE should eliminate that bias because of the correct model used for g_0. The results (Fig. 8.1) confirm the double robustness property of the TMLE, and thus its value for rectifying bias that can result from nontargeted initial estimates of $\bar{Q}_0$.

8.4 Data Analysis

We use data on 9-month faculty salaries at two schools at the University of California, Irvine, for the academic year 2007–08. There were 579 male and 269 female faculty members. The W variables were as follows: Ph.D. degree, years of UC service (in any position), years since earning highest degree, and department. From a causal direct effect point of view, one should use other measures of performance as

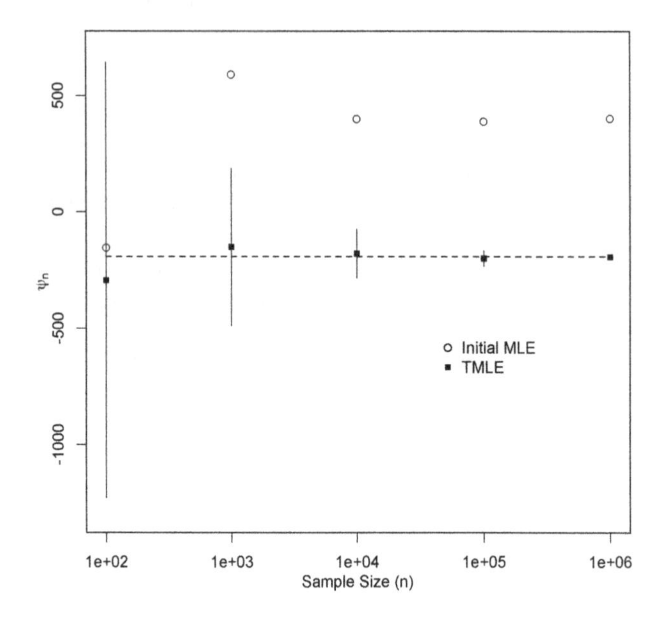

Fig. 8.1 Simulation results for the NDE. *Vertical bars* represent 95% confidence intervals based on standard errors derived from the influence curve (8.5); the *dotted line* is the true value, $\psi_{NDE}(Q_0, g_0)$

well, but there is great controversy in defining academic merit (which itself might be subject to biases, including gender biases), and thus only the most noncontroversial variables associated with salary are typically used.

8.4.1 Unadjusted Mean Difference in Salary

We first carried out a standard least squares regression analysis in which we only have gender (females are $A = 1$) in the regression. Assuming our SCM, and again suppressing the dependence on hiring, H, the coefficient on A is an estimate of the total additive effect due to gender: $\psi^F_{0,Total} \equiv E_0[Y_1 - Y_0]$, where now $Y(a)$ represents the outcome when, possibly contrary to fact, $A = a$, or, using our system of SCM above, $Y(a) = f_Y(a, f_W(a, U_W), U_Y)$. Under our SCM, and the assumption that U_A is independent of U_Y, this is identifiable as a mapping of P_0 as $\psi_{0,Total} = E_0(Y \mid A = 1) - E_0(Y \mid A = 0)$. The corresponding plug-in estimator is simply the difference in average salary among the women ($A = 1$) vs. the men ($A = 0$). This analysis resulted in an estimate $\psi_{n,Total}$ of $-\$13{,}853$ and a 95% confidence interval given by (−\$18,510, −\$9,197). Thus, the salary among women is on average \$13,000 less than the average salary among men, and this difference is statistically significant. These results are also displayed in Table 8.1.

8.4.2 Adjusted Mean Difference in Salary: $\Psi_{NDE}(P_0)$

As is evident from representation (8.6) of the TMLE, the only distinction between the TMLE and the standard approach is the choice of estimator of $\bar{Q}_0(1, W)$, i.e., the conditional mean of the salaries among men as a function of the intermediate variables W. This regression function is then used to predict the salary for the females, and one takes the average of the prediction errors among all the females in the sample. The standard approach uses a simple multivariate linear regression to fit $\bar{Q}_0(1, W)$ among the males ($A = 1$). This main term linear regression includes as main terms the indicator of having earned a Ph.D., years of service, years since highest degree, and nine dummy variables representing the ten departments. To obtain robust standard errors, we used a nonparametric bootstrap. This analysis resulted in an estimate of the estimand given by −\$2,235, with a 95% confidence interval (−\$5,228, \$756).

We then used a TMLE that acknowledges that the model for both $\bar{Q}_0$ and g_0 are unknown (and thus uses a data-adaptive estimator) but targets these adaptive estimators to optimize the estimate of $\psi_{NDE,0}$. However, we must start with initial estimates $\bar{Q}_n^0$ of $\bar{Q}_0$ and g_n^0 of g_0. For $\bar{Q}_n^0$, we used a super learner with three linear regression candidate estimators (one with all covariates entered linearly, one with only the covariates besides the dummy variables indicating the department, and one with only gender), polymars, and DSA. The latter two algorithms are machine learning procedures, and for both we enforced the inclusion of gender in the model fit. As initial estimate g_n^0 of the conditional distribution of gender given W, we used simple multivariate linear logistic regression with all covariates entered as main terms. In order to estimate the variance of the TMLE, we used both the empirical variance of the estimated influence curve (8.5), plugging in the final fits, $(\bar{Q}_n^*, g_n^*, \Psi(Q_n^*, g_n^*))$, as well as a more conservative cross-validated empirical variance of the estimated influence curve using a 10-fold cross-validation, where the training sample was used to estimate the influence curve, while the validation sample was used to estimate the variance of this influence curve (van der Laan and Gruber 2010).

In Table 8.1, we display estimates of the unadjusted effect, the naive direct effect, and the TMLE direct effect. Neither estimate of the direct effect of gender is statistically significantly different from the null value. It is of interest to note that the TMLE had a much smaller estimate of the variability: the estimate of the variance of the TMLE was 30% smaller than the estimate of the variance of the naive estimate. (We note that the more conservative CV-based variance of the TMLE was approximately 1400, still reflecting a significant gain in variance.) Thus, although the statistical model for P_0 for the TMLE was much larger than the main term linear regression model of the naive approach, and the TMLE carried out a subsequent tar-

Table 8.1 Analysis results for University of California, Irvine salary gender equity study estimates for the average salary difference between genders, as well as estimates of ψ_{NDE} using both the naive estimator and the TMLE

Parameter	Approach	Estimate	SE	95% CI
ψ_{Unadj}		–$13,853	2,372	(–$18,510, –$9,197)
ψ_{NDE}	Naive	–$2,235	1,526	(–$5,228, $756)
ψ_{NDE}	TMLE	–$2,212	1,336	(–$4,830, $406)

geted bias reduction as well, the variability of the TMLE was still lower. Regarding data analysis, the bottom line is what appeared to be very strong evidence of salary inequity based on a simple difference in average salaries; the naive and TMLE direct effects of gender, controlling for some intermediate variables, show that these data do not support the presence of salary inequality, but it can be stated that the estimated salary gap is around $2,200, and, with a 95% confidence level, the salary gap is at most $4,800.

8.5 Discussion

The road map for assessing a causal direct effect (1) states explicitly the causal model and causal direct effect ψ_0^F of interest, (2) states explicitly the identifiability assumptions required to identify the causal direct effect from the observed data distribution, P_0, thereby defining a statistical target parameter mapping, $\Psi(P_0)$, (3) defines the statistical model $\mathcal{M}$ for P_0 based on what is truly known about P_0, (4) estimates the required components of P_0 respecting the statistical model $\mathcal{M}$ using loss-based machine learning, (5) targets the estimation of these components of P_0 for optimizing estimation of $\Psi(P_0)$, where this definition of optimal is based on efficiency theory for estimators. This salary equity example serves as a useful exercise in demonstrating how current ad hoc approaches are more a function of traditional practice than a rigorous methodology used to derive as much information about a scientific question as possible from the data at hand. As discussed, when the covariates W are confounders of a treatment variable A of interest, the *average treatment effect among the treated* (Heckman et al. 1997) is identified by the identical statistical estimand that is the focus of this chapter. Thus, this discussion also applies to situations where the estimand is the same, but the interpretation is different based on a different causal model. We note that much has been written about the average treatment effect among the treated, being a common parameter of interest in fields such as economics and political science. The approach emphasized here has significant relevance to current practice in several disciplines.

8.6 Notes and Further Reading

A popular class of methods for estimation of the treatment effect among the treated is semiparametric matching methods, including propensity score matching algorithms (Rosenbaum and Rubin 1983), and the more recently developed genetic matching algorithms (Sekhon 2006). However, these methods are somewhat inefficient, i.e., the stratification of the sample in clusters of matched treated and nontreated subjects is only informed by the data on (W, A), ignoring the outcome. Attempts to rectify this (Hansen 2008) have failed to provide useful solutions. One can think of such an estimator as an NPMLE that stratifies on W according to an unsupervised method. Two disadvantages of such a method are the lack of smoothing in estimation of $\bar{Q}_0$, and the lack of targeting of the stratification strategy with respect to the target parameter. For example, a treated person might be considered similar to a nontreated person based on similarity in variables that are nonpredictive of the outcome. (C-)TMLE resolves both of these issues.

There is considerable literature on pay equity studies in the academy. In particular, the American Association of University Professors (AAUP) has published a guidebook on implementation of pay equity studies (Haignere 2002). The naive approach presented for ψ_{NDE} is in fact the recommended AAUP approach. Interpretation of these studies is complicated by the absence of adequate measures of the quality and quantity of an individual's performance in terms of research, teaching, and public and professional service despite the fact that it is these very attributes that are presumably the predominant factors in the salary reward system in academia. Without such factors available, gender comparisons are usually adjusted solely by various demographic factors, largely reflecting the "academic age" of individuals. The two principal variables of this type that are associated with current salaries are (1) the number of years since receipt of the highest degree (usually the Ph.D.) and (2) the number of years since appointment to the current institution. The latter variable is important in capturing the influence of market forces in determining salary, almost always at play at the time an individual is hired.

In this chapter, we postulated the existence of an underlying counterfactual salary for an individual whose gender was different. However, this chapter was not focused on questions of the existence of such counterfactuals, and other ontological issues, but on defining sensible parameters of the data-generating distribution that aim to address gender equity. For debates on defining the "causal" effect of a variable such as gender, see, for instance, Holland (1988).

Chapter 9
Marginal Structural Models

Michael Rosenblum

In many applications, one would like to estimate the effect of a treatment or exposure on various subpopulations. For example, one may be interested in these questions:

- What is the effect of an antidepressant medication on Hamilton Depression Rating Scale (HAM-D) score for those who enter a study with severe depression, and for those who enter with moderate depression?
- What is the effect of a cancer therapy for those who test positive for overexpression of a particular gene and for those who test negative for overexpression of that gene?
- What is the impact of low adherence to antiretroviral therapy on viral load for HIV-positive individuals who have just achieved viral suppression and for those who have maintained continuous viral suppression for 1 year?

In this chapter, we present a method for estimating the effect of a treatment or exposure in various subpopulations in an HIV treatment application. We first present an analysis in which there are only two subpopulations of interest. Then we present an analysis with 12 subpopulations of interest, where we use a marginal structural model as a working model. Marginal structural models, an important class of causal models and target parameters, were introduced by Robins (1998).

9.1 Impact of Missing Doses on Virologic Failure

For HIV-positive individuals taking antiretroviral medication, a danger in missing doses is that the HIV virus may increase replication. A measure of the amount of circulating virus is called "viral load." It is of interest to understand how different levels of missed doses (e.g., missing 20% of doses in a month or 40% of doses in a month) are related to the probability of subsequent increases in viral load. Furthermore, we'd like to understand how the impact of missed doses on viral load may differ depending on patient history of viral suppression. The aspect of patient history of viral suppression we focus on is the number of consecutive months in the past, starting just before the current month, that a subject has had viral load below 50 copies/ml (which we refer to as "duration of continuous suppression"). As an example, we'd like to understand the impact of low adherence to antiretroviral therapy on viral load for HIV-positive individuals who have just achieved viral suppression and for those who have maintained continuous viral suppression for 1 year. We describe a particular data analysis that aimed to answer this question, which is fully described in Rosenblum et al. (2009).

The population we consider is HIV-positive individuals in the Research in Access to Care for the Homeless (REACH) cohort; subjects in the study consist of a systematic, community-based sample of HIV-positive urban poor individuals in San Francisco (Moss et al. 2004). Adherence to antiretroviral therapy was assessed based on unannounced pill counts, as described in Bangsberg et al. (2001).

We consider four levels of percent adherence to therapy in a given month: 0–49%, 50–74%, 75–89%, and 90–100%. The outcome we consider is whether a patient's viral load is less than 50 copies/ml in a given month. We say a patient experiences virologic failure if her viral load is at least 50 copies/ml.

Three hundred and fifty-seven subjects were monitored monthly for medication adherence. Each subject who had a viral load of less than 50 copies/ml over 2 consecutive months (which is an indicator of successful suppression of the HIV virus) was included in the study; a total of 221 subjects met this criterion. For each included subject, we found the earliest occurrence of 2 consecutive months with viral load less than 50 copies/ml; we let "month 0" denote the first of these two consecutive months.

The goal is to produce estimates of the risk of virologic failure at the end of a given month, under each of the four adherence levels, controlling for variables measured prior to that month. We will get such estimates for each of the following 12 groups:

1 Risk of virologic failure at the end of month 2 among subjects who remained continuously suppressed through month 1;
2 Risk of virologic failure at the end of month 3 among subjects who remained continuously suppressed through month 2;

⋮

12 Risk of virologic failure at the end of month 13 among subjects who remained continuously suppressed through month 12.

We point out that all 221 subjects included in the study contribute data to the estimate in group 1 above (since the inclusion criterion described above requires that subjects be suppressed during month 1). Fewer subjects directly contribute data to the estimates in the latter groups. We also used a nonsaturated marginal structural model in our analysis that "smoothed" estimates across the above 12 groups. In this case, data from each subject indirectly contributed to the estimates for each of the above groups. This is discussed further in Sect. 9.6.

Of special interest is to compare the relative risk of virologic failure between the highest adherence level (90–100%) and the lowest adherence level (0–49%) for each of the above 12 groups. We can then test for effect modification by comparing this relative risk across the 12 groups.

9.2 Data

Longitudinal data were collected on each subject in the REACH cohort. However, for clarity, we present a simplified data structure in which each subject contributes only a single time point of data. The extension to longitudinal data structures is described elsewhere (Rosenblum and van der Laan 2010a, Sect. 4.2). Longitudinal data structures are also discussed in Chaps. 24–26 of this book.

In our simplified data structure, each subject contributes a vector of data consisting of baseline variables (V, W) measured at the beginning of a month, percent adherence to antiretroviral medication during that month (A), and virologic failure at the end of the month (Y). The baseline variable V denotes duration of continuous viral suppression up to the current time point. The baseline variables W include the following potential confounders of the effect of adherence on virologic failure:

> prior adherence, prior duration of HAART, prior exposure to mono/dual nucleoside therapy, recent CD4+ T cell count (lagged 2 months), CD4+ T cell nadir (lagged 2 months), demographics (sex, ethnicity, age), years of education, past and current antiretroviral treatment characteristics, crack cocaine and alcohol use, calendar time, and homelessness (Rosenblum et al. 2009, p. 2).

Percent adherence A has four levels: $\mathcal{A} = \{0, 1, 2, 3\}$, representing adherence in a given month at 0–49%, 50–74%, 75–89%, and 90–100%, respectively. Y is a binary-valued indicator of virologic failure. Duration of past continuous suppression V takes levels $\mathcal{V} = \{0, 1, 2, \ldots, 11\}$. We denote this vector of data for each subject i by (V_i, W_i, A_i, Y_i). We assume that each subject's data vector is an independent draw from an unknown distribution P_0 of a random vector (V, W, A, Y).

9.3 Statistical Model

We assume a nonparametric statistical model for P_0; that is, we put no restrictions on the true data-generating distribution except that it can be represented as a density with respect to a known dominating measure. Since each distribution we consider has a corresponding density, with a slight abuse of notation, we sometimes refer to distributions such as P_0 as densities. The likelihood of the data at a candidate probability distribution P can be written

$$\prod_{i=1}^{n} P(Y_i, A_i, V_i, W_i) = \prod_{i=1}^{n} P_Y(Y_i \mid A_i, V_i, W_i) P_A(A_i \mid V_i, W_i) P_{V,W}(V_i, W_i).$$

9.4 Parameter of Interest

We are interested in the impact of percent adherence to antiretroviral therapy during a given month on virologic failure at the end of that month. We would furthermore like to know how this impact of adherence varies depending on duration of continuous viral suppression prior to that month.

Let Y_a denote the potential outcome that would have been observed had adherence been at level $a \in \mathcal{A}$. We'd like to learn the probability that $Y_a = 1$, within strata of duration of continuous, past suppression V, that is

$$P(Y_a = 1 \mid V = v), a \in \mathcal{A}, v \in \mathcal{V}. \tag{9.1}$$

We also would like to express the above display as a mapping from the distribution of the observed data (since for each subject three of the four potential outcomes $\{Y_a\}_{a \in \mathcal{A}}$ are unobserved). We make the following assumptions, described in Chap. 2, which we use to connect the potential outcomes to the observed data:

- Time-ordering assumption: W, V precede A, which precedes Y;
- Consistency assumption: For all $a \in \mathcal{A}$, $Y = Y_a$ on the event $A = a$;
- Randomization assumption (no unmeasured confounders): $\{Y_a\}_{a \in \mathcal{A}} \perp\!\!\!\perp A \mid W, V$; and
- Positivity assumption: $P(A = a \mid W = w, V = v) > 0$ for all $a \in \mathcal{A}$ and all (w, v) in the support of P_0.

Under these assumptions, we can equate function (9.1) of the potential outcomes we are interested in with a mapping from the distribution of the observed data, as follows:

$$P(Y_a = 1 \mid V = v) = E_{W|V=v} P(Y = 1 \mid A = a, V = v, W), a \in \mathcal{A}, v \in \mathcal{V},$$

where $E_{W|V=v}$ is expectation with respect to the distribution of baseline variables W given $V = v$.

We define our parameter of interest $\Psi(P)$ to be the mapping from the observed data distribution given on the right-hand side of the previous display:

$$\Psi(P)(a, v) = E_{W|V=v} P(Y = 1 \mid A = a, V = v, W). \tag{9.2}$$

If A and V each had only a couple levels, we could estimate $\Psi(P_0)(a, v)$ (where P_0 is the true, unknown data-generating distribution) directly for each value of a and v. As a stepping stone to the more complex case, we give such an estimator below in Sect. 9.5. Then, in Sect. 9.6, we handle the case described in Sect. 9.2 where there are 48 levels of (A, V) (that come from four possible values for A and 12 for V), and where we define a different parameter of interest using a marginal structural model as a working model.

9.5 Effect Modification: Simplified Case

We consider the case where both A and V are binary valued. The goal is to estimate (9.2) for all four of the possible combinations of a, v. This is a special case of the more general situation we consider in Sect. 9.6. Here we show an estimator for $\Psi(P_0)(0,0)$; the estimators for the parameter at the other values of a and v are similar. We note that it is also possible to construct an estimator of the vector of parameter values $(\Psi(P_0)(0,0), \Psi(P_0)(0,1), \Psi(P_0)(1,0), \Psi(P_0)(1,1))$ using a single iteration of the targeted maximum likelihood algorithm, but for clarity of exposition we do not present the details here, and instead focus on estimating just $\Psi(P_0)(0,0)$.

9.5.1 Obtaining Q_n^0, an Initial Estimate of Q_0

Parameter (9.2) depends on the data-generating distribution P only through the conditional distribution of Y given (A, V, W), and the marginal distribution of (V, W). We let $Q = (P(Y \mid A, V, W), P(V, W))$ denote these relevant parts of the density P. We let Q_0 denote these relevant parts of the true density P_0. There are many ways to construct an initial estimator Q_n^0 of Q_0. For example, one could fit a parametric statistical model. Here, for simplicity, we fit a parametric statistical model for the conditional distribution of virologic failure Y given (A, V, W), and use the empirical distribution for the baseline variables (V, W). We assume that for at least one subject i in our sample, $V_i = 0$.

We fit a logistic regression model for $P_0(Y \mid A, V, W)$ such as

$$P(Y = 1 \mid A, V, W) = \text{expit}\,(\alpha_0 + \alpha_1 A + \alpha_2 V + \alpha_3 W)\,.$$

Denote the model fit by $\bar{Q}_n(Y = 1 \mid A, V, W)$. There are no constraints on what model could be used, e.g., interaction terms could have been included as well. For the initial estimator of $P_0(V, W)$, we use the empirical distribution, which we denote by $Q_{V,W,n}$. Our initial estimator Q_n^0 is defined as the pair $\left(\bar{Q}_n(Y = 1 \mid A, V, W), Q_{V,W,n}(V, W)\right)$. Below, in constructing the fluctuation, we will use the substitution estimator at the initial density estimate Q_n^0:

$$\begin{aligned}\Psi(Q_n^0)(0,0) &= E_{Q_n^0}\left[\bar{Q}_n(Y = 1 \mid A = 0, V = 0, W) \mid V = 0\right] \\ &= \frac{1}{\sum_{i=1}^n I(V_i = 0)} \sum_{i=1}^n I(V_i = 0)\bar{Q}_n(Y = 1 \mid A = 0, V = 0, W_i), \quad (9.3)\end{aligned}$$

where $I(S)$ is the indicator function taking value 1 when S is true and 0 otherwise. The second equality follows since in Q_n^0 we set the distribution of (V, W) to be the empirical distribution, so that the corresponding expectation conditional on $V = 0$ is obtained by averaging over all data points with $V_i = 0$.

9.5.2 Calculating the Optimal Fluctuation

To compute the optimal fluctuation, we first need the efficient influence curve for the parameter $\Psi(P)(0,0)$ in the nonparametric model. This can be derived using the methods in Appendix A. The efficient influence curve is (up to a normalizing constant)

$$\begin{aligned} D_{0,0}(Y, A, V, W) = I(A = 0, V = 0)&\left(\frac{Y - P(Y = 1 \mid A = 0, V = 0, W)}{P(A = 0 \mid V = 0, W)}\right) \\ &+ I(V = 0)[P(Y = 1 \mid A = 0, V = 0, W) - \Psi(P)(0,0)]. \quad (9.4) \end{aligned}$$

We now construct a parametric model $\{P(\epsilon) : \epsilon\}$ that (1) contains the initial estimator Q_n^0 at $\epsilon = 0$ and (2) has a score at $\epsilon = 0$ whose linear span contains the efficient influence curve at Q_n^0. To do this, we first define the clever covariate $H_1^*(A, V, W)$ for fluctuation of the outcome-regression, and function $H_2^*(V, W)$ for fluctuation of the distribution of (V, W):

$$H_1^*(A, V, W) = \frac{I(A = 0, V = 0)}{g_n(A = 0 \mid V = 0, W)}$$

and

$$H_2^*(V, W) = I(V = 0)[\bar{Q}_n(Y = 1 \mid A = 0, V = 0, W) - \Psi(Q_n^0)(0,0)],$$

where $\Psi(Q_n^0)(0,0)$ is defined in (9.3) and $g_n(A \mid V, W)$, for example, is defined based on fitting a logistic regression model.

Let $\epsilon = (\epsilon_1, \epsilon_2)$. Define the parametric model $\{P(\epsilon) : \epsilon\}$:

$$\begin{aligned} P(\epsilon)(Y = 1 \mid A, V, W) &= \text{expit}\left(\epsilon_1 H_1^*(A, V, W) + \text{logit}\left(\bar{Q}_n(Y = 1 \mid A, V, W)\right)\right), \quad (9.5) \\ P(\epsilon)(A \mid V, W) &= g_n(A \mid V, W), \\ P(\epsilon)(V, W) &= s_{\epsilon_2} \exp(\epsilon_2 H_2^*(V, W)) Q_{V,W,n}(V, W), \end{aligned}$$

where the constant $s_{\epsilon_2} = 1/[\frac{1}{n}\sum_{i=1}^n \exp(\epsilon_2 H_2^*(V_i, W_i))]$ is chosen such that $P(\epsilon)(V, W)$ integrates to 1 for each ϵ. It is straightforward to verify that conditions (1) and (2) above are satisfied for the parametric model $\{P(\epsilon) : \epsilon\}$.

9.5.3 Obtaining Q_n^*, a Targeted Estimate of Q_0

We fit the above parametric model using maximum likelihood estimation to get estimates $\epsilon_n = (\epsilon_{1,n}, \epsilon_{2,n})$ of (ϵ_1, ϵ_2). We give arguments below to show that the maximum likelihood estimate $\epsilon_n = (\epsilon_{1,n}, \epsilon_{2,n})$ can be obtained simply as follows: to obtain $\epsilon_{1,n}$, fit the logistic regression model (9.5), which has a single term (H_1^*) and offset equal to $\text{logit}\left(\bar{Q}_n(Y = 1 \mid A, V, W)\right)$; we show below that $\epsilon_{2,n}$ must equal 0.

First, since the only term involved in the likelihood that depends on ϵ_1 is the term in (9.5), the ϵ_1 component of the maximum likelihood estimator is obtained by fitting logistic regression model (9.5). We now show that $\epsilon_{2,n} = 0$. The derivative of the log-likelihood with respect to ϵ_2 is zero at $\epsilon_2 = 0$; also, the second derivative of the log-likelihood with respect to ϵ_2 is everywhere strictly negative as long as the values $H_2^*(V_i, W_i)$, for i in $\{1, \ldots, n\}$, are not all equal. (If these values were all equal, the model $P(\epsilon)(V, W) = Q_{V,W,n}$ for all ϵ.) Therefore, the maximum likelihood estimator $\epsilon_{1,n}, \epsilon_{2,n}$ must have $\epsilon_{2,n} = 0$. This means $P(\epsilon_n)(V, W)$ equals the initial density estimator $Q_{V,W,n}$, which was chosen to be the empirical distribution of (V, W).

It is not necessary here to iterate the above steps, since a second iteration [involving fitting a parametric model as above, but now with clever covariates defined in terms of the density $P(\epsilon_n)$ instead of the initial density estimate Q_n^0] would lead to no update of the current density estimate $P(\epsilon_n)$. This follows since the covariate $H_1^*(A, V, W)$ only depends on g_n, which is not updated in the above model fitting; the covariate $H_2^*(V, W)$ does not lead to any update of the density as argued in the previous paragraph. Thus, a single iteration of the above step suffices for convergence. Our final estimator for the relevant part Q_0 of the density of the data-generating distribution is

$$Q_n^* = P(\epsilon_n) = \left(P(\epsilon_{1,n})(Y = 1 \mid A, V, W), Q_{V,W,n}\right). \tag{9.6}$$

9.5.4 Estimation of Parameter

Lastly, we compute the substitution estimator $\Psi(Q_n^*)(0, 0)$:

$$\psi_n(0, 0) = \frac{1}{\sum_{i=1}^n I(V_i = 0)} \sum_{i=1}^n I(V_i = 0) Q_n^*(Y = 1 \mid A = 0, V = 0, W_i). \tag{9.7}$$

This estimator was obtained by evaluating parameter (9.2) at the final density estimate Q_n^* defined in (9.6). This involved first taking the estimated conditional distribution $Q_n^*(Y = 1 \mid A = 0, V = 0, W)$ and computing its average given V, again according to Q_n^*. Since in Q_n^* we set the distribution of (V, W) to be the empirical distribution, this is obtained by averaging $Q_n^*(Y = 1 \mid A = 0, V = 0, W_i)$ over all data points with $V_i = 0$, as in (9.7). In summary, the above estimator involved obtaining initial estimators for $P_0(Y \mid A, V, W)$ and $P_0(A \mid V, W)$, then fitting a logistic regression involving clever covariates constructed from these initial estimators, and finally averaging this logistic regression fit over the empirical distribution of baseline variables as in (9.7).

A class of estimators that is a special case of the above class of estimators was given in a previous paper (Scharfstein et al. 1999, p. 1141). To the best of our knowledge, they were the first to include the inverse of the propensity score as a covariate in a parametric regression-based estimator for the parameter considered in this section. The estimators there are parametric regression estimators that include the inverse propensity score (H_1^*) as a term in the regression model; these estimators were shown to be double robust and locally efficient.

We next consider the case where V can take 12 values, rather than just 2 values as in this subsection. In that case, estimator (9.7) will not perform well, since for some values of V there may be very few data points contributing to the summation. We will use a marginal structural model to smooth across values of V.

9.6 Effect Modification: Marginal Structural Models

We consider the case introduced in Sect. 9.2, where adherence A can take four possible values, and the number of months of continuous viral suppression V can take 12 values. Here, instead of trying to estimate $\Psi(a, v)$ defined in (9.2) for all 48 possible combinations of (a, v), we will define a different parameter Ψ'. This involves a working statistical model (i.e., marginal structural model as working model) for $\Psi(a, v)$, which can be thought of as smoothing over (a, v). This approach of using marginal structural models as working models to define target parameters is presented in detail Neugebauer and van der Laan (2007) for general longitudinal data structures and multiple time point treatments. The following presentation in this section closely follows that in Rosenblum and van der Laan (2010a, Sect. 4.1).

Marginal Structural Models

For a given treatment level a and duration of past suppression v, the TMLE above for the parameter $\psi_0(a, v)$ defined in (9.2) involves the clever covariate:

$$\frac{I(A = a, V = v)}{g_n(a \mid v, W)}.$$

As a consequence, this estimator may become unstable if there are few subjects in the sample with $A = a$ and $V = v$. In particular, the variance of the estimator will depend on the number of subjects in the category defined by $A = a$ and $V = v$. We present two possible approaches for dealing with this, both of which involve smoothing over the different values of a and v.

The first approach is to assume a statistical model for the parameter $\psi_0(a, v)$ such as:

$$\text{logit}\, \psi_0(a, v) = \beta_0(a, v),$$

indexed by a Euclidean parameter β_0 of lower dimension than $\{\psi_0(a,v), a \in \mathcal{A}, v \in \mathcal{V}\}$. Such a model allows one to focus on estimating the parameter β_0, and the TMLE of β_0 will smooth across all the observations. However, this requires making a model assumption, and if this model assumption is incorrect (i.e., if there is model misspecification, which may be difficult to rule out), then β_0 (and thereby ψ_0) is not defined.

The second approach, which we take here, is to define our target parameter as a summary measure of the parameters $\{\psi_0(a,v) : a, v\}$. For example, for a given adherence level a, one could define our target parameter as the minimizer (β_0, β_1) of the expectation (with respect to the true data-generating distribution) of the squared residuals $(\psi_0(a,V) - \beta_0 - \beta_1 V)^2$. In this case $\beta_0 + \beta_1 V$ represents the least squares projection of the true treatment-specific mean at level a as a function of V onto a linear trend.

The choice of working statistical model, such as the linear statistical model $\beta_0 + \beta_1 V$, defines the target parameter of interest, but it does not represent a statistical assumption.

The parameter $\Psi(P)$ is now well defined for any probability distribution P, including the true distribution P_0. One could also define a whole collection of such summary measures as target parameters, thereby allowing the investigation of a whole collection of features of the true response curve $\psi_0(a,v)$ as a function of a and v.

Define the working model m as follows:

$$m(a, v, \Psi') = \text{expit}(\Psi^{(0)'} + \Psi^{(1)'} a_1 + \Psi^{(2)'} a_2 + \Psi^{(3)'} a_3 + \Psi^{(4)'} v),$$

where a_1, a_2, a_3 are indicator variables for the first three (out of four total) adherence levels defined in Sect. 9.2. The parameter we will estimate throughout this section, in terms of the potential outcomes Y_a, is

$$\Psi'_0 = \arg\max_{\Psi'} \sum_{a \in \mathcal{A}} E_{P_0} h(a, V) \log\left[m(a, V, \Psi')^{Y_a}(1 - m(a, V, \Psi'))^{1-Y_a}\right], \tag{9.8}$$

for some bounded, measurable weight function $h(a,V) \geq 0$ that we specify. When the model m is correctly specified, this can be interpreted as the maximizer of a weighted log-likelihood, in terms of the potential outcomes Y_a. When the model m is misspecified, the parameter is still well defined.

We assume there is a unique maximizer Ψ' to the expression on the right-hand side of (9.8). In this case, the parameter Ψ'_0 is the unique solution of

$$\sum_{a \in \mathcal{A}} E_{P_0} h(a, V)(Y_a - m(a, V, \Psi'))(1, a_1, a_2, a_3, V)' = 0. \tag{9.9}$$

Under the assumptions in Sect. 9.4 linking potential outcomes to a mapping of the observed data, we have that Ψ' is also the unique solution to

$$\sum_{a \in \mathcal{A}} E_{P_0} h(a, V)(P_0(Y = 1 \mid A = a, V, W) - m(a, V, \Psi'))(1, a_1, a_2, a_3, V)' = 0. \quad (9.10)$$

This last display involves a mapping from the distribution of the observed data, and no reference to potential outcomes Y_a; we will use it below in constructing the TMLE for Ψ'.

9.6.1 Obtaining Q_n^0, an Initial Estimate of Q_0

Just as in Sect. 9.5, parameter (9.8), which is the solution to (9.10), depends on the data-generating distribution only through the conditional distribution of Y given A, V, W and the marginal distribution of (V, W). We let $Q = (P(Y \mid A, V, W), P(V, W))$ denote those relevant parts of the density P, and let Q_0 denote those relevant parts of the density at the true data-generating distribution P_0. There are many ways to construct an initial estimator Q_n^0 of Q_0. Just as in Sect. 9.5, for simplicity, here we fit a single logistic regression model to obtain an estimator for the first component of Q_0 and use the empirical distribution as estimator for the second component of Q_0. The resulting initial estimator Q_n^0 is denoted by $\left(\bar{Q}_n(Y = 1 \mid A, V, W), Q_{V,W,n}(V, W)\right)$. We fit a multinomial logistic regression model for $P_0(A \mid V, W)$, which we denote by g_n. Below we will use the substitution estimator at the initial density estimate Q_n^0, denoted by $\Psi'(Q_n^0)$, which satisfies [by property (9.10) above]

$$\sum_{a \in \mathcal{A}} \sum_{i=1}^{n} h(a, V_i)(\bar{Q}_n^0(Y = 1 \mid A = a, V_i, W_i) - m(a, V_i, \Psi'(Q_n^0))(1, a_1, a_2, a_3, V_i)' = 0. \quad (9.11)$$

We assume there is a unique solution $\Psi'(Q_n^0)$ to the above display.

9.6.2 Calculating the Optimal Fluctuation

To compute the optimal fluctuation, we need the efficient influence curve for the parameter Ψ' in the nonparametric model. The efficient influence curve is (up to a normalizing matrix) given by

$$D^*(P)(Y, A, V, W) = \left[\frac{h(A, V)(Y - P(Y = 1 \mid A, V, W))}{P(A \mid V, W)} (1, A_1, A_2, A_3, V)' \right.$$
$$\left. + \sum_{a \in \mathcal{A}} h(a, V) \left(P(Y = 1 \mid A = a, V, W) - m(a, V, \Psi')\right) (1, a_1, a_2, a_3, V)' \right],$$

where A_1, A_2, A_3 are indicator variables of adherence levels $A = 1, A = 2$, and $A = 3$, respectively. Note that the above efficient influence function reduces to its counterpart (9.4) for the simpler case in Sect. 9.5, for the special case where the weight function $h(a, v)$ is the indicator that $a = 0, v = 0$ and the working model m has only an intercept term.

We now construct a parametric model $\{P(\epsilon) : \epsilon\}$ that (1) contains the initial estimator Q_n^0 at $\epsilon = 0$ and (2) has a score at $\epsilon = 0$ whose linear span contains the efficient influence function at Q_n^0. To do this, we first define the clever covariates $H_1^*(A, V, W)$ and $H_2^*(V, W)$:

$$H_1^*(A, V, W) = \frac{h(A, V)}{g_n(A \mid V, W)}(1, A_1, A_2, A_3, V)'$$

and

$$H_2^*(V, W) = \sum_{a \in \mathcal{A}} h(a, V)\left(\bar{Q}_n(Y = 1 \mid A = a, V, W) - m(a, V, \Psi'(Q_n^0))\right)(1, a_1, a_2, a_3, V)'.$$

Here H_1^* and H_2^* are each column vectors with five components.

Let $\epsilon = (\epsilon_1, \epsilon_2)$, where ϵ_1 and ϵ_2 are each row vectors with five components (so as to have the same length as H_1^* and H_2^*, respectively). Define the parametric model $\{P(\epsilon) : \epsilon\}$:

$$\begin{aligned} P(\epsilon)(Y = 1 \mid A, V, W) &= \text{expit}\left(\epsilon_1 H_1^*(A, V, W) + \text{logit}\left(\bar{Q}_n(Y = 1 \mid A, V, W)\right)\right), \quad (9.12) \\ P(\epsilon)(A \mid V, W) &= g_n(A \mid V, W), \\ P(\epsilon)(V, W) &= s_{\epsilon_2} \exp(\epsilon_2 H_2^*(V, W)) Q_{V,W,n}(V, W), \end{aligned}$$

where the constant $s_{\epsilon_2} = 1/[\frac{1}{n}\sum_{i=1}^n \exp(\epsilon_2 H_2^*(V_i, W_i))]$ is chosen such that $P(\epsilon)(V, W)$ integrates to 1 for each ϵ. It is straightforward to verify that conditions (1) and (2) above are satisfied for the parametric model $\{P(\epsilon) : \epsilon\}$.

9.6.3 Obtaining Q_n^*, a Targeted Estimate of Q_0

We fit the above parametric model using maximum likelihood estimation to get the estimate $\epsilon_n = (\epsilon_{1,n}, \epsilon_{2,n})$ of (ϵ_1, ϵ_2). One can show (using slight extensions of the arguments in Sect. 9.5.3) that the maximum likelihood estimate $\epsilon_n = (\epsilon_{1,n}, \epsilon_{2,n})$ can be obtained by fitting the logistic regression model (9.12), which has five terms (one for each component of H_1^*) and offset equal to $\text{logit}\left(\bar{Q}_n(Y = 1 \mid A, V, W)\right)$, to obtain $\epsilon_{1,n}$; arguments as in Sect. 9.5.3 can be used to show $\epsilon_{2,n}$ must equal 0 and that no iteration is necessary, since convergence occurs in a single step. Our final estimator for the relevant part Q_0 of the density of the observed data is

$$Q_n^* = P(\epsilon_n) = (P(\epsilon_{1,n})(Y = 1 \mid A, V, W), Q_{V,W,n}). \quad (9.13)$$

9.6.4 Estimation of Parameter

We compute the substitution estimator $\Psi'(Q_n^*)$, which by property (9.10) solves

$$\sum_{a\in\mathcal{A}}\sum_{i=1}^{n} h(a,V_i)(\bar{Q}_n^*(Y=1\mid A=a,V_i,W_i)-m(a,V_i,\Psi'(Q_n^*))(1,a_1,a_2,a_3,V_i)'=0. \tag{9.14}$$

We assume there is a unique solution to the above equation. The solution $\Psi'(Q_n^*)$ to the above equation can be computed using iteratively reweighted least squares, where the set of outcomes is $\bar{Q}_n^*(Y = 1 \mid A = a, V_i, W_i)$ for each $a \in \mathcal{A}$ and each subject i, which are regressed on the working model $m(a, V_i, \Psi')$ using weights $h(a, V_i)/[m(a, V_i, \Psi')(1 - m(a, V_i, \Psi'))]$.

This iteratively reweighted least squares solution can be implemented in the statistical programming language R with the generalized linear statistical model (glm) function. This involves first constructing a new data set where there are four rows for each subject, one for each possible level of adherence $a \in \mathcal{A}$. For subject i and adherence level $a \in \mathcal{A}$, the following entries make up the corresponding row of this new data set:

1. $\bar{Q}_n^*(Y = 1 \mid A = a, V_i, W_i)$ (which is the "outcome" in the new data set);
2. a (the adherence level under consideration; note that this is not the subject's observed adherence level);
3. V_i (the number of continuous months of past viral suppression);
4. $h(a, V_i)$ (the weight).

One regresses the first column (the new "outcome") on the model $m(a, V_i, \Psi')$ using the glm function with family binomial and logistic link function and using weights $h(a, V_i)$ (from the fourth column of the new data set). Even though the new "outcome" is not binary valued but lies in the interval [0, 1], the glm function computes the desired iteratively reweighted least squares solution, as long as the algorithm converges. It is shown in Rosenblum and van der Laan (2010a) that if this algorithm converges to a value Ψ'_n, then this is the unique solution to (9.14).

We now summarize the steps in constructing the TMLE for parameter (9.8). First, we obtained the initial estimators of the conditional densities $P_0(Y = 1 \mid A, V, W)$ and $P_0(A \mid V, W)$. Next, we fit a logistic regression model for Y, with terms H_1^* and offset both depending on the initial density estimators and the formula for the efficient influence function for the parameter. Lastly, we used iterated reweighted least squares to solve Eq. (9.14), yielding the final estimate Ψ'_n.

An important special case of the class of TMLEs given above was previously given in the Rejoinder to Comments in Scharfstein et al. (1999), on p. 1142. To the best of our knowledge, their class of parametric regression-based estimators for the parameter defined by (9.10) is the first to include the covariate H_1^*. Their class of parametric regression-based estimators is double robust and locally efficient.

9.7 Constructing Confidence Intervals

We constructed separate 95% confidence intervals for $m(a, v, \Psi')$, for each $a \in \mathcal{A}, v \in \mathcal{V}$, using the nonparametric bootstrap bias-corrected and accelerated (BCa) method (Efron 1987), with 10,000 iterations. The entire procedure, including refitting the initial regressions, was iterated for each bootstrap replicate. Note that these are not simultaneous 95% confidence intervals. It is also possible to use the nonparametric bootstrap to construct simultaneous confidence intervals. In addition, the asymptotic multivariate normal distribution or the bootstrap distribution of the estimator of $(m(a, v, \Psi') : a, v)$ can be used to carry out multiple testing procedures, controlling a user-supplied type I error rate such as the familywise error rate using methods in Dudoit and van der Laan (2008).

9.8 Results

We now apply the method from Sects. 9.6 and 9.7 to the data from the REACH cohort described in Sect. 9.1. The analysis in Sect. 9.6 was implemented using a working model $m(a, V, \Psi')$ with main terms and interaction terms. Unlike the simplified description above, in which each subject contributed a single time point of data, in the actual analysis subjects contributed multiple time points of data. Overall there were 1201 patient-months of data used in the analysis. The parameter of interest involved a generalization of (9.8) to this setting, as described in Rosenblum and van der Laan (2010a).

For the initial density estimator $Q_n^0 = \left(\bar{Q}_n(Y = 1 \mid A, V, W), Q_{V,W,n}(V, W)\right)$, we let $\bar{Q}_n$ be the fit of a logistic regression model, which included the following terms:

- Intercept;
- Indicator variables for the first three levels of adherence (A_1, A_2, A_3);
- Duration of continuous suppression (V);
- Interactions of (A_1, A_2, A_3) and V;
- Main terms for each confounder variable from Sect. 9.2.

We let $Q_{V,W,n}(V, W)$ be the empirical distribution of (V, W). We fit a multinomial logistic regression model for adherence level A given V, W, which included as terms: intercept, duration of continuous suppression (V), V^2, and main terms for each confounder variable from Sect. 9.2. We denote this by g_n. Similarly, we fit a multinomial logistic regression model for adherence level A given just V, which included as terms intercept, duration of continuous suppression (V), and V^2, which we denote by h_n.

We chose the weight function $h(a, V)$ in the definition of parameter (9.8) to be an approximation to $g_0(a \mid V)$. The motivation behind such a choice was to help stabilize the inverse weights in the clever covariate $H_1^*(A, V, W)$ defined in Sect. 9.6.2. The approximation to $g_0(a \mid V)$ that we use in defining $h(a, V)$ is the limit in probability, as $n \to \infty$, of h_n. Having thus defined $h(a, V)$, we still need to be able to

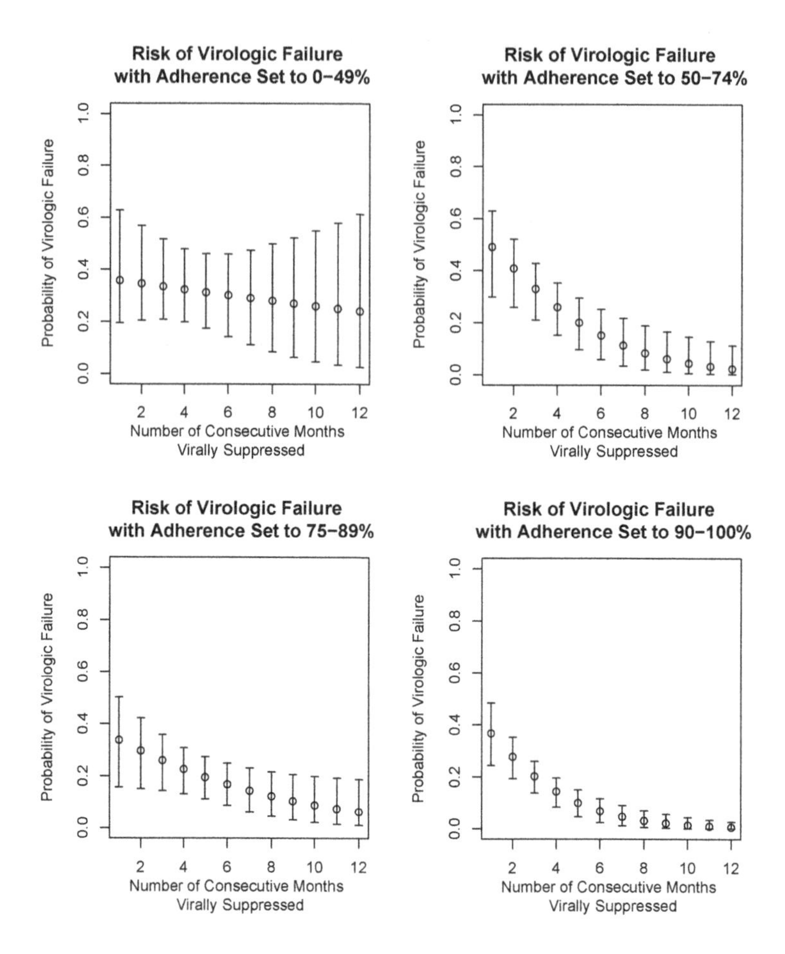

Fig. 9.1 "Estimates and 95% Confidence Intervals for the Risk of Virologic Failure, at Four Ranges of Adherence, Given Duration of Continuous Viral Suppression." This figure and caption are reproduced from Rosenblum et al. (2009)

compute it, or at least approximate it, based on the data we have to work with. In implementing the targeted maximum likelihood algorithm, as in Sect. 9.6, we substitute h_n for h in the definition of $H_1^*(A, V, W)$. We point out that super learning could have been used to construct density estimators in this problem.

The resulting estimate Ψ'_n corresponds to the following working model fit:

$$m(a, v, \Psi'_n) = \text{expit}[-0.5 - 0.04A_1 + 0.6A_2 - 0.13A_3 \\ - 0.4V + 0.36A_1V + 0.07A_2V + 2.3A_3V].$$

We show a plot of this function of a, v, along with 95% confidence intervals computed with the nonparametric bootstrap, in Fig. 9.1. The null hypothesis of no effect modification on the relative risk scale, comparing lowest to highest adherence levels was tested.

$$H_0 : \frac{m(0, v, \Psi')}{m(3, v, \Psi')} = \frac{m(0, v', \Psi')}{m(3, v', \Psi')} \text{ for all } v, v' \in \mathcal{V}.$$

The test involved computing substitution estimates of the relative risks

$$RR(v) = \frac{m(0, v, \Psi')}{m(3, v, \Psi')}$$

for all $v \in \mathcal{V}$ (where the final estimator Ψ'_n was substituted for Ψ'), and then regressing $\log RR(V)$ on the model $\alpha_0 + \alpha_1 V$. The hypothesis of no effect modification on the relative risk scale is rejected if the confidence interval (based on the nonparametric bootstrap) for the coefficient α_1 excludes 0. This hypothesis was rejected at a p-value of 0.001. This hypothesis-testing procedure relies on the consistency and asymptotic normality of the estimator Ψ'_n. To be interpretable in terms of causal relative risks, we additionally need the assumptions given above relating potential outcomes to observed data, and also the assumption that the working model m is a correctly specified marginal structural model.

9.9 Discussion

Under the assumptions given above, and under weak regularity conditions, the TMLEs from Sects. 9.5 and 9.6 are doubly robust, locally efficient. In contrast to this, standard propensity score methods, regression-based methods, and inverse probability weighted methods are generally not doubly robust. Since our goal was to look at effect modification by number of months of continuous suppression (V), we are, by design, comparing effects across different subpopulations. These subpopulations are the 12 groups listed in Sect. 9.1. Observed differences do not, therefore, point to any causal mechanism. However, the results of our analysis are relevant in predicting the impact of missed doses for patients, based on the number of months of continuous viral suppression. Due to the relatively small sample size of the study, and the set of assumptions required by the analysis (which are common to many such analyses), any conclusions from this single study should be made with care.

9.10 Notes and Further Reading

We focused on an application in HIV treatment that can be found in Rosenblum et al. (2009). The content of this chapter is based on work previously published in Rosenblum and van der Laan (2010a). The seminal paper promoting the use of marginal structural working models to define a parameter is Neugebauer and van der Laan (2007). As previously mentioned, a special case of the class of TMLEs presented in this chapter for the parameter of a marginal structural model was previously given in the Rejoinder to Comments in Scharfstein et al. (1999), on p. 1142. A description of the estimator of Scharfstein et al. (1999) and its relationship to the estimators in this chapter is given in Appendix 2 of Rosenblum and van der Laan (2010a).

We started this chapter with several motivating examples for the estimation of effects in subpopulations. Kirsch et al. (2008) found that there was a difference between the effect of an antidepressant medication on HAM-D score for those entering a study with severe depression vs. less severe depression. An example of the effect of a cancer therapy differing among those with and without overexpression of a particular gene is given in Baselga (2001).

Chapter 10
Positivity

Maya L. Petersen, Kristin E. Porter, Susan Gruber, Yue Wang,
Mark J. van der Laan

The identifiability of causal effects requires sufficient variability in treatment or exposure assignment within strata of confounders. The causal inference literature refers to the assumption of adequate exposure variability within confounder strata as the assumption of positivity or experimental treatment assignment. Positivity violations can arise for two reasons. First, it may be theoretically impossible for individuals with certain covariate values to receive a given exposure of interest. For example, certain patient characteristics may constitute an absolute contraindication to receipt of a particular treatment. The threat to causal inference posed by such structural or theoretical violations of positivity does not improve with increasing sample size. Second, violations or near violations of positivity can arise in finite samples due to chance. This is a particular problem in small samples but also occurs frequently in moderate to large samples when the treatment is continuous or can take multiple levels, or when the covariate adjustment set is large or contains continuous or multilevel covariates. Regardless of the cause, causal effects may be poorly or nonidentified when certain subgroups in a finite sample do not receive some of the treatment levels of interest. In this chapter we will use the term "sparsity" to refer to positivity violations and near-violations arising from either of these causes, recognizing that other types of sparsity can also threaten valid inference.

Data sparsity can increase both the bias and variance of a causal effect estimator; the extent to which each is impacted will depend on the estimator. An estimator-specific diagnostic tool is thus needed to quantify the extent to which positivity violations threaten the validity of inference for a given causal effect parameter (for a given model, data-generating distribution, and finite sample). Wang et al. (2006) proposed such a diagnostic based on the parametric bootstrap. Application of a candidate estimator to bootstrapped data sampled from the estimated data-generating distribution provides information about the estimator's behavior under a data-generating distribution that is based on the observed data. The true parameter value in the bootstrap data is known and can be used to assess estimator bias. A large bias estimate can alert the analyst to the presence of a parameter that is poorly identified, an important warning in settings where data sparsity may not be reflected in the variance of the causal effect estimate.

Once bias due to violations in positivity has been diagnosed, the question remains how best to proceed with estimation. We review several approaches. Identifiability can be improved by extrapolating based on subgroups in which sufficient treatment variability does exist; however, such an approach requires additional parametric model assumptions. Alternative approaches to responding to sparsity include the following: restriction of the sample to those subjects for whom the positivity assumption is not violated (known as trimming); redefinition of the causal effect of interest as the effect of only those treatments that do not result in positivity violations (estimation of the effects of "realistic" or "intention to treat" dynamic regimes); restriction of the covariate adjustment set to exclude those covariates responsible for positivity violations; and, when the target parameter is defined using a marginal structural working model, use of a projection function that focuses estimation on areas of the data with greater support.

As we discuss, all of these approaches change the parameter being estimated by trading proximity to the original target of inference for improved identifiability. We advocate incorporation of this tradeoff into the effect estimator itself. This requires defining a family of parameters whose members vary in their proximity to the initial target and in their identifiability. An estimator can then be defined that selects among the members of this family according to some prespecifed criterion.

10.1 Framework for Causal Effect Estimation

We proceed from the basic premise that model assumptions should honestly reflect investigator knowledge. The SCM framework provides a systematic approach for translating background knowledge into a causal model and corresponding statistical model, defining a target causal parameter, and assessing the identifiability of that parameter. We illustrate this approach using a simple point treatment data structure $O = (W, A, Y) \sim P$ and a nonparametric statistical model augmented with possibly additional causal assumptions, with the SCM given by (2.1), which we restate as follows: $W = f_W(U_W)$, $A = f_A(W, U_A)$, $Y = f_Y(W, A, U_Y)$. Again, let W denote a set of baseline covariates, A denote a treatment or exposure variable, Y denote an outcome, and $U = (U_W, U_A, U_Y) \sim P_U$ denotes the set of background factors that deterministically assign values to (W, A, Y) according to functions (f_W, f_A, f_Y). We minimize notation by focusing on discrete-valued random variables.

Target parameter. A causal effect can be defined in terms of the joint distribution of the observed data under an intervention on one or more of the structural equations in the corresponding SCM or, equivalently, under an intervention on the corresponding causal graph. For example, consider the postintervention distribution of Y under an intervention on the structural model to set $A = a$. Such an intervention corresponds to replacing $A = f_A(W, U_A)$ with $A = a$ in the structural model (2.1) presented in

Chap. 2. The counterfactual outcome that a given subject with background factors u would have had if he or she were to have received treatment level a is denoted $Y_a(u)$. This counterfactual can be derived as the solution to the structural equation f_Y in the modified equation system with f_A set equal to a and with input $U = u$.

Let F_X denote the distribution of $X = (W, (Y_a : a \in \mathcal{A}))$, where $\mathcal{A}$ denotes the possible values that the treatment variable can take (e.g. $\{0, 1\}$ for a binary treatment). F_X describes the joint distribution of the baseline covariates and counterfactual outcomes under a range of interventions on treatment variable A. A causal effect can be defined as some function of F_X. For example, a common target parameter for binary A is the average treatment effect:

$$E_{F_X}(Y_1 - Y_0), \tag{10.1}$$

or the difference in expected counterfactual outcome if every subject in the population had received vs. had not received treatment.

Alternatively, an investigator may be interested in estimating the average treatment effect separately within certain strata of the population or for nonbinary treatments. Specification of a marginal structural model (a model on the conditional expectation of the counterfactual outcome given effect modifiers of interest) provides one option for defining the target causal parameter in such cases (Chap. 9). Marginal structural models take the following form: $E_{F_X}(Y_a \mid V) = m(a, V \mid \beta)$, where $V \subset W$ denotes the strata in which one wishes to estimate a conditional causal effect. For example, one might specify the following model:

$$m(a, V \mid \beta) = \beta_1 + \beta_2 a + \beta_3 V + \beta_4 aV.$$

For a binary treatment $\mathcal{A} \in \{0, 1\}$, such a model implies an average treatment effect within stratum $V = v$ equal to $\beta_2 + \beta_4 v$.

The true functional form of $E_{F_X}(Y_a \mid V)$ will generally not be known. One option is to assume that the parametric model $m(a, V \mid \beta)$ is correctly specified, or in other words that $E_{F_X}(Y_a \mid V) = m(a, V \mid \beta)$ for some value β. Such an approach, however, can place additional restrictions on the allowed distributions of the observed data and thus change the statistical model. In order to respect the premise that the statistical model should faithfully reflect the limits of investigator knowledge and not be altered in order to facilitate definition of the target parameter, we advocate an alternative approach in which the target causal parameter is defined using a marginal structural working model. Under this approach the target parameter β is defined as the projection of the true causal curve $E_{F_X}(Y_a \mid V)$ onto the specified model $m(a, V \mid \beta)$ according to some projection function $h(a, V)$:

$$\beta(F_X, m, h) = \underset{\beta}{\operatorname{argmin}}\, E_{F_X}\left[\sum_{a \in \mathcal{A}} (Y_a - m(a, V \mid \beta))^2 h(a, V)\right]. \tag{10.2}$$

When $h(a, V) = 1$, the target parameter β corresponds to an unweighted projection of the entire causal curve onto the working model $m(a, V \mid \beta)$; alternative choices of h correspond to placing greater emphasis on specific parts of the curve [i.e., on certain (a, V) values].

Use of a marginal structural working model such as (10.2) is attractive because it allows the target causal parameter to be defined within the original statistical model. However, this approach by no means absolves the investigator of careful consideration of marginal structural working model specification. A poorly specified working model $m(a, V \mid \beta)$ may result in a target parameter that provides a poor summary of the features of the true causal relationship that are of interest.

In the following sections we discuss the parameter $\beta(F_X, m, 1)$ as the target of inference, corresponding to estimation of the treatment-specific mean for all levels $a \in \mathcal{A}$ within strata of V as projected onto working model m, with projection $h(a, V) = 1$ chosen to reflect a focus on the entire causal curve. To simplify notation we use β to refer to this target parameter unless otherwise noted.

Identifiability. We assess whether the target parameter β of the counterfactual data distribution F_X is identified as a parameter of the observed data distribution P under causal model (2.1). Because the background factors U are assumed to be jointly independent in SCM (2.1), or in other words the model is assumed to be Markov, we have that

$$P_{F_X}(Y_a = y) = \sum_w P(Y = y \mid W = w, A = a)P(W = w), \tag{10.3}$$

identifying the target parameter β according to projection (10.2) (Pearl 2009). This identifiability result is often referred to as the g-computation formula or g-formula (Robins 1986, 1987a,b). The weaker assumption of randomization (10.4), or the assumption that A and Y_a are conditionally independent given W, is also sufficient for identifiability result (10.3) to hold:

$$A \coprod Y_a \mid W \text{ for all } a \in \mathcal{A}. \tag{10.4}$$

Whether or not a given structural model implies that assumption (10.4) holds can be assessed from the graph using the backdoor criterion.

The need for experimentation in treatment assignment. The g-formula (10.3) is valid only if the conditional distributions in the formula are well defined. Let $g(a \mid W) = P(A = a \mid W), a \in \mathcal{A}$ denote the conditional distribution of treatment variable A under the observed data distribution P. If one or more treatment levels of interest do not occur within some covariate strata, the conditional probability $P(Y = y \mid A = a, W = w)$ will not be well defined for some value(s) (a, w) and the identifiability result (10.3) will break down.

A simple example provides insight into the threat to parameter identifiability posed by sparsity of this nature. Consider an example in which $W = I(woman)$, A is a binary treatment, and no women are treated ($g(1 \mid W = 1) = 0$). In this data-generating distribution there is no information regarding outcomes among treated women. Thus, as long as there are women in the target population (i.e., $P(W = 1) >$

0), the average treatment effect $E_{F_X}(Y_1 - Y_0)$ will not be identified without additional parametric assumptions.

This simple example illustrates that a given causal parameter under a given model may be identified for some joint distributions of the observed data but not for others. An additional assumption beyond (10.4) is thus needed to ensure identfiability. We begin by presenting the strong version of this assumption, needed for the identification of $P_{F_X}((Y_a = y, W = w) : a, y, w)$ in a nonparametric model.

Strong Positivity Assumption

$$\inf_{a \in \mathcal{A}} g(a \mid W) > 0, \; P\text{-a.e.} \tag{10.5}$$

The strong positivity assumption states that each possible treatment level occurs with some positive probability within each stratum of W.

Parametric model assumptions may allow the positivity assumption to be weakened. In the example above, an assumption that the treatment effect is the same among treated men and women would result in identification of the average treatment effect (10.1) based on extrapolation from the treatment effect among men (assuming that other identifiability assumptions were met). Parametric model assumptions of this nature are dangerous, however, because they extrapolate to regions of the joint distribution of (A, W) that are not supported by the data. Such assumptions should be approached with caution and adopted only when they have a solid foundation in background knowledge.

In addition to being model-specific, the form of the positivity assumption needed for identifiability is parameter-specific. Many target causal parameters require much weaker versions of positivity than (10.5). To take one simple example, if the target parameter is $E(Y_1)$, the identifiability result only requires that $g(1 \mid W) > 0$ hold; it doesn't matter if there are some strata of the population in which no one was treated. Similarly, the identifiability of $\beta(F_X, m, h)$, defined using a marginal structural working model, relies on a weaker positivity assumption.

Positivity Assumption for $\beta(F_X, h, m)$

$$\sup_{a \in \mathcal{A}} \frac{h(a, V)}{g(a \mid W)} < \infty, \; P\text{-a.e.} \tag{10.6}$$

The choice of projection function $h(a, V)$ used to define the target parameter thus has implications for how strong an assumption about positivity is needed for identifiability. In Sect. 10.4 we consider specification of alternative target parameters that allow for weaker positivity assumptions than (10.5), including parameters indexed by alternative choices of $h(a, V)$. For now we focus on the target parameter β indexed by the choice $h(a, V) = 1$ and note that (10.5) and (10.6) are equivalent for this parameter.

10.2 Estimator-Specific Behavior Under Positivity Violations

Let $\Psi(P_0)$ denote the target parameter of the observed data distribution P_0 of O, which under the assumptions of randomization (10.4) and positivity (10.6) equals the target causal parameter $\beta(F_{X,0}, m, h)$. Estimators of this parameter are denoted $\hat{\Psi}(P_n)$, where P_n is the empirical distribution of a sample of n i.i.d. observations from P_0. We use $Q_{W,0}(w) \equiv P_0(W = w)$, $Q_{Y,0}(y \mid A, W) = P_0(Y = y \mid A, W)$, $\bar{Q}_0 = E_0(Y \mid A, W)$, and $Q_0 \equiv (Q_{W,0}, \bar{Q}_0)$. Recall that $g_0(a \mid W) = P_0(A = a \mid W)$. See Chaps. 1–6 for an introductory presentation of the estimators in this section.

We focus our discussion on bias in the point estimate of the target parameter β_0. While estimates of the variance of estimators of β_0 can also be biased when data are sparse, methods exist to improve variance estimation or to provide upper bounds for the true variance. The nonparametric or semiparametric bootstrap provides one straightforward approach to variance estimation in settings where the central limit theorem may not apply as a result of sparsity; alternative approaches to correct for biased variance estimates are also possible (Rosenblum and van der Laan 2009b). These methods will not, however, protect against misleading inference if the point estimate itself is biased.

10.2.1 MLE

MLEs provide a mapping from the empirical data distribution P_n to a parameter estimate $\hat{\beta}_{MLE}$. The estimator $\hat{\Psi}_{MLE}(P_n)$ is a substitution estimator based on identifiability result (10.3). It is implemented based on an estimator of Q_0 and its consistency relies on the consistency of this estimator. $Q_{W,0}$ can generally be estimated based on the empirical distribution of W. However, even when positivity is not violated, the dimension of (A, W) is frequently too large for $\bar{Q}_0$ to be estimated simply by evaluating the mean of Y within strata of (A, W). Given an estimator $\bar{Q}_n$ of $\bar{Q}_0$, MLE can be implemented by generating a predicted counterfactual outcome for each subject under each possible treatment: $\hat{Y}_{a,i} = \bar{Q}_n(a, W_i)$ for $a \in \mathcal{A}$, $i = 1, ..., n$. The estimate $\hat{\beta}_{MLE}$ is then obtained by regressing $\hat{Y}_a$ on a and V according to the model $m(a, V \mid \beta)$, with weights based on the projection function $h(a, V)$. When all treatment levels of interest are not represented within all covariate strata [i.e., assumption (10.5) is violated], some of the conditional probabilities in the nonparametric g-formula (10.3) will not be defined. A given estimate $\bar{Q}_n$ may allow the MLE to extrapolate based on covariate strata in which sufficient experimentation in treatment level does exist. Importantly, however, this requires extrapolation of the fit $\bar{Q}_n$ into areas not supported by the data, and the resulting effect estimates will be biased if the extrapolation used to estimate $\bar{Q}_0$ is misspecified.

10.2.2 IPTW Estimator

The IPTW estimator $\hat{\Psi}_{IPTW}(P_n)$ provides a mapping from the empirical data distribution P_n to a parameter estimate $\hat{\beta}_{IPTW}$ based on an estimator g_n of $g_0(A \mid W)$. The estimator is defined as the solution in β to the following estimating equation:

$$0 = \sum_{i=1}^{n} \frac{h(A_i, V_i)}{g_n(A_i \mid W_i)} \frac{d}{d\beta} m(A_i, V_i \mid \beta)(Y_i - m(A_i, V_i \mid \beta)),$$

where $h(A, V)$ is the projection function used to define the target causal parameter $\beta(F_X, m, h)$ according to (10.2). The IPTW estimator of the true value β_0 can be implemented as the solution to a weighted regression of the outcome Y on treatment A and effect modifiers V according to model $m(A, V \mid \beta)$, with weights equal to $h(A, V)/g_n(A \mid W)$. Consistency of $\hat{\Psi}_{IPTW}(P_n)$ requires that g_0 satisfy positivity and that g_n be a consistent estimator of g_0. Depending on the choice of projection function, implementation may further require estimation of $h(A, V)$; if one defines the desired projection function as the estimand of the estimator h_n then a consistent estimator of $h(A, V)$ is not required to ensure consistency of the IPTW estimator.

The IPTW estimator is particularly sensitive to bias due to data sparsity. Bias can arise due to structural positivity violations (positivity may not hold for g_0) or may occur by chance because certain covariate and treatment combinations are not represented in a given finite sample [$g_n(a \mid W = w)$ may have values of zero or close to zero for some (a, w) even when positivity holds for g_0 and g_n is consistent] (Wang et al. 2006; Neugebauer and van der Laan 2005; Bembom and van der Laan 2007a; Cole and Hernan 2008; Moore et al. 2009). In the latter case, as fewer individuals within a given covariate stratum receive a given treatment, the weights of those rare individuals who do receive the treatment become more extreme. The disproportionate reliance of the causal effect estimate on the experience of a few unusual individuals can result in substantial finite sample bias.

While values of $g_n(a \mid W)$ remain positive for all $a \in \mathcal{A}$, elevated weights inflate the variance of the effect estimate and can serve as a warning that the data may poorly support the target parameter. However, as the number of individuals within a covariate stratum who receive a given treatment level shifts from few (each of whom receives a large weight and thus elevates the variance) to none, estimator variance can decrease while bias increases rapidly. In other words, when $g_n(a \mid W = w) = 0$ for some (a, w), the weight for a subject with $A = a$ and $W = w$ is infinity; however, as no such individuals exist in the data set, the corresponding threat to valid inference will not be reflected in either the weights or in estimator variance.

Weight truncation. Weights are commonly truncated or bounded in order to improve the performance of the IPTW estimator in the face of data sparsity (Wang et al. 2006; Moore et al. 2009; Cole and Hernan 2008; Kish 1992; Bembom and van der Laan 2008). Weights are truncated at either a fixed or relative level (e.g., at the 1st and 99th percentiles), thereby reducing the variance arising from large weights and limiting the impact of a few possibly nonrepresentative individuals on the effect estimate. This advantage comes at a cost, however, in the form of increased bias due to misspecification of the treatment model g_n, a bias that does not decrease with increasing sample size.

Stabilized weights. The use of projection function $h(a, V) = 1$ implies the use of unstabilized weights. In contrast, stabilized weights, corresponding to a choice of $h(a, V) = g_0(a \mid V)$ [where $g_0(a \mid V) = P_0(A = a \mid V)$] are generally recommended for the implementation of marginal structural-model-based effect estimation. The choice of $h(a, V) = g_0(a \mid V)$ results in a weaker positivity assumption by (10.6). It is important to stress the contrast between assuming a marginal structural model vs. using it as a working model. For example, if A is an ordinal variable with multiple levels, $V = \{\}$, and the target parameter is defined as the true β_0 of a linear marginal structural model $m(a, V \mid \beta) = \beta_{(0)} + \beta_{(1)}a$, it is possible to identify this parameter by using a weight function h that is only nonzero at two values of a chosen such that $g_0(a \mid W) > 0$ for these two values. The corresponding IPTW estimator will extrapolate to levels of A that are sparsely represented in the data by assuming a linear relationship between E_0Y_a and a for $a \in \mathcal{A}$. However, when the target parameter β is defined using a marginal structural working model according to (10.2) [an approach that acknowledges that the model $m(A, V \mid \beta)$ may be misspecified], the choice of h, including the choice of stabilized vs. unstabilized weights, corresponds to a choice of the target parameter (Neugebauer and van der Laan 2007).

10.2.3 Double Robust Estimators

Double robust approaches to estimation of β include the A-IPTW estimator and the TMLE we focus on in this text. Implementation of double robust estimators requires estimators of both Q_0 and g_0. Double robust estimators remain consistent if either (1) g_n is a consistent estimator of g_0 and g_0 satisfies positivity or (2) Q_n is a consistent estimator of Q_0 and g_n converges to a distribution g^* that satisfies positivity. Thus when positivity holds, these estimators are truly double robust, in the sense that consistent estimation of either g_0 or Q_0 results in a consistent estimator. When positivity fails, however, the consistency of the double robust estimators relies entirely on consistent estimation of Q_0. In the setting of positivity violations, double robust estimators are thus faced with the same vulnerabilities as MLE.

In addition to illustrating how positivity violations increase the vulnerability of double robust estimators to bias resulting from inconsistent estimation of Q_0, these asymptotic results have practical implications for the implementation of the double robust estimators. Specifically, they suggest that the use of an estimator g_n that yields predicted values in $[0+\gamma, 1-\gamma]$ (where γ is some small number) can improve finite sample performance. One way to achieve such bounds is by truncating the predicted probabilities generated by g_n, similar to the process of weight truncation described for the IPTW estimator.

10.3 Diagnosing Bias Due to Positivity Violations

Positivity violations can result in substantial bias, with or without a corresponding increase in variance, regardless of the causal effect estimator used. Practical methods are thus needed to diagnose and quantify estimator-specific positivity bias for a given model, parameter, and sample. Basic descriptive analyses of treatment variability within covariate strata can be helpful; however, this approach quickly becomes unwieldy when the covariate set is moderately large and includes continuous or multilevel variables. Cole and Hernan (2008) suggest a range of informal approaches to diagnose and quantify estimator specific positivity bias when the IPTW estimator is applied. As they note, well-behaved weights are not sufficient to ensure the absence of positivity violations. An alternative formulation is to examine the distribution of the estimated propensity score values given by $g_n(a \mid W)$ for $a \in \mathcal{A}$. However, while useful in diagnosing the presence of positivity violations, examination of the estimated propensity scores does not provide any quantitative estimate of the degree to which such violations result in estimator bias and may pose a threat to inference. The parametric bootstrap can be used to provide an optimistic bias estimate specifically targeted at bias caused by positivity violations and near-violations (Wang et al. 2006).

10.3.1 The Parametric Bootstrap as a Diagnostic Tool

We focus on the bias of estimators that target a parameter of the observed data distribution; this target observed data parameter is equal under the randomization assumption (10.4) to the target causal parameter. [Divergence between the target observed data parameter and target causal parameter when (10.4) fails is a distinct issue not addressed by the proposed diagnostic.] The bias in an estimator is the difference between the true value of the target parameter of the observed data distribution and the expectation of the estimator applied to a finite sample from that distribution:

$$\mathrm{Bias}(\hat{\Psi}, P_0, n) = E_{P_0}\hat{\Psi}(P_n) - \Psi(P_0),$$

where we recall that $\Psi(P_0)$ is the target observed data parameter, $\hat{\Psi}(P_n)$ is an estimator of that parameter (which may be a function of g_n or Q_n or both), and P_n

denotes the empirical distribution of a sample of n i.i.d. observations from the true observed data distribution P_0.

Bias in an estimator can arise due to a range of causes. First, the estimators g_n and Q_n may be inconsistent. Second, g_0 may not satisfy the positivity assumption. Third, consistent estimators g_n and Q_n may still have substantial finite sample bias. This latter type of finite sample bias arises in particular due to the curse of dimensionality in a nonparametric or semiparametric model when g_n or Q_n is a data-adaptive estimator, although it can also be substantial for parametric estimators. Fourth, estimated values of g_n may be equal or close to zero or one, despite use of a consistent estimator g_n and a distribution g_0 that satisfies positivity. The relative contribution of each of these sources of bias will depend on the model, the true data-generating distribution, the estimator, and the finite sample.

The parametric bootstrap provides a tool that allows the analyst to explore the extent to which bias due to any of these causes is affecting a given parameter estimate. The parametric bootstrap-based bias estimate is defined as

$$\widehat{\text{Bias}}_{PB}(\hat{\Psi}, \hat{P}_0, n) = E_{\hat{P}_0} \hat{\Psi}(P_n^{\#}) - \Psi(\hat{P}_0),$$

where $\hat{P}_0$ is an estimate of P_0 and $P_n^{\#}$ is the empirical distribution of a bootstrap sample obtained by sampling from $\hat{P}_0$. In other words, the parametric bootstrap is used to sample from an estimate of the true data-generating distribution, resulting in multiple simulated data sets. The true data-generating distribution and target parameter value in the bootstrapped data are known. A candidate estimator is then applied to each bootstrapped data set and the mean of the resulting estimates compared with the known "truth" (i.e., the true parameter value for the bootstrap data-generating distribution).

We focus on a particular algorithm for parametric bootstrap-based bias estimation, which specifically targets the component of estimator-specific finite sample bias due to violations and near-violations of the positivity assumption. The goal is not to provide an accurate estimate of total bias, but rather to provide a diagnostic tool that can serve as a "red flag" warning that positivity bias may pose a threat to inference. The distinguishing characteristic of the diagnostic algorithm is its use of an estimated data-generating distribution $\hat{P}_0$ that both approximates the true P_0 as closely as possible and is compatible with the estimators $\bar{Q}_n$ and g_n used in $\hat{\Psi}(P_n)$. In other words, $\hat{P}_0$ is chosen such that the estimator $\hat{\Psi}$ applied to bootstrap samples from $\hat{P}_0$ is guaranteed to be consistent unless g_0 fails to satisfy the positivity assumption or g_n is truncated. As a result, the parametric bootstrap provides an optimistic estimate of finite sample bias, in which bias due to model misspecification other than truncation is eliminated.

We refer informally to the resulting bias estimate as Bias_{ETA} because in many settings it will be predominantly composed of bias from the following sources: (1) violation of the positivity assumption by g_0; (2) truncation, if any, of g_n in response to positivity violations; and (3) finite sample bias arising from values of g_n close to zero or one (sometimes referred to as practical violations of the positivity assumption). The term Bias_{ETA} is imprecise because the bias estimated by the proposed algorithm will also capture some of the bias in $\hat{\Psi}(P_n)$ due to finite sample bias of the estimators g_n and $\bar{Q}_n$ (a form of sparsity only partially related to positivity). Due to the curse of dimensionality, the contribution of this latter source of bias may be substantial when g_n or Q_n is a data-adaptive estimator in a nonparametric or semi-parametric model. However, the proposed diagnostic algorithm will only capture a portion of this bias because, unlike P_0, $\hat{P}_0$ is guaranteed to have a functional form that can be well approximated by the data-adaptive algorithms employed by g_n and Q_n. The diagnostic algorithm for Bias_{ETA} is implemented as follows.

Step 1: Estimate P_0. Estimation of P_0 requires estimation of $Q_{W,0}$, g_0, and $Q_{Y,0}$. We define $Q_{\hat{P}_0,W} = Q_{P_n,W}$ (or, in other words, use an estimate based on the empirical distribution of the data), $g_{\hat{P}_0} = g_n$, and $\bar{Q}_{\hat{P}_0} = \bar{Q}_n$. Note that the estimators $Q_{P_n W}$, g_n, and $\bar{Q}_n$ were all needed for implementation of the IPTW, MLE, and double robust estimators; the same estimators can be used here. Additional steps may be required to estimate the entire conditional distribution of Y given (A, W) (beyond the estimate of its mean given by $\bar{Q}_n$). The true target parameter for the known distribution $\hat{P}_0$ is only a function of $Q_n = (Q_{P_n W}, \bar{Q}_n)$, and $\Psi(\hat{P}_0)$ is the same as the MLE (using Q_n) applied to the observed data:

$$\Psi(\hat{P}_0) = \hat{\Psi}_{MLE}(P_n).$$

Step 2: Generate $P_n^{\#}$ by sampling from $\hat{P}_0$. In the second step, we assume that $\hat{P}_0$ is the true data-generating distribution. Bootstrap samples $P_n^{\#}$, each with n i.i.d. observations, are generated by sampling from $\hat{P}_0$. For example, W can be sampled from the empirical distribution, a binary A might be generated as a Bernoulli with probability $g_n(1 \mid W)$, and a continuous Y can be generated by adding a $N(0, 1)$ error to $\bar{Q}_n(A, W)$ (alternative approaches are also possible).

Step 3: Estimate $E_{\hat{P}_0}\hat{\Psi}(P_n^{\#})$. Finally, the estimator $\hat{\Psi}$ is applied to each bootstrap sample. Depending on the estimator being evaluated, this step involves applying the estimators g_n or Q_n or both to each bootstrap sample. If Q_n or g_n is a data-adaptive estimator, the corresponding data-adaptive algorithm should be rerun in each bootstrap sample; otherwise, the coefficients of the corresponding models should be refit. Bias_{ETA} is calculated by comparing the mean of the estimator $\hat{\Psi}$ across bootstrap samples $[E_{\hat{P}_0}\hat{\Psi}_{IPTW}(P_n^{\#})]$ with the true value of the target parameter under the bootstrap data-generating distribution $[\Psi(\hat{P}_0)]$. Application of the bootstrap to the IPTW estimator offers one particularly sensitive assessment of positivity bias because, unlike the MLE and double robust estimators, the IPTW estimator cannot extrapolate based on $\bar{Q}_n$. However, this approach can be applied to any causal effect estimator, including estimators introduced in Sect. 10.4 that trade off identifiability for proximity to the target parameter. In assessing the threat posed by positivity violations, the bootstrap should ideally be applied to both the IPTW estimator and the estimator of choice.

Remarks on interpretation of the bias estimate. We caution against using the parametric bootstrap for any form of bias correction. The true bias of the estimator is $E_{P_0}\hat{\Psi}(P_n) - \Psi(P_0)$, while the parametric bootstrap estimates $E_{\hat{P}_0}\hat{\Psi}(P_n^{\#}) - \Psi(\hat{P}_0)$.

The performance of the diagnostic thus depends on the extent to which $\hat{P}_0$ approximates the true data-generating distribution. This suggests the importance of using flexible data-adaptive algorithms to estimate P_0. Regardless of estimation approach, however, when the target parameter $\Psi(P_0)$ is poorly identified due to positivity violations, $\Psi(\hat{P}_0)$ may be a poor estimate of $\Psi(P_0)$. In such cases one would not expect the parametric bootstrap to provide a good estimate of the true bias. Further, the Bias_{ETA} implementation of the parametric bootstrap provides a deliberately optimistic bias estimate by excluding bias due to model misspecifcation for the estimators g_n and $\bar{Q}_n$.

Rather, the parametric bootstrap is proposed as a diagnostic tool. Even when the data-generating distribution is not estimated consistently, the bias estimate provided by the parametric bootstrap remains interpretable in a world where the estimated data-generating mechanism represents the truth. If the estimated bias is large, an analyst who disregards the implied caution is relying on an unsubstantiated hope that first, he or she has inconsistently estimated the data-generating distribution but still done a reasonable job estimating the causal effect of interest; and second, the true data-generating distribution is less affected by positivity (and other finite sample) bias than is the analyst's best estimate of it.

The threshold level of Bias_{ETA} that is considered problematic will vary depending on the scientific question and the point and variance estimates of the causal effect. With that caveat, we suggest the following two general situations in which Bias_{ETA} can be considered a "red flag" warning: (1) when Bias_{ETA} is of the same magnitude as (or larger than) the estimated standard error of the estimator and (2) when the interpretation of a bias-corrected confidence interval would differ meaningfully from initial conclusions.

10.3.2 Simulations

Data were simulated using a data-generating distribution published by Freedman and Berk (2008). Two baseline covariates, $W = (W_1, W_2)$, were generated bivariate normal, $N(\mu, \Sigma)$, with $\mu_1 = 0.5$, $\mu_2 = 1$, and

$$\Sigma = \begin{bmatrix} 2 & 1 \\ 1 & 1 \end{bmatrix}.$$

Y was generated as $1 + A + W_1 + 2W_2 + N(0, 1)$, and $g_0(1 \mid W)$ was given by $\Phi(0.5 + 0.25W_1 + 0.75W_2)$, where Φ is the CDF of the standard normal distribution. With this treatment mechanism $g_0 \in [0.001, 1]$. The target parameter was $E_0(Y_1 - Y_0)$ [corresponding to $\beta_{(1)}$ marginal structural model $m(a \mid \beta) = \beta_{(0)} + \beta_{(1)}a)$]. The true value of the target parameter $\Psi(P_0) = 1$.

The bias, variance, and mean squared error of the MLE, IPTW, A-IPTW, and TMLE estimators were estimated by applying each estimator to 250 samples of size 1000 drawn from this data-generating distribution. The four estimators were implemented with each of the following three approaches: (1) correctly specified model to estimate both $\bar{Q}_0$ and g_0 (CC), (2) correctly specified model to estimate $\bar{Q}_0$ and a misspecified model to estimate g_0 obtained by omitting W_2 from g_n (CM), and (3) correctly specified model to estimate g_0 and a misspecified model to estimate $\bar{Q}_0$ obtained by omitting W_2 from $\bar{Q}_n$ (MC). The double robust and IPTW estimators were further implemented using the following sets of bounds for the values of g_n: $[0, 1]$ (no bounding), $[0.025, 0.975]$, $[0.050, 0.950]$, and $[0.100, 0.900]$. For the IPTW estimator, the latter three bounds correspond to truncation of the unstabilized weights at $[1.03, 40]$, $[1.05, 20]$, and $[1.11, 10]$.

The parametric bootstrap was then applied using the Bias_{ETA} algorithm to 10 of the 250 samples. For each sample and for each model specification, Q_n and g_n were used to draw 1000 parametric bootstrap samples. Specifically, W was drawn from the empirical distribution for that sample, A was generated given the bootstrapped values of W as a series of Bernoulli trials with probability $g_n(1 \mid W)$, and Y was generated given the bootstrapped values of A, W by adding an $N(0, 1)$ error to $\bar{Q}_n(A, W)$. Each candidate estimator was then applied to each bootstrap sample. In this step, the parametric models g_n and $\bar{Q}_n$ were held fixed and their coefficients refit. Bias_{ETA} was calculated for each of the 10 samples as the difference between the mean of the bootstrapped estimator and the initial MLE estimate $\Psi(\hat{P}_0) = \hat{\Psi}_{MLE}(P_n)$ in that sample.

Table 10.1 displays the effect of positivity violations and near-violations on estimator behavior across 250 samples. MSE remained minimally biased when the estimator $\bar{Q}_n$ was consistent; use of inconsistent $\bar{Q}_n$ resulted in bias. Given consistent estimators $\bar{Q}_n$ and g_n, the IPTW estimator was more biased than the other three estimators, as expected given the practical positivity violations present in the simulation. The finite sample performance of the A-IPTW and TMLE estimators was also affected by the presence of practical positivity violations. The double robust estimators achieved the lowest MSE when (1) $\bar{Q}_n$ was consistent and (2) g_n was inconsistent but satisfied positivity (as a result either of truncation or of omission of W_2, a major source of positivity bias). Interestingly, in this simulation TMLE still did quite well when $\bar{Q}_n$ was inconsistent and the model used for g_n was correctly specified but its values bounded at $[0.025, 0.925]$.

The choice of bound imposed on g_n affected both the bias and variance of the IPTW estimator, A-IPTW estimator, and TMLE. As expected, truncation of the IPTW weights improved the variance of the estimator but increased bias. Without additional diagnostic information, an analyst who observed the dramatic decline in the variance of the IPTW estimator that occurred with weight truncation might have concluded that truncation improved estimator performance; however, in this simulation weight truncation increased MSE. In contrast, and as predicted by theory, use of bounded values of g_n decreased MSE of the double robust estimators despite the inconsistency introduced into g_n.

Table 10.2 shows the mean of Bias_{ETA} across 10 of the 250 samples; the variance of Bias_{ETA} across the samples was small [results available in Petersen et al. (2010)]. Based on the results shown in Table 10.1, a red flag was needed for the IPTW estimator with and without bounded g_n and for the TMLE without bounded g_n. (The

Table 10.1 Performance of estimators in 250 simulated data sets of size 1000; rows for each estimator indicate the bound on g_n. *CC* is correctly specified $\bar{Q}_n$ and g_n, *CM* is correctly specified $\bar{Q}_n$ and misspecified g_n, and *MC* is misspecified $\bar{Q}_n$ and correctly specified g_n

	CC			*CM*			*MC*		
	Bias	Var	MSE	Bias	Var	MSE	Bias	Var	MSE
MLE									
	0.007	0.009	0.009	0.007	0.009	0.009	1.145	0.025	1.336
IPTW									
[0.000, 1.000]	0.544	0.693	0.989	1.547	0.267	2.660	0.544	0.693	0.989
[0.025, 0.975]	1.080	0.090	1.257	1.807	0.077	3.340	1.080	0.090	1.257
[0.050, 0.950]	1.437	0.059	2.123	2.062	0.054	4.306	1.437	0.059	2.123
[0.100, 0.900]	1.935	0.043	3.787	2.456	0.043	6.076	1.935	0.043	3.787
A-IPTW									
[0.000, 1.000]	0.080	0.966	0.972	−0.003	0.032	0.032	−0.096	16.978	16.987
[0.025, 0.975]	0.012	0.017	0.017	0.006	0.017	0.017	0.430	0.035	0.219
[0.050, 0.950]	0.011	0.014	0.014	0.009	0.014	0.014	0.556	0.025	0.334
[0.100, 0.900]	0.009	0.011	0.011	0.008	0.011	0.011	0.706	0.020	0.519
TMLE									
[0.000, 1.000]	0.251	0.478	0.540	0.026	0.059	0.060	−0.675	0.367	0.824
[0.025, 0.975]	0.016	0.028	0.028	0.005	0.021	0.021	−0.004	0.049	0.049
[0.050, 0.950]	0.013	0.019	0.020	0.010	0.016	0.017	0.163	0.027	0.054
[0.100, 0.900]	0.010	0.014	0.014	0.009	0.013	0.013	0.384	0.018	0.166

Table 10.2 Finite sample bias and mean of Bias_{ETA} across ten simulated data sets of size 1000

		Bound on g_n			
		[0.000, 1.000]	[0.025, 0.975]	[0.050, 0.950]	[0.100, 0.900]
MLE					
Finite sample bias	*CC*	7.01e−03	–	–	–
Mean(Bias_{ETA})	*CC*	−8.51e−04	–	–	–
Mean(Bias_{ETA})	*CM*	2.39e−04	–	–	–
Mean(Bias_{ETA})	*MC*	5.12e−04	–	–	–
IPTW					
Finite sample bias	*CC*	5.44e−01	1.08e+00	1.44e+00	1.93e+00
Mean(Bias_{ETA})	*CC*	4.22e−01	1.04e+00	1.40e+00	1.90e+00
Mean(Bias_{ETA})	*CM*	1.34e−01	4.83e−01	7.84e−01	1.23e+00
Mean(Bias_{ETA})	*MC*	2.98e−01	7.39e−01	9.95e−01	1.35e+00
A-IPTW					
Finite sample bias	*CC*	7.99e−02	1.25e−02	1.07e−02	8.78e−03
Mean(Bias_{ETA})	*CC*	1.86e−03	2.80e−03	5.89e−05	1.65e−03
Mean(Bias_{ETA})	*CM*	−3.68e−04	−6.36e−04	2.56e−05	5.72e−04
Mean(Bias_{ETA})	*MC*	−3.59e−04	1.21e−04	−1.18e−04	−1.09e−03
TMLE					
Finite sample bias	*CC*	2.51e−01	1.60e−02	1.31e−02	9.98e−03
Mean(Bias_{ETA})	*CC*	1.74e−01	4.28e−03	2.65e−04	1.84e−03
Mean(Bias_{ETA})	*CM*	2.70e−02	−3.07e−04	2.15e−04	7.74e−04
Mean(Bias_{ETA})	*MC*	1.11e−01	9.82e−04	−2.17e−04	−1.47e−03

A-IPTW estimator without bounded g_n exhibited a small to moderate amount of bias; however, the variance would likely have alerted an analyst to the presence of sparsity.) The parametric bootstrap correctly identified the presence of substantial finite sample bias in the IPTW estimator for all truncation levels and in the TMLE with unbounded g_n. Bias_{ETA} was minimal for the remaining estimators.

For correctly specified $\bar{Q}_n$ and g_n (g_n unbounded), the mean of Bias_{ETA} across the ten samples was 78% and 69% of the true finite sample bias of the IPTW estimator and TMLE, respectively. The fact that the true bias was underestimated in both cases illustrates a limitation of the parametric bootstrap: its performance, even as an intentionally optimistic bias estimate, suffers when the target estimator is not asymptotically normally distributed. Bounding g_n improved the ability of the bootstrap to accurately diagnose bias by improving estimator behavior (in addition to adding a new source of bias due to truncation of g_n). This finding suggests that practical application of the bootstrap to a given estimator should at minimum generate Bias_{ETA} estimates for a single low level of truncation of g_n in addition to any unbounded estimate. When g_n was bounded, the mean of Bias_{ETA} for the IPTW estimator across the 10 samples was 96 to 98% of the true finite sample bias; the finite sample bias for the TMLE with bounded g_n was accurately estimated to be minimal. Misspecification of g_n or $\bar{Q}_n$ by excluding a key covariate led to an estimated data-generating distribution with less sparsity than the true P_0, and as a result the parametric bootstrap underestimated bias to a greater extent for these model specifications.

While use of an unbounded g_n resulted in an underestimate of the true degree of finite sample bias for the IPTW and TMLE, in this simulation the parametric bootstrap would still have functioned well as a diagnostic in each of the ten samples considered. Table 10.3 reports the output that would have been available to an analyst applying the parametric bootstrap to the unbounded IPTW and TMLE for each of the ten samples. In all samples Bias_{ETA} was of roughly the same magnitude as the estimated standard error of the estimator, and in most was of significant magnitude relative to the point estimate of the causal effect.

The simulation demonstrates how the parametric bootstrap can be used to investigate the tradeoffs between bias due to weight truncation/bounding of g_n and positivity bias. The parametric bootstrap accurately diagnosed both an increase in the bias of the IPTW estimator with increasing truncation and a reduction in the bias of the TMLE with truncation. When viewed in light of the standard error estimates under different levels of truncation, the diagnostic would have accurately suggested that truncation of g_n for the TMLE was beneficial, while truncation of the weights for the IPTW estimator was of questionable benefit. The parametric bootstrap can also be used to provide a more refined approach to choosing an optimal truncation constant based on estimated MSE (Bembom and van der Laan 2008).

These results further illustrate the benefit of applying the parametric bootstrap to the IPTW estimator in addition to the analyst's estimator of choice. Diagnosis of substantial bias in the IPTW estimator due to positivity violations would have alerted an analyst that MLE was relying heavily on extrapolation and that the double

Table 10.3 Estimated causal treatment effect, standard error, and Bias_{ETA} in ten simulated datasets of size 1000; g_n and Q_n correctly specified, g_n unbounded

	IPTW			**TMLE**		
Sample	$\hat{\beta}_{IPTW}$	$\widehat{\text{SE}}$	Bias_{ETA}	$\hat{\beta}_{TMLE}$	$\widehat{\text{SE}}$	Bias_{ETA}
1	0.207	0.203	0.473	0.827	0.197	0.172
2	1.722	0.197	0.425	0.734	0.114	0.153
3	1.957	0.184	0.306	1.379	0.105	0.087
4	1.926	0.206	0.510	0.237	0.089	0.252
5	2.201	0.192	0.565	2.548	0.182	0.245
6	0.035	0.236	0.520	0.533	0.228	0.234
7	1.799	0.180	0.346	1.781	0.184	0.150
8	0.471	0.215	0.420	1.066	0.114	0.188
9	2.749	0.184	0.391	1.974	0.114	0.161
10	0.095	0.228	0.263	0.628	0.173	0.099

robust estimators were sensitive to bias arising from misspecification of the model used to estimate $\bar{Q}_0$.

10.3.3 HIV Data Application

We analyzed an observational cohort of HIV-infected patients in order to estimate the effect of mutations in the HIV protease enzyme on viral response to the antiretroviral drug lopinavir. The question, data, and analysis have been described previously (Bembom et al. 2009). Here, a simplified version of prior analyses was performed and the parametric bootstrap was applied to investigate the potential impact of positivity violations on results.

Baseline covariates, mutation profiles prior to treatment change, and viral response to therapy were collected for 401 treatment change episodes (TCEs) in which protease-inhibitor-experienced subjects initiated a new antiretroviral regimen containing the drug lopinavir. We focused on 2 target mutations in the protease enzyme: p82AFST and p82MLC (present in 25% and 1% of TCEs, respectively). The data for each target mutation consisted of $O = (W, A, Y)$, where A was a binary indicator that the target mutation was present prior to treatment change, W was a set of 35 baseline characteristics including summaries of past treatment history, mutations in the reverse transcriptase enzyme, and a genotypic susceptibility score for the background regimen (based on the Stanford scoring system). The outcome Y was the change in $\log_{10}$(viral load) following initiation of the new antiretroviral regimen. The target observed data parameter was $E_0[E_0(Y \mid A = 1, W) - E(Y \mid A = 0, W)]$, equal under (10.4) to the average treatment effect $E_0(Y_1 - Y_0)$.

Effect estimates were obtained for each mutation using the IPTW estimator and TMLE with a logistic fluctuation (Chap. 7). $\bar{Q}_0$ and g_0 were estimated with stepwise forward selection of main terms based on the AIC criterion. Estimators were implemented using both unbounded values for $g_n(A \mid W)$ and values truncated at $[0.025, 0.975]$. Standard errors were estimated using the influence curve treating the values of g_n as fixed. The parametric bootstrap was used to estimate bias for each estimator using 1000 samples and the Bias_{ETA} algorithm.

Results for both mutations are presented in Table 10.4. p82AFST is known to be a major mutation for lopinavir resistance (Johnson et al. 2009). The current results support this finding; the IPTW and TMLE point estimates were similar and both suggested a significantly more positive change in viral load (corresponding to a less effective drug response) among subjects with the mutation as compared to those without it. The parametric-bootstrap-based bias estimate was minimal, raising no red flag that these findings might be attributable to positivity bias.

The role of mutation p82CLM is less clear based on existing knowledge; depending on the scoring system used it is either not considered a lopinavir resistance mutation, or given an intermediate lopinavir resistance score (http://hivdb.stanford.edu, Johnson et al. 2009). Initial inspection of the point estimates and standard errors in the current analysis would have suggested that p82CLM had a large and highly significant effect on lopinavir resistance. Application of the parametric-bootstrap-based diagnostic, however, would have suggested that these results should be interpreted with caution. In particular, the bias estimate for the unbounded TMLE was larger than the estimated standard error, while the bias estimate for the unbounded IPTW estimator was of roughly the same magnitude. While neither bias estimate was of sufficient magnitude relative to the point estimate to change inference, their size relative to the corresponding standard errors would have suggested that further investigation was warranted.

In response, the nonparametric bootstrap (based on 1000 bootstrap samples) was applied to provide an alternative estimate of the standard error. Using this alternative approach, the standard errors for the unbounded TMLE and IPTW estimator of the effect of p82MLC were estimated to be 2.77 and 1.17, respectively. Nonparametric-bootstrap-based standard error estimates for the bounded TMLE and IPTW estimator were lower (0.84 and 1.12, respectively), but still substantially higher than the initial naive standard error estimates. These revised standard error estimates dramatically changed interpretation of results, suggesting that the current analysis was unable to provide essentially any information on the presence, magnitude, or direction of the p82CLM effect. (Nonparametric-bootstrap-based standard error estimates for p82AFST were also somewhat larger than initial estimates but did not change inference).

In this example, Bias_{ETA} is expected to include some nonpositivity bias due to the curse of dimensionality. However, the resulting bias estimate should be interpreted as highly optimistic (i.e., as an underestimate of the true finite sample bias). The parametric bootstrap sampled from estimates of g_0 and $\bar{Q}_0$ that had been fit using the forward stepwise algorithm. This ensured that g_n and $\bar{Q}_n$ (which applied the same stepwise algorithm) would do a good job approximating $g_{\hat{P}_0}$ and $\bar{Q}_{\hat{P}_0}$ in each bootstrap sample. Clearly, no such guarantee exists for the true P_0. This simple example further illustrates the utility of the nonparametric bootstrap for standard error estimation in the setting of sparse data and positivity violations. In this particular

Table 10.4 Point estimate, standard error, and parametric-bootstrap-based bias estimates for the effect of two HIV resistance mutations on viral response

	TMLE			IPTW		
	$\hat{\beta}_{TMLE}$	$\widehat{\text{SE}}$	Bias_{ETA}	$\hat{\beta}_{IPTW}$	$\widehat{\text{SE}}$	Bias_{ETA}
p82AFST						
[0.000, 1.000]	0.65	0.13	−0.01	0.66	0.15	−0.01
[0.025, 0.975]	0.62	0.13	0.00	0.66	0.15	−0.01
p82MLC						
[0.000, 1.000]	2.85	0.14	−0.37	1.29	0.14	0.09
[0.025, 0.975]	0.86	0.10	−0.01	0.80	0.23	0.08

example, the improved variance estimate provided by the nonparametric bootstrap was sufficient to prevent positivity violations from leading to incorrect inference. As demonstrated in the simulations, however, in other settings even accurate variance estimates may fail to alert the analyst to threats posed by positivity violations.

10.4 Practical Approaches to Positivity Violations

Approach #1: Change the projection function $h(A, V)$. Throughout this chapter we have focused on the target causal parameter $\beta(F_X, m, h)$ defined according to (10.2) as the projection of the $E_{F_X}(Y_a \mid V)$ on the working marginal structural model $m(a, V \mid \beta)$. Choice of function $h(a, V)$ both defines the target parameter by specifying which values of (A, V) should be given greater weight when estimating β_0 and, by assumption (10.6), defines the positivity assumption needed for β_0 to be identifiable.

We have focused on parameters indexed by $h(a, V) = 1$, a choice that gives equal weight to estimating the counterfactual outcome for all values (a, v) (Neugebauer and van der Laan 2007). Alternative choices of $h(a, V)$ can significantly weaken the needed positivity assumption. For example, if the target of inference only involves counterfactual outcomes among some restricted range $[c, d]$ of possible values $\mathcal{A}$, defining $h(a, V) = I(a \in [c, d])$ weakens the positivity assumption by requiring sufficient variability only in the assignment of treatment levels within the target range. In some settings, the causal parameter defined by such a projection over a limited range of $\mathcal{A}$ might be of substantial a priori interest. For example, one may wish to focus estimation of a drug dose response curve only on the range of doses considered reasonable for routine clinical use, rather than on the full range of doses theoretically possible or observed in a given data set.

An alternative approach, commonly employed in the context of IPTW estimation and introduced in Sect. 10.2.2, is to choose $h(a, V) = g(a \mid V)$, where $g(a \mid V) = P(A = a \mid V)$ is the conditional probability of treatment given the covariates included in the marginal structural model. In the setting of IPTW estimation this choice corresponds to the use of stabilizing weights, a common approach to reducing both the variance of the IPTW estimator in the face of sparsity (Robins et al. 2000a). When the target causal parameter is defined using a marginal structural working model, use of $h(a, V) = g(a, V)$ corresponds to a decision to define a target parameter that gives greater weight to those regions of the joint distribution of (A, V) that are well supported and that relies on smoothing or extrapolation to a greater degree in areas that are not (Neugebauer and van der Laan 2007).

Use of a marginal structural working model makes clear that the utility of choosing $h(a, V) = g(a \mid V)$ as a method to approach data sparsity is not limited to the IPTW estimator. Recall that MLE can be implemented by regressing predicted values for Y_a on (a, V) according to model $m(a, V \mid \beta)$ with weights provided by $h(a, V)$. When the projection function is chosen to be $g_0(a \mid V)$, this corresponds to a weighted regression in which weights are proportional to the degree of support in the data.

Even when one is ideally interested in the entire causal curve [implying a target parameter defined by choice $h(a, V) = 1$], specification of alternative choices for h offers a means of improving identifiability, at a cost of redefining the target parameter. For example, one can define a family of target parameters indexed by $h_\delta(a, V) = I(a \in [c(\delta), d(\delta)])$, where an increase in δ corresponds to progressive restriction on the range of treatment levels targeted by estimation. Fluctuation of δ thus corresponds to trading a focus on more limited areas of the causal curve for improved parameter identifiability. Selection of the final target from among this family can be based on an estimate of bias provided by the parametric bootstrap. For example, the bootstrap can be used to select the parameter with the smallest δ below some prespecified threshold for allowable Bias_{ETA}.

Approach #2: Restrict the adjustment set. Exclusion of problematic Ws (i.e., those covariates resulting in positivity violations or near-violations) from the adjustment set provides a means to trade confounding bias for a reduction in positivity violations (Bembom et al. 2008). In some cases, exclusion of covariates from the adjustment set may come at little or no cost to bias in the estimate of the target parameter. In particular, a subset of W that excludes covariates responsible for positivity violations may still be sufficient to control for confounding. In other words, a subset $W' \subset W$ may exist for which both identifying assumptions (10.4) and (10.5) hold [i.e., $Y_a \coprod A \mid W'$ and $g_0(a \mid W') > 0, a \in \mathcal{A}$], while positivity fails for the full set of covariates. In practice, this approach can be implemented by first determining candidate subsets of W under which the positivity assumption holds, and then using causal graphs to assess whether any of these candidates is sufficient to control for confounding. Even when no such candidate set can be identified, background knowledge (or sensitivity analysis) may suggest that problematic Ws represent a minimal source of confounding bias (Moore et al. 2009). Often, however, those covariates that are most problematic from a positivity perspective are also strong confounders.

As suggested with respect to the choice of projection function $h(a, V)$ in the previous section, the causal effect estimator can be fine-tuned to select the degree of restriction on the adjustment set W according to some prespecified rule for eliminating covariates from the adjustment set, and the parametric bootstrap used to select the minimal degree of restriction that maintains Bias_{ETA} below an acceptable threshold (Bembom et al. 2008). In the case of substantial positivity violations, such an approach can result in small covariate adjustment sets. While such limited covariate adjustment accurately reflects a target parameter that is poorly supported by the available data, the resulting estimate can be difficult to interpret and will no longer carry a causal intepretation.

Approach #3: Restrict the sample. An alternative, sometimes referred to as "trimming," discards classes of subjects for whom there exists no or limited variability in observed treatment assignment. A causal effect is then estimated in the remaining subsample. This approach is popular in econometrics and social science (Crump et al. 2006; LaLonde 1986; Heckman et al. 1997; Dehejia and Wahba 1999).

When the subset of covariates responsible for positivity violations is low- or one-dimensional, such an approach can be implemented simply by discarding subjects with covariate values not represented in all treatment groups. For example, say that one aims to estimate the average effect of a binary treatment and, in order to control for confounding, one needs to adjust for W, a covariate with possible levels $\{1, 2, 3, 4\}$. However, inspection of the data reveals that no one in the sample with $W = 4$ received treatment [i.e., $g_n(1 \mid W = 4) = 0$]. The sample can be trimmed by excluding those subjects for whom $W = 4$ prior to applying a given causal effect estimator for the average treatment effect. As a result, the target parameter is shifted from $E_0(Y_1 - Y_0)$ to $E_0(Y_1 - Y_0 \mid W < 4)$, and positivity assumption (10.5) now holds (as $W = 4$ occurs with zero probability).

Often W is too high-dimensional to make this straightforward implementation feasible; in such a case matching on the propensity score provides a means to trim the sample. There is an extensive literature on propensity score-based effect estimators; however, such estimators are beyond the scope of the current review. Several potential problems arise with the use of trimming methods to address positivity violations. First, discarding subjects responsible for positivity violations shrinks sample size and thus runs the risk of increasing the variance of the effect estimate. Further, sample size and the extent to which positivity violations arise by chance are closely related. Depending on how trimming is implemented, new positivity violations can be introduced as sample size shrinks. Second, restriction of the sample may result in a causal effect for a population of limited interest. In other words, as can occur with alternative approaches to improving identifiability by shifting the target of inference, the parameter actually estimated may be far from the initial target. Further, when the criterion used to restrict the sample involves a summary of high-dimensional covariates, such as is provided the propensity score, it can be difficult to interpret the parameter estimated. Finally, when treatment is longitudinal, the covariates responsible for positivity violations may themselves be affected by past treatment. Trimming to remove positivity violations in this setting amounts to conditioning on posttreatment covariates and can thus introduce new bias.

Crump proposes an approach to trimming that falls within the general strategy of redefining the target parameter in order to explicitly capture the tradeoff between parameter identifiability and proximity to the initial target (Crump et al. 2006). In addition to focusing on the treatment effect in an a priori specified target population, he defines an alternative target parameter corresponding to the average treatment effect in that subsample of the population for which the most precise estimate can be achieved. Crump further suggests the potential for extending this approach to achieve an optimal (according to some user-specified criterion) tradeoff between the representativeness of the subsample in which the effect is estimated and the variance of the estimate.

Approach #4: Change the intervention of interest. A final alternative for improving the identifiability of a causal parameter in the presence of positivity violations is to redefine the intervention of interest. Realistic rules rely on an estimate of the propensity score $g_0(a \mid W)$ to define interventions that explicitly avoid positivity violations. This ensures that the causal parameter estimated is sufficiently supported by existing data.

Realistic interventions avoid positivity violations by first identifying subjects for whom a given treatment assignment is not realistic (i.e., subjects whose propensity score for a given treatment is small or zero) and then assigning an alternative treatment with better data support to those individuals. Such an approach is made possible by focusing on the causal effects of dynamic treatment regimes (van der Laan and Petersen 2007a; Robins et al. 2008). The causal parameters described thus far are summaries of the counterfactual outcome distribution under a fixed treatment applied uniformly across the target population. In contrast, a dynamic regime assigns treatment in response to patient covariate values. This characteristic makes it possible to define interventions under which a subject is only assigned treatments that are possible (or "realistic") given a subject's covariate values.

To continue the previous example in which no subjects with $W = 4$ were treated, a realistic treatment rule might take the form "treat only those subjects with W less than 4." More formally, let $d(W)$ refer to a treatment rule that deterministically assigns a treatment $a \in \mathcal{A}$ based on a subject's covariates W and consider the rule $d(W) = I(W < 4)$. Let Y_d denote the counterfactual outcome under the treatment rule $d(W)$, which corresponds to treating a subject if and only if his or her covariate W is below 4. In this example $E_0(Y_0)$ is identified as $\sum_w E_0(Y \mid W = w, A = 0)P_0(W = w)$; however, since $E_0(Y \mid W = w, A = 1)$ is undefined for $W = 4$, $E_0(Y_1)$ is not identified (unless we are willing to extrapolate based on $W < 4$). In contrast, $E_0(Y_d)$ is identified by the nonparametric g-formula: $\sum_w E_0(Y = y \mid W = w, A = d(W))P_0(W = w)$. Thus the average treatment effect $E_0(Y_d - Y_0)$, but not $E_0(Y_1 - Y_0)$, is identified. The redefined causal parameter can be interpreted as the difference in expected counterfactual outcome if only those subjects with $W < 4$ were treated as compared to the outcome if no one were treated.

More generally, realistic rules indexed by a given static treatment a assign a only to those individuals for whom the probability of receiving a is greater than some user-specified probability α (such as $\alpha > 0.05$). Let $d(a, W)$ denote the rule indexed by static treatment a. If A is binary, then $d(1, W) = 1$ if $g(1 \mid W) > \alpha$, otherwise $d(1, W) = 0$. Similarly, $d(0, W) = 0$ if $g(0 \mid W) > \alpha$; otherwise $d(0, W) = 1$. Realistic causal parameters are defined as some parameter of the distribution of $Y_{d(a,W)}$ (possibly conditional on some subset of baseline covariates $V \subset W$). Estimation of the causal effects of dynamic rules $d(W)$ allows the positivity assumption to be relaxed to $g(d(W) \mid W) > 0$, a.e (i.e., only those treatments that would be assigned based on rule d to patients with covariates W need to occur with positive probability within strata of W). Realistic rules $d(a, W)$ are designed to satisfy this assumption by definition. When a given treatment level a is unrealistic [i.e., when $g(a \mid W) < \alpha$], realistic rules assign an alternative from among viable (well-supported) choices. The choice of an alternative is straightforward when treatment is binary. When treatment has more than two levels, however, a rule for selecting the alternative treatment level is needed. One option is to assign a treatment level that is as close as possible to the original assignment while still remaining realistic. For example, if high doses of drugs occur with low probability in a certain subset of the population, a realistic rule might assign the maximum dose that occurs with probability $> \alpha$ in that subset. An alternative class of dynamic regimes, referred to as "intent-to-treat" rules, instead assigns a subject to his or her observed treatment value if an initial assignment is deemed unrealistic. Moore et al. (2009) and Bembom and van der Laan (2007a) provide illustrations of these types of realistic rules using simulated and real data.

The causal effects of realistic rules clearly differ from their static counterparts. The extent to which the new target parameter diverges from the initial parameter of interest depends on both the extent to which positivity violations occur in the finite sample (i.e., the extent of support available in the data for the initial target parameter) and on a user-supplied threshold α. The parametric bootstrap approach presented in Sect. 10.3 can be employed to data-adaptively select α based on the level of Bias_{ETA} deemed acceptable (Bembom and van der Laan 2007a).

Selection among a family of parameters. Each of the methods described for estimating causal effects in the presence of data sparsity corresponds to a particular strategy for altering the target parameter in exchange for improved identifiability. In each case, we have outlined how this tradeoff could be made systematically based on some user-specified criterion such as the bias estimate provided by the parametric bootstrap. We now summarize this general approach in terms of a formal method for estimation in the face of positivity violations.

1. Define a family of parameters. The family should include the initial target of inference together with a set of related parameters, indexed by γ in index set I, where γ represents the extent to which a given family member trades improved identifiability for decreased proximity to the initial target. In the examples given in the previous section, γ could be used to index a set of projection functions $h(a, V)$ based on an increasingly restrictive range of the possible values $\mathcal{A}$, degree to which the adjustment covariate set or sample is restricted, or choice of a threshold for defining a realistic rule.
2. Apply the parametric bootstrap to generate an estimate Bias_{ETA} for each $\gamma \in I$. In particular, this involves estimating the data-generating distribution, simulating new data from this estimate, and then applying an estimator to each target indexed by γ.

3. Select the target parameter from among the set that falls below a prespecified threshold for acceptable Bias_{ETA}. In particular, select the parameter from within the set that is indexed by the value γ that corresponds to the greatest proximity to the initial target.

This approach allows an estimator to be defined in terms of an algorithm that identifies and estimates the parameter within a candidate family that is as close to the initial target of inference as possible while remaining within some user-supplied limit on the extent of tolerable positivity violations.

10.5 Discussion

The identifiability of causal effects relies on sufficient variation in treatment assignment within covariate strata. The strong version of positivity requires that each possible treatment occur with positive probability in each covariate stratum; depending on the model and target parameter, this assumption can be relaxed to some extent. In addition to assessing identifiability based on measurement of and control for sufficient confounders, data analyses should directly assess threats to identifiability based on positivity violations. The parametric bootstrap is a practical tool for assessing such threats, and provides a quantitative estimator-specific estimate of bias arising due to positivity violations.

This chapter has focused on the positivity assumption for the causal effect of a treatment assigned at a single time point. Extension to a longitudinal setting in which the goal is to estimate the effect of multiple treatments assigned sequentially over time introduces considerable additional complexity. First, practical violations of the positivity assumption can arise more readily in this setting. Under the longitudinal version of the positivity assumption the conditional probability of each possible treatment history should remain positive regardless of covariate history. However, this probability is the product of time-point-specific treatment probabilities given the past. When the product is taken over multiple time points, it is easy for treatment histories with very small conditional probabilities to arise. Second, longitudinal data make it harder to diagnose the bias arising due to positivity violations. Implementation of the parametric bootstrap in longitudinal settings requires Monte Carlo simulation both to implement the MLE and to generate each bootstrap sample. In particular, this requires estimating and sampling from the time-point-specific conditional distributions of all covariates and treatment given the past. Additional research on assessing the impact of positivity bias on longitudinal causal parameters is needed, including investigation of the parametric bootstrap in this setting.

When positivity violations occur for structural reasons rather than due to chance, a causal parameter that avoids these positivity violations will often be of substantial interest. For example, when certain treatment levels are contraindicated for certain types of individuals, the average treatment effect in the population may be of less interest than the effect of treatment among that subset of the population without contraindications, or, alternatively, than the effect of an intervention that assigns treatment only to those subjects without contraindications. Similarly, the effect of a multilevel treatment may be of greatest interest for only a subset of treatment levels.

In other cases researchers may be happy to settle for a better estimate of a less interesting parameter. Sample restriction, estimation of realistic parameters, and change in projection function $h(a, V)$ all change the causal effect being estimated; in contrast, restriction of the covariate adjustment set often results in estimation of a noncausal parameter. However, all of these approaches can be understood as means to shift from a poorly identified initial target toward a parameter that is less ambitious but more fully supported by the available data. The new estimand is not determined a priori by the question of interst, but rather is driven by the observed data distribution in the finite sample at hand. There is thus an explicit tradeoff between identifiability and proximity to the initial target of inference. Ideally, this tradeoff will be made in a systematic way rather than on an ad hoc basis at the discretion of the investigator. Definition of an estimator that selects among a family of parameters according to some prespecified criteria is a means to formalize this tradeoff. An estimate of bias based on the parametric bootstrap can be used to implement the tradeoff in practice.

In summary, we offer the following advice for applied analyses. First, define the causal effect of interest based on careful consideration of structural positivity violations. Second, consider estimator behavior in the context of positivity violations when selecting an estimator. Third, apply the parametric bootstrap to quantify the extent of estimator bias under data simulated to approximate the true data-generating distribution. Fourth, when positivity violations are a concern, choose an estimator that selects systematically from among a family of parameters based on the tradeoff between data support and proximity to the initial target of inference.

10.6 Notes and Further Reading

While perhaps less well-recognized than confounding bias, violations and near-violations of the positivity assumption can increase both the variance and bias of causal effect estimates, and if undiagnosed can seriously threaten the validity of causal inference. The dangers of causal effect estimation in the absence of adequate data support have long been understood (Cochran 1957). More recent causal inference literature refers to the need for adequate exposure variability within confounder strata as the assumption of positivity or experimental treatment assignment (Robins 1986, 1987a, 2000). A summary of estimator behavior in the face of positivity violations is also discussed in previous work (Neugebauer and van der Laan 2005, 2007; Bembom and van der Laan 2007a; Moore et al. 2009; Cole and Hernan 2008). Additional simulations are discussed in Petersen et al. (2010), the article from which this chapter was adapted.

Part III
TMLE and Parametric Regression in RCTs

Chapter 11
Robust Analysis of RCTs Using Generalized Linear Models

Michael Rosenblum

It is typical in RCTs for extensive information to be collected on subjects prior to randomization. For example, age, ethnicity, socioeconomic status, history of disease, and family history of disease may be recorded. Baseline information can be leveraged to obtain more precise estimates of treatment effects than the standard unadjusted estimator. This is often done by carrying out model-based analyses at the end of the trial, where baseline variables predictive of the primary study outcome are included in the model. As shown in Moore and van der Laan (2007), such analyses have potential to improve precision and, if carried out in the appropriate manner, give asymptotically unbiased, locally efficient estimates of the marginal treatment effect even when the model used is arbitrarily misspecified.

In this chapter, we extend the results of Moore and van der Laan (2007) for linear and logistic regression models to a wider range of generalized linear models. Our main result implies that a large class of generalized linear models, such as linear regression models (for continuous outcomes), logistic regression models (for binary outcomes), Poisson regression models (for count data), and gamma regression models (for positive-valued outcomes), can be used to produce estimators that are asymptotically unbiased even when the model is arbitrarily misspecified. The estimators that we show to have this property are TMLEs that use the fits of such generalized linear models as initial density estimators. The results hold when the canonical link function for the family of generalized linear models is used, which is commonly the default link function used.

In this chapter we describe (1) a class of model-based estimators particularly useful in analyzing RCT results and (2) a relatively simple and useful application of TMLE. We also show a new robustness property of Poisson regression models when used in RCTs; this result is the log-linear analog to the robustness to model misspecification of ANCOVA for linear models when used in RCTs.

The TMLEs we present below are examples of parametric MLEs, double robust estimators (Scharfstein et al. 1999; Robins 2000; Robins and Rotnitzky 2001; van der Laan and Robins 2003), and estimators in Tsiatis (2006) and Zhang et al. (2008). The estimators we present are special cases of a class of estimators in the Comments to the Rejoinder to Scharfstein et al. (1999, p. 1141), for RCTs. Their arguments involving parametric generalized linear models with canonical link functions imply that the estimators given in this chapter are asymptotically unbiased under arbitrary model misspecification, and are locally efficient.

11.1 Summary of Main Result

We are interested in estimating the marginal treatment effect of a randomized treatment or intervention. We want to compare the average of the outcomes for the population of interest under the following two scenarios: (1) had everyone in the population received the treatment and (2) had everyone in the population received the control. These treatment-specific marginal means can be contrasted in many ways. For example, we could be interested in the risk difference, the relative risk, the log relative risk, log odds ratio, etc. Such marginal contrasts are often the goal of RCTs and enter into the decision-making process of the FDA in approving new drugs. We focus on estimating the marginal risk difference, but the methods can be modified to robustly estimate any of these other contrasts, as we describe in Sect. 11.3.1.

Robustness property. We show that a class of TMLEs is robust to misspecification of the working model.

We use the term *working model* to refer to a parametric statistical model that is used in computing an estimator, but that we don't assume to be correctly specified; that is, we don't assume it contains the true data-generating distribution. Here we use generalized linear models as working models.

The robustness property we demonstrate for a class of TMLEs is that these estimators are asymptotically unbiased and asymptotically normal, under arbitrary misspecification of the working model used, under mild regularity conditions. That is, even when the true data-generating distribution is not captured by a generalized linear model at all, the class of estimators we present will be consistent and asymptotically normal. If the generalized linear model used as working model is correctly specified, then the resulting estimator will in addition be efficient; that is, it will attain the semiparametric efficiency bound. These robustness properties require that data come from an RCT. Extensions to observational studies are discussed in Rosenblum and van der Laan (2010b).

Data, statistical model, and target parameter. For each subject i, we denote their baseline variables by W_i, treatment assignment by A_i, and outcome by Y_i. We assume that each triple (W_i, A_i, Y_i) is an independent draw from an unknown data-generating distribution P_0 on the random vector (W, A, Y). [We note that this often-made assumption is not guaranteed by randomization (Freedman 2008c). However, this, or a slightly weaker assumption, is often needed in order to prove even that the standard unadjusted estimator is asymptotically unbiased and asymptotically normal.] We also assume that A is binary, with $A = 1$ indicating assignment to the treatment arm and $A = 0$ indicating assignment to the control arm. Additionally, we assume A is independent of baseline variables W, which is guaranteed by randomization. The prerandomization variables W can take various values (e.g., they may be continuous, categorical, etc.). The outcome Y can also take various values. This defines the statistical model $\mathcal{M}$ for P_0.

Consider estimation of the risk difference $E_{P_0}(Y \mid A = 1) - E_{P_0}(Y \mid A = 0)$. In an RCT, this target parameter identifies the additive causal effect as defined by the SCM. Due to the independence between A and W assumed by the model $\mathcal{M}$, this statistical parameter is equivalent to the parameter $\Psi : \mathcal{M} \to \mathbb{R}$ defined by $\Psi(P) = E_P[E_P(Y \mid A = 1, W) - E_P(Y \mid A = 0, W)]$. There are n total subjects.

The choice of generalized linear (working) model that defines the estimators below will in part depend on the possible values taken by the outcome variable Y. For example, if Y is a count variable (nonnegative integer), then a Poisson regression model may (but won't necessarily) be appropriate.

Class of estimators with robustness property. We refer to the following estimator as the unadjusted estimator of the risk difference:

$$\frac{1}{N_A}\sum_{i=1}^{n} Y_i A_i - \frac{1}{N_{A^c}}\sum_{i=1}^{n} Y_i(1 - A_i),$$

where $N_A = \sum_{i=1}^{n} A_i$ and $N_{A^c} = n - N_A$. This is the difference in sample averages between the treatment and control arms. No baseline variables are used.

The class of TMLEs that we will show to have the robustness property defined above is constructed as follows. First, fit a generalized linear model m, resulting in an estimate $\bar{Q}_n(A, W) = \mu(A, W, \beta_n)$ for $E_{P_0}(Y \mid A, W)$. Then compute the following estimator based on this model fit:

$$\psi_n = \frac{1}{n}\sum_{i=1}^{n} \mu(1, W_i, \beta_n) - \frac{1}{n}\sum_{i=1}^{n} \mu(0, W_i, \beta_n). \tag{11.1}$$

This can be thought of as the difference in the average of the predicted outcomes based on a model fit of m, using the baseline variables W, had all subjects been assigned to the treatment arm vs. had all subjects been assigned to the control arm. We show below that such estimators result from applying the TMLE when using the model fit of m as initial density estimator.

When the generalized linear model is one of the models we describe below, estimator (11.1) will be asymptotically unbiased, even when the model is arbitrarily misspecified, under the mild regularity conditions given below. It will be asymptotically unbiased regardless of whether the true data-generating distribution $P_0(Y \mid A, W)$ is an element of model m. It will be asymptotically unbiased even when $P_0(Y \mid A, W)$ is not in an exponential family at all.

The well-known robustness of analysis of covariance (ANCOVA) to model misspecification in RCTs [as described, e.g., by Yang and Tsiatis (2001) and Leon et al. (2003)] is a special case of the results here and in Moore and van der Laan (2007). This follows since ANCOVA is equivalent to estimator (11.1) when the generalized linear model used is from the normal family with identity link function, and only an intercept and main terms are included in the linear part.

Similarly, ANCOVA II has been shown to be robust to model misspecification (Yang and Tsiatis 2001; Leon et al. 2003); this too is a special case of estimator (11.1), using the same generalized linear model as just described for ANCOVA, except also including an interaction term in the linear part. The definition of the ANCOVA II estimator in Yang and Tsiatis (2001) and Leon et al. (2003) involves ordinary least squares regression of the centered outcome on an intercept, the centered treatment indicator, the centered baseline variable, and a corresponding interaction term involving centered variables; the estimated coefficient of the centered treatment indicator is the ANCOVA II estimator. This estimator is identical to estimator (11.1) when the generalized linear model used is from the normal family with identity link function, and only an intercept, main terms A and W, and an interaction term $A \times W$ are included in the linear part.

11.2 The Generalized Linear (Working) Models

We briefly summarize several facts we use below concerning generalized linear models. More information can be found in, for example, McCullagh and Nelder (1989). We then give examples of generalized linear models that can be used as working models in constructing the estimators (11.1) that are robust to model misspecification in RCTs.

Generalized linear models are a special class of parametric models for the conditional distribution of an outcome (or sequence of outcomes) Y conditional on predictor variables. Here, we use study arm assignment A and baseline variables W as the predictor variables. We only consider generalized linear models with canonical link functions below. Generalized linear models with canonical link functions relate the density p of the outcome Y to the predictors through a linear part η and functions b and c that depend on the generalized linear model family as follows:

$$P(Y \mid A, W) = \exp(Y\eta - b(\eta(A, W)) + c(Y, \phi)),$$

where $\eta(A, W) = \sum_{i=1}^{k} \beta_i h_i(A, W)$, for some functions $h_i(A, W)$, and where ϕ is a dispersion parameter. We require that $h_1(A, W) = 1$ (which gives an intercept term) and that $h_2(A, W) = A$ (which gives a main term A) in the linear part. (Actually, it suffices that these two terms are in the linear span of the terms $h_i(A, W)$.) The link function f_{link} relates the conditional mean $E(Y \mid A, W)$ under the model to the linear part η as follows:

$$f_{\text{link}}[E(Y \mid A, W)] = \eta(A, W).$$

A canonical link function f_{link} satisfies $\dot{b}(\eta) = f_{\text{link}}^{-1}(\eta)$, where $\dot{b}$ is the first derivative of b. When the above model is fit, the coefficients β, ϕ are estimated by maximum likelihood estimation. We denote the conditional mean $E(Y \mid A, W)$ corresponding to the model fit by $\mu(A, W, \beta_n)$ (where, for simplicity, we suppress the fit of the dispersion parameter ϕ_n in our notation). For ease of exposition, we sometimes refer to the generalized linear model as the parameterization "$\beta \to \mu(A, W, \beta)$," even though this only represents a model for the conditional mean of Y given A, W (and not the full conditional distribution of Y given A, W implied by the generalized linear model). We will also use the notation μ_β for the function $(A, W) \to \mu(A, W, \beta)$.

The results in this chapter hold for generalized linear models from the following families: normal, binomial, Poisson, gamma, and inverse normal. We provide below a list of example generalized linear models with canonical links that can be used as working models to construct the TMLEs (11.1). Each example corresponds to a particular choice of the functions b, c, and h_i, $1 \le i \le k$, in the definition above.

Examples of Working Models Satisfying Given Requirements

1. **Least squares regression:** For Y continuous, the normal model assuming $E(Y \mid A, W)$ has the form $\mu_1(A, W, \beta) = \beta_0 + \beta_1 A + \beta_2 W + \beta_3 AW + \beta_4 W^2$.
2. **Logistic regression:** For Y binary and $\text{logit}(x) = \log(x/(1-x))$, the following model for $P(Y = 1 \mid A, W)$: $\mu_2(A, W, \beta) = \text{logit}^{-1}(\beta_0 + \beta_1 A + \beta_2 W)$.
3. **Poisson regression:** For Y a "count" (that is, Y a nonnegative integer), the Poisson (log-linear) model with mean of Y given A, W of the form $\mu_3(A, W, \beta) = \exp(\beta_0 + \beta_1 A + \beta_2 W)$.
4. **Gamma regression:** For Y positive, real valued, the gamma model with mean of Y given A, W modeled by
$$\mu_4(A, W, \beta) = 1/\left(\beta_0 + \beta_1(1 + A) + \beta_2 \exp(W) + \beta_3 \exp(AW)\right),$$
where all coefficients β_j are assumed to be positive and bounded away from 0 by some $\delta > 0$.
5. **Inverse normal regression:** For Y positive, real valued, the inverse normal model with mean of Y given A, W modeled by
$$\mu_5(A, W, \beta) = 1/\sqrt{\beta_0 + \beta_1 \exp(A) + \beta_2 \exp(W)},$$
where all coefficients β_j are assumed to be positive and bounded away from 0 by some $\delta > 0$.

The additional restrictions in the gamma and inverse normal regression examples above are needed to ensure the corresponding $\mu(A, W \mid \beta)$ is bounded. We make two assumptions that, along with the assumptions above, guarantee that the maximum likelihood estimator for the generalized linear model is well defined and converges to a value β^* as sample size goes to infinity. The first assumption guarantees the design matrix will have full rank, with probability 1, as long as sample size is greater than the number of terms in the linear part of the model. The second assumption guarantees convergence of the maximum likelihood estimator to a value β^*.

Assumption 1: If a set of constants c_j satisfies $\sum_j c_j h_j(A, W) = 0$ with probability 1, then $c_j = 0$ for all j.

Assumption 2: There exists a maximizer β^* of the expected log-likelihood

$$E_{P_0}[Y\eta - b(\eta) + c(Y, \phi)] = E_{P_0}\left[Y \sum_j \beta_j h_j(A, W) - b\left(\sum_j \beta_j h_j(A, W)\right) + c(Y, \phi)\right],$$

and the maximum likelihood estimator β_n of the generalized linear model converges in probability to β^*. In addition, we assume each component of β^* has absolute value smaller than some prespecified bound M.

These two assumptions imply there is a unique maximizer β^* of the expected log-likelihood give above, which follows by concavity of the expected log-likelihood for these generalized linear model families when using canonical links.

11.3 TMLE Using Generalized Linear Model in Initial Estimator

We are interested in estimating the marginal effect of assignment to treatment vs. control in an RCT. We make no assumptions on the unknown, true data-generating distribution P_0, except the following two assumptions. (1) Study arm assignment A is independent of baseline variables and takes values 1 with probability $g_0(1)$ and 0 with probability $g_0(0)$, which is enforced by design in an RCT. (2) P_0 has a smooth density with respect to some dominating measure. The likelihood of the data at a candidate density P can be written

$$\begin{aligned}\prod_{i=1}^{n} P(Y_i, A_i, W_i) &= \prod_{i=1}^{n} P_Y(Y_i \mid A_i, W_i) P_A(A_i \mid W_i) P_W(W_i) \\ &= \prod_{i=1}^{n} P_Y(Y_i \mid A_i, W_i) P_W(W_i) g_0(A_i).\end{aligned}$$

The second equality follows by the first assumption above.

11.3.1 Parameter as a Mapping from the Distribution of the Data

The target parameter is the risk difference. In an RCT, where study arm assignment A is independent of baseline variables W, we have

$$\Psi(P_0) = E_{P_0}(Y \mid A = 1) - E_{P_0}(Y \mid A = 0) \quad (11.2)$$
$$= E_{P_0}\left[E_{P_0}(Y \mid A = 1, W) - E_{P_0}(Y \mid A = 0, W)\right]. \quad (11.3)$$

We note that parameter (11.2) is a function of the data-generating distribution P_0 only through the conditional mean $\bar{Q}_0(A, W) = E_{P_0}(Y \mid A, W)$ and the marginal distribution $Q_{W,0}$ of W. We denote this relevant part of the data-generating distribution by $Q_0 = (\bar{Q}_0, Q_{W,0})$, and we also denote the target parameter by $\Psi(Q_0)$. As in previous chapters, $D^*(Q_0, g_0)$ denotes the efficient influence curve of the risk difference $\Psi : \mathcal{M} \rightarrow \mathbb{R}$ at P_0, which will also be defined below. Let $D_1^*(Q_0, g_0)$ and $D_0^*(Q_0, g_0)$ denote the efficient influence curves of the statistical parameters $\psi_0^{(1)} = E_0[E_0(Y \mid A = 1, W)]$ and $\psi_0^{(0)} = E_0[E_0(Y \mid A = 0, W)]$, respectively.

The adjusted estimator (11.1) is the substitution estimator of (11.3) at the generalized linear model fit for $E_{P_0}(Y \mid A, W)$, and using the empirical distribution for the marginal distribution of the baseline variables. Denoting these choices for $E_{P_0}(Y \mid A, W)$ and $Q_{W,0}$ by Q_n, we then have the estimator ψ_n defined in (11.1) equals the substitution estimator $\Psi(Q_n)$.

Note that we can also use Q_n to obtain the substitution estimators $\psi_n^{(1)} = \Psi^{(1)}(Q_n)$ and $\psi_n^{(0)} = \Psi^{(0)}(Q_n)$ of the two treatment-specific means. We have $\psi_n = \psi_n^{(1)} - \psi_n^{(0)}$.

Normally the TMLE involves computing a substitution estimator at a density that is an updated version (via iteratively fitting suitably chosen parametric models) of the initial density estimator. As we show below, for the target parameter ψ_0 and model we consider in this chapter, the updating step of the TMLE always leaves the initial density estimator unchanged. This is due to the initial density estimator already being a maximum likelihood estimator for a parametric working model that happens to have a score that equals the efficient influence curve (at the maximum likelihood estimator) for our parameter of interest ψ_0: that is, $P_n D^*(Q_n, g_0) = 0$, and, also $P_n D^*(Q_n, g_n) = 0$ if $g_n(1) = \sum_i A_i/n$ is the empirical proportion. In fact, we also have $P_n D_1^*(Q_n, g_0) = P_n D_0^*(Q_n, g_0) = 0$ so that $\psi_n^{(1)}$ and $\psi_n^{(0)}$ are also TMLEs of $\psi_0^{(1)}$ and $\psi_0^{(0)}$. In other words, Q_n equals the estimate of the relevant part of the data-generating distribution obtained by the TMLE that targets the parameter $(\psi_0^{(0)}, \psi_0^{(1)})$. This property of generalized linear models with canonical link functions was, to the best of our knowledge, first noted in the Comments to the Rejoinder to Scharfstein et al. (1999, Sect. 3.2.3, p. 1141). This property can be used to show the consistency, asymptotic normality, and local efficiency of the simple estimator (11.1).

A TMLE of any smooth functions of treatment-specific means $[E_{P_0}(Y \mid A = 0), E_{P_0}(Y \mid A = 1)]$ is obtained by substitution of Q_n. For example, for a count variable Y, we might be interested in the marginal log rate ratio

$$\log\left[E_{P_0}(Y \mid A = 1)/E_{P_0}(Y \mid A = 0)\right], \quad (11.4)$$

which we could estimate by the substitution estimator

$$\log\left[\frac{1}{n}\sum_{i=1}^{n}\mu(1,W_i,\beta_n)\bigg/\left\{\frac{1}{n}\sum_{i=1}^{n}\mu(0,W_i,\beta_n)\right\}\right]. \tag{11.5}$$

Below we focus on estimating the risk difference (11.2), but analogous arguments apply to other smooth functions of the treatment-specific means.

11.3.2 Obtaining Q_n^0, an Initial Estimate of Q_0

We set the initial estimate $\bar{Q}_n(A,W)$ of $E_{P_0}(Y \mid A,W)$ to be the fit $\mu(A,W,\beta_n)$ of the generalized linear model we are using. This is the maximum likelihood estimate based on using the generalized linear model as a parametric working model. We set the initial density estimate $Q_{W,n}$ of the marginal density $Q_{W,0}$ to be the empirical distribution of $W_1,\ldots,W_n$. Summarizing, we have our initial estimate $Q_n^0 = (\bar{Q}_n, Q_{W,n})$, which also implies an initial density estimate of P_0, according to the generalized linear model, given by $P_n^0 = P_{Q_n^0}$.

11.3.3 Loss Function for TMLE Step

One possible loss function to use is minus the log-likelihood $L(P)(O) = -\log P_Y(Y \mid A,W)P_A(A \mid W)P_W(W)$. Here, however, we use a loss function that only depends on the part Q_0 of the data-generating distribution that is relevant to the parameter of interest. We use $L(Q)(O) = -\log P_{\bar{Q}}(Y \mid A,W) - \log Q_W(W)$ as the loss function for Q_0, where $P_{\bar{Q}}(Y \mid A,W)$ is defined as

$$P_{\bar{Q}}(Y \mid A,W) = \exp(Y f_{\text{link}}(\bar{Q}(A,W)) - b(f_{\text{link}}(\bar{Q}(A,W))) + c(Y)),$$

which is the conditional distribution of Y, given (A,W), implied by the conditional mean function $\bar{Q}$ and the generalized linear working model defined in Section 11.2 (where we omit the dispersion parameter ϕ). This is a valid loss function, i.e., for any of the generalized linear working models we allow, the expected value of the loss function is minimized at the true Q_0.

11.3.4 Calculating the Optimal Fluctuation/Submodel

We now determine a parametric model $\{P_n^0(\epsilon) = P_{Q_n^0(\epsilon)} : \epsilon\}$ that (1) equals the initial density at $\epsilon = 0$ and (2) has a score at $\epsilon = 0$ whose linear span contains the efficient influence function at the initial density estimate $P_n^0 = P_{Q_n^0}$. Given the definition of the loss function $L(Q)$ above, this is equivalent to stating that we determine a submodel $\{Q_n^0(\epsilon) : \epsilon\}$ so that $Q_n^0 = Q_n^0(0)$, and $d/d\epsilon L(Q_n^0(\epsilon))$ at $\epsilon = 0$ equals the efficient influence curve at $P_n^0 = P_{Q_n^0}$.

The efficient influence function for $\Psi(P)$ defined in (11.2) is

$$D^*(P) = H^*_{g_0}(A)(Y - E_P(Y \mid A, W)) + E_P(Y \mid A = 1, W) - E_P(Y \mid A = 0, W) - \Psi(P),$$

where $H^*_{g_0}(A) = (2A - 1)/g_0(A)$. Note that the function $D^*(P)$ only depends on the relevant part $Q = Q(P)$ of the joint density P since g_0 is known. We sometimes write $D(P) = D^*(Q, g_0)$ as $D(Q)$ below. Let $\epsilon = (\epsilon_1, \epsilon_2, \epsilon_3)$. Define the scalar covariates: $H_1^* = 1$, $H_2^*(A) = A$, and $H_3^*(P)(W) = E_P(Y \mid A = 1, W) - E_P(Y \mid A = 1) - [E_P(Y \mid A = 0, W) - E_P(Y \mid A = 0)]$. Let $H_3^*(Q_n^0)$ be the covariate at the initial estimator Q_n^0. The two covariates (H_1^*, H_2^*) can be replaced by $H_1^*(A) = A/g_0(A)$ and $H_2^*(A) = (1 - A)/g_0(A)$, which are the clever covariates that define the TMLE that targets $(\psi_0^{(0)}, \psi_0^{(1)})$ in general, as in Chaps. 4 and 5. This follows since the linear span of $(1, A)$ is identical to the linear span of $(A/g_0(A), (1-A)/g_0(A))$, so that these different choices do not affect the TMLE.

Recall that f_{link} is the canonical link function for the generalized linear model family used in the initial density estimator. For example, if the generalized linear model family is the Poisson family, then we have $f_{\text{link}} = \log$. We define the following function, which will be used to construct the parametric fluctuation:

$$\eta(\epsilon, A, W) = \epsilon_1 H_1^* + \epsilon_2 H_2^*(A) + f_{\text{link}}\left(\bar{Q}_n(A, W)\right).$$

Here η will be the linear part (including offset) of a generalized linear model. The offset guarantees that at $\epsilon = 0$ we have $\eta(\epsilon, A, W)$ equals $f_{\text{link}}(\bar{Q}_n(A, W))$, which is the linear part corresponding to the initial density estimator $P_n^0 = P_{Q_n^0}$. This can also be stated as a submodel $\{\bar{Q}_n(\epsilon) : \epsilon\}$ defined as

$$f_{\text{link}}\left(\bar{Q}_n(\epsilon)\right) = f_{\text{link}}\left(\bar{Q}_n(A, W)\right) + \epsilon_1 H_1^* + \epsilon_2 H_2^*(A).$$

Define the parametric model $\{P_n^0(\epsilon) : \epsilon\}$:

$$\begin{aligned} P_n^0(\epsilon)(Y \mid A, W) &= \exp(Y\eta_n^0(\epsilon, A, W) - b(\eta_n^0(\epsilon, A, W)) + c(Y, \phi)), \\ P_n^0(\epsilon)(A \mid W) &= g_0(A), \\ P_n^0(\epsilon)(W) &= Q_{W,n}(\epsilon)(W) = s_{\epsilon_3} \exp(\epsilon_3 H_3^*(Q_n^0)(W)) Q_{W,n}(W), \end{aligned}$$

where the constant $s_{\epsilon_3} = 1/[\frac{1}{n}\sum_{i=1}^n \exp(\epsilon_3 H_3^*(Q_n^0)(W_i))]$ is chosen such that $P_n^0(\epsilon)(W)$ integrates to 1 for each ϵ. This also implies a corresponding submodel $\{Q_n^0(\epsilon) = (\bar{Q}_n(\epsilon), Q_{W,n}(\epsilon)) : \epsilon\}$ that equals Q_n^0 at $\epsilon = 0$, so that condition (1) above is satisfied. It is straightforward to verify that condition (2) above is satisfied for the parametric model $\{P_n^0(\epsilon) : \epsilon\}$, or, equivalently, $d/d\epsilon L(Q_n^0(\epsilon))$ at $\epsilon = 0$ equals $D^*(Q_n^0)$.

11.3.5 Obtaining Q_n^*, a Targeted Estimate of Q_0

Consider the maximum likelihood estimator $\epsilon_n = \arg\max P_n \log P_n^0(\epsilon)$ for the parametric model $\{P_n^0(\epsilon) = P_{Q_n^0(\epsilon)} : \epsilon\}$. Note that we also have $\epsilon_n = \arg\min_\epsilon P_n L(Q_n^0(\epsilon))$. The TMLE of P_0 is defined by $P_n^* = P_n^0(\epsilon_n)$. Let $Q_n^* = Q_n^0(\epsilon_n)$, so that $P_n^* = P_{Q_n^*}$. We have $\epsilon_n = (\epsilon_{1,n}, \epsilon_{2,n}, \epsilon_{3,n}) = (0, 0, 0)$. The components $\epsilon_{1,n}, \epsilon_{2,n}$ of the maximum likelihood estimator are found by fitting the generalized linear model $P_n^0(\epsilon)(Y \mid A, W)$. Since the initial density estimator was assumed to have an intercept term and main term A, and was itself fit by maximum likelihood estimation, we must have $(\epsilon_{1,n}, \epsilon_{2,n}) = (0, 0)$. Since $Q_{W,n}$ is the empirical distribution and thereby also a nonparametric maximum likelihood estimator, it follows that $\epsilon_3 = 0$. Thus, the targeted estimate $P_n^* = P_{Q_n^*}$ is identical to the initial density estimate P_n^0, and $Q_n^* = Q_n^0$.

11.3.6 Estimation of Marginal Treatment Effect

The TMLE is the substitution estimator of the risk difference (11.2) evaluated at the targeted density $P_n^* = P_{Q_n^*}$. This density, as described above, consists of the maximum likelihood estimate of the generalized linear model, and the empirical distribution of the baseline variables W. The substitution estimator $\Psi(P_n^*) = \Psi(Q_n^*)$ is given by estimator (11.1). Since Q_n^* is the final density estimate for the TMLE that targets both $(\psi_0^{(0)}, \psi_0^{(1)})$, we also have that Q_n^* maps into the TMLEs of the two treatment specific means $(\psi_0^{(0)}, \psi_0^{(1)})$.

11.4 Main Theorem

The following theorem about the performance of estimator (11.1) under possible misspecification of the working model is a special case of the theorem proved in Rosenblum and van der Laan (2010b).

Theorem 1. *Let $\mu(A, W, \beta)$ be the generalized linear regression model for $E_0(Y \mid A, W)$ implied by a generalized linear model from the normal, binomial, Poisson, gamma, or inverse Gaussian family, with canonical link function, in which the linear part contains the treatment variable A as a main term and also contains an intercept (and possibly contains other terms as well). Under the assumptions in the previous sections, estimator (11.1) is an asymptotically consistent and asymptotically linear estimator of the risk difference ψ_0 defined in (11.2), under arbitrary misspecification of the working model $\mu(A, W, \beta)$. Its influence curve is given by $D^*(Q^*, g_0)$, where $Q^* = (\mu_{\beta^*}, Q_{W,0})$, and $\bar{Q}^* = \mu_{\beta^*}$ denotes the limit of $\bar{Q}_n = \mu_{\beta_n}$. It is locally efficient, meaning that if the working model is correctly specified, then its influence curve $D^*(Q^*, g_0) = D^*(Q_0, g_0)$ is the efficient influence curve, so that the asymptotic vari-*

ance of estimator (11.1) achieves the semiparametric efficiency bound.

Since we showed that μ_{β_n} is also the TMLE that targets both treatment-specific means, it follows that the same theorem applies to any parameter defined as a function of $(E_0(Y \mid A = 0), E_0(Y \mid A = 1))$. See Rosenblum and van der Laan (2010b) for the more general version of Theorem 1.

11.5 Special Robustness of Poisson Model with Only Main Terms

Consider the Poisson regression model given as the third example in Sect. 11.2:

$$\mu_3(A, W, \beta) = \exp(\beta_0 + \beta_1 A + \beta_2 W) . \tag{11.6}$$

Denote the maximum likelihood estimator for coefficient β_1 at sample size n by $\beta_{1,n}$. This can be found by simply fitting the above Poisson regression model using standard statistical software. It follows from the generalization of Theorem 1 that $\beta_{1,n}$ is an asymptotically consistent and linear estimator for the marginal log rate ratio (11.4), under arbitrary misspecification of the working model (11.6). To see this, note that the generalization of Theorem 1 discussed above implies that

$$\log\left\{\frac{1}{n}\sum_{i=1}^{n}\mu_3(1, W_i, \beta_n)\right\} \Bigg/ \left\{\frac{1}{n}\sum_{i=1}^{n}\mu_3(0, W_i, \beta_n)\right\}$$

is an asymptotically consistent and asymptotically linear estimator for the marginal log rate ratio (11.4). But in the special case here, where the Poisson model has only main terms, we have that the above display simplifies to coefficient estimate $\beta_{1,n}$. This can be seen from the following chain of equalities:

$$\begin{aligned}
&\log\left\{\frac{1}{n}\sum_{i=1}^{n}\mu_3(1, W_i, \beta_n)\right\} \Bigg/ \left\{\frac{1}{n}\sum_{i=1}^{n}\mu_3(0, W_i, \beta_n)\right\} \\
&= \log\left\{\frac{1}{n}\sum_{i=1}^{n}\exp(\beta_{0,n} + \beta_{1,n} + \beta_{2,n} W_i)\right\} \Bigg/ \left\{\frac{1}{n}\sum_{i=1}^{n}\exp(\beta_{0,n} + \beta_{2,n} W_i)\right\} \\
&= \log \exp(\beta_{1,n})\left\{\frac{1}{n}\sum_{i=1}^{n}\exp(\beta_{0,n} + \beta_{2,n} W_i)\right\} \Bigg/ \left\{\frac{1}{n}\sum_{i=1}^{n}\exp(\beta_{0,n} + \beta_{2,n} W_i)\right\} \\
&= \beta_{1,n},
\end{aligned}$$

where $\beta_n = (\beta_{0,n}, \beta_{1,n}, \beta_{2,n})$ is the maximum likelihood estimator for β at sample size n. Thus, $\beta_{1,n}$ is an asymptotically unbiased estimator for the marginal log rate ratio (11.4). This is the log-linear analog of the ANCOVA estimator (discussed briefly in Sect. 11.1) being robust to arbitrary model misspecification. This result for the above Poisson model was shown by Gail (1986) under stronger model assumptions than used here.

11.6 Standard Errors and Confidence Intervals

The asymptotic variance σ^2 of the estimator ψ_n defined in (11.1) can be estimated based on its influence curve evaluated at the limit Q^* of Q_n^*. Let β^* be the probability limit of β_n, where β_n is the maximum likelihood estimator for the generalized linear model being used. Then $\bar{Q}^* = \mu_{\beta^*}$. The variance of $\sqrt{n}(\psi_n - \psi_0)$ converges to $\sigma^2 = E_{P_0}\{D(Q^*, g_0)(O)\}^2$. We can estimate σ^2 by replacing E_{P_0} with the empirical mean E_{P_n} and substituting $D(Q_n^*, g_0)$ for $D(Q^*, g_0)$ to get

$$\begin{aligned}\sigma_n^2 &= E_{P_n}(D(Q_n^*, g_0)(O))^2 \\ &= \frac{1}{n}\sum_{i=1}^{n}\left\{H_{g_0}(A_i)(Y_i - \mu(A_i, W_i, \beta_n)) + \mu(1, W_i, \beta_n) - \mu(0, W_i, \beta_n) - \psi_n\right\}^2.\end{aligned}$$

The standard error of ψ_n can then be approximated by $\sigma_n/\sqrt{n}$ and 95% confidence intervals can be constructed as $(\psi_n - 1.96\sigma_n/\sqrt{n}, \psi_n + 1.96\sigma_n/\sqrt{n})$, which has coverage probability that converges to 95% as sample size tends to infinity.

For parameters other than the risk difference, it is just as easy to compute the asymptotic variance σ^2 of the corresponding TMLE defined above. This follows since, in general, the efficient influence curve of a parameter $f(\psi_0^{(0)}, \psi_0^{(1)})$ for some real-valued function f is given by $d/d\psi_0^{(0)} f(\psi_0^{(0)}, \psi_0^{(1)})D_0^* + d/d\psi_0^{(1)} f(\psi_0^{(0)}, \psi_0^{(1)})D_1^*$, where D_j^* is the efficient influence curve of $\psi_0^{(j)}$, $j = 0, 1$. The influence curve of $f(\psi_n^{(0)}, \psi_n^{(1)})$ is determined with the delta method accordingly as a linear combination of the influence curves $D_j^*(Q^*, g_0)$ of $\psi_n^{(j)}$, $j = 0, 1$. For example, the asymptotic variance σ^2 of estimator (11.5) of the marginal log rate ratio can be derived from its influence curve (Rosenblum and van der Laan 2010b, Sect. 4) and can be estimated by

$$\begin{aligned}\sigma_n^2 = \frac{1}{n}\sum_{i=1}^{n}\Bigg(&-\frac{1}{\psi_n^{(0)}}\left\{\frac{1-A_i}{g_0(A_i)}(Y_i - \mu(0, W_i, \beta_n)) + \mu(0, W_i, \beta_n) - \psi_n^{(0)}\right\} \\ &+ \frac{1}{\psi_n^{(1)}}\left\{\frac{A_i}{g_0(A_i)}(Y_i - \mu(1, W_i, \beta_n)) + \mu(1, W_i, \beta_n) - \psi_n^{(1)}\right\}\Bigg)^2,\end{aligned}$$

where $\psi_n^{(0)} = \frac{1}{n}\sum_{i=1}^{n}\mu(0, W_i, \beta_n)$ and $\psi_n^{(1)} = \frac{1}{n}\sum_{i=1}^{n}\mu(1, W_i, \beta_n)$. Inference for $f(\psi_0^{(0)}, \psi_0^{(1)})$ based on $f(\psi_n^{(0)}, \psi_n^{(1)})$ proceeds as above.

11.7 Discussion

We showed an application of the targeted maximum likelihood algorithm for estimating marginal treatment effects in RCTs. These estimators use generalized linear models as working models. The resulting estimators are simple to compute, and have the robustness property that they are asymptotically unbiased and asymptotically normal even under arbitrary misspecification of the working model used. If the working model is correctly specified, then these estimators are also asymptotically efficient. For the linear normal error regression model and $g_0(0) = g_0(1) = 0.5$, the TMLE is always at least as efficient, asymptotically, as the unadjusted estimator. In general, the TMLEs considered here may have more precision than the unadjusted estimator for misspecified working models, but there is no guarantee of such an improvement, and it is possible that the TMLE given here could be less efficient than the unadjusted estimator. In the next chapter, we will show how TMLE based on generalized linear regression models can be constructed to provide such guaranteed improvement.

11.8 Notes and Further Reading

The material in this chapter is based on Rosenblum and van der Laan (2010b). Proofs of these results are given in that paper. Previous work related to estimators in RCTs (and in general in observational studies with known probabilities of treatment) that are robust to model misspecification include, for example, Robins (1994), Robins et al. (1995), Scharfstein et al. (1999), van der Laan and Robins (2003), Leon et al. (2003), Tan (2006), Tsiatis (2006), Moore and van der Laan (2007), Zhang et al. (2008), Rubin and van der Laan (2008), Freedman (2008a,b), and Rosenblum and van der Laan (2009a).

As noted in the introduction, the estimators (11.1) are special cases of the class of parametric regression-based estimators in the Comments to the Rejoinder to Scharfstein et al. (1999, Sect. 3.2.3, p. 1141). Scharfstein et al. (1999, Sect. 3.2.3, p. 1141) construct simple, parametric regression-based estimators of the risk difference. These estimators are double robust and locally efficient. Some of these estimators involve generalized linear models with canonical link functions, in which certain simple functions of the inverse of the propensity score are included as terms in the linear part of the model. These estimators take a special form for RCTs; in this case, including the additional terms of Scharfstein et al. (1999) is equivalent to including a treatment variable and an intercept. It follows that their estimator is equal to ours in the special case of estimating the risk difference in an RCT. Their arguments imply that this estimator is consistent under arbitrary model misspecification, and locally efficient. Also, the class of estimators we give is not identical but asymptotically equivalent to the class of estimators given in Tsiatis (2006, Sect. 5.4, p. 132).

Chapter 12
Targeted ANCOVA Estimator in RCTs

Daniel B. Rubin, Mark J. van der Laan

In many randomized experiments the primary goal is to estimate the average treatment effect, defined as the difference in expected responses between subjects assigned to a treatment group and subjects assigned to a control group. Linear regression is often recommended for use in RCTs as an attempt to increase precision when estimating an average treatment effect on a (nonbinary) outcome by exploiting baseline covariates. The coefficient in front of the treatment variable is then reported as the estimate of the average treatment effect, assuming that no interactions between treatment and covariates were included in the linear regression model.

In this setting, regression is actually not necessary but can lead to efficiency gains relative to the unadjusted estimator if the covariates are predictive of subject responses, and the consistency and asymptotic normality of the estimator of the average treatment effect does not depend on the linear model being correctly specified. However, we show that the usual least squares approach is a suboptimal way to fit a linear model in randomized experiments for the purpose of estimating the average treatment effect. A simple alternative linear regression fit utilizing TMLE guarantees that the average treatment effect estimator will be asymptotically efficient among a large class of popular methods. In addition, we argue and show that this TMLE often outperforms other proposed techniques if the sample size is small or moderate relative to the number of covariates, so that one can safely adjust for more predictors.

For a subject in the study, let W denote a vector of such baseline covariates. Let variable A be an indicator of treatment assignment, so that $A = 0$ signifies assignment to the control group, and $A = 1$ signifies assignment to the treatment group. Finally, let Y denote the primary outcome measurement that is taken on the subject at the end of the study. For our purposes it will not matter if Y is a continuous measurement, is restricted to some range, or even is a binary indicator.

It will be convenient to use counterfactuals, described in Chap. 2 as a consequence of the SCM. For a subject in the study, let Y_1 denote the response that the subject would have realized if he or she had been assigned to treatment. Likewise, let Y_0 be the response if the subject had been assigned to control. In reality each subject is assigned to only one group, either treatment or control, so one of these counterfactual outcomes will be missing. The observed response is $Y = AY_1 + (1 - A)Y_0$. The full data we would have liked to measure about a subject are $X = (W, Y_0, Y_1)$, while what we actually measure is $O = (W, A, Y)$. As this is an RCT, we assume the treatment assignment indicator A is independent of the full data (W, Y_0, Y_1).

For defining parameters we assume a superpopulation statistical model in which the study subjects are drawn with replacement from some larger population of subjects. That is, we assume the full data $(W_i, Y_{0,i}, Y_{1,i})$, $i = 1, ..., n$, are independent and identically distributed random triples. This assumption is mainly for simplicity. Freedman (2008a) shows how regression asymptotics can be analyzed in sequences of finite population statistical models, where the only randomness is that induced by the random assignment of subjects to treatment or control groups. The probability distribution of the full data structure (W, Y_0, Y_1) is unspecified. In addition, let $g_0(A \mid X)$ denote the probability distribution of treatment A, given X: by assumption, $g_0(1 \mid X) = g_0(1)$. Let P_0 denote the probability distribution of the observed data structure $(W, A, Y = Y_A)$.

The mean of the counterfactuals can be identified as a parameter of the probability distribution P_0:

$$\psi_0^{(1)} = E_0(Y \mid A = 1) = E_0(Y_1)$$

and

$$\psi_0^{(0)} = E_0(Y \mid A = 0) = E_0(Y_0),$$

the expected responses of subjects assigned to treatment or control. For quantifying the treatment effect, a parameter can then be defined as the contrast $\psi_0 = \psi_0^{(1)} - \psi_0^{(0)}$ between the mean responses among those assigned to the two arms (i.e., the average treatment effect). Note that we also have $\psi_0 = E_0(E_0(Y \mid A = 1, W) - E_0(Y \mid A = 0, W))$.

The statistical model for the probability distribution P_0 of $O = (W, A, Y)$ is identified by the nonparametric model for the full-data distribution, and that A is independent of the full-data structure. Thus the only testable assumption is that A is independent of W. This defines now the statistical model $\mathcal{M}$, and target parameter mapping $\Psi : \mathcal{M} \to \mathbb{R}$, $\Psi(P) = E_P(E_P(Y \mid A = 1, W) - E_P(Y \mid A = 0, W))$, and thereby the estimation problem.

The usual ANCOVA approach for using covariates to estimate this treatment effect ψ_0 on a continuous outcome is to use linear least squares to regress response Y on the treatment assignment indicator A and covariates W and then report the estimated coefficient in front of the treatment indicator.

In this chapter we propose an alternative to least squares fitting based on the TMLE algorithm such that:

- The treatment effect estimator generally becomes more efficient when $g(0) \neq 0.5$;

- The estimator tends to perform better with small or moderate samples than other common estimators with equivalent asymptotic efficiency, so more covariates can safely be used for the adjustment;
- The treatment effect estimator is the coefficient in front of A of a parsimonious fitted linear regression model. The technique should therefore be acceptable to nonstatistician investigators who are already familiar with interpreting regression coefficients in textbook linear models.

Two-sample problem, or one i.i.d. sample? Suppose there are n subjects in the study, and a randomly selected subgroup of m of them are assigned to treatment, with the random selection not depending on covariates. Here n and m are fixed. Let $g = m/n$ represent the proportion assigned treatment. In many studies $m = n/2$, so g will be $1/2$.

In our statistical formulation above we assume that A is a Bernoulli random variable. If in truth A is Bernoulli with probability (say) 0.5, then by chance the treatment group will not be of the same size as the control group. However, by design, the study often arranges the treatment and control groups to be of the same size, showing that it is not completely accurate to state that the sample is an i.i.d. sample from (W, A, Y) with $P_0(A = 1) = 0.5$.

This suggests another description of the data-generating distribution of the actual observed data structure. Suppose that $O = (W, A, Y) \sim P_0$ is the random variable in which A is random with $P_0(A = 1) = 0.5$, and the causal effect is identified by $\Psi(P_0)$ defined above, but that our observed data consist of a sample of n observations from (W, Y), conditional on $A = 1$, and a sample of n observations from (W, Y), given $A = 0$. That is, we took a "biased" "case-control" sample from P_0, where a case is defined as "$A = 1$." (This type of sampling has been referred to in other literature as a particular type of cohort sampling, and we note that the "case-control" terminology we use here is not typically applied to sampling conditional on A.) The results for semiparametric estimation based on case-control data (van der Laan 2008a; Rose and van der Laan 2008) state that, without loss of consistency or efficiency, we can apply an estimator developed for an i.i.d. sample from P_0, *but* we have to assign weights $q_0 = P_0(A = 1)$ to the observations with $A = 1$ and $1 - q_0$ for the observations with $A = 0$ in the pooled case-control sample. We also refer the interested reader to Chaps. 13 and 14.

As a consequence, the case-control-weighted TMLE is identical to the nonweighted TMLE. Therefore one can simply apply the estimators developed under i.i.d. sampling from P_0 and act as if the two-sample problem was an i.i.d. sample from O. Indeed, in this article, we proceed under our posed statistical model and suffice with the remark that all our estimators and results apply by letting $g_n(1)$ play the role of this set g.

12.1 Previously Proposed Estimators

In this section we review the strengths and weaknesses of common methods for estimating the treatment effect previously defined.

Unadjusted estimation. The simplest approach is to ignore baseline covariates altogether. Then, the obvious estimator of the expected response in the treatment group is the empirical mean of responses for subjects assigned to treatment, and analogously for the control subjects. Estimators for $\psi_0^{(0)}$, $\psi_0^{(1)}$, and ψ_0 become

$$\psi_n^{(0)} = \frac{1}{n}\sum_{i=1}^{n} \frac{(1-A_i)}{g_n(0)} Y_i,$$

$$\psi_n^{(1)} = \frac{1}{n}\sum_{i=1}^{n} \frac{A_i}{g_n(1)} Y_i,$$

and $\psi_n = \psi_n^{(1)} - \psi_n^{(0)}$.

The unadjusted estimator of treatment effect is consistent, and it is also asymptotically normal, in that $\sqrt{n}(\psi_n - \psi_0)$ will converge in law to an $N(0, \sigma^2)$ distribution (e.g., Yang and Tsiatis 2001). The influence curve of this estimator is given by $IC(Q, g_0) = h_{g_0}(A)(Y - \bar{Q}(A))$, where $\bar{Q}(A) = E_0(Y \mid A)$ and $h_{g_0}(A) = (2A-1)/g_0(A)$, so that $\sigma^2 = P_0 IC(Q, g_0)^2$ is the variance of this influence curve.

The asymptotic variance σ^2 of this limiting normal distribution can be used to gauge the precision of this estimator, and compare it to other estimators. Unfortunately, it is known that the unadjusted estimator can be much less efficient than other techniques when covariates are predictive of the response. This is because only one of the two counterfactual responses can be measured for a subject, while the covariates may contain information about what the missing response would have been.

ANCOVA. As noted earlier, the most popular way to adjust for covariates is to use linear least squares in fitting the regression model:

$$Y = \alpha + \psi_0 A + \gamma^\top W + \text{error}.$$

The least squares fit of ψ_0 then estimates the average treatment effect defined earlier. Let $\bar{Q}_I$ denote the limit of the linear regression ANCOVA estimator of $\bar{Q}_0(A, W) = E_0(Y \mid A, W)$. This ANCOVA estimator of ψ_0 will also generally be asymptotically normal, even if $E_0(Y \mid A, W)$ is not actually linear in (A, W), or if the errors are not homoscedastic or exogenous (Yang and Tsiatis 2001; Leon et al. 2003; Tsiatis et al. 2008). See the previous chapter for a more general presentation and proof of this result for RCTs based on the observation that the TMLE of ψ_0 that takes as initial estimator a maximum likelihood estimator according to a (possibly misspecified) generalized linear regression model will result in no update in the TMLE step. As a consequence, the ANCOVA estimator is a TMLE targeting $(E_0(Y_0), E_0(Y_1))$, corresponding with squared error loss and linear fluctuation

$\bar{Q}_n^0(\epsilon) = \bar{Q}_n^0 + \epsilon_1 A/g_n(1) + \epsilon_2(1-A)/g_n(0)$. Note that the targeting step in the TMLE corresponds with adding $\epsilon(1, A)$ and that $\epsilon_n = 0$ since $(1, A)$ is already included in the working linear regression model. Invoking the known asymptotics of the TMLE, it follows that it is asymptotically linear with influence curve

$$IC(Q, g_0)(O) = D^*(Q_l, g_0)(O) - C(A),$$

where

$$D^*(Q, g_0) = h_{g_0}(A)(Y - \bar{Q}(A, W)) + \bar{Q}(1, W) - \bar{Q}(0, W) - \psi_0$$

is the efficient influence curve of Ψ at (Q, g_0), and C is a correction term, due to g_n being an estimator of g_0, defined as $C(A) = E_0(D^*(Q, g_0)(O) \mid A)$. It is easy to verify that, if Q is such that $\Psi^{(1)}(Q) = \psi_0^{(1)}$, $\Psi^{(0)}(Q) = \psi_0^{(0)}$, then it follows that $C = 0$. This holds for the limit Q of a TMLE that targets both $E_0(Y_1)$ and $E_0(Y_0)$ such as this ANCOVA estimator. As a consequence, the ANCOVA estimator is asymptotically linear with influence curve $D^*(Q, g_0)$.

The only real additional assumption for the asymptotic linearity of this estimator is that the distributions of W and Y do not have overly heavy tails. The linear model can thus be viewed as a working model, used in an intermediate step to estimate the average treatment effect.

However, Freedman (2008a) shows that unless $g_0(1) = 0.5$, this ANCOVA estimator can be less efficient than the unadjusted estimator, in terms of asymptotic variance. It might also be biased in finite samples under model misspecification, although the $n^{-1/2}$-scale asymptotic normality result suggests that this bias will quickly become negligible relative to the variance.

The properties of this method are not fully understood when the number of covariates is large relative to the sample size, as the asymptotic approximations may begin to break down. Therefore, the usual recommendation is to simply adjust for an a priori specified handful of covariates that are considered to be the most important predictors.

ANCOVA II. A simple extension of ANCOVA is to add interaction terms and fit the model

$$Y = \theta_1 + \theta_2 A + \theta_3^T W + \theta_4^T (A \times W) + \text{error}$$

with linear least squares. The estimate of the treatment effect is no longer a coefficient fit, but the value obtained when using the fitted model $\bar{Q}_n$ of $\bar{Q}_0$ to impute missing counterfactuals, i.e.,

$$\psi_n = \Psi(Q_n) = \frac{1}{n} \sum_{i=1}^{n} \{\bar{Q}_n(1, W_i) - \bar{Q}_n(0, W_i)\}.$$

Again, as remarked above, this estimator of ψ_0 equals the same TMLE mentioned above, but now using as initial estimator the least squares regression fit of this parametric working model.

By the same arguments as above, this estimator is asymptotically linear with influence curve $D^*(Q_{II}, g_0)$, where Q_{II} denotes the limit of this linear regression ANCOVA II estimator of $\bar{Q}_0$. The ANCOVA II estimator is also asymptotically normal under the same minimal conditions we have discussed, and its asymptotic variance is guaranteed to be at least as small as the ANCOVA estimator and unadjusted estimator, while under many data-generating distributions it is asymptotically more efficient (Yang and Tsiatis 2001).

In fact, the ANCOVA II approach possesses an optimality property (Tsiatis et al. 2008). To appreciate this optimality property, one must know about the following alternative representation of $D^*(Q, g_0)$ for Q satisfying $\Psi(Q) = \psi_0$:

$$D^*(Q, g_0)(O) = h_{g_0}(A)(Y - f(Q)(W)) - \psi_0 \equiv D_{f(Q)}(\psi_0)(O), \tag{12.1}$$

where

$$f(Q)(W) \equiv g_0(1)\bar{Q}(0, W) + g_0(0)\bar{Q}(1, W)$$

and $h_{g_0}(A_i) = A_i/g_0(1) - (1 - A_i)/g_0(0)$. This representation defines a class of estimators $\psi_n(f) = 1/n \sum_i h_{g_0}(A_i)(Y_i - f(W_i))$ as solutions of the estimating equation $P_n D_f(\psi) = 0$, indexed by a choice f. These estimators are consistent and asymptotically linear with influence curve $h_{g_0}(A)(Y - f(W))$. Suppose two estimators are asymptotically equivalent if their difference is of order $o(n^{-1/2})$ in probability, under the distribution P_0 governing (W, A, Y). The asymptotic variance of the ANCOVA II estimator is no larger than that of any regular asymptotically normal estimator that is asymptotically equivalent to one of the form

$$\psi_n(f) = \frac{1}{n} \sum_{i=1}^{n} \left(\frac{A_i}{g_0} - \frac{1 - A_i}{1 - g_0} \right) (Y_i - f(W_i)) \tag{12.2}$$

for $f(W) = \eta^{\top}(1, W)$ linear in the components of W. The unadjusted, ANCOVA, and ANCOVA II estimators are all asymptotically equivalent to estimators in this class corresponding with functions $f(W)$ that are linear in W.

However, the ANCOVA II estimator is based on a less parsimonious model than the usual ANCOVA. It essentially fits separate linear regressions in the treatment and control arms and thus can be less stable with small or moderate samples due to loss of degrees of freedom. An analyst using the ANCOVA II method might therefore adjust for fewer covariates than someone using the regular ANCOVA technique, and thus make less use of potentially informative predictors.

Interestingly, in the special case that $g_0(1) = 0.5$, it happens that $f(Q_I) = f(Q_{II})$, so that the ANCOVA estimator and the ANCOVA II estimator have identical influence curves ($D^*(Q_I, g_0) = D^*(Q_{II}, g_0)$) (Yang and Tsiatis 2001; Leon et al. 2003; Tsiatis et al. 2008). Apparently the simple ANCOVA estimator achieves the same asymptotic efficiency as the more data-adaptive ANCOVA II estimator, and should thus be favored in small samples.

Koch estimator. Koch et al. (1998) introduced the treatment effect estimator defined by

$$\psi_n = \frac{1}{n}\sum_{i=1}^{n}\left(\frac{A_i}{g_n(1)} - \frac{1-A_i}{1-g_n(1)}\right)Y_i + \frac{n}{m(n-m)}V^\top U^{-1}\sum_{i=1}^{n}(A_i - g_n(1))W_i.$$

Here $m = \sum_{i=1}^n A_i$, $V = V^{(0)}/(n-m) + V^{(1)}/m$ and $U = U^{(0)}/(n-m) + U^{(1)}/m$. Matrices $U^{(0)}$ and $U^{(1)}$ are unbiased sample estimates of covariance matrices of W in the control and treatment groups. Vectors $V^{(0)}$ and $V^{(1)}$ are likewise unbiased sample estimates of covariances between elements of W and the response Y in the control and treatment groups.

This estimator is also asymptotically normal, with the same asymptotic variance as the ANCOVA II estimator (Tsiatis et al. 2008), although it is motivated from a different perspective. Hence, it also has the optimality property of being asymptotically efficient among estimators asymptotically equivalent to those in (12.2).

This estimator appears to not be consistent with fitting a regression model for the response on both covariates and treatment assignment, i.e., it is not a substitution estimator. Additionally, like the ANCOVA II method, it requires estimating covariances between the outcome and each element of the covariate vector within each of the two treatment arms. If the sample size is small relative to the number of covariates, this might lead to more instability than the unadjusted or standard ANCOVA estimators.

Leon estimator. Leon et al. (2003) discuss a general class of estimators asymptotically equivalent to those of the form of (12.2), but with f a linear combination of given basis functions of W, and they mention using quadratic or cross product terms. We consider the reduction of their method when $f(W)$ must be a linear combination of the elements of W, along with an intercept. The estimator is defined by

$$\psi_n = \frac{1}{n}\sum_{i=1}^{n}\left(\frac{A_i}{g_n(1)} - \frac{1-A_i}{1-g_n(1)}\right)Y_i - n(S_1/m^2 + S_2/(n-m)^2)^\top S_3^{-1}S_4.$$

To explain the definition, let $F = [1, W]^\top$ be the addition of constant 1 to a subject's covariate vector. Here,

$$S_3 = \sum_{i=1}^{n} F_i F_i^\top,$$

$$S_4 = \sum_{i=1}^{n}(A_i - g_n(1))F_i,$$

$$S_1 = \sum_{i=1}^{n} A_i(Y_i - \bar{Y}_{1,n})F_i,$$

and

$$S_2 = \sum_{i=1}^{n}(1 - A_i)(Y_i - \bar{Y}_{0,n})F_i,$$

where $\bar{Y}_{1,n}$ and $\bar{Y}_{0,n}$ are the empirical means of response Y in the treatment and control groups.

This estimator is asymptotically equivalent to the ANCOVA II and Koch estimators. Like these two estimators, in both treatment arms it requires computing covariances between the outcome and each element of the covariate vector. This is not a computational issue, but it causes instability in small samples. Also, the method does not seem to correspond with fitting a simple linear regression model for the outcome on treatment assignments and covariates, and is thus not a substitution estimator.

12.2 Targeted ANCOVA

We now introduce a new treatment effect estimator. Recall the linear model

$$Y = \alpha + \psi_0 A + \gamma^\top W + \text{error}$$

used in the ANCOVA approach. Rather than fit coefficients with linear least squares, we proceed as follows. First, we let δ_n and γ_n minimize:

$$\sum_{i=1}^{n} \left(\frac{A_i}{g_n(1)} - \frac{1 - A_i}{1 - g_n(1)} \right)^2 |Y_i - \delta - \gamma^\top W_i|^2.$$

This is a weighted linear least squares regression of the response on the covariates, with an intercept, weighting subjects in the treatment group by $g_n(1)^{-2}$ and subjects in the control group by $(1 - g_n(1))^{-2}$. We have thus fitted γ. Next, let α_n and ψ_n minimize the sum of squares:

$$\sum_{i=1}^{n} |Y_i - \gamma_n^\top W_i - \alpha - \psi_0 A_i|^2.$$

That is, we regress response Y on an intercept and A, using the initial weighted least squares regression as offset. The targeted ANCOVA estimate of the treatment effect is ψ_n^*. Let $\bar{Q}_n^*$ be the targeted ANCOVA regression fit. Note that $\psi_n^* = \Psi(Q_n^*)$. One can also estimate expected responses in the treatment and control arms by using the fitted regression model $\bar{Q}_n^*$ to impute missing counterfactuals and obtain $\psi_n^{(0)} = \Psi^{(0)}(Q_n^*) = n^{-1} \sum_{i=1}^n (\alpha_n + \gamma_n^\top W_i)$ and $\psi_n^{(1)} = \Psi^{(1)}(Q_n^*) = \psi_n^{(0)} + \psi_n^*$.

This estimator equals the TMLE using the squared error loss and linear regression submodel $\bar{Q}_n^0(\epsilon) = \bar{Q}_n^0 + \epsilon(1, A)$, with the additional feature that the initial estimator $\bar{Q}_n^0$ is a *weighted* least squares estimator according to a linear regression model of Y in W. Specifically,

- The initial estimator $\bar{Q}_n^0$ of $\bar{Q}_0(A, W) = E_0(Y \mid A, W)$ is targeted by minimizing a weighted least squares criterion, and $Q_{W,0}$ is estimated with the empirical distribution $Q_{W,n}$. This defines the initial estimator Q_n^0 of $Q_0 = (Q_{W,0}, \bar{Q}_0)$. The weighted least squares loss function $L_{g_n}(\bar{Q})(O) = h^2_{g_n}(A)(Y - \bar{Q}(A,W))^2$ is still a valid loss function for $\bar{Q}_0$ but is tailored to correspond with minimizing the asymptotic variance of the resulting TMLE.

- For the TMLE step, we use a squared error loss function $L(\bar{Q})(O) = (Y - \bar{Q}(A,W))^2$ for $\bar{Q}_0$ and a log-likelihood loss function $L(Q_W) = -\log Q_W$ for $Q_{W,0}$. This results in a loss function $L(Q) = L(\bar{Q}) + L(Q_W)$ for $Q_0 = (Q_{W,0}, \bar{Q}_0)$ for the TMLE step.
- For the TMLE step, we use the linear regression submodel $\bar{Q}^0_n(\epsilon_2) = \bar{Q}^0_n + \epsilon_2 H^*$, where $H^*(A,W) = (1, A)$, or, equivalently, $H^*(A,W) = (A/g_n(1), (1-A)/g_n(0))$, is chosen so that the score $d/d\epsilon_2 L(\bar{Q}^0_n(\epsilon_2))$ at $\epsilon_2 = 0$ spans the component $D^*_Y(\bar{Q}^0_n, g_n)(O) = (2A-1)/g_n(A)(Y - \bar{Q}^0_n(W))$ of the efficient influence curve $D^*(Q^0_n, g_n) = D^*_Y(\bar{Q}^0_n, g_n) + D^*_W(Q^0_n)$. The empirical distribution of W is separately fluctuated with a submodel $Q_{W,n}(\epsilon_1) = (1 + \epsilon_1 D^*_W(Q^0_n))Q_{W,n}$ with score $D^*_W(Q^0_n)(O) = \bar{Q}^0_n(1,W) - \bar{Q}^0_n(0,W) - \Psi(Q^0_n)$. Since $Q_{W,n}$ is a nonparametric maximum likelihood estimator, the maximum likelihood estimators of ϵ_1 in the TMLE algorithm equals zero. The score of $L(Q(\epsilon_1, \epsilon_2))$ at $\epsilon_1 = \epsilon_2 = 0$ spans the efficient influence curve $D^*(Q^0_n, g_n)$.

12.2.1 Asymptotic Optimality

What are the statistical properties of this estimator $\Psi(Q^*_n)$ of the additive causal effect of treatment ψ_0? Since the targeted ANCOVA estimator is a TMLE targeting $(E_0(Y_1), E_0(Y_0))$, we can refer to asymptotic linearity theorems established for such estimators. Since $\bar{Q}^*_n$ is a simple linear regression estimator, all the empirical process conditions and convergence rate conditions are trivially met. As a consequence, $\psi^{(0)}_n$, $\psi^{(1)}_n$, and ψ^*_n will all be consistent and asymptotically normal estimators of the respective target parameters under minimal conditions, such as W and Y not having overly heavy tails.

Moreover, we claim that the asymptotic variance of treatment effect estimator $\psi^*_n = \Psi(Q^*_n)$ will equal that of the ANCOVA II estimator, Koch estimator, and Leon estimator. Thus, we achieve the optimality bound discussed for estimators of the form (12.2) with linear $f(W)$ and are guaranteed to be at least as asymptotically efficient as the unadjusted and standard ANCOVA techniques.

This is shown as follows. The TMLE $Q^*_n = (Q_{W,n}, \bar{Q}^*_n)$ solves the efficient influence curve estimating equation $P_n D^*(Q^*_n, g_n, \psi^*_n) = 0$, where we denoted the efficient influence curve $D^*(Q, g_0)$ as an estimating function $D^*(Q, g_0, \Psi(Q))$ in ψ. By (12.1) this can also be represented as $P_n D_{f(Q^*_n)}(\psi^*_n) = 0$, and thereby

$$\psi^*_n = \frac{1}{n} \sum_i h_{g_n}(A_i)(Y_i - f(Q^*_n)(W_i)).$$

Recall that $\bar{Q}^*_n = \bar{Q}^0_n + \epsilon_n(1, A)$, so that $f(Q^*_n) = f(Q^0_n) + c$ for some constant c. However, this constant c cancels out since $P_n h_{g_n} c = P_n h_{g_n} = 0$. Thus, it follows that

$$\psi_n^* = \frac{1}{n}\sum_i h_{g_n}(A_i)(Y_i - f(Q_n^0)).$$

Standard analysis now shows that ψ_n^* is asymptotically linear with influence curve

$$IC(O) = D_{f(Q)}(\psi_0)(O) - E_0(D_{f(Q)}(\psi_0)(O) \mid A),$$

where $D_{f(Q)}(\psi_0)$ can also be represented as $D^*(Q, g_0, \psi_0)$, Q denotes the limit of Q_n^0, and the additional projection term is due to the estimation of g_0 with g_n. However, by definition of $\bar{Q}_n^0$ as the linear regression that minimizes the empirical variance of $D_f^*(\psi_0)$ over all linear functions $f(W) = \eta^\top(1, W)$, we know that

$$\text{var } D_{f(Q)}(\psi_0) = \arg\min_\eta \text{var}\{h_{g_0}(A)(Y - \eta^\top(1, W)) - \psi_0\}.$$

The additional term in IC can only reduce the variance, which proves that the variance of IC is smaller than or equal to the variance of all the influence curves $D_f^*(\psi_0)$ with $f(W) = \eta^\top(1, W)$ for some η. Since the additional term only changes the intercept in f, it also follows that the additional term will not affect the variance relative to the already optimal $f(Q)$. Thus, $IC = D_{f(Q)}^*(\psi_0) = D^*(Q, g_0, \psi_0)$.

12.2.2 Targeted ANCOVA Is a Substitution Estimator

A byproduct of our method is a fit of a parsimonious linear model. Hence, targeted ANCOVA could be easier to use than the Koch or Leon methods for nonstatistician investigators who are already used to fitting parametric linear regression models. If the linear ANCOVA model is a good approximation to the unknown data-generating distribution, then, like linear least squares, our fit should accurately approximate the regression function $(A, W) \rightarrow E_0(Y \mid A, W)$. To see this, note that by first fitting the coefficient vector γ of covariates W and then fixing it in the next step, we are merely implementing forward stagewise modeling with weights in one of the stages, which is a well-known regression technique (Hastie et al. 2001, Sect. 10.3). Since A and W are independent, the separation of the two stages does not harm the fit of $\bar{Q}_0$.

12.2.3 Small and Moderate Sample Performance

While we have noted that our targeted ANCOVA technique will perform similarly in large samples to the ANCOVA II, Koch, and Leon methods, we claim that asymptotics will often kick in more quickly for the targeted ANCOVA estimator, so we could safely adjust for more predictors. Simulations in the following sections will be used to investigate this issue in more depth, but for now we give an explanation for our confidence.

Table 12.1 Summary of ANCOVA methods and their properties

	Unadjusted	ANCOVA	ANCOVA II	Koch	Leon	Targeted ANCOVA
Meets asymptotic bound of (12.2)			×	×	×	×
Parametric regression model		×	×			×
Doesn't estimate $2p$ parameters	×	×				×

Suppose that the covariate vector is p-dimensional. The ANCOVA II estimator reduces to performing two linear regressions of the response on the covariate vector, one in each arm. Hence, fits in each model are based on fewer observations than with ordinary ANCOVA. Similarly, the Koch and Leon estimators both involve estimating the $2p$ quantities corresponding to how each of the p baseline predictors covaries with the response in each treatment arm. The optimal linear $f(W)$ in (12.2) involves a mixture of two p-dimensional vectors: the vector of covariances between predictors and the response in the treatment arm, and likewise for controls (Tsiatis et al. 2008, Eq. 11). While earlier methods attaining the efficiency bound fit both vectors, we try to directly fit the optimal linear $f(W)$ in (12.2) and implicitly just estimate the relevant mixture $f(Q_0)(W) = g_0(1)\bar{Q}_0(0, W)+g_0(0)\bar{Q}_0(1, W)$ according to a linear working model. A related way of viewing targeted ANCOVA is that relative to ANCOVA II and other techniques, we improve finite sample performance by sacrificing asymptotic efficiency for our separate estimators of expected responses $\psi_0^{(0)}$ and $\psi_0^{(1)}$ in the two arms, as the treatment effect contrast will usually be of primary importance. There is subjectivity in these statements, just as there are many ways to represent estimators and how many parameters they fit in intermediate steps. Still, Table 12.1 seems to summarize the added value of our method.

12.3 Standard Error Estimation

Yang and Tsiatis (2001), Leon et al. (2003), and Tsiatis et al. (2008) give semiparametric representations of asymptotic variances for estimators in this problem, and this framework can be applied to our method. Alternatively, we use that our targeted ANCOVA estimator $\psi_n^* = \Psi(Q_n^*)$ is a TMLE that solves the efficient influence curve estimating equation $0 = P_n D^*(Q_n^*, g_0, \psi_n^*) = 0$, so that inference can proceed accordingly. Specifically, the TMLE $\Psi(Q_n^*)$ is asymptotically linear with an influence curve given by

$$D^*(Q^*, g_0)(O) = \frac{2A-1}{g_0(A)}(Y - \bar{Q}^*(A,W)) + \bar{Q}^*(1,W) - \bar{Q}^*(0,W) - \psi_0,$$

where Q^* denotes the limit of the TMLE Q_n^*.

Let α_n, ψ_n^*, and γ_n denote the fitted coefficients from targeted ANCOVA, with α, ψ_0, and γ the corresponding large sample limits. We have that $\bar{Q}_n^*(A,W) = \alpha_n + \gamma_n W + \psi_n^* A$, which converges to $\bar{Q}^*(A,W) = \alpha + \gamma + \psi_0 A$. The variance of $\psi_n = \Psi(Q_n^*)$ can thus be estimated as

$$\sigma^2_{\psi_n,n} = \frac{1}{n^2}\sum_{i=1}^{n} D^*(Q_n^*, g_0)(O_i)^2.$$

The same variance formulas can be applied to estimate the variance of the TMLE of E_0Y_1 and E_0Y_0. These formulas correspond with the formulas in the above referenced articles.

Confidence intervals and test statistics can now be constructed based on the normal approximation of $\psi_n^* - \psi_0$. Although the consistency and asymptotic normality properties of the standard ANCOVA estimator of the treatment effect do not depend on the linear model's being correctly specified, the usual nominal variance formulas produced by the software can be incorrect (Freedman 2008a). The above standard error estimators for targeted ANCOVA here do not depend on any parametric modeling assumptions since they are based on the influence curve of the estimator in the posed semiparametric model that only assumed the randomization assumption.

12.4 Simulations

We investigated the performance of targeted ANCOVA through simulating four data-generating distributions studied in Yang and Tsiatis (2001). For each distribution we evaluated estimators in simulated experiments with sample sizes $n = 20$, $n = 50$, and $n = 100$. In addition to redoing the original Yang and Tsiatis simulations, in which each subject had a single covariate W, we also considered scenarios with more covariates. For each subject, three additional covariates were generated from the same marginal distribution originally used, but independently of all the subject's other measurements. This was to simulate clinical trial settings where substantial baseline information is available yet "most covariates are not strongly related to the outcome" (Pocock et al. 2002).

For each of the four data-generating distributions, each of the three sample sizes, and both choices of including one covariate or four covariates, we ran 100,000 Monte Carlo simulations of randomized experiments. The true treatment effect in all cases was $\psi_0 = 1/2$, and the Monte Carlo replications allowed us to estimate the root mean squared errors (RMSEs) of different estimators. Although the results that follow do not present estimates of simulation error, the number of replications was chosen to be large enough so that this simulation error can be ignored.

Table 12.2 Simulation 1: RMSE

Extra covariates	n	Unadjusted	ANCOVA	ANCOVA II	Koch	Leon	Targeted ANCOVA
No	20	0.69	0.59	0.60	0.59	0.59	0.56
	50	0.43	0.37	0.38	0.37	0.37	0.37
	100	0.31	0.26	0.26	0.26	0.26	0.26
Yes	20	0.69	0.65	0.69	0.65	0.62	0.53
	50	0.44	0.39	0.39	0.39	0.38	0.36
	100	0.31	0.27	0.27	0.27	0.27	0.26

Table 12.3 Simulation 2: RMSE

Extra covariates	n	Unadjusted	ANCOVA	ANCOVA II	Koch	Leon	Targeted ANCOVA
No	20	0.46	0.47	0.47	0.47	0.47	0.45
	50	0.29	0.29	0.29	0.29	0.29	0.29
	100	0.21	0.21	0.21	0.21	0.21	0.20
Yes	20	0.46	0.52	0.56	0.52	0.49	0.43
	50	0.29	0.30	0.30	0.30	0.30	0.28
	100	0.21	0.21	0.21	0.21	0.21	0.20

Table 12.4 Simulation 3: RMSE

Extra covariates	n	Unadjusted	ANCOVA	ANCOVA II	Koch	Leon	Targeted ANCOVA
No	50	0.51	0.42	0.43	0.43	0.43	0.42
	100	0.36	0.30	0.30	0.30	0.30	0.30
Yes	50	0.51	0.44	0.47	0.45	0.45	0.42
	100	0.36	0.30	0.31	0.31	0.31	0.30

Table 12.5 Simulation 4: RMSE

Extra covariates	n	Unadjusted	ANCOVA	ANCOVA II	Koch	Leon	Targeted ANCOVA
No	20	0.99	0.81	0.84	0.81	0.80	0.77
	50	0.63	0.53	0.55	0.53	0.53	0.52
	100	0.45	0.39	0.39	0.39	0.39	0.38
Yes	20	0.99	0.90	0.96	0.90	0.85	0.72
	50	0.63	0.55	0.56	0.55	0.55	0.51
	100	0.45	0.39	0.40	0.39	0.39	0.38

Simulation 1. For the initial simulation the covariate followed a standard normal distribution. Half of the subjects were assigned to treatment, meaning that $g_0 = 1/2$. Responses were generated through

$$Y = (-1/4 + \psi_0 A) + (\beta_1 + \beta_2 A)W + (\beta_3 + \beta_4 A)(W^2 - \mathrm{var}(W)) + U,$$

where $(\beta_1, \beta_2, \beta_3, \beta_4) = (1/2, 3/5, 2/5, 3/10)$. The error U followed a standard normal distribution, independently of covariates. RMSEs are shown in Table 12.2. Targeted ANCOVA appeared slightly more accurate than other methods, particularly as the sample size got smaller or the number of baseline covariates got larger. The unadjusted estimator was noticeably less efficient than all covariate-adjusted estimators, as the covariate was strongly predictive of the response for this artificial data-generating distribution.

Simulation 2. In the second simulation we took $(\beta_1, \beta_2, \beta_3, \beta_4) = (1/10, 1/10, 1/10, 1/10)$, making the baseline covariate less predictive of the response. Recall that in settings where three extra covariates were added, these were unrelated to the outcome. RMSEs are reported in Table 12.3. For this distribution the unadjusted estimator performed more favorably. All methods were mostly similar, but it was notable that targeted ANCOVA had the best performance across each of these six independent Monte Carlo settings.

Simulation 3. The third simulation was identical to the first, except that the proportion of subjects assigned treatment was $g_0 = 3/10$ instead of $1/2$. Following Yang and Tsiatis (2001), we don't report results for the $n = 20$ sample size as too few subjects were assigned treatment to make meaningful generalizations. RMSE results are shown in Table 12.4. The unadjusted estimator appeared slightly worse than the others. Adjusted estimators were all similar, with targeted ANCOVA consistently having slightly smaller RMSEs than its competitors over these four settings.

Simulation 4. The final simulation was identical to simulation 1, except covariates W and error U were drawn from t-distributions with seven degrees of freedom instead of standard normal distributions. Table 12.5 shows RMSEs. Once more, we found that targeted ANCOVA performed best, particularly when the sample size became small or when the three extra covariates were added. An unusual feature of the simulations was that, unlike the other estimators, targeted ANCOVA occasionally seemed to perform better with the three extra covariates than without them, even though they were unrelated to the treatment or response.

12.5 Discussion

We have introduced a new alternative to least squares for fitting linear models in RCTs. Our estimator of the average treatment effect generally increases the asymptotic efficiency of the usual ANCOVA approach and still produces a regression fit. It may also often outperform estimators with similar asymptotic efficiency if the sample size is moderate relative to the number of covariates, so that one could safely adjust for more predictors. Our work is a special case of a TMLE, which is based on the idea that fitting a regression model isn't always an end in itself. Rather, it is an intermediate step in estimating the target parameter of interest, which in our case is the average causal effect. In such circumstances it may be suboptimal to use standard parametric maximum likelihood or least squares for model fitting of the initial estimator in the TMLE and advantageous to keep the final desired estimand in mind while targeting the initial regression fit accordingly. This approach has beneficial applications in a variety of problems, including RCTs. In this chapter we focused on using a parametric regression working model. Instead, the initial estimator $\bar{Q}_n^0$ in the targeted ANCOVA could be replaced by a super learner based on the weighted squared error loss function $L_{g_n}(\bar{Q}) = (Y - f(\bar{Q}))^2 h_{g_n}^2$. We also refer the interested reader to Appendix A.19.

To summarize, in the TMLE one has the option to select a loss function for the initial estimator, separate from the loss function selected for the targeting step in the TMLE. For example, this loss function can be selected so that minimizing its empirical risk over candidate TMLEs $Q_n^*(Q^0)$ indexed by different initial estimators Q^0 (or values such as regression functions) corresponds with minimizing the variance of the efficient influence curve $D^*(Q_n^*(Q^0), g_0)$ at these TMLEs over a working model for Q^0. As a result of such a procedure, the variance of the influence curve of the TMLE will be the variance of $D^*(Q^*, g_0)$, where Q^* has been tailored to minimize the variance of these influence curves over a specified set of candidate functions for Q^*. In this chapter's example, this loss function was the weighted least squares loss $L_{g_n}(\bar{Q}) = (Y - f(\bar{Q}))^2 h_{g_n}^2$ and the working model was linear regression functions in W for $\bar{Q}$. To conclude, we showed that TMLE can accommodate the incorporation of additional targeting of the initial estimator through empirical efficiency maximization (Rubin and van der Laan 2008), so that additional optimality properties, such as having an influence curve that is more optimal than a user-supplied class of influence curves, can be guaranteed.

Disclaimer

This work concerns only the views of the authors and does not necessarily represent the position of the Food and Drug Administration.

Part IV
Case-Control Studies

Chapter 13
Independent Case-Control Studies

Sherri Rose, Mark J. van der Laan

Case-control study designs are frequently used in public health and medical research to assess potential risk factors for disease. These study designs are particularly attractive to investigators researching rare diseases, as they are able to sample known cases of disease vs. following a large number of subjects and waiting for disease onset in a relatively small number of individuals.

Case-control sampling is a biased design. Bias occurs due to the disproportionate number of cases in the sample vs. the population.

Researchers commonly employ the use of logistic regression in a parametric statistical model, ignoring the biased design, and estimate the conditional odds ratio of having disease given the exposure of interest A and measured covariates W.

Our proposed case-control-weighted TMLE for case-control studies relies on knowledge of the true prevalence probability, or a reasonable estimate of this probability, to eliminate the bias of the case-control sampling design. We use the prevalence probability in case-control weights, and our case-control weighting scheme successfully maps the TMLE for a random sample into a method for case-control sampling. The case-control-weighted TMLE (CCW-TMLE) is an efficient estimator for the case-control sample when the TMLE for the random sample is efficient. In addition, the CCW-TMLE inherits the robustness properties of the TMLE for the random sample.

13.1 Data, Model, and Target Parameter

Let us define a simple example with $X = (W, A, Y) \sim P_{X,0}$ as the full-data experimental unit and corresponding distribution $P_{X,0}$ of interest, which consists of baseline covariates W, exposure variable A, and a binary outcome Y that defines case or

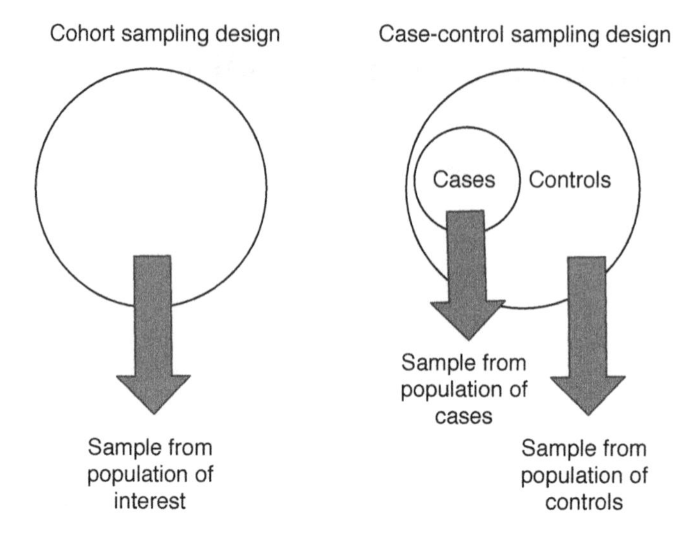

Fig. 13.1 Case-control sampling design

control status. In previous chapters, our target parameter of interest was the causal risk difference, which we now denote

$$\begin{aligned}\psi^F_{RD,0} = \Psi^F(P_{X,0}) &= E_{X,0}[E_{X,0}(Y \mid A=1,W) - E_{X,0}(Y \mid A=0,W)] \\ &= E_{X,0}(Y_1) - E_{X,0}(Y_0) \\ &= P_{X,0}(Y_1=1) - P_{X,0}(Y_0=1)\end{aligned}$$

for binary A, binary Y, and counterfactual outcomes Y_0 and Y_1, where F indicates "full data." Other common parameters of interest include the causal relative risk and the causal odds ratio, given by

$$\psi^F_{RR,0} = \frac{P_{X,0}(Y_1=1)}{P_{X,0}(Y_0=1)}$$

and

$$\psi^F_{OR,0} = \frac{P_{X,0}(Y_1=1)P_{X,0}(Y_0=0)}{P_{X,0}(Y_1=0)P_{X,0}(Y_0=1)}.$$

We describe the case-control design as first sampling (W_1, A_1) from the conditional distribution of (W, A), given $Y = 1$ for a case. One then samples J controls (W_0^j, A_0^j) from (W, A), given $Y = 0, j = 1, \ldots, J$. The observed data structure in independent case-control sampling is then defined by

$$O = \big((W_1, A_1), (W_0^j, A_0^j : j = 1, \ldots, J)\big) \sim P_0, \text{ with}$$

$$(W_1, A_1) \sim (W, A \mid Y = 1),$$
$$(W_0^j, A_0^j) \sim (W, A \mid Y = 0),$$

where the cluster containing one case and J controls is considered the experimental unit. Therefore, a case-control data set consists of n independent and identically distributed observations $O_1, \ldots, O_n$ with sampling distribution P_0 as described above. The statistical model $\mathcal{M}^F$, where the prevalence probability $P_{X,0}(Y = 1) \equiv q_0$ may or may not be known, implies a statistical model for the distribution of O consisting of (W_1, A_1) and controls (W_2^j, A_2^j), $j = 1, \ldots, J$.

This coupling formulation is useful when proving theoretical results for the case-control weighting methodology (van der Laan 2008a), and those results show that the following is also true. If independent case-control sampling is described as sampling nC cases from the conditional distribution of (W, A), given $Y = 1$, and sampling nCo controls from (W, A), given $Y = 0$, the value of J used to weight each control is then nCo/nC. This simple ratio $J = nCo/nC$ can be used effectively in practice. We also stress that this formulation does not describe *individually matched* case-control sampling, which we describe in Chap. 14.

13.2 Prevalence Probability

The population under study should be clearly defined. As such, the prevalence probability q_0 is then truly basic information about a population of interest. The use of the prevalence probability to eliminate the bias of a case-control sampling design as an update to a logistic regression intercept in a parametric statistical model was first discussed in Anderson (1972). This update enforces the intercept to be equal to $\log(q_0/(1 - q_0))$.

13.3 CCW-TMLE

In this section we build on the readers familiarity with the TMLE as described in detail in Chaps. 4 and 5. We discuss a CCW-TMLE for the causal risk difference with $X = (W, A, Y) \sim P_{X,0}$ and $O = \big((W_1, A_1), (W_0^j, A_0^j : j = 1, \ldots, J)\big) \sim P_0$. The full-data efficient influence curve $D^F(Q_0, g_0)$ at $P_{X,0}$ is given by

$$D^F(Q_0, g_0) = \left(\frac{I(A = 1)}{g_0(1 \mid W)} - \frac{I(A = 0)}{g_0(0 \mid W)}\right)(Y - \bar{Q}_0(A, W))$$
$$+ \bar{Q}_0(1, W) - \bar{Q}_0(0, W) - \Psi^F(Q_0), \tag{13.1}$$

where $Q_0 = (\bar{Q}_0, Q_{W,0})$, $Q_{W,0}$ is the true full-data marginal distribution of W, $\bar{Q}_0(A, W) = E_{X,0}(Y \mid A, W)$, and $g_0(a \mid W) = P_{X,0}(A = a \mid W)$. The first term will be denoted by D_Y^F and the second term by D_W^F, since these two terms represent components of the full-data efficient influence curve that are elements of the tangent space of the conditional distribution of Y, given (A, W), and the marginal distribution of W, respectively. That is, D_Y^F is the component of the efficient influence curve that equals a score of a parametric fluctuation model of a conditional distribution of Y, given (A, W), and D_W^F is a score of a parametric fluctuation model of the marginal distribution of W. Note that $D_Y^F(Q, g)$ equals a function $H^*(A, W)$ times the residual $(Y - \bar{Q}(A, W))$, where

$$H^*(A, W) = \left(\frac{I(A = 1)}{g(1 \mid W)} - \frac{I(A = 0)}{g(0 \mid W)} \right).$$

13.3.1 Case-Control-Weighted Estimators for Q_0 and g_0

We can estimate the marginal distribution of $Q_{W,0}$ with case-control-weighted maximum likelihood estimation:

$$Q_{W,n}^0 = \arg\min_{Q_W} \sum_{i=1}^{n} \left(q_0 L^F(Q_W)(W_{1,i}) + \frac{1 - q_0}{J} \sum_{j=1}^{J} L^F(Q_W)(W_{2,i}^j) \right),$$

where $L^F(Q_W) = -\log Q_W$ is the log-likelihood loss function for the marginal distribution of W. If we maximize over all distributions, this results in a case-control-weighted empirical distribution that puts mass q_0/n on the cases and $(1 - q_0)/(nJ)$ on the controls in the sample.

Suppose that based on a sample of n i.i.d. observations X_i we would have estimated $\bar{Q}_0$ with loss-based learning using the log-likelihood loss function $L^F(\bar{Q})(X) = -\log \bar{Q}(A, W)^Y (1 - \bar{Q}(A, W))^{1-Y}$. Given the actual observed data we can estimate $\bar{Q}_0$ with super learning and the case-control weights for observations $i = 1, \ldots, n$, which corresponds with the same super learner but now based on the case-control-weighted loss function:

$$L(\bar{Q})(O) \equiv q_0 L^F(\bar{Q})(W_1, A_1, 1) + \frac{1 - q_0}{J} \sum_{j=1}^{J} L^F(\bar{Q})(W_2^j, A_2^j, 0).$$

Let $L^F(Q) = L^F(Q_W) + L^F(\bar{Q})$ be the full-data loss function for $Q = (\bar{Q}, Q_W)$, and let $L(Q, q_0) = q_0 L^F(Q)(W_1, A_1, 1) + ((1 - q_0)/J) \sum_{j=1}^{J} L^F(Q)(W_2^j, A_2^j, 0)$ be the corresponding case-control-weighted loss function. We have $Q_0 = \arg\min_Q E_{P_0} L(Q, q_0)(O)$, so that indeed the case-control-weighted loss function for Q_0 is a valid loss function. Similarly, we can estimate g_0 with loss-based super learning based on the case-control-weighted log-likelihood loss function:

$$L(g)(O) \equiv -q_0 \log g(A_1 \mid W_1) - \frac{1 - q_0}{J} \sum_{j=1}^{J} \log g(A_2^j \mid W_2^j).$$

We now have an initial estimator $Q_n^0 = (Q_{W,n}^0, \bar{Q}_n^0)$ and g_n^0.

13.3.2 Parametric Submodel for Full-Data TMLE

Let $Q^0_{W,n}(\epsilon_1) = (1 + \epsilon_1 D^F_W(Q^0_n))Q^0_{W,n}$ be a parametric submodel through $Q^0_{W,n}$, and let

$$\bar{Q}^0_n(\epsilon_2)(Y = 1 \mid A, W) = \text{expit}\left(\log \frac{\bar{Q}^0_n}{(1 - \bar{Q}^0_n)}(A, W) + \epsilon_2 H^*_n(A, W)\right)$$

be a parametric submodel through the conditional distribution of Y, given A, W, implied by $\bar{Q}^0_n$. This describes a submodel $\{Q^0_n(\epsilon) : \epsilon\}$ through Q^0_n with a two-dimensional fluctuation parameter $\epsilon = (\epsilon_1, \epsilon_2)$. We have that $d/d\epsilon L^F(Q^0_n(\epsilon))$ at $\epsilon = 0$ yields the two scores $D^F_W(Q^0_n)$ and $D^F_Y(Q^0_n, g^0_n)$, and thereby spans the full-data efficient influence curve $D^F(Q^0_n, g^0_n)$, a requirement for the parametric submodel for the full-data TMLE. This parametric submodel and the loss function $L^F(Q)$ now defines the full data TMLE, and this same parametric submodel with the case-control loss function defines the CCW-TMLE.

13.3.3 Obtaining a Targeted Estimate of Q_0

We define

$$\epsilon_n = \arg\min_{\epsilon} \sum_{i=1}^{n} q_0 L^F(Q^0_n(\epsilon))(W_{1i}, A_{1i}) + \frac{1 - q_0}{J} \sum_{j=1}^{J} L^F(1 - Q^0_n(\epsilon))(W^j_{2i}, A^j_{2i})$$

and let $Q^1_n = Q^0_n(\epsilon_n)$. Note that $\epsilon_{1,n} = 0$, which shows that the case-control-weighted empirical distribution of W is not updated. Note also that $\epsilon_{2,n}$ is obtained by performing a case-control-weighted logistic regression of Y on $H^*_n(A, W)$, where $\bar{Q}^0_n(A, W)$ is used as an offset, and extracting the coefficient for $H^*_n(A, W)$. We then update $\bar{Q}^0_n$ with $\text{logit}\bar{Q}^1_n(A, W) = \text{logit}\bar{Q}^0_n(A, W) + \epsilon^1_n H^*_n(A, W)$. This updating process converges in one step in this example, so that the CCW-TMLE is given by $Q^*_n = Q^1_n$.

13.3.4 Estimator of the Target Parameter

Lastly, one evaluates the target parameter $\psi^*_n = \Psi^F(Q^*_n)$, where $Q^*_n = (\bar{Q}^1_n, Q^0_{W,n})$, by plugging $\bar{Q}^1_n$ and $Q^0_{W,n}$ into our substitution estimator to get the CCW-TMLE of ψ^F_0:

$$\psi^*_n = \left\{ \frac{1}{n} \sum_{i=1}^{n} \left(q_0 \bar{Q}^1_n(1, W_{1,i}) + \frac{1 - q_0}{J} \sum_{j=1}^{J} \bar{Q}^1_n(1, W^j_{2,i}) \right) - \left(q_0 \bar{Q}^1_n(0, W_{1,i}) + \frac{1 - q_0}{J} \sum_{j=1}^{J} \bar{Q}^1_n(0, W^j_{2,i}) \right) \right\}.$$

13.3.5 Calculating Standard Errors

Recall from Part I that the variance of our estimator is well approximated by the variance of the influence curve, divided by sample size n. Let IC^F be the influence curve of the full-data TMLE. We also showed that one can define IC^F as the full-data efficient influence curve given in (13.1). The case-control-weighted influence curve for the risk difference is then estimated by

$$IC_n(O) = q_0 IC_n^F(W_1, A_1, 1) + (1 - q_0)\frac{1}{J}\sum_{j=1}^{J} IC_n^F(W_2^j, A_2^j, 0).$$

Just as in Chap. 4, an estimate of the asymptotic variance of the standardized TMLE viewed as a random variable, using the estimate of the influence curve $IC_n(O)$, is given by $\sigma_n^2 = \frac{1}{n}\sum_{i=1}^{n} IC_n^2(O_i)$.

13.4 Simulations

In the following simulation studies, we compare the CCW-TMLE to two other estimators to examine finite sample performance.

CCW-MLE. Case-control-weighted estimator of $\bar{Q}_0$ mapped to causal effect estimators by averaging over the case-control-weighted distribution of W. This is a case-control-weighted maximum likelihood substitution estimator of the g-formula (CCW-MLE) first discussed in van der Laan (2008a) and Rose and van der Laan (2008).

CCW-TMLE. The targeted case-control-weighted maximum likelihood substitution estimator of the g-formula discussed in the chapter.

IPTW estimator. Robins (1999a) and Mansson et al. (2007) discuss, under a rare disease assumption, the use of an "approximately correct" IPTW method for case-control study designs. It uses the estimated exposure mechanism among control subjects to update a logistic regression of Y on A. This estimator targets a nonparametrically nonidentifiable parameter, which indicates strong sensitivity to model misspecification for the exposure mechanism. Estimates of the risk difference and relative risk cannot be obtained using this method.

We limit our simulations in this chapter to the odds ratio since the IPTW estimator can only estimate this parameter.

Simulation 1. This first simulation study was based on a population of $N = 120{,}000$ individuals, where we simulated a one-dimensional covariate W, a binary exposure A, and an indicator Y. These variables were generated according to the following rules: $W \sim U(0, 1)$, $P_{X,0}(A \mid W) = \text{expit}(W^2 - 4W + 1)$, and $P_{X,0}(Y = 1 \mid A, W) = \text{expit}(1.2A - \sin W^2 + A \sin W^2 + 5A \log W + 5 \log W - 1)$. The resulting population had a prevalence probability of $q_0 = 0.035$, and exactly 4,165 cases. We sampled the population using a varying number of cases and controls, and for each sample size we ran 1,000 simulations. The true value for the odds ratio was given by $OR = 2.60$.

For methods requiring an initial estimator of the conditional mean of Y, it was estimated using a correctly specified logistic regression and also a misspecified logistic regression with A and W as main terms. For methods requiring a fit for exposure mechanism, it was estimated using a correctly specified logistic regression and also a misspecified logistic regression with only the main term W.

Since we realistically generated A dependent on W, this led to substantial increases in efficiency in the targeted estimator when the initial estimator was misspecified and sample size grew, as it also adjusts for the exposure mechanism. This emphasizes the double robustness of the targeted estimators, and suggests that one should always target in practice. It is not surprising that when $\bar{Q}_n(A, W)$ was correctly specified, the relative efficiency of the targeted estimator (CCW-TMLE) was similar to its nontargeted counterpart (CCW-MLE). One should recall that correct specification in practice is unlikely and also note that this data structure is overly simplistic compared to real data. Even with this simple data structure, the IPTW estimators had the poorest overall efficiency. MSEs and relative efficiencies for the causal odds ratio are provided in Table 13.1.

When examining bias, it is clear that the IPTW estimators had the highest level of bias across all sample sizes, as observed in the bias plot displayed in Fig. 13.2. The CCW-MLE and CCW-TMLE with misspecified initial $\bar{Q}_n(A, W)$ had more bias than their correctly specified counterparts.

Table 13.1 Simulation results for the odds ratio. M is for misspecified $\bar{Q}_n(A, W)$ or $g_n(A \mid W)$ fit, C is for correctly specified $\bar{Q}_n(A, W)$ or $g_n(A \mid W)$. When two letters are noted in the "Fit" column, the first letter refers to $\bar{Q}_n(A, W)$ and the second to $g_n(A \mid W)$

		nC	250	500	500	1000	1000
Simulation 1	Fit	nCo	250	500	1000	1000	2000
IPTW MSE	M		1.76	1.75	3.39	1.80	3.40
IPTW RE	C		0.91	0.89	1.69	0.89	1.69
CCW-MLE RE	C		1.27	3.65	14.64	8.44	32.12
	M		3.07	5.72	14.54	7.83	18.93
CCW-TMLE RE	CC		1.27	3.62	14.58	8.40	32.03
	CM		1.26	3.62	14.57	8.40	31.97
	MC		1.96	4.63	16.68	9.52	31.91

		nC	100	250	250	500
Simulation 2	Fit	nCo	250	250	500	500
IPTW MSE	M		404.40	3667.56	306.42	2433.62
IPTW RE	C		1.0	1.2	1.0	1.2
CCW-MLE RE	C		290	4200	570	5800
CCW-TMLE RE	CC		280	4100	570	5700
	CM		290	4100	570	5700

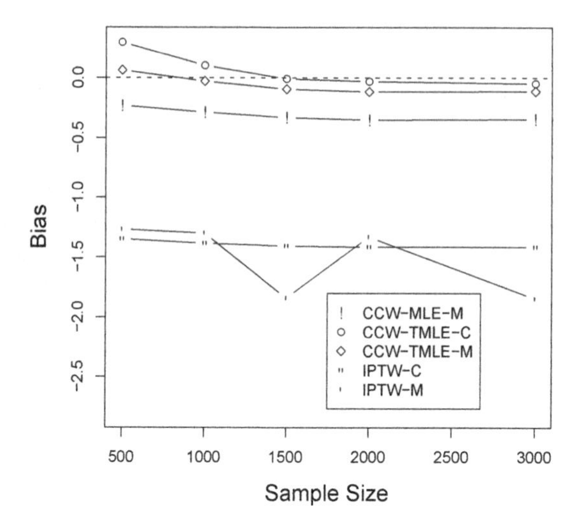

Fig. 13.2 Simulation 1 bias results. Bias results for the CCW-TMLE with misspecified $g_n(A \mid W)$ and the correctly specified CCW-MLE were excluded since values were the same as those for the TMLE with correctly specified $\bar{Q}_n(A, W)$ and $g_n(A \mid W)$.

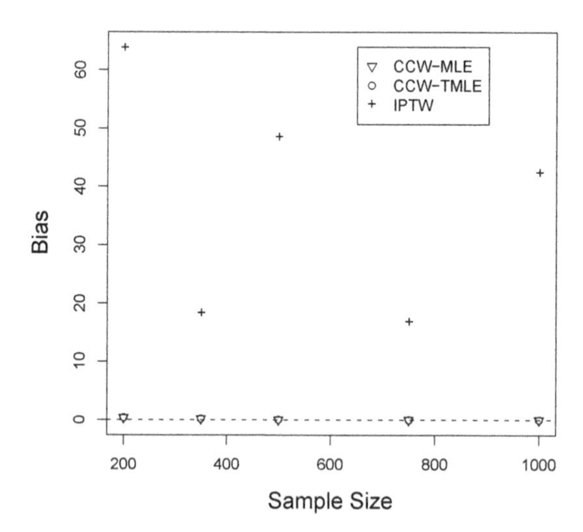

Fig. 13.3 Simulation 2 bias results. Bias results for the CCW-TMLE with misspecified $g_n(A \mid W)$ were excluded since those values were the same as those for the CCW-TMLE with correctly specified $\bar{Q}_n(A, W)$ and $g_n(A \mid W)$

Simulation 2. Our second set of simulations was based on a population of N = 80,000 individuals. The population had a binary exposure A, binary disease status Y, and a one-dimensional covariate W. These variables were generated according to the following rules: $W \sim U(0, 1)$, $P_{X,0}(A \mid W) = \text{expit}(-5 \sin W)$, and $P_{X,0}(Y = 1 \mid A, W) = \text{expit}(2A - 25W + A \times W)$. The resulting population had a prevalence probability of $q_0 = 0.053$, exactly 4,206 cases. The true value for the odds ratio was given by $OR = 3.42$. The parameter was estimated using the same general methods as in the previous section, albeit with different fits for $\bar{Q}_n(A, W)$ and $g_n(A \mid W)$. The initial fit for each method requiring an estimate of $\bar{Q}_0(A, W)$ was estimated using a correctly specified logistic regression. For methods requiring a fit for exposure mechanism, it was estimated using a correctly specified logistic regression and also a misspecified logistic regression with W as a main term.

Results across the two case-control-weighted methods for the odds ratio were nearly identical, indicating again that when $\bar{Q}_n(A, W)$ is correct and q_0 is known, one may be well served by either of these methods. However, the IPTW method for odds ratio estimation was extremely inefficient in comparison. We theorized in van der Laan (2008a), and Mansson et al. (2007) demonstrated, that the IPTW procedure has a strong sensitivity to model misspecification. This result was observed in simulation 1, although the results in simulation 2 are more extreme. Results can be seen in Table 13.1 and Fig. 13.3.

13.5 Discussion

Case-control weighting provides a framework for the analysis of case-control study designs using TMLEs. We observed that the IPTW method was outperformed in conditions similar to a practical setting by CCW-TMLE in two simulation studies. The CCW-TMLE yields a fully robust and locally efficient estimator of causal parameters of interest. Model misspecification within this framework, with known or consistently estimated exposure mechanism, still results in unbiased and highly efficient CCW-TMLE. Further, in practice we recommend the use of super learner for the estimation of $\bar{Q}_0$. We showed striking improvements in efficiency and bias in all methods incorporating knowledge of the prevalence probability over the IPTW estimator, which does not use this information.

13.6 Notes and Further Reading

As previously discussed, conditional estimation of the odds ratio of disease given the exposure and baseline covariates is the prevalent method of analysis in case-control study designs. Key publications in the area of logistic regression in parametric statistical models for independent case-control study designs are Anderson (1972), Prentice and Pyke (1979), Breslow and Day (1980), and Breslow (1996). Greenland (1981) and Holland and Rubin (1988) discuss another model-based method: the use of log-linear statistical models to estimate the marginal odds ratio. There are also multiple references for standardization in case-control studies, which estimates marginal effects with population or person-time averaging, including Rothman and Greenland (1998) and Greenland (2004). We also refer the interested reader to Newman (2006) for a related IPTW-type method. This procedure builds on the standardization approach in order to weight exposed and unexposed controls using a regression of A on W.

Given the availability of city, state, and national databases for many diseases, including many cancers, knowledge of the prevalence probability is now increasingly realistic. The literature, going back to the 1950s, supports this. See, for example, Cornfield (1951, 1956). If the prevalence probability is not known, an estimate can be used in the CCW-TMLE, and this additional uncertainty can be incorporated into the standard errors. In situations where data on the population of interest may be sparse, the use of a range for the prevalence probability is also appropriate.

Other papers, in addition to Anderson (1972), discuss the use of $\log(q_0/(1-q_0))$ as an update to the intercept of a logistic regression, including Prentice and Breslow (1978), Greenland (1981), Morise et al. (1996), Wacholder (1996), and Greenland (2004). However, its use in practice remains limited. The adjustment is sometimes presented as a ratio of sampling fractions: $\log(P(\text{sampled} \mid Y = 1)/P(\text{sampled} \mid Y = 0))$, which reduces to $\log(q_0/(1-q_0))$.

This chapter was adapted from a previously published paper (Rose and van der Laan 2008). We refer readers to this paper for additional simulations where q_0 is estimated, and for a demonstration of the use of the influence curve for standard error estimation in a single simulated data set. We also refer readers to van der Laan (2008a) for the theoretical development of CCW-TMLE, as well as a formal discussion of the "approximately correct" IPTW estimator. The appendix of van der Laan (2008a) also discusses in detail the incorporation of the additional uncertainty from an estimated q_0 into the standard errors.

The complexity of a case-control study can vary. Additional designs include individually matched, incidence-density, and nested. Individually matched case-control studies are discussed in the next chapter, and prediction in nested case-control studies is discussed in Chap. 15. A TMLE for general two-stage designs, including so-called nested case-control designs, is presented in Rose and van der Laan (2011). Adaptations for incidence-density designs are discussed briefly in van der Laan (2008a) and will be further developed in future work.

Chapter 14
Why Match? Matched Case-Control Studies

Sherri Rose, Mark J. van der Laan

Individually matched case-control study designs are common in public health and medicine, and conditional logistic regression in a parametric statistical model is the tool most commonly used to analyze these studies. In an individually matched case-control study, the population of interest is identified, and cases are randomly sampled. Each of these cases is then matched to one or more controls based on a variable (or variables) *believed* to be a confounder. The main potential benefit of matching in case-control studies is a gain in efficiency, not the elimination of confounding. Therefore, when are these study designs truly beneficial?

Given the potential drawbacks, including extra cost, added time for enrollment, increased bias, and potential loss in efficiency, the use of matching in case-control study designs warrants careful evaluation.

In this chapter, we focus on individual matching in case-control studies where the researcher is interested in estimating a causal effect, and certain prevalence probabilities are known or estimated. In order to eliminate the bias caused by the matched case-control sampling design, this technique relies on knowledge of the true prevalence probability $q_0 \equiv P_{X,0}(Y = 1)$ and an additional value:

$$\bar{q}_0(M) \equiv q_0 \frac{P_{X,0}(Y = 0 \mid M)}{P_{X,0}(Y = 1 \mid M)},$$

where M is the matching variable. We will compare the use of CCW-TMLEs in matched and unmatched case-control study designs as we explore which design yields the most information for the causal effect of interest. We assume readers have knowledge of the information presented in the previous chapter on independent case-control study designs.

14.1 Data, Model, and Target Parameter

We define $X = (W, M, A, Y) \sim P_{X,0}$ as the experimental unit and corresponding distribution $P_{X,0}$ of interest. Here X consists of baseline covariates W, an exposure variable A, and a binary outcome Y, which defines case or control status. We can define $\psi_0^F = \Psi^F(P_{X,0}) \in \mathbb{R}^d$ of $P_{X,0} \in \mathcal{M}^F$ as the causal effect parameter, and for binary exposure $A \in \{0,1\}$ we define the risk difference, relative risk, and odds ratio as in the previous chapter. The observed data structure in matched case-control sampling is defined by

$$O = \Big((M_1, W_1, A_1), (M_0^j = M_1, W_0^j, A_0^j : j = 1, \ldots, J)\Big) \sim P_0, \text{ with}$$

$$(M_1, W_1, A_1) \sim (M, W, A \mid Y = 1) \text{ for cases and}$$

$$(M_0^j, W_0^j, A_0^j) \sim (M, W, A \mid Y = 0, M = M_1) \text{ for controls.}$$

Here $M \subset W$, and M is a categorical matching variable. The sampling distribution of data structure O is described as above with P_0. Thus, the matched case-control data set contains n independent and identically distributed observations $O_1, \ldots, O_n$ with sampling distribution P_0. The cluster containing one case and the J controls is the experimental unit, and the marginal distribution of the cluster is specified by the population distribution $P_{X,0}$. The model $\mathcal{M}^F$, which possibly includes knowledge of q_0 or $\bar{q}_0(M)$, then implies models for the probability distribution of O consisting of cases (M_1, W_1, A_1) and controls (M_1, W_2^j, A_2^j), $j = 1, \ldots, J$.

14.2 CCW-TMLE for Individual Matching

CCW-TMLEs for individually matched case-control studies incorporate knowledge of q_0 and $\bar{q}_0(M)$, where $\bar{q}_0(M)$ is defined as

$$\bar{q}_0(M) \equiv q_0 \frac{P_{X,0}(Y = 0 \mid M)}{P_{X,0}(Y = 1 \mid M)} = q_0 \frac{q_0(0 \mid M)}{q_0(1 \mid M)}.$$

Implementation of CCW-TMLE in individually matched studies echos the procedure for independent (unmatched) case-control studies, with the exception that the weights now differ. We summarize this procedure assuming the reader is already familiar with the material in the previous chapter. We focus on the risk difference $\psi_{RD,0}^F = E_{X,0}[E_{X,0}(Y \mid A = 1, W) - E_{X,0}(Y \mid A = 0, W)]$ as an illustrative example.

Implementing CCW-TMLE for Individually Matched Data

Step 0. Assign weights q_0 to cases and $\bar{q}_0(M)/J$ to the corresponding J controls.

Step 1. Estimate the conditional probability of Y given A and W using super learning and assigned weights. The estimate of $P_{X,0}(Y = 1 \mid A, W, M) \equiv \bar{Q}_0(A, W, M)$ is $\bar{Q}_n^0(A, W, M)$. Let Q_n^0 be the estimate of the conditional mean and the case-control-weighted empirical distribution for the marginal distribution of W, representing the estimator of $Q_0 = (\bar{Q}_0, Q_{W,0})$.

Step 2. Estimate the exposure mechanism using super learning and weights. The estimate of $P_{X,0}(A \mid W, M) \equiv g_0(A \mid W, M)$ is $g_n(A \mid W, M)$.

Step 3. Determine a parametric family of fluctuations $Q_n^0(\epsilon)$ of Q_n^0 with fluctuation parameter ϵ, and a case-control-weighted loss function $L_{q_0}(Q) = q_0 L^F(Q)(M_1, W_1, A_1, 1) + (\bar{q}_0(M)/J) \sum_{j=1}^J L^F(Q)(M_1, W_2^j, A_2^j, 0)$ such that the derivative of $L^F(Q_n^0(\epsilon))$ at $\epsilon = 0$ equals the full-data efficient influence curve at any initial estimator $Q_n^0 = (\bar{Q}_n^0, Q_{W,n}^0)$ and g_n. Since initial Q_{Wn}^0 is the empirical distribution (i.e., case-control-weighted nonparametric maximum likelihood estimation), one only needs to fluctuate $\bar{Q}_n^0$ and the fluctuation function involves a choice of clever covariate chosen such that the above derivative condition holds. Calculate the clever covariate $H_n^*(A, W, M)$ for each subject as a function of $g_n(A \mid W, M)$:

$$H_n^*(A, W, M) = \left(\frac{I(A = 1)}{g_n(1 \mid W, M)} - \frac{I(A = 0)}{g_n(0 \mid W, M)} \right).$$

Step 4. Update the initial fit $\bar{Q}_n^0(A, W, M)$ from step 1 using the covariate $H_n^*(A, W, M)$. This is achieved by holding $\bar{Q}_n^0(A, W, M)$ fixed while estimating the coefficient ϵ for $H_n^*(A, W, M)$ in the fluctuation function using case-control-weighted maximum likelihood estimation. Let ϵ_n be this case-control-weighted parametric maximum likelihood estimator. The updated regression is given by $\bar{Q}_n^1 = \bar{Q}_n^0(\epsilon_n)$. No iteration is necessary since the next ϵ_n will be equal to zero. The CCW-TMLE of Q_0 is now $Q_n^* = (\bar{Q}_n^1, Q_{Wn}^0)$, where only the conditional mean estimator $\bar{Q}_n^0$ was updated.

Step 5. Obtain the substitution estimator of the target parameter by application of the target parameter mapping to Q_n^*:

$$\psi_n^* = \left\{ \frac{1}{n} \sum_{i=1}^n \left(q_0 \bar{Q}_n^1(1, W_{1,i}, M_{1,i}) + \frac{\bar{q}_0(M)}{J} \sum_{j=1}^J \bar{Q}_n^1(1, W_{2,i}^j, M_{1,i}) \right) \right.$$
$$\left. - \left(q_0 \bar{Q}_n^1(0, W_{1,i}, M_{1,i}) + \frac{\bar{q}_0(M)}{J} \sum_{j=1}^J \bar{Q}_n^1(0, W_{2,i}^j, M_{1,i}) \right) \right\}.$$

Step 6. Calculate standard errors, p-values, and confidence intervals based on the influence curve of the CCW-TMLE ψ_n^*. The influence curve can be selected to be the case-control-weighted full-data efficient influence curve (just as we defined the case-control-weighted full-data loss function).

14.3 Simulations

In the following simulation studies, we compare the CCW-TMLE in independent and individually matched study designs.

Simulation 1. Our first simulation study is designed to illustrate the differences between independent case-control sampling and matched case-control sampling in "ideal" situations where control information is not discarded (e.g., data collection is expensive, and covariate information is only collected when a control is a match). The population contained $N = 35{,}000$ individuals, where we simulated a 9-dimensional covariate $W = (W_i : i = 1, \ldots, 9)$, a binary exposure (or "treatment") A, and an indicator Y. These variables were generated according to the following rules: $P_{X,0}(W_i = 1) = 0.5$, $P_{X,0}(A = 1 \mid W) = \text{expit}(W_1 + W_2 + W_3 - 2W_4 - 2W_5 + 2W_6 - 4W_7 - 4W_8 + 4W_9)$, and $P_{X,0}(Y = 1 \mid A, W) = \text{expit}(1.5A + W_1 - 2W_2 - 4W_3 - W_4 - 2W_5 - 4W_6 + W_7 - 2W_8 - 4W_9)$.

Both the exposure mechanism and the conditional mean of Y given its parents were generated with varied levels of association with A and Y in order to investigate the role of weak, medium, and strong association between a matching variable W_i and A and Y. The corresponding associations can be seen in Table 14.1. For example, W_1 was weakly associated with both A and Y. Matching is only potentially beneficial when the matching variable is a true confounder.

Another illustration of the varied association levels can be seen in Table 14.2, where we display the probability an individual in the population was a case given $W_i = w$, all the nonmatching covariates (Z), and A. For example, let's say matching variable W_2 is *age* with 1 representing <50 years old and 0 representing ≥ 50 years old. In this population, it was not very likely (0.013) that someone who is <50 years old will become a case, while someone who is ≥ 50 years old has a much higher chance of becoming a case (0.047), given Z and A. Therefore, W_2, W_5, and W_8 represent situations where the distribution of W_i among cases and controls is very different. The covariates W_3, W_6, and W_9 represent situations where this difference is even more extreme.

The simulated population had a prevalence probability of $q_0 = 0.030$ and exactly 1,045 cases, and the true value of the odds ratio was given by $OR = 2.302$. We sampled the population using a varying number of cases $nC = (200, 500, 1000)$ in both matched and unmatched designs, and for each sample size we ran 1000 simulations. In each sample, the same cases were used for both designs. Controls were matched to cases in our matched simulations based on one variable (W_i) for both 1:1 and 1:2 designs. The causal odds ratio was estimated using a CCW-TMLE with correctly specified case-control-weighted logistic regressions.

The matched and unmatched designs performed similarly with respect to bias for the nine covariates (results not shown; Rose and van der Laan 2009). There were consistent increases in efficiency when the association between W_i and Y was high (W_3, W_6, and W_9), when comparing matched to independent. Results when the association with W_i and Y was medium (W_2, W_5, and W_8) were not entirely consistent, although covariates W_5 and W_8 did show increases in efficiency for the matched

Table 14.1 Simulated covariates

		Y		
	Association	Weak	Medium	Strong
	Weak	W_1	W_2	W_3
A	Medium	W_4	W_5	W_6
	Strong	W_7	W_8	W_9

Table 14.2 Simulated covariates: probabilities

W_i	$P_{X,0}(Y = 1 \mid W_i = 1, Z, A)$	$P_{X,0}(Y = 1 \mid W_i = 0, Z, A)$
W_1	0.039	0.021
W_2	0.013	0.049
W_3	0.003	0.060
W_4	0.021	0.040
W_5	0.013	0.047
W_6	0.003	0.061
W_7	0.040	0.023
W_8	0.013	0.046
W_9	0.004	0.066

Table 14.3 Simulation 1: MSE is mean squared error, RE is relative efficiency, and *nC* is number of cases

		1:1			**1:2**		
	nC	200	500	1000	200	500	1000
W_1	Matched MSE	2.67	0.77	0.30	0.98	0.32	0.14
	Independent RE	1.09	1.05	1.03	0.97	0.97	1.00
W_2	Matched MSE	2.63	0.70	0.33	1.07	0.40	0.15
	Independent RE	1.01	0.93	1.18	1.00	1.21	1.07
W_3	Matched MSE	1.95	0.59	0.23	0.93	0.29	0.13
	Independent RE	0.80	0.78	0.79	0.90	0.88	1.00
W_4	Matched MSE	2.20	0.64	0.30	1.05	0.32	0.14
	Independent RE	0.77	1.07	1.11	1.00	0.94	0.93
W_5	Matched MSE	2.10	0.61	0.28	0.98	0.30	0.14
	Independent RE	0.82	0.80	0.93	0.91	0.83	1.00
W_6	Matched MSE	2.28	0.61	0.24	0.92	0.27	0.12
	Independent RE	0.74	0.97	0.80	0.95	0.84	0.86
W_7	Matched MSE	2.55	0.69	0.30	1.08	0.32	0.16
	Independent RE	1.11	0.96	1.00	0.98	1.00	1.23
W_8	Matched MSE	2.00	0.61	0.22	0.86	0.25	0.11
	Independent RE	0.78	0.88	0.76	0.90	0.78	0.85
W_9	Matched MSE	1.77	0.58	0.24	0.71	0.24	0.12
	Independent RE	0.72	0.91	0.77	0.63	0.75	0.92

design for all or nearly all sample sizes. These results are in line with the consensus found in the literature: that matching may produce gains in efficiency when the distribution of the matching variable differs drastically between the cases and the controls. Efficiency results for the odds ratio can be seen in Table 14.3.

Simulation 2. The second simulation study was designed to address less ideal more common situations where control information is discarded. Controls were sampled from the population of controls in simulation 1 until a match on covariate W_i was found for each case. Nonmatches were returned to the population of controls. The number of total controls sampled to find sufficient matches was recorded for each simulation. This was the number of randomly sampled controls that was used for the corresponding independent case-control simulation. The mean number of controls sampled to achieve 1:1 and 1:2 matching at each sample size is noted in Table 14.4 as nCo. For example, in order to obtain 200 controls matched on covariate W_1 in a 1:1 design, an average of 404 controls had to be sampled from the population. Thus,

Table 14.4 Simulation 2: MSE is mean squared error, RE is relative efficiency, nC is number of cases, and nCo is mean number of controls for the independent case-control design

		1:1			**1:2**		
	nC	200	500	1000	200	500	1000
	nCo	404	1006	2010	804	2011	4026
W_1	Matched MSE	2.90	0.76	0.28	1.00	0.27	0.14
	Independent RE	2.89	2.24	2.14	2.12	1.70	2.16
	nCo	404	1009	2016	808	2016	4031
W_2	Matched MSE	2.91	0.77	0.30	1.15	0.36	0.16
	Independent RE	2.91	2.72	2.13	2.32	2.21	2.49
	nCo	406	1016	2033	812	2034	4065
W_3	Matched MSE	1.99	0.48	0.22	0.84	0.28	0.11
	Independent RE	1.82	1.43	1.65	1.81	1.78	1.85
	nCo	403	1006	2010	806	2012	4023
W_4	Matched MSE	2.47	0.67	0.29	1.09	0.28	0.13
	Independent RE	2.38	2.09	2.20	2.29	1.91	2.03
	nCo	406	1010	2019	810	2019	4040
W_5	Matched MSE	2.41	0.63	0.25	0.92	0.29	0.12
	Independent RE	2.24	2.00	1.92	1.95	1.89	2.10
	nCo	411	1025	2046	819	2045	4094
W_6	Matched MSE	2.08	0.64	0.23	0.88	0.27	0.13
	Independent RE	2.13	1.99	1.69	1.92	1.70	2.23
	nCo	402	1001	2000	801	1999	4000
W_7	Matched MSE	2.71	0.72	0.30	1.09	0.34	0.15
	Independent RE	2.54	2.42	2.18	2.19	2.25	2.18
	nCo	407	1014	2028	811	2027	4055
W_8	Matched MSE	2.28	0.56	0.23	0.97	0.25	0.11
	Independent RE	2.35	1.76	1.71	1.99	1.59	1.68
	nCo	413	1030	2059	824	2061	4121
W_9	Matched MSE	1.97	0.54	0.22	0.80	0.26	0.12
	Independent RE	1.91	1.77	1.69	1.62	1.69	1.84

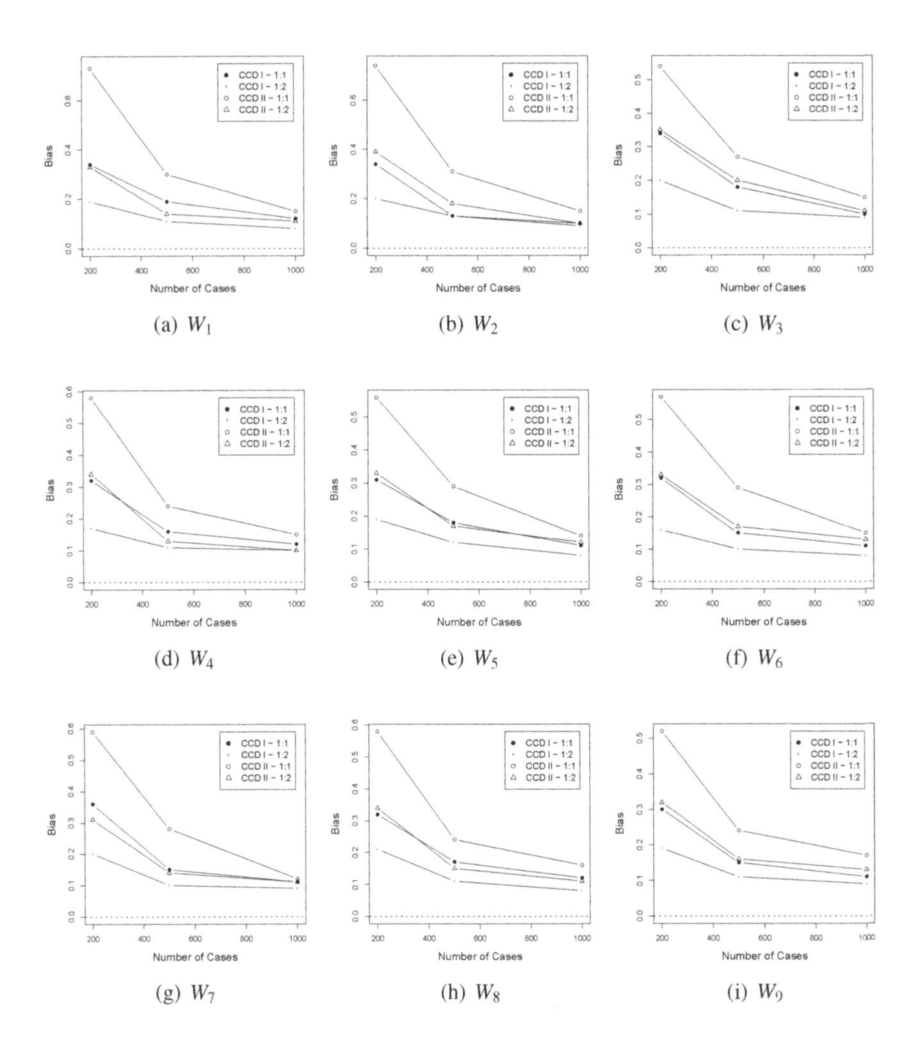

Fig. 14.1 Simulation 2 bias. CCD I is "Case-Control Design I" referring to the independent case-control design and CCD II is "Case-Control Design II" referring to the matched case-control design

an average of 404 controls were used in the corresponding independent case-control design.

CCW-TMLE was performed for both designs with correctly specified case-control-weighted logistic regression estimators for the exposure mechanism and conditional mean of Y given A and W. The independent design outperformed the matched design with respect to efficiency and bias for all sample sizes and both 1:1 and 1:2 matching. This was not surprising given the mean number of controls in each of the independent unmatched designs was, on average, about two times the number of controls for the matched design. Additionally, as association between W_i

and Y increased, there was a trend that the number of controls necessary for complete matching also increased. A similar trend between A and W_i was not apparent. Bias results do not vary greatly with association between W_i and A or Y. Efficiency results can be seen in Table 14.4. Bias results are displayed in Fig. 14.1.

14.4 Discussion

The main benefit of a matched case-control study design is a potential increase in efficiency. However, an increase in efficiency is not automatic. If one decides to implement a matched case-control study design, selection of the matching variable is crucial. In practice, it may be difficult to ascertain the strength of the association between the matching variable, the exposure of interest, and the outcome. Our simulations confirmed the consensus in the existing literature: that in situations where the distribution of the matching covariate is drastically different between the case and control populations, matching may provide an increase in efficiency. Our simulations indicated that $P_{X,0}(Y = 1 \mid W_i = 1, Z, A)$, for matching variable W_i and covariate vector Z, may need to be very small for an increase in efficiency using a matched design. These results were true, however, only for simulations where *no control subjects were discarded*; it is very common for matched study designs to discard controls (Freedman 1950; Cochran 1965; Billewicz 1965; McKinlay 1977). We showed that in practical situations (e.g., when controls are discarded), an unmatched design is likely to be a more efficient, less biased study design choice.

14.5 Notes and Further Reading

There is a collection of literature devoted to the topic of individual matching in case-control study designs, and discussion of the advantages and disadvantages of matching goes back more than 40 years. While some literature cites the purpose of matching as improving validity, later publications (Kupper et al. 1981; Rothman and Greenland 1998) demonstrate that matching has a greater impact on efficiency over validity. Costanza (1995) notes that matching on confounders in case-control studies does nothing to remove the confounding. Similarly, Rothman and Greenland (1998) discuss that matching cannot control confounding in case-control study designs but can, in fact, introduce bias. Methodologists in the literature stress that it is often possible and preferred for confounders to be *adjusted for* in the analysis instead of matching in case-control designs (Schlesselman 1982; Vandenbrouke et al. 2007).

Matching has a substantial impact on the study sample; most notably, it creates a sample of controls that is not representative of exposure in the population or the population as a whole. The effect of the matching variable can no longer be studied directly, and the exposure frequency in the control sample will be shifted towards that of the cases (Rothman and Greenland 1998).

Matched sampling leads to a balanced number of cases and controls across the levels of the selected matching variables. This balance can reduce the variance in the parameter of interest, which improves statistical efficiency. A study with a randomly selected control group may yield some strata with an imbalance of cases and controls. It is important to add, however, that matching in case-control studies can lead to gains *or* losses in efficiency (Kupper et al. 1981; Rothman and Greenland 1998). Matching variables are chosen a priori on the belief that they confound the relationship between exposure and disease. If controls are matched to cases based on a variable that is not a true confounder, this can impact efficiency. For example, if the matching variable is associated not with disease but with the exposure, this will increase the variance of the estimator compared to an unmatched design. Here, the matching leads to larger numbers of exposure-concordant case-control pairs, which are not informative in the analysis, leading to an increase in variance. If the matching variable is only associated with disease, there is often a loss of efficiency as well (Schlesselman 1982). If the matching variable is along the causal pathway between disease and exposure, then matching will contribute bias that cannot be removed in the analysis (Vandenbrouke et al. 2007). The number of matching variables should also be reduced to as few as possible. As the number of matching variables grows, the cases and controls will become increasingly similar with respect to the exposure of interest, and the study may produce a spurious result or provide no information (Breslow and Day 1980). Additionally, when matching on more than one variable, matching variables should not be strongly correlated with each other (Schlesselman 1982). This chapter was adapted from Rose and van der Laan (2009). We refer readers to this paper for additional discussion of the implications of individually matched designs.

Cochran (1953) demonstrates the efficiency of matched designs. However, as noted by McKinlay (1977), Cochran's result can be misleading. Comparisons between matched and unmatched study designs are often made with *equal* sample sizes and no other method of covariate adjustment. In a matched design, controls may be discarded if they do not match a particular case on the variable or variables of interest. Multiple controls may be discarded per case, depending on the variables of interest (Freedman 1950; Cochran 1965; McKinlay 1977). In many cases, if the discarded controls were available to be rejected in the matched study, they would be available for an unmatched design in the same investigation (Billewicz 1965; McKinlay 1977). Therefore, it is often more appropriate to compare the efficiencies of matched case-control studies of size n to randomly selected case-control studies of size n+*number of discarded controls*.

The predominant method of analysis in individually matched case-control studies is conditional logistic regression in a parametric statistical model. The logistic regression model for matched case-control studies differs from unmatched studies in that it allows the intercept to vary among the matched units of cases and controls. The matching variable is not included in the model (Breslow et al. 1978; Holford et al. 1978; Breslow and Day 1980; Schlesselman 1982). In order to estimate an effect of exposure A with conditional logistic regression, the case and control must be discordant on A. Rothman and Greenland (1998) and Greenland (2004) demonstrate the use of standardization in case-control studies, which estimate marginal effects with population or person-time averaging.

Chapter 15
Nested Case-Control Risk Score Prediction

Sherri Rose, Bruce Fireman, Mark J. van der Laan

Risk scores are calculated to identify those patients at the highest level of risk for an outcome. In some cases, interventions are implemented for patients at high risk. Standard practice for risk score prediction relies heavily on parametric regression. Generating a good estimator of the function of interest using parametric regression can be a significant challenge. As discussed in Chap. 3, high-dimensional data are increasingly common in epidemiology, and researchers may have dozens, hundreds, or thousands of potential predictors that are possibly related to the outcome.

The analysis of full cohort data for risk prediction is frequently not feasible, often due to the cost associated with purchasing access to large comprehensive databases, storage and memory limitations in computer hardware, or other practical considerations. Thus, researchers frequently conduct nested case-control studies instead of analyzing the full cohort, particularly when their prediction research question involves a rare outcome. This type of two-stage design introduces bias since the proportion of cases in the sample is not the same as the population. This complication may have contributed to the relative lack of prediction studies for rare diseases.

We consider a two-stage sampling design in which one takes a random sample from a target population and measures Y, the outcome, on each subject in the first stage. The second stage involves drawing a subsample from the original sample, collecting additional data on the subsample. The decision regarding selection into the subsample is influenced by Y. This data structure can be viewed as a missing-data structure on the full data structure X collected in the second stage of the study. Using nested case-control data from a Kaiser Permanente database, we generate a function for mortality risk score prediction using super learner and inverse probability of missingness weights to correct the bias introduced by the sampling design.

15.1 Data, Model, and Parameter

Kaiser Permanente Northern California provided medical services to approximately 3 million members during the study period. They served 345,191 persons over the age of 65 in the 2003 calendar year, and 13,506 of these subjects died the subsequent year. The death outcome was ascertained from California death certificate filings. Disease and diagnosis variables, which we refer to in this paper simply as medical flags, were obtained from Kaiser Permanente clinical and claims databases. There are 184 medical flags covering a variety of diseases, treatments, conditions, and other reasons for visits. Gender and age variables were obtained from Kaiser Permanente administrative databases.

A nested case-control sample was extracted from the Kaiser Permanente database for computational ease. All 13,506 cases from the 2003–2004 data were sampled with probability 1, and an equal number of controls were sampled from the full database with probability 0.041 for a total of 27,012 subjects. Approval from the institutional review board at Kaiser Permanente Northern California for the protection of human subjects was obtained.

Formally, we define the full data structure as $X = (W, Y) \sim P_{X,0}$, with covariate vector $W = \{W_1, \ldots W_{186}\}$ and binary outcome Y, indicating death in 2004. The observed data structure for a randomly sampled subject is $O = (Y, \Delta, \Delta X) \sim P_0$, where Y is included in X and Δ denotes the indicator of inclusion in the second-stage sample (nested case-control sample). The parameter of the full-data distribution of X is given by $\bar{Q}_0 = E_{X,0}(Y \mid W)$ and the full-data statistical model $\mathcal{M}^F$ is nonparametric.

15.2 Loss Function

Had our sample been comprised of n i.i.d. observations X_i, we would have estimated $\bar{Q}_0 = E_{X,0}(Y \mid W)$ with loss-based learning using loss function $L^F(X, \bar{Q})$. Given the actual observed data, we can estimate $\bar{Q}_0$ with super learning and weights $\Delta_i / P_{X,n}(\Delta_i = 1 \mid Y_i)$ for observations $i = 1, \ldots, n$, which corresponds with the same super learner, but now based on the inverse probability of missingness (censoring) weighted loss function:

$$L(O, \bar{Q}) = \frac{\Delta}{P_{X,n}(\Delta = 1 \mid Y)} L^F(X, \bar{Q}).$$

We define our parameter of interest as: $\bar{Q}_0 = \arg\min_{\bar{Q}} E_0 L(O, \bar{Q})$, where $\bar{Q}$ is a possible function in the parameter space of functions that map an input W into a predicted value for Y. $E_0 L(O, \bar{Q})$, the expected loss, evaluates the candidate $\bar{Q}$, and it is minimized at the optimal choice of $\bar{Q}_0$.

15.3 Data Analysis

We implemented super learning with observation weighting in R to obtain our estimate of $\bar{Q}_0$ using our observed data. Observation weights within the super learner were assigned based on the inverse probability of missingness, $w_i = \Delta_i / P_{X,n}(\Delta_i = 1 \mid Y_i)$ thus cases were given observation weights equal to 1 and controls were given observation weights of $1/0.041 = 24$. One could further stabilize the weights by standardizing them to sum to 1: in other words, we would divide the above w_i by $\sum_{i=1}^{n} \Delta_i / P_{X,n}(\Delta = 1 \mid Y_i)$. Any algorithm that allows observation weighting can be used with super learner in nested case-control data.

The collection of 16 algorithms included in this analysis can be found in Table 15.1. We implemented dimension reduction among the covariates as part of each algorithm, retaining only those covariates associated with Y in a univariate regression ($p < 0.10$). After screening, 135 covariates remained. Algorithms with different options (e.g., degree, size, etc.) were considered distinct algorithms. The selection of these algorithms was based on investigator knowledge, the ability to take observation weights, and computational speed. The super learner algorithm is explained in detail in Chap. 3, and we refer readers to this chapter for an intuitive understanding of the procedure. Demonstrations of the super learner's superior finite sample performance in simulations and publicly available data sets, as well as asymptotic results, are also discussed in Chap. 3.

A summary of the nested case-control variables can be found in Table 15.2. All 187 variables, except death, were evaluated from 2003 records. The majority of the sample is female, with 45.2% male. The age category with the largest num-

Table 15.1 Collection of algorithms

Algorithm	Description
glm.1	Main terms logistic regression
glm.2	Main terms logistic regression with gender × age interaction
glm.3	Main terms logistic regression with gender × age^2 interaction
glm.4	Main terms logistic regression with gender × age^3 interaction
glm.5	Main terms logistic regression with age^2 term
glm.6	Main terms logistic regression with age^3 term
glm.7	Main terms logistic regression with age × covariate interaction for remaining main terms
glm.8	Main terms logistic regression with gender × covariate interaction for remaining main terms
glm.9	Main terms logistic regression with age × covariate and gender × covariate interaction
bayesglm	Bayesian main terms logistic regression
glmnet.1	Elastic net, $\alpha = 1.00$
glmnet.5	Elastic net, $\alpha = 0.50$
gam.2	Generalized additive regression, degree = 2
gam.3	Generalized additive regression, degree = 3
nnet.2	Neural network, size = 2
nnet.4	Neural network, size = 4

ber of members was 70 to 79, with 41.0%. (For presentation, age is summarized categorically in Table 15.2, although the variable is continuous and was analyzed as a continuous variable. All other variables are binary.) The top ten most prevalent medical flags in the sample were: screening/observation/special exams, other endocrine/metabolic/nutritional, hypertension, minor symptoms, postsurgical status/aftercare, major symptoms, history of disease, other musculoskeletal/connective tissue, cataract, and other dermatological disorders. The majority of medical flags (47.2%) had a prevalence of less than 1%. Twenty medical flags had a prevalence of 0%. These variables were excluded from our analysis as they provide no information. We remind the reader that these percentages do not reflect estimates of prevalence in the *population* given the biased sampling design.

The super learning algorithm for predicting death (risk score) in the nested case-control sample performed as well as or outperformed all single algorithms in the collection of algorithms. With a cross-validated MSE (i.e., the cross-validated risk, not to be confused with *risk score*) of 3.336e-2, super learner improved upon the

Table 15.2 Characteristics of Northern California Kaiser Permanente members aged 65 years and older in nested case-control sample, 2003

Variables	No.	%
Death (in 2004)	13,506	50.0
Male	12,213	45.2
Age, years[a]		
65 to <70	5,193	19.2
70 to <80	11,077	41.0
80 to <90	8,525	31.6
≥ 90	2,217	8.2
Most prevalent medical flags	No.	%
Screening/observation/special exams	23,597	87.4
Other endocrine/metabolic/nutritional	10,633	39.4
Hypertension	10,612	39.3
Minor symptoms, signs, findings	9,748	36.1
Postsurgical status/aftercare	9,447	35.0
Major symptoms, abnormalities	8,251	30.5
History of disease	7,376	27.3
Other musculoskeletal/connective tissue	7,359	27.2
Cataract	5,976	22.1
Other dermatological disorders	5,692	21.1
Medical flag prevalence	No.	%
Zero	20	10.8
$0 < x < 1\%$	67	36.4
$1 \leq x < 10\%$	72	39.1
≥10%	25	13.6

[a] Age is summarized categorically although the variable is continuous.

Table 15.3 Results from super learner analysis

Algorithm	CV MSE	RE	R^2
SuperLearner	3.336e-2	–	0.113
glm.1	3.350e-2	1.004	0.109
glm.2	3.350e-2	1.004	0.109
glm.3	3.349e-2	1.004	0.109
glm.4	3.348e-2	1.004	0.109
glm.5	3.348e-2	1.004	0.109
glm.6	3.348e-2	1.004	0.109
glm.7	3.458e-2	1.037	0.080
glm.8	3.443e-2	1.032	0.084
glm.9	3.533e-2	1.059	0.060
bayesglm	3.778e-2	1.132	-0.005
glmnet.1	3.337e-2	1.000	0.112
glmnet.5	3.336e-2	1.000	0.112
gam.2	3.349e-2	1.004	0.109
gam.3	3.349e-2	1.004	0.109
nnet.2	3.913e-2	1.173	-0.041
nnet.4	3.913e-2	1.173	-0.041

worst algorithms by 17% with respect to estimated cross-validated MSE. MSEs in the collection of algorithms ranged from 3.336e-2 to 3.913e-2. While the collection of algorithms was somewhat limited, which isn't optimal from a theoretical perspective, we see some benefits in relative efficiency. Results are presented in Table 15.3 where relative efficiency for each of the k algorithms is defined as RE=cross validated MSE(k)/cross validated MSE(*super learner*).

When examining R^2 values, the super learner had the largest R^2 compared to the collection of algorithms with an $R^2 = 0.113$, although ten of the algorithms approached this value. Super learner had an 11.3% gain relative to using the marginal probability (i.e., assigning probability of death 0.039 to each observation). The algorithms in the collection had R^2 values ranging from 0.112 to -0.041. (Negative R^2 values indicate that the marginal prevalence probability is a better predictor of mortality than the algorithm. Values for R^2 can fall outside the range [0,1] when calculated in cross-validated data.) See Table 15.3. While the performance of the super learner improved upon the collection of algorithms with respect to R^2 values, it should be noted that the overall prediction power of this data set is somewhat limited with the best $R^2 = 0.113$.

15.4 Discussion

Alternatives to parametric approaches to risk score prediction include the flexible approach super learning. The algorithm provides a system to combine many estimators into an improved estimator and returns a function we can use for prediction in new data sets. Cross-validation of the individual algorithms and the super learner prevents overfitting and the selection of a fit that is too biased. Our criterion for estimator selection is based on an a priori established benchmark (e.g., cross-validated MSE).

Super learning allows for the use of observation weighting in order to generate prediction functions with nested case-control data, as well as data from other two-stage sampling designs, case-control designs, and general biased sampling designs. In our nested case-control Kaiser Permanente data, super learner performed as well as or outperformed all algorithms in the collection of algorithms. While the overall predictive power of this data set was limited ($R^2 = 0.113$), the utility of super learning is still apparent. In Chap. 3, larger improvements in cross-validated MSE were seen in other real data sets. The minimal improvement of the super learner in this analysis is not unexpected since the outcome is rare in the population of interest. This can be understood intuitively since any large improvement in predicting death by an algorithm among "case" subjects is averaged over the entire sample.

It is not possible to know with certainty a priori which single algorithm will perform the best in any given data set. Even when the result is a negligible improvement relative to the best algorithms in the collection, the super learner provides a tool for researchers to run many algorithms and return a prediction function with the best cross-validated MSE, avoiding the need to commit to a single algorithm.

For example, even in this analysis, had the logistic regression with main terms and age covariate and gender covariate interactions for each covariate (glm.9) been the a priori selected single algorithm, with $R^2 = 0.060$, its performance is poor compared to that of the super learner. Several other algorithms were considerably worse thanglm.9 and also could have been the single a priori selected algorithm. In other words, the use of the super learner prevents poor a priori algorithm choices.

15.5 Notes and Further Reading

Prediction has been used most notably to generate tables for risk of heart disease (Kannel et al. 1976; Anderson et al. 1991; Ramsay et al. 1995, 1996; Wilson et al. 1998; Jackson 2000) and breast cancer (Gail et al. 1989; Costantino et al. 1999; Tyrer et al. 2004; Barlow et al. 2006). An existing method for prediction in parametric statistical models with nested case-control samples is intercept adjustment. The addition of $\log(P_{X,0}(\Delta = 1 \mid Y = 1)/P_{X,0}(\Delta = 1 \mid Y = 0))$, or equivalently $\log(q_0/(1 - q_0))$, to the intercept in a logistic regression yields the true logistic regression function $P_{X,0}(Y = 1 \mid W)$, assuming the statistical model is correctly specified. Here Δ denotes the indicator of inclusion in the nested case-control sample, and the value q_0 is the prevalence probability $P_{X,0}(Y = 1) = q_0$ (Anderson 1972;

Prentice and Breslow 1978; Greenland 1981; Wacholder 1996; Morise et al. 1996; Greenland 2004).

We introduced a more flexible method for prediction in two-stage nested case-control data. This method is an application of the general loss-based super learner, the appropriate loss function is selected. It corresponds with an inverse probability of missingness full-data loss function. The method involves observation weights $w_i = \Delta_i / P_n(\Delta_i = 1 \mid Y_i)$ to eliminate the bias of the sampling design, where these weights are determined by the inverse probability of missingness. For nested case-control studies, this is equalivalent to using case-control weights, with cases assigned the weight q_n (an estimate of q_0 obtained from the full cohort) and controls assigned a weight of $(1 - q_n)/J$, where J is the average number of controls per case. Thus the choice of loss function can also be presented as the case-control-weighted loss function presented in the preceding two chapters, van der Laan (2008a), and Rose and van der Laan (2008, 2009).

One might also be interested in the effect of each medical flag on mortality, controlling for all other medical flags. This is a variable-importance research question, one where we can use a TMLE. In a recent paper, Rose and van der Laan (2011) describe the TMLE for two-stage designs. We also refer readers to Appendix A.

Part V
RCTs with Survival Outcomes

Chapter 16
Super Learning for Right-Censored Data

Eric C. Polley, Mark J. van der Laan

The super learner was introduced in Chap. 3 as a loss-based estimator of a parameter of the data-generating distribution, defined as the minimizer of the expectation (risk) of a loss function over all candidate parameter values in the parameter space. This chapter demonstrates how the super learner framework can also be applied to estimate parameters such as conditional hazards or survival functions of a failure time, given a vector of baseline covariates, based on right-censored data. We strongly advise readers to familiarize themselves with the concepts presented in Chap. 3 before reading this chapter, as we assume the reader has a firm grasp of that material.

If the outcome of interest is time-to-event, then one is often interested in the survival function of the time-to-event. This allows one to answer questions such as, "What is the probability of having a recurrence of cancer within 5 years?" A survival function at a time point, such as 5 years, is defined as the probability that the survival time exceeds 5 years. Thus, the survival function is a monotone decreasing function in time, starting at 1 at time 0 ($t = 0$), and typically ending at 0 (assuming that every subject will eventually experience the event). Since survival functions will change as a function of characteristics of the subject, it is often of interest to understand the effect of treatment and baseline covariates on the conditional survival function at one particular time point, or on the whole conditional survival curve.

The hazard is defined as the instantaneous probability of the event occurring at time t, given the event has not occurred yet by time t. One inescapable feature of survival time data is that the time-to-event is almost always subject to right censoring: some subjects will drop out before the event can occur, or, at the endpoint of the study, a subject has not failed yet. The (conditional) hazard function provides the (conditional) survival function, and the conditional hazard can be estimated in the same manner as if there was no censoring. These two reasons provide an important motivation for the construction of estimators of the (conditional) hazard. As we will see, indeed, we can provide convenient loss functions for the hazard that naturally handle right censoring, without the requirement of incorporating an estimate of a censoring mechanism.

Since many target parameters, such as causal effects of a treatment on a survival time, are functions of the conditional hazard, the TMLE requires an initial estimator of the conditional hazard, and a corresponding targeted update of this conditional hazard, before mapping it into the desired target parameter. As a consequence, in order to obtain a TMLE of causal effects based on right-censored data structures, data-adaptive estimation of the conditional hazard is needed. In some applications, one might be interested in the density or hazard itself as well, as in this chapter.

In fact, the probability distribution of any longitudinal data structure can be expressed in terms of a product over time t of conditional probabilities of binary outcomes/indicators at time t, given a past string of events. The TMLE of a causal effect of a multiple-time-point intervention requires estimation of such conditional probabilities (for the nonintervention nodes of the SCM). Super learner for the conditional hazard presented here applies more generally to the estimation of such conditional probability functions for binary indicators. Longitudinal data are handled rigorously in Part VIII.

This provides more than enough motivation to devote a chapter to super learning of the conditional hazard in this book. As we learned in Chap. 3, the super learner requires defining a valid loss function, building a collection of candidate estimators, proposing a parametric family consisting of weighted combinations of the estimators in the collection, and computing the optimal weighted combination by minimizing the cross-validated risk of the loss function over all candidate weighted combinations of estimators.

16.1 Data Structure

Let T be the survival time and $W = (W_1, W_2, \ldots, W_p)$ a set of p baseline covariates. The full data structure is defined as $X = (T, W)$, and let $P_{X,0}$ denote its probability distribution known to belong to the statistical model $\mathcal{M}^F$. The survival time is possibly right censored by the censoring time C. The observed data structure is defined as

$$O = \left(W, \tilde{T} = \min(T, C), \Delta = \mathrm{I}(\tilde{T} = T)\right).$$

Let P_0 denote the true probability distribution of O. Note that the probability distribution of O is determined by the distribution $P_{X,0}$ of $X = (T, W)$ and the conditional distribution of C, given X.

We denote the conditional survival function of C by $G_0(t \mid X) = P_0(C > t \mid X)$ and its conditional density by $g_0(t \mid X) = P_0(C = t \mid X)$. We assume that the time scale is discretized and we denote the time points by $t = 1, \ldots, \tau$. Let $N(t) = I(\tilde{T} \leq t, \Delta = 1)$ and $A(t) = I(\tilde{T} \leq t, \Delta = 0)$ be the counting processes that indicate if a failure time event and censoring event is observed at time t, respectively. Note that $N(t)$ is a process that starts at 0 at time $t = 0$, and jumps to 1 at time $\tilde{T}$ if a failure is observed (i.e., if $\Delta = 1$). Similarly, $A(t)$ jumps to 1 at time $\tilde{T}$ if a censoring event is observed (i.e., if $\Delta = 0$).

The likelihood of the data can be represented as a product over time t of the conditional probability of events one observes at time t, conditional on all the data observed up till time t. Thus, such a likelihood involves conditional probabilities of observing a jump of N (or A) at time t, conditional on the history up till time t, which we often refer to as the parents of $N(t)$ (or parents of $A(t)$). We will denote such an indicator of N (or A) jumping from 0 to 1 at time t by $dN(t)$ (or $dA(t)$) and its parents by $Pa(N(t))$ (or $Pa(A(t))$).

Let $Q_{dN(t)}$ denote the conditional distribution of $dN(t)$, given its parents $Pa(N(t)) = (\bar{N}(t-1), \bar{A}(t-1), W)$, and let $g_{dA(t)}$ denote the conditional distribution of $dA(t)$, given its parents $Pa(A(t)) = (\bar{N}(t), \bar{A}(t-1), W)$. The true probability distribution of O factorizes as

$$P_0(O = o) = P_{W,0}(W) \prod_{t=1}^{\tau} Q_{dN(t),0}(dN(t) \mid Pa(N(t))) \prod_{t=1}^{\tau} g_{dA(t),0}(dA(t) \mid Pa(A(t))).$$

The conditional distribution $Q_{dN(t),0}$ of the binary indicator $dN(t)$ is determined by $P_0(dN(t) = 1 \mid Pa(N(t))) = E_0(dN(t) \mid Pa(N(t)))$.

In the counting process literature, for counting processes that jump in continuous time, one refers to the instantaneous conditional probabilities $E(dN(t) \mid Pa(N(t))$, conditional on the history right before $N(t)$, as an intensity. Therefore, we will refer to $E_0(dN(t) \mid Pa(N(t))$ as a discrete intensity, since we assumed that events only occur on a discrete time scale. Note that these discrete intensities equal zero if $Pa(N(t))$ imply that $N(t)$ cannot jump anymore, i.e., if $\tilde{T} < t$. Let $\bar{Q}_0(t \mid W) = E_0(dN(t) \mid W, \tilde{T} \geq t)$, and $\bar{g}_0(t \mid W) = E_0(dA(t) \mid N(t) = A(t-1) = 0, W)$ denote the discrete intensities (conditioning on histories for which the counting process is at risk of jumping) of these two counting processes $N(t)$ and $A(t)$.

The statistical model for P_0 is implied by the statistical model $\mathcal{M}^F$ and a statistical model $\mathcal{G}$ for g_0. We assume coarsening at random (CAR) for the conditional distribution of C, given $X = (T, W)$, which will be referred to as the censoring mechanism. CAR is implied by the assumption that C is independent of T, given W. We note that, under CAR, these discrete intensities equal the conditional hazard of T, given W, and C, given W, respectively:

$$\bar{Q}_0(t \mid W) = P_0(T = t \mid T \geq t, W),$$
$$\bar{g}_0(t \mid W) = P_0(C = t \mid C \geq t, W).$$

Thus, under CAR we can also refer to these intensities as conditional hazards.

16.2 Parameters of Interest

For the remainder of this chapter, we consider the case that prediction is the target parameter of interest, not a causal effect; thus we use Ψ notation to refer to this function. We consider two common parameter of interests for survival outcomes.

1. The first is a conditional expectation of a user-supplied function of T, given the baseline covariates, $\psi_0(W) = E_0(m(T) \mid W)$ for a user-supplied function $m(T)$. Here possible choices for $m(T)$ are given by $m(T) = T$, $m(T) = \log T$, and $m(T) = I(T > t_0)$ for some time point t_0. Since many distributions of a survival time T are skewed, and since T is often not observed in the tail of its distribution due to right censoring, it is often argued that the mean of T is not as much of interest as other location parameters such as the median of T or a truncated mean. A truncated mean can be obtained by defining $m(T)$ as a truncated version of T. One can also simply truncate T and focus on the mean of the truncated T. Since the density of a log-survival time T is often more symmetrically distributed, the mean of $\log T$ is often viewed as an interesting parameter, possibly transformed back to the T-scale. The choice $m(T) = I(T > t_0)$ is naturally of interest since it provides the conditional survival function.
2. The second parameter of interest we consider is the conditional hazard (or conditional density) $\psi_0(t \mid W) = \bar{Q}_0(t \mid W)$, even though its main application might be to map it into its corresponding survival function.

In both cases ψ_0 is a parameter of the full-data distribution $P_{X,0}$, and only through the Q_0-factor, so that $\Psi(P_0) = \Psi^F(Q_0)$. The parameter space for this parameter is implied by the full-data model $\mathcal{M}^F$: $\mathbf{\Psi} = \{\Psi(P) : P \in \mathcal{M}\} = \{\Psi^F(Q(P_X)) : P_X \in \mathcal{M}^F\}$.

16.3 Cross-Validation for Censored Data Structures

Estimator selection based on cross-validation for censored data structures is extensively examined in van der Laan and Dudoit (2003). Suppose the parameter ψ_0 of the full-data distribution can be defined as a minimizer of the expectation of a full-data loss function:

$$\psi_0 = \text{argmin}_{\psi} \int L(x, \psi)\, dP_{X,0}(x).$$

In order to apply loss-based cross-validation and, in particular, the loss-based super learner, we need to construct an observed data loss function $L(O, \psi)$ of the observed data structure O so that $E_0 L(O, \psi) = E_0 L(X, \psi)$.

If the parameter of interest is the conditional mean, $\psi_0 = E(m(T) \mid W)$, a commonly used loss function is the IPCW squared error loss function:

$$L(O, \psi) = \frac{\Delta}{\bar{G}_0(T \mid X)} \{m(T) - \psi(W)\}^2, \tag{16.1}$$

where $\bar{G}_0(T \mid W) = P_0(C > t \mid W)$ is the conditional survival function of censoring time C, given W. Since the censoring mechanism is often not known, $\bar{G}_0$ is an unknown nuisance parameter for the loss function. If the parameter of interest is the conditional hazard function, $\psi_0 = \bar{Q}_0(\cdot \mid W)$, we have the following two possible loss functions:

$$L_{loglik}(O, \psi) = \sum_t \mathrm{I}(\widetilde{T} \geq t) \log(\psi(t \mid W))^{dN(t)} \log(1 - \psi(t \mid W))^{1-dN(t)},$$

$$L_{L_2}(O, \psi) = \sum_t \mathrm{I}(\widetilde{T} \geq t) \{dN(t) - \psi(t \mid W)\}^2 .$$

In this case, neither loss function is indexed by an unknown nuisance parameter.

Given an observed data loss function, the cross-validation selector to select among candidate estimators $\hat{\Psi}_k$ of ψ_0, $k = 1, \ldots, K$, is defined as before in Chap. 3, with the only remark that, if the loss function depends on a nuisance parameter, then one needs to plug in an estimator of this nuisance parameter. If censoring is known to be independent, then one could estimate the marginal survivor function $\bar{G}_0(t) = P(C > t)$ with the Kaplan–Meier estimator defined as:

$$\bar{G}_{KM,n}(t) = \prod_{s \leq t} \left(1 - \frac{\sum_{i=1}^n I(\tilde{T}_i = s, \Delta_i = 0)}{\sum_{i=1}^n I(\tilde{T}_i \geq s)}\right).$$

If, on the other hand, such knowledge is not available, then one can use a machine learning algorithm, such as a super learner, to estimate the conditional hazard $\bar{g}_0(t \mid W)$ of C, given W, using one of the two loss functions $L_{loglik}(O, \bar{g}_0)$ or $L_{L_2}(O, \bar{g}_0)$, to construct a data-adaptive estimator of $\bar{g}_0(t \mid W)$.

To construct the super learner to estimate our parameter of interest we require the following ingredients:

1. A collection of candidate estimators of the parameter of interest ψ_0,
2. A loss function $L(O, \psi)$,
3. A parametric statistical model for combining the estimators in the collection.

The candidate estimators are not restricted to being based on the loss function used in the cross-validation selector. However, for the cross-validation one wishes to use a loss function whose dissimilarity

$$d(\psi, \psi_0) = E_0 L(O, \psi) - E_0 L(O, \psi_0),$$

directly measures a discrepancy between the true target parameter ψ_0 and candidate ψ. For example, if one is concerned with estimation of the conditional survival function $\psi_0(W) = P_0(T > t_0 \mid W)$, then the IPCW loss function presented in (16.1) provides a more direct measure of fit of ψ_0 than the log-likelihood or squared error loss function for the conditional hazard, even though all three loss functions are valid loss functions.

This may seem like common sense, but researchers often use a hazard loss function when the interest is on the survival probability at a specific time point (e.g., 10-year survival). The loss function should be chosen with respect to the problem you are trying to solve.

The oracle inequality results for the cross-validation selector, and thereby for the super learner, assume the loss function is bounded. Therefore, the parametric statistical model for combining the estimators in the collection needs to be chosen to maintain a bounded loss function among all candidates that can be constructed as weighted combinations of the candidate estimators. We propose constraints on the parametric statistical model for combining the algorithms to maintain a bounded loss function.

For the L_2 loss function, we can use as parametric statistical model

$$\left\{\sum_k \alpha_k \psi_k : \sum_k \alpha_k = 1, \alpha_k \geq 0\right\}.$$

Here we constrained the space for the weight vector α to be $\alpha_k \geq 0$ and $\sum_k \alpha_k = 1$. In this case, it is easy to show that the loss function is uniformly bounded by the bound on the parameter space $\boldsymbol{\Psi}$ and the number of time points τ.

For the log-likelihood loss function we propose using the logit link function:

$$g(x) = \text{logit}(x) = \log\left(\frac{x}{1-x}\right),$$

using the convex combination on the logit scale, and then transforming it back into a probability with the inverse logit function. That is, given a candidate estimator of the conditional hazard, $\psi_{k,n}$, we transform it into

$$g(\psi_{k,n}) = \log \frac{\psi_{k,n}}{1-\psi_{k,n}},$$

and we consider combinations $\sum_k \alpha_k g(\psi_{k,n})$, which corresponds with a hazard estimator $g^{-1}(\sum_k \alpha_k g(\psi_{k,n}))$. The advantage of this approach is that the logit of hazards, $g(\psi_{k,n})$, are not subject to any constraint, so that the α-vector does not need to be constrained to positive weights. In addition, it has numeric advantages since the minimizer of the cross-validated risk is now an interior point.

In our implementation of the super learner, enforcing $\sum_k \alpha_k = 1$ and $\alpha_k \geq 0$ is an option. In this case, the parametric family for combining the candidate estimators is given by:

$$\left\{g^{-1}\left(\sum_k \alpha_k g(\psi_k)\right) : \quad \text{with} \sum_k \alpha_k = 1 \ \& \ \alpha_k \geq 0 \, \forall k\right\}.$$

A problem occurs when the conditional hazard ψ_k approaches either 0 or 1, in which case logit(ψ) approaches $\pm\infty$. To avoid this problem, we will use the symmetric truncated logit link,

$$g^*(x, c) = \begin{cases} g(c) & \text{if } x < c, \\ g(x) & \text{if } c \leq x \leq 1 - c, \\ g(1 - c) & \text{if } x > 1 - c, \end{cases}$$

for a small constant c. It follows that, as long as c is selected such that $g(1-c) < M/\tau$, the loss will be bounded by M. In current implementations, we enforce small levels of truncations such as $c = 0.01$. It is of interest for future research to investigate data-adaptive strategies for setting such global bounds on the loss function.

16.4 Super Learner for Hazard Estimation in Lung Cancer

In this censored-data demonstration, we focus on the case where the full-data statistical model is nonparametric, and estimate the conditional hazard. We examined the North Central Cancer Treatment Group lung cancer data set (Loprinzi et al. 1994), available in the survival package in R (Therneau and Lumley 2009).

The data set contains the survival time (in days) for 228 patients with advanced lung cancer. In addition to the survival time, information on the patient's age, sex, and three performance scores was included. The parameter of interest was the hazard function given the patient's age, sex, and performance scores. Five patients were removed from the analysis set due to incomplete information on the covariates. With the 223 patients in the analysis set, 63 were right censored and 160 had observed death times. We used the squared error loss function on the hazard for the super learner:

$$L_{L_2}(O, \psi) = \sum_t \mathrm{I}\left(\widetilde{T} \geq t\right) \{dN(t) - \psi(W)\}^2 .$$

The first step was to convert the right-censored data structure $(W, \Delta, \tilde{T})$ into a longitudinal data structure collecting at time t the change in counting processes, $dN(t)$, $dA(t)$: $(W, (dN(t), dA(t) : t))$. A grid of 30 time points was created using the quantiles of the observed death times, and then $dN(t)$ was defined as the number of observed failures in the window containing t, and, similarly, $dA(t)$ was defined as the number of observed censoring events in this window.

The collection of estimators consisted of logistic regression, random forests, generalized additive models (gam), polyclass, deletion/substitution/addition algorithm (DSA), neural networks (nnet) , and a null statistical model using only time and no covariates. For most hazard estimation problems, time is one of the most important variables in the estimator. We considered the variable time with a few approaches. One was to use an indicator for each time point. Logistic regression in a parametric statistical model with an indicator for each time point will approximate the Cox proportional hazards model if one uses an increasingly finer grid of time points. Another approach added an additional step of smoothing in time using a generalized additive statistical model. These estimators in the collection involved a two-stage estimation procedure.

In the first step, one of the algorithms is applied to fit the hazard as a function of time t and covariates W. This results in an estimator $\bar{Q}^0_{k,n}(t \mid W)$ for the kth estimator of the conditional hazard $\bar{Q}_0(t \mid W)$. Subsequently, these predicted probabilities $\bar{Q}^0_{k,n}(t \mid W)$ were used as an offset in a generalized additive logistic regression statistical model with m degrees of freedom for time:

$$\text{logit}P(dN(t) \mid \tilde{T} \geq t, W) = \bar{Q}_{k,n}(t \mid W) + s(t, m).$$

The degrees-of-freedom tuning parameter m for the smoothing spline $s(t, m)$ is not known a priori, but different values of m simply represent different estimators in the collection of algorithms defining the super learner. The estimators in the super learner collection of algorithms are the candidate estimators for binary outcome repeated measures regression, coupled with the generalized additive statistical models estimator for the time trend.

Table 16.1 contains a list of the estimators used in the super learner. The first column is the algorithm used for the covariates (including time t as one covariate), and the second column indicates if any additional step was taken to estimate the effect of time. For the sake of comparison, we also report the results for a regression fit in a parametric statistical model for the conditional hazard according to the Weibull proportional hazards model:

$$P(T = t \mid T \geq t, W) = \alpha t^{\alpha-1} \exp(\beta^\top W).$$

This parametric model assumes, in particular, that the hazard function is monotone in time t, and it includes the exponential distribution (i.e., constant hazard) as a special case.

The honest cross-validated risks are provided for each of the estimators in the collection of algorithms, and for the super learner algorithms. The reported risk of the Weibull estimator of the hazard was also cross-validated. An estimate of the standard error of this honest V-fold cross-validated risk is also provided, based on the variance estimator

$$\frac{1}{n^2} \sum_{v=1}^{V} \sum_{i \in \text{Val}(v)} \left(L(O_i, \hat{\Psi}(P_{n,\text{Tr}(v)}) - \bar{L} \right)^2,$$

where Val(v) and Tr(v) are a partition of $\{1, \ldots, n\}$ indicating the observations in the validation sample and training sample, respectively, for the vth split, and

$$\bar{L} = \frac{1}{n} \sum_{v} \sum_{i \in \text{Val}(v)} L(O_i, \hat{\Psi}(P_{n,\text{Tr}(v)})$$

Table 16.1 Honest 10-fold cross-validated risk estimates for the super learner, each algorithm in the collection, and the Weibull proportional hazards statistical model. All algorithms included time as a covariate. The second column (Time) denotes if any additional smoothing for time was part of the given estimator, and the value for the degrees of freedom, if used

Algorithm	Time	CV Risk	SE
Super learner		0.6548	0.0258
Discrete SL		0.6589	0.0261
glm	No smoothing	0.6534	0.0260
glm	df = 1	0.6534	0.0260
glm	df = 2	0.6541	0.0260
glm	df = 3	0.6548	0.0261
glm	df = 4	0.6556	0.0261
glm	df = 5	0.6564	0.0261
glm	Indicator	0.6700	0.0266
glm (2-way interactions)	df = 5	0.6569	0.0261
randomForest	No smoothing	0.7628	0.0313
randomForest	df = 2	1.0323	0.0607
randomForest	df = 3	1.0364	0.0627
randomForest	df = 4	1.0483	0.0628
randomForest	df = 5	1.0362	0.0608
gam	df = 2	0.6558	0.0260
gam	df = 3	0.6563	0.0260
gam	df = 4	0.6570	0.0261
gam	df = 5	0.6577	0.0261
gam(df = 2)	No smoothing	0.6554	0.0260
gam(df = 3)	No smoothing	0.6579	0.0261
gam(df = 4)	No smoothing	0.6619	0.0263
gam(df = 5)	No smoothing	0.6554	0.0260
gam (only time, df = 3)	No smoothing	0.6548	0.0257
gam (only time, df = 4)	No smoothing	0.6556	0.0257
gam (only time, df = 5)	No smoothing	0.6541	0.0256
polyclass	No smoothing	0.6570	0.0258
DSA	No smoothing	0.6671	0.0270
DSA	df = 5	0.6669	0.0269
nnet	No smoothing	0.7175	0.0302
Weibull PH model		0.7131	0.0300

denotes the cross-validated risk of the estimator $\hat{\Psi}$ (Dudoit and van der Laan 2005, Theorem 3).

The estimated coefficients for the super learner were

$$\begin{aligned}\Psi_{SL,n} &= 0.182\Psi_{n,\text{glm, no}} + 0.182\Psi_{n,\text{gam only time,df = 5}}\\ &\quad +0.581\Psi_{n,\text{polyclass, no}} + 0.056\Psi_{n,\text{glm 2-way, df = 5}},\end{aligned}$$

where $\Psi_{n,a,b}$ represents the fit of algorithm a using the smoothing in time method b. The only estimators to receive nonzero weight in the final super learner fit were logistic regression using main terms and no smoothing, a gam statistical model using only time and 5 degrees of freedom, polyclass with no additional smoothing, and a logistic regression in a parametric statistical model with all two-way interaction (including time) combined with smoothing time using df = 5. Thus, of the 29 estimators in the library, only 4 received a nonzero weight.

16.5 Notes and Further Reading

Selection among candidate estimators of a target parameter for survival outcomes has received less attention compared to estimator selection for continuous and categorical (noncensored) outcomes. Notable examples of estimator selection for censored data include the cross-validation selector based on a double robust IPCW full-data loss function (van der Laan and Dudoit 2003). In van der Laan et al. (2004), the cross-validation selector based on the IPCW loss function is analyzed in detail.

A variety of methods have been proposed for nonparametric estimation of a conditional hazard based on right-censored data, involving likelihood-based cross-validation or penalized log-likelihood [e.g., LASSO in Tibshirani (1997) and Zhang and Lu (2007), or other penalties such as Akaike's information criterion in Akaike (1973)] to select fine-tuning parameters. For example, Hastie and Tibshirani (1990) proposed using additive Cox proportional hazards models with smoothing splines for the covariates. Kooperberg et al. (1995) similarly used polynomial splines to approximate the conditional hazard. Tree-based approximations of the conditional hazard have also been proposed, often referred to as survival trees or survival forests (LeBlanc and Crowley 1992; Segal 1988; Hothorn et al. 2006; Ishwaran et al. 2008). Cross-validated Cox regression is described in the context of penalized partial likelihoods in van Houwelingen et al. (2006). All these algorithms can be included in the library of the super learner to maximize its performance.

Chapter 17
RCTs with Time-to-Event Outcomes

Kelly L. Moore, Mark J. van der Laan

RCTs are often designed with the goal of investigating a causal effect of a new treatment drug vs. the standard of care on a time-to-event outcome. Possible outcomes are time to death, time to virologic failure, and time to recurrence of cancer. The data collected on a subject accumulates over time until the minimum of the time of analysis (end of study), the time the subject drops out of the study, or until the event of interest is observed. Typically, for a large proportion of the subjects recruited into the trial, the subject is right censored before the event of interest is observed, i.e., the time of analysis or the time the subject drops out of the study occurs before the time until the event of interest. The dropout time of the subject can be related to the actual time to failure one would have observed if the person had not dropped out prematurely. In this case, the standard unadjusted estimator of a causal effect of treatment on a survival time, such as the difference of the treatment-specific Kaplan–Meier survival curves at a particular point in time, is not only inefficient by not utilizing the available covariate information, but it is also biased due to informative dropout.

The TMLE can be applied to the estimation of the causal effect of the treatment on a survival outcome in an RCT, incorporating covariates for the purpose of more efficient estimation, without the risk of inducing bias, and reducing bias due to informative dropout. In this chapter we only consider the utilization of the baseline covariates. We present the TMLE of a causal effect of treatment on survival, as well as a simulation study. In the next chapter, we will present an RCT data analysis, including more complicated target parameters incorporating effect modification, but based on the same right-censored data structure. This next data application chapter also provides a detailed discussion of the flaws of current practice based on applications of Cox proportional hazards statistical models. We also encourage readers to study the previous chapter, which introduces many topics related to right censoring and time-to-event data.

17.1 Data, Likelihood, and Model

We assume that in the study protocol, each patient is monitored at K clinical visits. At each visit, an outcome is evaluated as having occurred or not occurred. Let T represent the first visit at which the event was reported and thus can take values $\{1, ..., \tau\}$. The censoring time C is the first visit when the subject is no longer enrolled in the study. Let $A \in \{0, 1\}$ represent the treatment assignment at baseline and W represent a vector of baseline covariates. The observed data structure is: $O = (W, A, \tilde{T}, \Delta) \sim P_0$, where $\tilde{T} = \min(T, C)$, $\Delta = I(T \leq C)$ is the indicator that subject was not censored, and P_0 denotes the true probability distribution of O.

Let $N(t) = I(\tilde{T} \leq t, \Delta = 1)$ and $A(t) = I(\tilde{T} \leq t, \Delta = 0)$ denote the indicators that jumps at an observed failure time and observed censoring time, respectively. We can represent O as the following longitudinal data structure: $O = (W, A, (N(t), A(t) : t = 1, \ldots, K))$. The likelihood of O can be represented accordingly, and is given by

$$\begin{aligned} P_0(O) &= Q_{W,0}(W) g_{A,0}(A \mid W) \\ &\quad \times \prod_{t=1}^{\tau} Q_{dN(t),0}(dN(t) \mid Pa(dN(t))) \prod_{t=1}^{\tau} g_{dA(t),0}(dA(t) \mid Pa(A(t))), \end{aligned}$$

where $Pa(dN(t)) = (W, A, \bar{N}(t-1), \bar{A}(t-1))$ denotes the history available before $dN(t)$ is realized, and similarly, $Pa(A(t)) = (W, A, \bar{N}(t), \bar{A}(t-1))$ denotes the parent set for the censoring indicator $A(t)$. Here $Q_{dN(t),0}$ and $g_{A(t),0}$ denote the conditional probability distributions of the binary indicators $dN(t)$ and $dA(t)$, respectively.

The intensity of the counting process $N()$ is defined as $E_0(dN(t) \mid Pa(dN(t)))$, and can be represented as

$$E_0(dN(t) \mid Pa(dN(t)) = I(\tilde{T} \geq t)\bar{Q}_0(t \mid A, W),$$

where $\bar{Q}_0(t \mid A, W) = E_0(dN(t) \mid \tilde{T} \geq t, A, W)$. Similarly, the intensity of $A(t)$, $E_0(dA(t) \mid Pa(dA(t)))$, can be represented as

$$E_0(dA(t) \mid Pa(dA(t))) = I(A(t-1) = 0, N(t) = 0)\bar{g}_0(t \mid A, W),$$

where $\bar{g}_0(t \mid A, W) = E_0(dA(t) \mid N(t) = A(t-1) = 0, W, A)$. Thus, $Q_{dN(t),0}$ and $g_{A(t),0}$ are identified by $\bar{Q}_0(t \mid A, W)$ and $\bar{g}_0(t \mid A, W)$, respectively. To conclude, the likelihood of O is parameterized by the marginal distribution of W, the treatment mechanism $g_{A,0}$, the conditional probabilities $\bar{Q}_0$ for the binary indicator $dN(t)$, and censoring mechanism $g_{A(t),0}$. Let $Q_0 = (Q_{W,0}, \bar{Q}_0)$.

The statistical model for P_0 is defined by possible knowledge of the censoring mechanism $g_{A(t),0}$, a known treatment mechanism $g_{A,0}$, and a nonparametric statistical model for $Q_0 = (Q_{W,0}, \bar{Q}_0)$. We assume an SCM:

$$\begin{aligned} W &= f_W(U_W), \\ A &= f_A(W, U_A), \end{aligned}$$

$$dN(t) = f_{dN(t)}(Pa(dN(t)), U_{dN(t)}), t = 1, \ldots, K,$$
$$dA(t) = f_{dA(t)}(Pa(dA(t)), U_{dA(t)}), t = 1, \ldots, K.$$

This SCM allows us to define counterfactual failure times $T_a = T_{a,\bar{A}=\bar{0}}$ corresponding with the intervention $A = a$ and $A(t) = 0$ for all $t = 1, \ldots, \tau$. Thus T_1 represent a patient's time to the occurrence of the failure event had the patient, possibly contrary to fact, been assigned to the treatment group, and was also not right censored. Let T_0 likewise represent the time to the occurrence of the event had the patient been assigned to the control group, also not right censored.

17.2 Causal Quantity, Identifiability, and Statistical Parameter

We can then define our causal effect of treatment on survival at time t_0 as

$$\psi_0^F = P_0(T_1 > t_0) - P_0(T_0 > t_0) \equiv S_1(t_0) - S_0(t_0).$$

We assume that treatment A is randomized in the sense that A is conditionally independent of (T_0, T_1), given W, and that $\min_a g_{A,0}(a \mid W) > 0$ a.e., which is true in an RCT. In addition, we assume that for each $t = 1, \ldots, \tau$, the censoring indicator $A(t)$ is conditionally independent of (T_0, T_1), given $Pa(A(t))$ (e.g., for each t, the unobserved exogenous error $U_{dA(t)}$ is independent of the exogenous errors $(U_{dN(s)} : s > t)$), and the following positivity assumption holds:

$$\bar{G}_0(t_0 \mid A, W) \equiv \prod_{t=1}^{t_0} (1 - \bar{g}_0(t \mid A, W)) > 0 \text{ a.e.}$$

Under these assumptions, it follows that the causal effect is identified from the true observed data distribution P_0:

$$\psi_0^F = \Psi(Q_0) \equiv E_{W,0}[S_0(t_0 \mid A = 1, W) - S_0(t_0 \mid A = 0, W)],$$

where $S_0(t_0 \mid A, W) = P_0(T > t_0 \mid A, W)$ is the conditional survival function of T, given A, W. The latter conditional survival function $S_0(t_0 \mid A, W)$ is identified by the conditional hazard $\bar{Q}_0(t \mid A, W) = P_0(T = t \mid T \geq t, A, W)$ through the product-integral relation between a survival function and a hazard:

$$S_0(t_0 \mid A, W) = \prod_{t=1}^{t_0} (1 - \bar{Q}_0(t \mid A, W)).$$

Here we used that under the stated sequential independence assumption on the censoring indicators, the conditional hazard of T, given (A, W), is indeed given by $\bar{Q}_0$.

Let $\Psi_a(P_0) = S_a(t_0)$ denote the target parameters of P_0 that map into the desired treatment-specific survival function $S_a(t_0)$, indexed by treatment group $a \in \{0, 1\}$.

The additive causal effect on survival at t_0 is thus given by

$$\Psi(P_0) = \Psi_1(P_0) - \Psi_0(P_0) = S_1(t_0) - S_0(t_0).$$

Similarly, the causal relative risk at t_0 is given by

$$\frac{S_1(t_0)}{S_0(t_0)},$$

and the causal odds ratio at t_0 is given by

$$\frac{S_1(t_0)(1 - S_0(t_0))}{S_0(t_0)(1 - S_1(t_0))},$$

where these parameters are all defined as simple functions of $\Psi_a(P_0)$. We will present the TMLE targeting both $(S_0(t_0), S_1(t_0))$, so that this also yields the TMLE procedure for these other causal measures of the treatment effect on survival.

Positivity

It is important to note that the TMLE, like other estimators, relies on the assumption that each subject has a positive probability of being observed (i.e., not censored) up till time t_0+. More formally, this assumption is $\bar{G}(t_0 \mid A, W) > 0$ a.e. This identifiability assumption for the target parameter $S_1(t_0) - S_0(t_0)$ has been addressed as an important assumption for right-censored data (Robins and Rotnitzky 1992). One is alerted to such violations by observing very small probabilities of remaining uncensored based on the estimated censoring mechanism, i.e., there are patients with a probability of censoring of almost one given their observed past at a time $t < t_0$. We recommend the parametric bootstrap method for assessing bias in the estimator due to practical or theoretical violation of the positivity assumption, as presented in Chap. 10.

17.3 Efficient Influence Curve

The efficient influence curve of $\Psi_a : \mathcal{M} \to \mathbb{R}$ at P_0, for any model on the treatment mechanism and censoring mechanism, is given by

$$D_a^*(P_0) = \sum_{t=1}^{T} I(\tilde{T} \geq t) H_a^*(t, A, W)(dN(t) - \bar{Q}_0(t \mid A, W)) \\ + S_0(t_0 \mid A = 1, W) - S_0(t_0 \mid A = 0, W) - \Psi_a(P_0),$$

where, for $a \in \{0, 1\}$,

$$H_a^*(t, A, W) = -\left(\frac{I(A = a)}{g_{A,0}(a \mid W)\bar{G}_0(t_- \mid A = a, W)}\right)\left(\frac{S_0(t_0 \mid A = a, W)}{S_0(t \mid A = a, W)}\right) I(t \leq t_0).$$

Note that the efficient influence curve for parameters that are a function of $S_1(t_0)$ and $S_0(t_0)$ can be obtained by application of the δ-method to the efficient influence curves D_1^* and D_0^*. For example, the efficient influence curve for the parameter $\Psi(P_0) = S_1(t_0) - S_0(t_0)$ is given by $D_1^* - D_0^*$.

This formula for the efficient influence curve is derived in van der Laan and Rubin (2007) and Moore and van der Laan (2009a). We also refer readers to Appendix A, and Chapter 3 in van der Laan and Robins (2003). The general formula for this time-dependent covariate $H_0^*(t, A, W)$ to update an initial hazard fit was provided in van der Laan and Rubin (2007) and is given by

$$H^*(t, A, W) = \frac{D^{FULL}(A, W, t \mid P_0) - E_{P_0}[D^{FULL}(A, W, T \mid P_0) \mid A, W, T > t)]}{\bar{G}_0(t_0 \mid A, W)},$$

where D^{FULL} is the efficient influence curve of the parameter of interest in the nonparametric model for the full-data structure (W, A, T) in which there is no right censoring. For example, the full-data estimating function for $\Psi_1(P_0)(t_0)$ and $\Psi_0(P_0)(t_0)$ is given by $I(T_1 > t_0) - S_1(t_0)$ and $I(T_0 > t_0) - S_0(t_0)$. Substitution of this full-data estimating function for D^{FULL} in the general formula yields the expression above.

17.4 TMLE of Additive Effect on Survival at a Fixed End Point

The first step of the TMLE involves determining an initial estimator P_n^0 of the P_0 of O, identified by an estimator $\bar{Q}_n^0(t \mid A, W)$, an estimator $g_{A,n}(A \mid W)$ of the treatment mechanism, an estimator $\bar{g}_n(t \mid A, W)$ of the censoring mechanism, and the empirical probability distribution $Q_{W,n}$ of $W_1, ..., W_n$. The second step involves defining a loss function $L(P)$, and a fluctuation parametric working model $P_n^0(\epsilon)$ whose score (with respect to the loss function) at $\epsilon = 0$ equals the efficient influence curve $D_a^*(P_n^0)$ of the target parameter $\Psi_a(Q_0)$. As loss function we select the log-likelihood loss function $-\log P$. We recommend the use of super learning in the estimator $\bar{Q}_n(t \mid A, W)$ of the hazard $\bar{Q}_0(t \mid A, W)$. The marginal distribution of W is estimated with the empirical probability distribution of $W_1, \ldots, W_n$.

In order to fluctuate $\bar{Q}_n^0$, we will use as fluctuation parametric working model

$$\text{logit}\bar{Q}_n^0(\epsilon)(t \mid A, W) = \text{logit}\ \bar{Q}_n^0(t \mid A, W) + \epsilon H_{a,n}^*(t, A, W),$$

where the estimated time-dependent clever covariate is given by

$$H_{a,n}^*(t, A, W) = \left(\frac{I(A = a)}{g_{A,n}(a \mid W)\bar{G}_n(t_0 \mid A = a, W)}\right)\left(\frac{S_n^0(t_0 \mid A = a, W)}{S_n^0(t \mid A = a, W)}\right) I(t \leq t_0).$$

In addition, let $Q_{W,n}(\epsilon) = (1 + \epsilon Q^0_{W,n}) D_2(Q^0_n)$ be a parametric working fluctuation model with score at $\epsilon = 0$ equal to $D_2(Q^0_n) = S^0_n(t_0 \mid 1, W) - S^0_n(t_0 \mid 0, W) - \Psi_a(Q^0_n)$. The corresponding fluctuation parametric working model for P^0_n is given by

$$P^0_n(\epsilon)(O) = Q^0_{W,n}(\epsilon_1)(W) g_{A,n}(A \mid W) \times \prod_t g_{A(t),n}(A(t) \mid Pa(A(t))) \prod_t Q^0_{dN(t),n}(\epsilon_2)(dN(t) \mid Pa(dN(t))),$$

where

$$\{Q^0_{dN(t),n}(\epsilon_2) : \epsilon_2\}$$

is the fluctuation working model implied by the fluctuation model $\{\bar{Q}^0_n(\epsilon) : \epsilon\}$ through the hazard fit $\bar{Q}^0_n$.

The TMLE procedure is now defined. One computes the maximum likelihood estimator $\epsilon_n = (\epsilon_{1,n}, \epsilon_{2,n})$, which maximizes $\epsilon \rightarrow P_n \log P^0_n(\epsilon)$. Since the empirical distribution of W is a nonparametric maximum likelihood estimator, it follows that $\epsilon_{1,n} = 0$. The maximum likelihood estimator $\epsilon_{2,n}$ can be estimated with univariate logistic regression software, using $\bar{Q}^0_n$ as an offset, applied to a pooled repeated measures sample in which each subject contributes a line of data for each time point t with $t \leq \tilde{T}$. The univariate logistic regression software can be invoked simply ignoring the repeated measures structure of the data. This now defines an updated estimator $P^1_n = P^0_n(\epsilon_n)$, defined by the update $Q^1_n = Q^0_n(\epsilon_n)$ of Q^0_n.

The above steps for evaluating ϵ_n, and thereby obtaining the updated hazard fit $\bar{Q}^1_n(t \mid A, W)$, correspond with a single iteration of the targeted maximum likelihood algorithm. In the second iteration, the updated $\bar{Q}^1_n(t \mid A, W)$ now plays the role of the initial fit, and the clever time-dependent covariate $H^*_a(t, A, W)$ is then reevaluated with the updated $S^1_n(t \mid A, W)$ based on $\bar{Q}^1_n(t \mid A, W)$, and ϵ_n is estimated again.

This updating process for $\bar{Q}_n$ is iterated until $\epsilon_{2,n} \approx 0$; let's denote its limit by $\bar{Q}^*_n$. The latter represents the TMLE of the conditional hazard $\bar{Q}_0$. Let $Q^*_n = (Q_{W,n}, \bar{Q}^*_n)$ be the corresponding TMLE of Q_0, and P^*_n is defined as the updated data-generating distribution corresponding with Q^*_n and the initial (nonupdated) estimator $g_n = (g_{A,n}, \bar{g}_n)$ of the treatment mechanism and right-censoring mechanism. The TMLE of $\psi_{a,0} = S_a(t_0)$ is the corresponding substitution estimator

$$\psi^*_{a,n} = \Psi_a(P^*_n) = \Psi_a(Q^*_n) = \frac{1}{n} \sum_{i=1}^{n} S^*_n(t_0 \mid A = a, W_i).$$

The TMLE can now be implemented separately for each treatment group $a \in \{0, 1\}$. The TMLE of the bivariate parameter $(S_0(t_0), S_1(t_0))$ follows the same algorithm as described above for $S_a(t_0)$, but one now adds both time-dependent clever covariates $H^*_{0,n}$ and $H^*_{1,n}$ to the logistic regression working model for fluctuating $\bar{Q}^0_n$:

$$\text{logit}(\bar{Q}^0_n(\epsilon_2)(t \mid A, W)) = \text{logit}\bar{Q}^0_n(t \mid A, W) + \epsilon_{2,1} H^*_{1,n}(t, A, W) + \epsilon_{2,0} H^*_{0,n}(t, A, W).$$

The fluctuation fit $\epsilon_{2,n} = \{\epsilon_{2,1,n}, \epsilon_{2,0,n}\}$ is now obtained by fitting a logistic regression in the covariates logit$\bar{Q}^0_n(t \mid A, W)$, $H^*_{1,t_0}(t, A, W)$ and $H^*_{0,t_0}(t, A, W)$, where the coefficient in front of logit$\bar{Q}^0_n$ is fixed at one, and the intercept is set to zero. Again, the updating of $Q_{W,n}$ does not occur. This TMLE $Q^*_n = (Q_{W,n}, \bar{Q}^*_n)$, whose hazard fit $\bar{Q}^*_n$ is now targeted to both treatment-specific survival functions, results in targeted maximum likelihood substitution estimators for any function of $(S_1(t_0), S_0(t_0))$.

For example, the TMLE of $\psi_0 = S_1(t_0) - S_0(t_0)$ is defined as the substitution estimator

$$\psi^*_n = \Psi(Q^*_n) = \frac{1}{n} \sum_{i=1}^{n} [S^*_n(t_0 \mid 1, W_i)) - S^*_n(t_0 \mid 0, W_i)] .$$

One can also target the TMLE directly toward the desired function $g(S_0(t_0), S_1(t_0))$ of $(S_0(t_0), S_1(t_0))$ by adding a single time-dependent clever covariate defined by

$$H^* = \frac{d}{dS_0(t_0)} g(S_0(t_0), S_1(t_0)) H^*_0 + \frac{d}{dS_1(t_0)} g(S_0(t_0), S_1(t_0)) H^*_1.$$

All three types of TMLEs of $S_1(t_0) - S_0(t_0)$ [target $S_a(t_0)$ separately, target both $(S_0(t_0), S_1(t_0))$, and target $S_1(t_0) - S_0(t_0)$] are double robust and asymptotically efficient, as stated below.

17.5 Statistical Properties

Consider the parameter $\Psi(Q_0)$. The targeted maximum likelihood estimate $P^*_n \in \mathcal{M}$ of P_0 solves the efficient influence curve estimating equation, given by

$$\sum_{i=1}^{n} D^*(g_n, Q^*_n, \Psi(Q^*_n))(O_i) = 0,$$

which is the optimal estimating equation for the parameter of interest. It has been shown that $E_0 D^*(g, Q, \Psi(Q_0)) = 0$ if either the conditional hazard $\bar{Q}$ and marginal Q_W is correctly specified, or the treatment g_A and censoring mechanism $\bar{g}$ is correctly specified: (1) $Q_W = Q_{W,0}$, $\bar{Q} = \bar{Q}_0$ or (2) $g = g_0$ (Moore and van der Laan 2009a). Since the treatment mechanism is known in an RCT and the marginal distribution of W is consistently estimated with the empirical distribution, the consistency of the TMLE $\psi^*_n(t_0)$ of $\Psi(Q_0)$ in an RCT relies only on consistent estimation of either the censoring survival function $\bar{G}_0(\cdot \mid A, W)$ or the conditional survivor function $S_0(\cdot \mid A, W)$. In particular, when there is no right censoring or censoring is independent so that $\bar{G}_0(t \mid A, W) = \bar{G}_0(t \mid A)$ can be consistently estimated with the Kaplan–Meier estimator, the TMLE ψ^*_n is consistent, even when the estimator $S^*_n(\cdot \mid A, W)$ of $S_0(\cdot \mid A, W)$ is inconsistent (e.g., if it relies on a misspecified statistical model).

17.6 Variance Estimator

Let P_n^* represent the TMLE of P_0 and $IC_n = D^*(P_n^*)$ be the corresponding estimate of the efficient influence curve. Under the assumption that the censoring mechanism is consistently estimated, one can conservatively estimate the asymptotic variance of $\sqrt{n}(\psi_n^* - \psi_0)$ with $\sigma_n^2 = 1/n \sum_{i=1}^n IC_n^2(O_i)$. In this case, the true influence curve of ψ_n^* is given by $D^*(Q^*, g_0, \psi_0)$ minus its projection onto the tangent space of the model used for g_0. Given a specified model for g_0, this influence curve can be explicitly determined as well. The bootstrap provides an alternative method for estimating the variance of the TMLE.

17.7 Simulations

Data were simulated to mimic an RCT in which the goal was to determine the effectiveness of a new drug in comparison to the current standard of care on survival as measured by an occurrence of an event (e.g., particular marker falling below a given level) at 6 months into treatment. For each recruited subject, the probability of receiving the new treatment was 0.5. At baseline, two covariates were measured, and both are negatively correlated with survival time with a univariate correlation of around −0.5 and −0.6. For example, these two covariates might represent age in years and weight gain in the year prior to baseline. Specifically, 1000 samples of size 500 were generated based on the following data-generating distribution, where time is discrete and takes values $t \in \{1, ..., 9\}$:

$$\begin{aligned} P(A = 1) &= 0.5, \\ W_1 &\sim U(2, 6), \\ W_2 &\sim N(10, 10), \\ \bar{Q}_0(t \mid A, W) &= \frac{I(t < 9)}{1 + \exp(-(-8 - 0.75A + 0.3W_1^2 + 0.25W_2))} + I(t = 9), \end{aligned}$$

where $\bar{Q}_0(t \mid A, W)$ is the conditional hazard of the survival time.

Censoring times were generated according to two different mechanisms, which we will refer to as uninformative censoring and informative censoring, respectively. The two censoring mechanisms were set such that approx. 27% and 20% of the observations were censored, respectively.

Under the uninformative censoring mechanism, the hazard for censoring is given by $\lambda_C(t) = 0.15$. Under the informative censoring mechanism, the hazard for censoring depends on A and W_1, where the treated subjects ($A = 1$) had a much higher hazard of censoring for high levels of W_1 than the untreated subjects, whereas the untreated subjects had a much higher hazard for censoring than the treated subjects for low levels of W_1. Specifically, the hazard of censoring is defined as follows: $\lambda_C(t = 1 \mid A, W) = 0$, and, for $t \in 2, ..., 9$

$$\lambda_C(t \mid A, W_1) = \begin{cases} 0.25 \text{ if } W_1 > 4.5 \text{ and } A = 1, \\ 0.20 \text{ if } 4.5 \leq W_1 > 3.5 \text{ and } A = 1, \\ 0.05 \text{ if } 3.5 \leq W_1 > 2.5 \text{ and } A = 1, \\ \quad 0 \text{ if } W_1 > 3.5 \text{ and } A = 0, \\ 0.25 \text{ if } 3.5 \leq W_1 > 2.5 \text{ and } A = 0, \\ 0.05 \text{ if } W_1 \leq 2.5. \end{cases}$$

If censoring and failure times were the same, the subject was considered uncensored. The target parameter of interest was the difference $S_1(6) - S_0(6)$ in survival at $t_0 = 6$. The TMLE was applied with three types of initial estimator for the conditional hazard. The first estimator was fitted with a correctly specified logistic regression. The second estimator was fitted according to a misspecified logistic regression, by including only a main term for A and W_1. The third estimator was fitted according to a misspecified logistic regression that only included a main term for A and W_2. In the uninformative censoring mechanism simulation, the censoring mechanism was consistently estimated with the Kaplan–Meier estimator. In the informative censoring mechanism simulation, the censoring mechanism was consistently estimated with a logistic regression model. For comparison, these TMLEs were compared with the the unadjusted estimator of the treatment effect defined as the difference of the two treatment-specific Kaplan–Meier estimators at $t = 6$.

The estimators were compared using a relative efficiency (RE) measure based on the MSE, computed as the MSE of the Kaplan–Meier estimates divided by the MSE of the targeted maximum likelihood estimates. Thus a value greater than one indicates a gain in efficiency of the TMLE over the unadjusted estimator. In addition, we report the percent bias, proportion of rejected tests (PR) for testing the null hypothesis of no treatment effect, and the coverage of the 95% confidence intervals.

Table 17.1 Power and efficiency comparison of TMLE and Kaplan–Meier estimator of additive causal effect on survival. The initial estimator of the failure time hazard was based on a correctly specified logistic regression (TMLE_C), misspecified logistic regression that included only a main term for treatment and W_1 (TMLE_{M1}), and misspecified logistic regression that included only a main term for treatment and W_2 (TMLE_{M2}). KM is unadjusted Kaplan–Meier estimate

Uninformative censoring	% Bias	PR	95%	RE
KM	2	0.32	0.95	1.00
TMLE_C	1	0.75	0.94	2.82
TMLE_{M1}	3	0.44	0.95	1.36
TMLE_{M2}	2	0.40	0.94	1.27
Informative censoring	**% Bias**	**PR**	**95%**	**RE**
KM	24	0.47	0.93	1.00
TMLE_C	−3	0.72	0.94	2.94
TMLE_{M1}	−3	0.38	0.94	1.45
TMLE_{M2}	−2	0.37	0.94	1.31

Table 17.1 provides the results for the simulations. In the uninformative censoring simulation, the results show the expected gain in efficiency of the TMLE relative to the unbiased unadjusted estimator. When the initial hazard is consistently estimated, the gain in power for the targeted maximum likelihood estimate was as high as 75% − 32% = 43%. Although the gains are more modest when the initial hazard is misspecified, the gain in power was still 12% for the TMLE over the unadjusted estimator. The relative efficiency is 2.8 for the targeted maximum likelihood estimate using a consistently estimated hazard over the Kaplan–Meier-based estimator, demonstrating the reduction in variance due to the full utilization of the available covariates. In the informative censoring simulation, the unadjusted estimate is severely biased ($\approx$24%), whereas the targeted maximum likelihood estimate remains consistent. In such a setting, one must account for the informative censoring as the results from the unadjusted method are completely unreliable.

17.8 Discussion

The TMLE is a robust and efficient estimator of the causal effect of treatment on survival in RCTs. Under uninformative censoring, the validity of the TMLE in an RCT does not require any assumptions. The advantage of the TMLE relative to the unadjusted estimator in an RCT is twofold. The first is the potential efficiency gains over the unadjusted estimator due to utilization of covariates. The second is that the TMLE accounts for informative censoring and is thereby a less biased estimator than the unadjusted estimator.

The simulation results demonstrate the importance of the initial estimator of the failure time hazard, and that, for full utilization of available covariate information, data-adaptive machine learning algorithms should be applied as long as the algorithm is specified a priori. However, even misspecified parametric regression working models for the conditional hazard of the failure time result in gains in efficiency and power. The ideal approach includes an aggressive machine learning algorithm such as super learning to obtain an initial estimator of the conditional hazard of the failure time, and the subsequent targeted maximum likelihood bias reduction step based on a data-adaptive estimator of the censoring mechanism within a realistic model for the censoring mechanism. These two steps combined provide valid statistical inference for the treatment effect with potentially large gains in power and bias over a procedure that ignores covariates.

17.9 Notes and Further Reading

Portions of this chapter were adapted from Moore and van der Laan (2009c), and the TMLE we present is also discussed in Moore and van der Laan (2009a). A general approach to constructing locally efficient double robust estimators that are guaranteed to improve on the unadjusted estimator can be found in van der Laan and Robins (2003), which is based on the original estimating equation methodology (Robins 1993; Robins and Rotnitzky 1992; Rubin and van der Laan 2008), grounded in empirical efficiency maximization. This reference also provides an overview of the literature on development of estimators based on right-censored data structures. In particular, we refer to Hubbard et al. (1999), who provide and implement nonparametric locally efficient estimation of the treatment-specific survival distribution with right-censored data and covariates in observational studies based on estimating equation methodology.

Covariate adjustment with time-to-event outcomes using Cox proportional hazards statistical models (e.g., Hernández et al. 2006), analogous to logistic linear regression for fixed-endpoint outcomes, relies on parametric assumptions for asymptotic validity of the effect estimates. In addition, the method estimates a conditional (on covariates W) effect rather than a marginal effect on survival. Lu and Tsiatis (2008) demonstrated how the efficiency of the logrank test in an RCT can be improved with covariate adjustment based on estimating equation methodology. Their method, which does not make assumptions beyond those of the logrank test, is more efficient and was shown to increase power over the logrank test. A nonparametric method for a covariate-adjusted method that uses logrank or Wilcoxon scores was proposed in Tangen and Koch (1999) and explored via simulation studies in Jiang et al. (2008). Adjusting for covariates instead of using the logrank test, with respect to power, is also discussed in Akazawa et al. (1997).

Chapter 18
RCTs with Time-to-Event Outcomes and Effect Modification Parameters

Ori M. Stitelman, Victor De Gruttola, C. William Wester, Mark J. van der Laan

Current methods used to evaluate effect modification in time-to-event data, such as the Cox proportional hazards model or its discrete time analog the logistic failure time model, posit highly restrictive parametric statistical models and attempt to estimate parameters that are specific to the model proposed. These methods, as a result of their parametric nature, tend to be biased and force practitioners to estimate parameters that are convenient rather than parameters they are actually interested in estimating. The TMLE improves on the currently implemented methods in both robustness, its ability to provide unbiased estimates, and flexibility, allowing practitioners to estimate parameters that directly answer their question of interest.

We apply the methods presented in the previous chapter, as well as introduce two new parameters of interest designed to quantify effect modification, to the Tshepo study. The Tshepo study is an open-label, randomized, 3×2×2 factorial design HIV study conducted at Princess Marina Hospital in Gaborone, Botswana, to evaluate the efficacy, tolerability, and development of drug resistance to six different first-line combination antiretroviral treatment (cART) regimens. We focus on the effect of two nonnucleoside reverse transcriptase inhibitor (NNRTI)-based cART therapies to which subjects were randomized. The two therapies of interest are efavirenz (EFV) and nevirapine (NVP).

Three statistical questions are of interest:

1. Is there a causal effect of EFV vs. NVP on time to viral failure, death, or treatment modification, or some combination of the three?
2. Does baseline CD4 level modify the effect of EFV vs. NVP on time to viral failure, death, or treatment modification, or some combination of the three?
3. Does the effect of EFV vs. NVP on time to viral failure, death, or treatment modification, or some combination of the three differ by sex?

Wester et al. (2010) performed an analysis of the Tshepo study using Cox proportional hazards analysis to address statistical questions 1 and 3 above. They concluded that there was no significant difference by assigned NNRTI in time to virological failure. They also presented a slightly less than significant result that women receiving NVP-based cART tended to have higher virological failure rates than the EFV-treated women. Furthermore, they concluded that individuals treated with NVP had shorter times to treatment modification than individuals treated with EFV (this result was highly statistically significant). Using the TMLE, we will readdress these questions as well as explore question 2. The TMLE results will be compared to results from a Cox proportional hazards analysis, and the advantages of using TMLE will be illustrated. This data analysis was originally presented in Stitelman and van der Laan (2011b). We conclude with an appendix presenting extensions of TMLE incorporating time-dependent covariates.

18.1 Data Structure

Time-to-event data capture information about the amount of time, T, it takes for a subject to experience a particular event. Usually one is interested in assessing the effect of a particular treatment, A, on the amount of time, T, it takes for the event of interest to occur. For the analysis performed here we are only concerned with binary levels of treatment, $A \in \{0, 1\}$, and a vector of baseline covariates W. We assume T is discrete and takes on the values $\{1, \ldots, \tau\}$, where τ is the last possible time the subjects are monitored. In the case where T is not discrete, one may discretize time into fine enough cut points as to not lose any signal in the data. The censoring time, C, is the last time at which a subject is observed, which might be marked by the end of the study, or an earlier dropout.

The observed data consist of n i.i.d. replicates of $O = (W, A, \tilde{T}, \Delta)$, where $\tilde{T} = \min(T, C)$ and $\Delta = I(T \le C)$. Thus $\tilde{T}$ is the last time point observed for a particular individual and Δ is an indicator variable that denotes whether or not the event was observed at that time point. In the observed data, each subject accounts for one line in the data set, and we will refer to this data structure as short-form data structure I. Data structure I in Fig. 18.1 is a sample data set displaying values for four subjects from this observed data structure, and W_1 and W_2 are two sample covariates measured at baseline.

An alternative representation of this data structure, which we refer to as long-form data structure II, is a more appropriate way of thinking about the data for our purposes. Define $N(t) = I(\tilde{T} \le t, \Delta = 1)$ as the counting process that denotes whether an event has occurred or not and $A(t) = I(\tilde{T} \le t, \Delta = 0)$ as the counting process that codes right-censoring events. Thus $dN(t) = 0$ for all time points up until there is an observed failure time event, and at time t of the observed event, $dN(t) = 1$. After a censoring event, $dN(t)$ can never jump from 0 to 1 since the event can no longer be observed. Similarly, $dA(t)$ remains 0 for all times the observation is uncensored and $dA(t) = 1$ at the time the observation becomes censored.

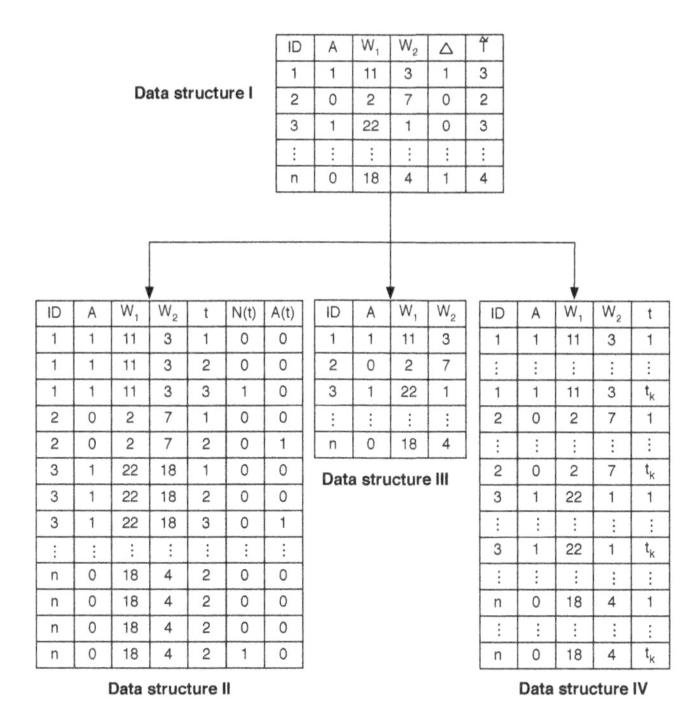

Data structure I

ID	A	W_1	W_2	Δ	$\tilde{T}$
1	1	11	3	1	3
2	0	2	7	0	2
3	1	22	1	0	3
⋮	⋮	⋮	⋮	⋮	⋮
n	0	18	4	1	4

ID	A	W_1	W_2	t	N(t)	A(t)
1	1	11	3	1	0	0
1	1	11	3	2	0	0
1	1	11	3	3	1	0
2	0	2	7	1	0	0
2	0	2	7	2	0	1
3	1	22	18	1	0	0
3	1	22	18	2	0	0
3	1	22	18	3	0	1
⋮	⋮	⋮	⋮	⋮	⋮	⋮
n	0	18	4	2	0	0
n	0	18	4	2	0	0
n	0	18	4	2	0	0
n	0	18	4	2	1	0

Data structure II

ID	A	W_1	W_2
1	1	11	3
2	0	2	7
3	1	22	1
⋮	⋮	⋮	⋮
n	0	18	4

Data structure III

ID	A	W_1	W_2	t
1	1	11	3	1
⋮	⋮	⋮	⋮	⋮
1	1	11	3	t_k
2	0	2	7	1
⋮	⋮	⋮	⋮	⋮
2	0	2	7	t_k
3	1	22	1	1
⋮	⋮	⋮	⋮	⋮
3	1	22	1	t_k
⋮	⋮	⋮	⋮	⋮
n	0	18	4	1
⋮	⋮	⋮	⋮	⋮
n	0	18	4	t_k

Data structure IV

Fig. 18.1 Data structures

Thus, the observed data may be represented in their long form as n i.i.d. observations of $O = (W, A, dN(t), dA(t) : t = 1, \ldots, \tau) \sim P_0$, where P_0 denotes the probability distribution of the observed data structure O. In this representation of the observed data structure, each subject contributes a line of data for each time point at which they were observed up until their event happens, or they are censored. Furthermore, the values measured at baseline, A and W, are just repeated at their initial values for each time point. Data structure II in Fig. 18.1 shows the exact same observations from data structure I, but in their long form.

The subject with ID 1 has $\tilde{T} = 3$ and $\Delta = 1$. This individual was observed for three time periods, and during the third time period the subject had the event of interest. As a result, subject 1 contributes three lines of data to the long form, as can be seen in data structure II in Fig. 18.1. The subject's event process, $N(t)$, remains zero up until time 3 when it jumps to 1, and the subject's censoring process, $A(t)$, remains 0 for all time points since the subject is never right censored. All covariates measured at baseline remain the same for all time points. Subject 2, on the other hand, was right censored at time point 2, so that this subject's event was never observed, resulting in $\tilde{T} = 2$ and $\Delta = 0$. Thus, subject 2 contributes two lines to the data in their long form and $N(t)$ is zero for all t, since the event was not observed, and the censoring-counting process, $A(t)$, jumps to 1 at time 2 since the subject was censored at that time. A, W_1, and W_2 remain constant at every time point. Contributions from subjects 3 and 4 to the data sets in both the short and long form are included in Fig. 18.1 as additional examples. The data in their long form may be thought of as being conditional on the failure time event or right censoring not having occurred before time t. So each observation contributes a line in the long form of the data for each time point at which the subject has neither experienced the event nor been censored. We also say that, at each time point at which the subject is still at risk of failing or being right censored, it contributes a line of data. Data structure III is used in estimating the treatment mechanism and data structure IV plays a special role in the evaluation of the target parameter. Both will be discussed further later in the chapter.

18.2 Cox Proportional Hazards and Failure Time Models

In 1972, Sir David Cox introduced the Cox proportional hazards model for the estimation of survival curves. The model is based on the proportional hazards assumption and assumes that the effect of treatment and covariates on a hazard follows a particular parametric form. The proportional hazards assumption states that survival curves for different strata must have hazard functions for which their ratio is constant in time.

Even though the Cox proportional hazards model represented a very important breakthrough for analyzing survival data, resulted in important theory, and beautifully generalized multiplicative intensity models for modeling intensities of general counting processes (Andersen et al. 1993), its stringent assumptions make these models susceptible to the same criticism as parametric regression models.

Over 35 years after the introduction of the model, the proportional hazards assumption is still assumed to hold for the majority of data analyses in survival analysis. In fact, there seems to be a common misconception that all semiparametric methods in survival analysis are susceptible to the shortcomings of the Cox proportional hazards model. In this section we will discuss the flaws of the discrete time analogue of the Cox proportional hazards model as well as the Cox proportional hazards model.

It is common in analyses that intend to test whether or not a treatment or exposure, A, has an effect on a particular time-to-event outcome, to assume an a priori specified model for the conditional hazard and to test if the coefficient in front of A in the specified model is different from zero. For continuous time, a Cox proportional hazards model is typically employed, and for discrete failure times, a logistic failure time model is used. It is common practice in both models to model the effect of time as flexibly as possible and to model the effect of the treatment and covariates, if they are adjusted for, with a linear parametric model.

The following is a typical model for modeling the conditional hazard in discrete time, $P(dN(t) = 1 \mid N(t-1) = 0, A(t-1) = 0, A, W)$:

$$\alpha_1 + \gamma_2 I(t = 2) + \ldots + \gamma_\tau I(t = \tau) + \beta_1 A + \beta_2 W. \tag{18.1}$$

The parameters in the above model for the conditional hazards are then estimated with maximum likelihood estimation, and the p-value for the null hypothesis $H_0 : \beta_1 = 0$ is examined to determine if one can conclude that β_1 is significantly different from zero. Such parameter estimates are contingent on how well the a priori specified model approximates the hazard. However, the model is highly restrictive, and, as a result, the estimate of β_1 may be highly biased with respect to its desired target (presumably, the logarithm of the relative hazard). In most cases, little work is done to assess how well the model does in approximating the true conditional hazard. Even if formal tests are carried out to test the validity of the Cox proportional hazards model, a procedure that reports the test for $H_0 : \beta_1 = 0$ if the null hypothesis of the model is correct is not rejected and reports something else is still subject to severe bias in estimation and assessment of uncertainty. The latter practice, though common, lacks any statistical foundation.

Similarly, the Cox proportional hazards model for continuous failure times specifies the effect due to A and W in terms of a linear model, while it models the baseline hazard as a function of time t nonparametrically. If the model is correct, the coefficient in front of A in the Cox proportional hazards model is the log-relative hazard (RH), where RH is defined as the ratio of the hazard at time t, conditional on $A = 1$, and the hazard at time t, conditional on $A = 0$, within a stratum defined by *any* particular value of W. The Cox proportional hazards model relates the hazard for a particular subject, $\lambda_i(t)$, with baseline data (W_i, A_i), to the baseline hazard, $\lambda_0(t)$, as follows:

$$\lambda_i(t) = \lambda_0(t) e^{\beta_1 A_i + \beta_2 W_i},$$

which may be rearranged in the following way:

$$\log\left[\frac{\lambda_i(t)}{\lambda_0(t)}\right] = \beta_1 A_i + \beta_2 W_i.$$

We will now show how the same parameter under the Cox proportional hazards assumption may be recast in terms of conditional survival probabilities. Let $f(t)$ equal the derivative of the cumulative distribution function $F(t)$ of a continuous survival time:

$$f(t) = \lim_{\delta \to 0}\left(\frac{F(t+\delta) - F(t)}{\delta}\right).$$

Since the survival probability, $S(t)$, equals $1 - F(t)$, the derivative of $S(t)$, $d/dt[S(t)]$, equals $-f(t)$. The hazard, λ, equals $f(t)/S(t)$, which may be rewritten as

$$\lambda(t) = -\frac{d}{dt}[\log S(t)]. \tag{18.2}$$

Solving Eq. (18.2) for $S(t)$ yields

$$S(t) = \exp(-\Lambda(t)), \tag{18.3}$$

where $\Lambda(t) = \int_0^t \lambda(u)\,du)$ is the cumulative hazard. It easily seen that, under the Cox proportional hazards assumption, the ratio of the conditional hazards is equal to the ratio of the conditional cumulative hazards, which is equal to the ratio of log survival probabilities [by (18.3)]. Thus, β_1 may be written in terms of survival probabilities as follows: for any time point t_k

$$\beta_1 = \log\left(\frac{\log S(t_k \mid A = 1, W)}{\log S(t_k \mid A = 0, W)}\right). \tag{18.4}$$

To conclude, β_1 can also be represented as an average over all time points t_k of (18.4) and all covariate values W. Most would agree that it is very difficult to comprehend what the average of the log ratio of log survival probabilities means in terms of the effect of A on the outcome. A parameter β_1 is a parameter only defined on the Cox model, but it can be extended as a parameter in a nonparametric model in many possible ways. It can be represented in terms of an average over time of log hazard ratios or the log of the ratio of the log conditional survival probabilities. These two extensions represent very different parameters for most conditional distributions of T, given (A, W), with very different interpretations, but they happen to be equal to each other for distributions that satisfy the constraints of the Cox proportional hazards model. If one believes the Cox proportional hazards model to be valid, then one also needs to believe that these different representations of β_1 as parameter of the distribution of the data are equal to each other.

In RCTs, the Cox proportional hazards analysis is typically implemented without adjusting for baseline covariates. In this case, the coefficient of the marginal structural Cox proportional hazards model, $\lambda_{T_a}(t) = \lambda_0(t)\exp(\beta a)$, can also be represented, for any weight function $w(t)$, as

$$\beta = \sum_{t_k} w(t_k) \log\left(\frac{\log S_1(t_k)}{\log S_0(t_k)}\right),$$

where $S_a(t_k) = P(T_a > t_k) = E_W S(t_k \mid A = a, W)$ is the treatment-specific survival function. The rationale for using a marginal Cox proportional hazards model $E(dN(t) \mid \tilde{T} \geq t, A) = \lambda_0(t)\exp(\beta A)$ is that (1) individuals have been randomized to treatment groups, and thus those two groups should be reasonably balanced with respect to the levels of all covariates, and (2) censoring is independent of (T, W). Under these assumptions, one indeed has that $E(dN(t) \mid \tilde{T} \geq t, A = a) = P(T_a = t \mid T_a \geq t)$, so that the Cox proportional hazards model for the conditional hazard of T, given A, is equivalent to a Cox proportional hazards marginal structural model for the causal hazard. So under these two assumptions the coefficient β in a Cox proportional hazards model for the conditional hazard of T, given A, represents a log causal relative hazard.

However, even though treatment/exposure is randomized in RCTs, dependent censoring is often informative, so that by ignoring covariates one may end up with a biased estimate of the causal effect of A on the event of interest. In addition, the estimate of the relative hazard is biased if the effect of A is not constant over time (a violation in the proportional hazards assumption). Thus these estimates can still be very biased, even under randomization, due to dependent censoring or violations in the proportional hazards assumption. In observational studies, practitioners may attempt to adjust for possible confounders by adding them as linear terms in the model. However, this is often done in an ad hoc way and many times covariates are added and removed solely based on how their inclusion in the model affects the estimate of the coefficient β_1 of the treatment A of interest.

Extensions of these methods are also commonly used to assess whether or not a variable V, a single baseline covariate within W, modifies the effect A on the outcome of interest. If the effect of A differs at different levels of V, then V is termed an effect modifier. A typical test for whether V is an effect modifier is to add an interaction term $A \times V$ to the above model and assess whether the coefficient on that term is significant in exactly the same way as was done above for just A.

Whether one adjusts for baseline covariates or not, these methods are usually biased due to the fact that they are dependent on highly restrictive parametric models that are typically not representative of the data-generating distribution. Furthermore, the parameters in these models are difficult to interpret even if the models are correct due to the fact that they were chosen because they are convenient to estimate, as opposed to natural parameters that directly address the questions practitioners are interested in answering.

18.3 Model and Parameters of Interest

We now examine the advantages of defining the parameter of interest as a function of the data-generating distribution, as well as introduce several interesting parameters of interest in time-to-event studies. Rather than choosing the parameter of interest because it is convenient within the chosen model, one can define the parameter of interest as a function of the data-generating distribution, $\Psi(P_0)$. By defining the parameter in this fashion, one can estimate the feature of the data-generating distribution that is of interest. Furthermore, by defining the parameter of interest in this way, it has meaning absent the validity of the Cox proportional hazards model.

The treatment-specific survival curve at a particular time point t_k is a simple example of this type of parameter, $Pr(T_a > t_k)$, where T_a is the counterfactual event time T one would have observed had an individual's treatment been set, possibly contrary to fact, to treatment level a. By formulating a set of causal assumptions through the use of a SCM, as visualized by a causal graph, one may define the distribution of the counterfactual outcomes indexed by an intervention on some treat-

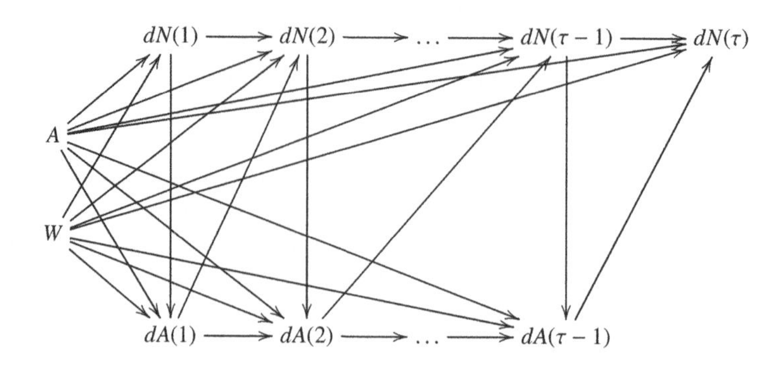

Fig. 18.2 Causal assumptions (exogenous errors omitted for simplicity)

ment and censoring nodes in the SCM. Then one may define a causal parameter as a difference between these counterfactual distributions of the outcome for different interventions on the treatment and censoring nodes.

In order to link the SCM to the observed data, the distribution of the observed data is assumed to be implied by the SCM. The SCM includes the distribution of the error/exogenous nodes and the deterministic functions that define each endogenous node as a function of its parents and a error. Typically, one assumes that the observed data structure corresponds with a subset of the nodes, such as all the endogenous nodes. Under certain causal assumptions one can then show that the causal effect of interest can be identified as a parameter of the distribution of the observed data, $\Psi(P_0)$. Figure 18.2 posits a set of causal assumptions in the form of a causal graph in which our data structure corresponds with the displayed nodes. Exogenous nodes are suppressed for simplicity. This is common practice for displaying that each displayed node has an exogenous node with an arrow going into it and no arrows going into any other nodes.

Necessary conditions typically stated to make causal parameters identifiable may be made through the use of this causal graph, namely, the consistency assumption and CAR assumption. The CAR assumption is arranged by assuming the strong sequential randomization assumption on the intervention nodes of the causal graph. In the analysis presented below, the treatment is in fact randomized; thus there is no arrow from W to A in the causal graph. Note, that simple unobserved nodes that only effect A or the censoring process $dA(t)$, but not the future outcome process $dN(t)$, do not violate these assumptions. This is because such nodes do not produce unblocked backdoor paths to the future outcome process, $dN(t)$.

Another assumption that may not be expressed within the causal graph is necessary in order for a parameter of interest to be identifiable from the observed data. This assumption is known as the positivity assumption, and was discussed in detail in Chap. 10. Suppose that the causal quantity of interest is the additive causal effect $P(T_1 > t_0) - P(T_0 > t_0)$ of treatment on survival at time t_0. The positivity assumption states, in particular, that there is no level of W that is completely predictive of treatment level A. However, since treatment is randomized, this is not an issue due to the design of the experiment in the Tshepo study. In addition, since we are only interested in the censoring nodes set at value 0, the positivity assumption also states that for all levels of the covariate W, at each time $t \leq t_0$, the conditional hazard of being censored at time t is bounded away from 1.

The causal graph in Fig. 18.2 suggests the following likelihood factorization:

$$P_0(O) = \overbrace{P_0(W)}^{Q_{W,0}} \overbrace{P_0(A)}^{g_{A,0}} \prod_{t=1}^{\tau} \overbrace{P_0(dN(t) \mid \bar{N}(t-1), \bar{A}(t-1), A, W)}^{Q_{dN(t),0}}$$
$$\prod_{t=1}^{\tau} \underbrace{P_0(dA(t) \mid \bar{N}(t), \bar{A}(t-1), A, W)}_{g_{dA(t),0}}.$$

Thus, the likelihood is factorized into a portion Q_0, corresponding to the conditional distributions of the nonintervention nodes, and a portion g_0, corresponding to the conditional distributions of the censoring and treatment nodes. Q_0 is composed of the distribution of the baseline covariates $Q_{W,0}$, and $Q_{dN(t),0}$ the conditional distribution of the binary indicators $dN(t)$, given its parents. We have that g_0 is further factorized into the treatment mechanism, $g_{A,0}$, and censoring mechanism, $g_{dA(t),0}$, which involves the conditional distributions of the binary censoring indicators $dA(t)$, given its parents.

We note that $Q_{dN(t),0}$ and $g_{dA(t),0}$ are identified by the discrete intensities $E_0(dN(t) \mid A, W, \bar{N}(t-1), \bar{A}(t-1)) = I(\tilde{T} \geq t)\bar{Q}_0(t \mid A, W)$ and $E_0(dA(t) \mid A, W, \bar{N}(t), \bar{A}(t-1)) = I(N(t) = 0, A(t-1) = 0)\bar{g}_0(t \mid A, W)$. Note that these two intensities of event process N and censoring process A indeed equal an indicator of being at risk times a function of t, A, W. Under CAR, it follows that $\bar{Q}_0(t \mid A, W) = P_0(T = t \mid T \geq t, A, W)$ equals the conditional hazard of the failure time T, and, similarly, $\bar{g}_0(t \mid A, W) = P_0(C = t \mid C \geq t, A, W)$ equals the conditional hazard of the censoring time C. Let's also define $S_0(t_k \mid A, W) = P_0(T > t_k \mid A, W)$, which is the conditional survival of the event of interest, and can be expressed as a function of the conditional hazard $\bar{Q}_0(t \mid A, W)$ under CAR as $S_0(t_k \mid A, W) = \prod_{t=1}^{t_k} \left(1 - \bar{Q}_0(t \mid A, W)\right)$.

By intervening in the SCM, as visualized by the causal graph, on A and $dA(t)$ by setting treatment A equal to the desired treatment a and setting $dA(t)$ equal to 0, or, equivalently, no censoring for all t, one obtains the distribution of the event process under the desired treatment and without censoring. This counterfactual distribution of the data structure under an intervention can be identified from the observed data, under the stated assumptions, in the g-formula. All of the nodes that are intervened upon in the causal graph are set to their intervened-upon level in the likelihood, and all the conditional distributions for those nodes are removed from the likelihood since they are no longer random variables. The following is the resulting g-computation formula, or distribution of the data (W, T_a) under the intervention:

$$Q_{W,0}(W) \prod_{t=1}^{\tau} Q_{dN(t),0}(dN(t) \mid \bar{N}(t-1), A(t-1) = 0, A = a, W).$$

We can now write the marginal treatment-specific survival probability, $P_0(T_a > t_k)$, in terms of the data-generating distribution, P_0:

$$\Psi_a(P_0)(t_k) = Pr(T_a > t_k) = E_0\left(S_0(t_k \mid A = a, W)\right).$$

Parameters that combine $\Psi_1(P_0)(t_k)$ and $\Psi_0(P_0)(t_k)$ allow one to quantify the effect of a change of A on T. Three examples are the marginal additive difference in the probability of survival, the log relative risk of survival, and the marginal log hazard of survival:

$$\begin{aligned}
\Psi_{RD}(P_0)(t_k) &= \Psi_1(P_0)(t_k) - \Psi_0(P_0)(t_k),\\
\Psi_{RR}(P_0)(t_k) &= \log\left(\frac{\Psi_1(P_0)(t_k)}{\Psi_0(P_0)(t_k)}\right),\\
\Psi_{RH}(P_0)(t_k) &= \log\left(\frac{\log(\Psi_1(P_0)(t_k))}{\log(\Psi_0(P_0)(t_k))}\right).
\end{aligned}$$

For ease of interpretation we prefer the first two of these parameters. However, for completeness, we show that the third parameter, which represents the parameter targeted by a marginal structural Cox proportional hazards model $P(T_a = t \mid T_a \geq t) = \lambda_0(t)\exp(\beta a)$, may also be estimated through the methods presented here. One should note that the parameter $\Psi_{RH}(P_0)(t_k)$ is undefined at t_k for which $P_0(T_a > t_k) = 1$. The above parameters quantify the effect of A at a particular time point, t_k; therefore, averages of the above parameters over a set of time points may also be of interest.

One possible method for estimating the mean counterfactual outcome as expressed in the parameters proposed above is MLE and construct the substitution estimator $\Psi(Q_n) = \psi_n^{MLE}$ according to the mapping $\Psi()$. Thus, it is necessary to estimate $Q_{W,0}$ and $\bar{Q}_0(t \mid A, W)$ and, consequently, its corresponding conditional survival function, $S_0(t_k \mid A, W)$. This estimator is consistent when both of these distributions are estimated consistently. We estimate $Q_{W,0}$ with nonparametric maximum likelihood estimation. In practice, several models have been used for $\bar{Q}_0(t \mid A, W)$. Many practitioners specify a parametric model a priori, often using main terms logistic regression, as in Eq. (18.1), and obtain the maximum likelihood estimate within this highly restrictive model. [Obtaining the estimates of the parameters in Eq. (18.1) can be done by using logistic regression with data structure II.]

This parametric approach almost certainly leads to biased estimates of $\bar{Q}_0(t \mid A, W)$, and thus a biased estimate of $\Psi(Q_0)$, since it is likely that the true $\bar{Q}_0$ is not contained in this highly restrictive model. If the model does not contain the true $\bar{Q}_0$, then the estimates of $\bar{Q}_0$ and $\Psi(Q_0)$ will generally not be consistent. For this reason a nonparametric model for $\bar{Q}_0$ often represents the realistic knowledge about $\bar{Q}_0$. Since this nonparametric model is very large, sieve-based (data-adaptive) maximum likelihood estimation (i.e., loss-based machine learning), involving fine-tuning of the amount of smoothing used, becomes necessary. Many different methods have been developed for estimating the effect of covariates on a binary outcome in the nonparametric model including regression trees, DSA, and k-nearest neigh-

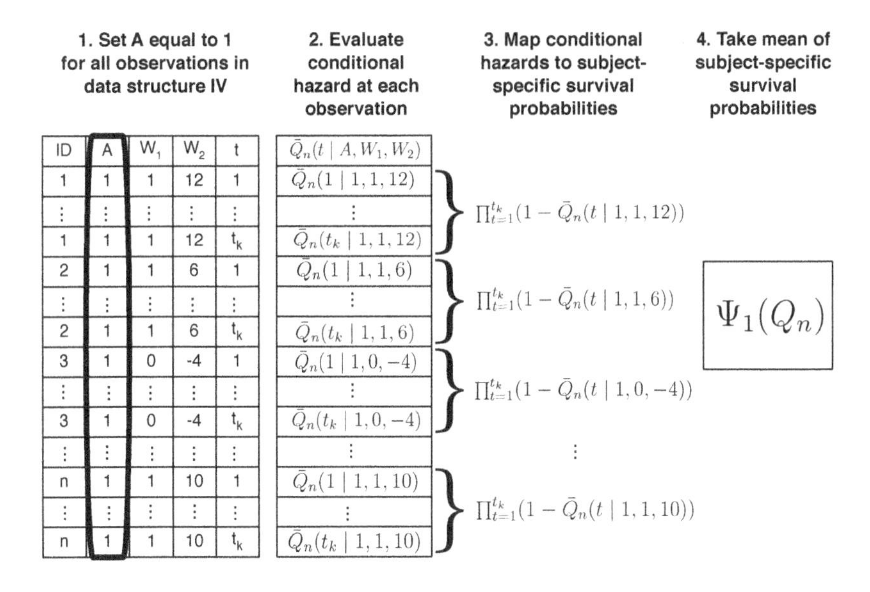

Fig. 18.3 Mapping $\bar{Q}_n$ and $Q_{W,n}$ into $\Psi(Q_n)$

bors. Rudser et al. (2008) used one of these methods, a nonparametric tree estimator, for estimating the survival distribution and subsequently $\Psi(Q_0)$. Even though a single estimator for estimating these distributions in the nonparametric model may yield consistent estimates, super learner will converge to the true distribution at a faster rate.

Once these estimates Q_n are obtained, the MLE of the treatment-specific survival, $\Psi_a(Q_0)(t_k)$ is the substitution estimator obtained by plugging in Q_n:

$$\Psi_a(Q_n)(t_k) = \frac{1}{n}\sum_{i=1}^{n} S_n(t_k \mid A = a, W_i).$$

Figure 18.3 demonstrates how to map $\bar{Q}_n$ and $Q_{W,n}$ into $\Psi_1(Q_n)$, an estimate of the treatment-specific survival curve at $a = 1$ using data structure IV from Fig. 18.1. The MLE of the parameters presented in this section can be generated by combining MLE estimates of the treatment-specific survival curves under alternative treatments.

18.4 Effect Modification Parameters

Parameters that quantify the level of effect modification due to another baseline variable V may also be of interest in studies aimed at assessing the effect of a treatment, A, at different levels of V. However, we must now consider an SCM with an explicit node for the effect modifier V, instead of collapsing it into a single node W. First, let's consider a V that occurs after the baseline covariates W but before treatment and the censoring and event processes. This SCM implies the following factorization of the likelihood:

$$\begin{aligned}P_0(O) = & P_0(W)P_0(V \mid W)P_0(A \mid V, W) \\ & \times \prod_{t=1}^{\tau} P_0(dN(t) \mid \bar{N}(t-1) = 0, \bar{A}(t-1), A, V, W) \\ & \times \prod_{t=1}^{\tau} P_0(dA(t) \mid \bar{N}(t), \bar{A}(t-1) = 0, A, V, W),\end{aligned}$$

and the corresponding g-formula for the intervention $A = a$, $V = v$, and all censoring nodes equal to zero:

$$P_0(W) \prod_{t=1}^{\tau} P_0(dN(t) \mid \bar{N}(t-1), \bar{A}(t-1) = 0, A = a, V = v, W).$$

As before, the MLE only requires an estimate of the marginal distribution of W, and $\bar{Q}_0(t \mid A, W)$. We will define the following parameters of interest to measure the causal effect modification when the effect modifier occurs after W:

$$\Psi_{RD}^{CEM}(P_0) = \sum_{t_k} w(t_k)[(\Psi_{11}(P_0)(t_k) - \Psi_{01}(P_0)(t_k)) - (\Psi_{10}(P_0)(t_k) - \Psi_{00}(P_0)(t_k))], \quad (18.5)$$

$$\Psi_{LR}^{CEM}(P_0) = \sum_{t_k} w(t_k) \left[\log \frac{\log(\Psi_{11}(P_0)(t_k))}{\log(\Psi_{01}(P_0)(t_k))} - \log \frac{\log(\Psi_{10}(P_0)(t_k))}{\log(\Psi_{00}(P_0)(t_k))} \right], \quad (18.6)$$

where $\Psi_{11}(P_0)(t_k)$ is counterfactual survival at t_k setting V to 1 and A to 1, and so on. That is, the first and second subscript code the level a and v for treatment and effect modifier, respectively. Here, $w(t_k)$ are time-varying weights. These weights may be dependent on the question of interest, or they may be set to the reciprocal of an estimate of the variance of the parameter estimate at the particular time, or simply be set to 1. We will weight each time-point-specific estimator by the reciprocal of its estimated variance, to put more emphasis on those time points with more information.

In situations where V is realized before the baseline covariates W, a different SCM must be considered. This SCM implies the following likelihood factorization:

$$\begin{aligned}P_0(O) = & P_0(V)P_0(W \mid V)P_0(A \mid V, W) \\ & \times \prod_{t=1}^{\tau} P_0(dN(t) \mid \bar{N}(t-1), \bar{A}(t-1), A, V, W)\end{aligned}$$

$$\times \prod_{t=1}^{\tau} P_0(dA(t) \mid \bar{N}(t), \bar{A}(t-1), A, V, W),$$

with the resulting g-formula

$$P_0(W \mid V = v) \prod_{t=1}^{\tau} P_0(dN(t) \mid \bar{N}(t-1), \bar{A}(t-1) = 0, A = a, V = v, W).$$

Characteristics such as sex and gender, which are set at birth, are examples of variables for which V is realized before W. In order to asses the level of effect modification in these situations, an estimate of $P_0(W \mid V = v)$ is needed instead of the marginal distribution $P_0(W)$ of W. The conditional hazard $\bar{Q}_0(t \mid A, W)$ may be estimated as before. The empirical distribution among $V = v$ will be used to estimate $P_0(W \mid V = v)$. We will refer to these causal effect modification parameters as stratified effect modification (SEM) parameters, as they can be expressed as follows:

$$\Psi_{RD}^{SEM}(P_0) = \left[\sum_{t_k} w(t_k)(S_{1|1}(t_k) - S_{0|1}(t_k))\right] - \left[\sum_{t_k} w(t_k)(S_{1|0}(t_k) - S_{0|0}(t_k))\right], \quad (18.7)$$

$$\Psi_{LR}^{SEM}(P_0) = \sum_{t_k} w(t_k) \left[\log\left(\frac{\log(S_{1|1}(t_k))}{\log(S_{0|1}(t_k))}\right) - \log\left(\frac{\log(S_{1|0}(t_k))}{\log(S_{0|0}(t_k))}\right)\right], \quad (18.8)$$

where $S_{1|1}(t_k)$ denotes survival at t_k for individuals with $V = 1$ and treatment set to 1, and so on. These are also counterfactual survival probabilities corresponding with setting $A = a$ and $V = v$. However, we have expressed them as a counterfactual survival probability, $S_{a|v}(t_0)$, conditional on $V = v$, to emphasize the fact that they are different parameters of interest of the data-generating distribution, corresponding to the alternative SCM where V occurs before W.

18.5 The TMLE

The TMLE of the parameters presented in the previous sections improves on the MLE by being consistent when either g_0 or Q_0 is estimated consistently. Thus, the method is double robust. In the TMLE algorithm, an initial estimator of the conditional hazard is obtained, and the algorithm updates it by iteratively adding a time-dependent clever covariate chosen to reduce bias in the estimate of the parameter of interest. This time-dependent clever covariate is a function of time, treatment, and the baseline covariates and requires an estimate of the treatment and censoring mechanisms. The marginal distribution of the covariates is estimated with the empirical distribution and is not updated by the TMLE.

The TMLE involves the construction of an initial estimator P_n^0 of the probability distribution P_0 described by initial estimates $\bar{Q}_n^0(t \mid A, W)$, $g_{A,n}^0$ (using data structure

III), $\bar{g}_n^0(t \mid A, W)$, and the empirical distribution $Q_{W,n}$. The TMLE also requires defining a loss function $L(P)$ for P_0 and a parametric working model $\{P_n^0(\epsilon) : \epsilon\}$ through an initial estimator so that the score $d/d\epsilon L(P_n^0(\epsilon))$ at $\epsilon = 0$ spans the efficient influence curve $D^*(P_n^0)$ at P_n^0 of the target parameter of interest. Our loss function will be the log-likelihood loss function $L(P) = -\log P$. The parametric working model will be selected to only update Q_n^0.

The target parameters $\Psi_1(P_0)(t_k)$ and $\Psi_0(P_0)(t_k)$ have the following two efficient influence curves:

$$D_1^*(P_0) = \sum_{t \le t_k} H_1^*(t, A, W)\left[I(\tilde{T} = t, \Delta = 1) - I(\tilde{T} \ge t)\bar{Q}_0(t \mid A = 1, W)\right] + S_0(t_k \mid A = 1, W) - \Psi_1(P_0)(t_k) \text{ and}$$

$$D_0^*(P_0) = \sum_{t \le t_k} H_1^*(t, A, W)\left[I(\tilde{T} = t, \Delta = 1) - I(\tilde{T} \ge t)\bar{Q}_0(t \mid A = 0, W)\right] + S_0(t_k \mid A = 0, W) - \Psi_0(P_0)(t_k).$$

We select $Q_{W,n}(\epsilon_1) = (1+\epsilon_1 D^*_{a,W}(P_n^0))Q_{W,n}$ as parametric working model for fluctuating the empirical distribution of W, where $D^*_{a,W}(P_n^0) = S_n^0(t_k \mid A = a, W) - \Psi_a(P_n^0)(t_k)$. Note that $D^*_{a,W}(P_0)$ represents the projection of the efficient influence curve $D_a^*(P_0)$ onto the tangent space of the marginal distribution of W. We select the logistic regression model $\text{logit}\, \bar{Q}_n^0(\epsilon_2) = \text{logit}\, \bar{Q}_n^0 + \epsilon_2 H_a^*(P_n^0)$ as parametric working model for fluctuating the conditional hazard, where the clever covariate for the target parameter $\Psi_a(P_0)(t_k)$ is given by

$$H_1^*(P_n^0)(t, A, W) = -\frac{I(A = 1)}{g_{A,n}^0(1 \mid W)\prod_{i=1}^{t-}\left(1 - \bar{g}_n^0(i \mid A, W)\right)} \frac{S_n^0(t_k \mid A, W)}{S_n^0(t \mid A, W)} I(t \le t_k) \text{ and}$$

$$H_0^*(P_n^0)(t, A, W) = -\frac{I(A = 0)}{g_{A,n}^0(0 \mid W)\prod_{i=1}^{t-}\left(1 - \bar{g}_n^0(i \mid A, W)\right)} \frac{S_n^0(t_k \mid A, W)}{S_n^0(t \mid A, W)} I(t \le t_k).$$

This now defines a parametric working model through the conditional distributions $Q^0_{dN(t),n}$ for all $t = 1, \ldots, \tau$. These two working models through the marginal distribution $Q_{W,n}$ and the conditional hazard $\bar{Q}_n^0$ also imply a working parametric model $\{Q_n^0(\epsilon) : \epsilon\}$ through $Q_n^0 = (Q^0_{W,n}, \bar{Q}_n^0)$ indexed by a bivariate $\epsilon = (\epsilon_1, \epsilon_2)$. The working parametric model $\{P_n^0(\epsilon) = (Q_n^0(\epsilon), g_n^0) : \epsilon\}$ through P_n^0 only fluctuates Q_n^0:

$$P_n^0(\epsilon)(O) = Q^0_{W,n}(\epsilon_1)(W) \prod_t Q_{dN(t),n}(\epsilon_2)(dA(t) \mid Pa(A(t))) \times g^0_{A,n}(A \mid W) \prod_t g^0_{dA(t),n}(dA(t) \mid Pa(A(t))).$$

The TMLE of $\Psi_a(P_0)(t_k)$ is now defined by the TMLE algorithm implied by the log-likelihood loss function and this parametric working model $P_n^0(\epsilon)$. The first step of the algorithm computes the maximum likelihood estimator $\epsilon_n = \arg\max_\epsilon \log P_n^0(\epsilon)$. The maximum likelihood estimator of ϵ_1 equals zero. In practice, the maximum likelihood estimator of ϵ_2 is obtained by implementing a univariate logistic regression regressing the binary outcome $dN(t)$ on $H^*_{a,n}(t, A, W)$ using the initial estimate $\bar{Q}_n^0(t \mid A, W)$ as an offset, pooling across the time points t. This results in an update $\text{logit}\bar{Q}_n^1 = \text{logit}\bar{Q}_n^0 + \epsilon_{2n} H^*_{an}$. The first step TMLE of Q_0 is given by $Q_n^1 = (Q_{W,n}, \bar{Q}_n^1)$.

This updating process is iterated until $\epsilon_n \approx 0$. The final TMLE of Q_0 is denoted by $Q_n^* = (Q_{W,n}, \bar{Q}_n^*)$, and the corresponding $P_n^* = (Q_n^*, g_n^0)$ is the TMLE of P_0. The TMLE of $\Psi_a(P_0)(t_k)$ is the substitution estimators based on plugging in the targeted estimator Q_n^*:

$$\Psi_a(Q_n^*)(t_k) = \frac{1}{n} \sum_{i=1}^{n} S_n^*(t_k \mid A = a, W_i),$$

where $S_n^*(t_k \mid A = a, W_i)$ is the survival probability corresponding with $\bar{Q}_n^*$ and $\Psi_a(Q_n^*)(t_k)$ can be constructed as previously shown in Fig. 18.3.

The update is implemented by fitting a univariate logistic regression model of the event process, $N(t)$, on the clever covariate $H^*_{n,a}$ with the initial fit $\bar{Q}_n^0(t \mid A, W)$ as an offset. $\bar{Q}_n^0(\epsilon_n^1)$ is the first-step TMLE of $\bar{Q}_0$, where ϵ_n^1 is the fitted regression coefficient of the clever covariate. This defines the first-step TMLE update P_n^1. Since the time-dependent clever covariate, $H^*(P_n^1)(t, A, W)$, is different under P_n^1 than it is under P_n^0, due to being a function of the estimator of $\bar{Q}_0$, it is necessary to iterate the updating step. The TMLE updating process is detailed in Fig. 18.4.

The above TMLE can be implemented separately for the two target parameters $\Psi_a(P_0)(t_k)$, resulting in a TMLE of any function of these two treatment-specific survival functions. Alternatively, one can construct a single TMLE targeting both target parameters simultaneously. In this case, we select the logistic regression model $\text{logit}\bar{Q}_n^0(\epsilon_2) = \text{logit}\bar{Q}_n^0 + \epsilon_{20} H_0^*(P_n^0) + \epsilon_{21} H_1^*(P_n^0)$ as the parametric working model for fluctuating the conditional hazard. That is, we add the two clever covariates $H_1^*(P_n^0)$ and $H_0^*(P_n^0)$ to the initial estimator of the conditional hazard, one clever covariate for $\Psi_1(P_0)(t_k)$ and one for $\Psi_0(P_0)(t_k)$. The TMLE updates both components $(\epsilon_{20}, \epsilon_{21})$ simultaneously until both components have converged to zero.

The TMLE of $\Psi_{av}(t_k)$ needed for constructing the parameter estimates of target parameters (18.5) and (18.6) may be constructed by treating A and V together as a treatment variable. The treatment mechanism must be replaced by the joint probability of $A = a$ and $V = v$, and the resulting clever covariate is

$$H^*(P_n^0)(t, A, V, W) = -\frac{I(A = a, V = v)}{g^0_{A,n}(A = a, V = v \mid W) \prod_{i=1}^{t-} \left(1 - \bar{g}_n^0(i \mid A, V, W)\right)} \times \frac{S_n^0(t_k \mid A = a, V = v, W)}{S_n^0(t \mid A = a, V = v, W)} I(t \leq t_k),$$

and the TMLE is:

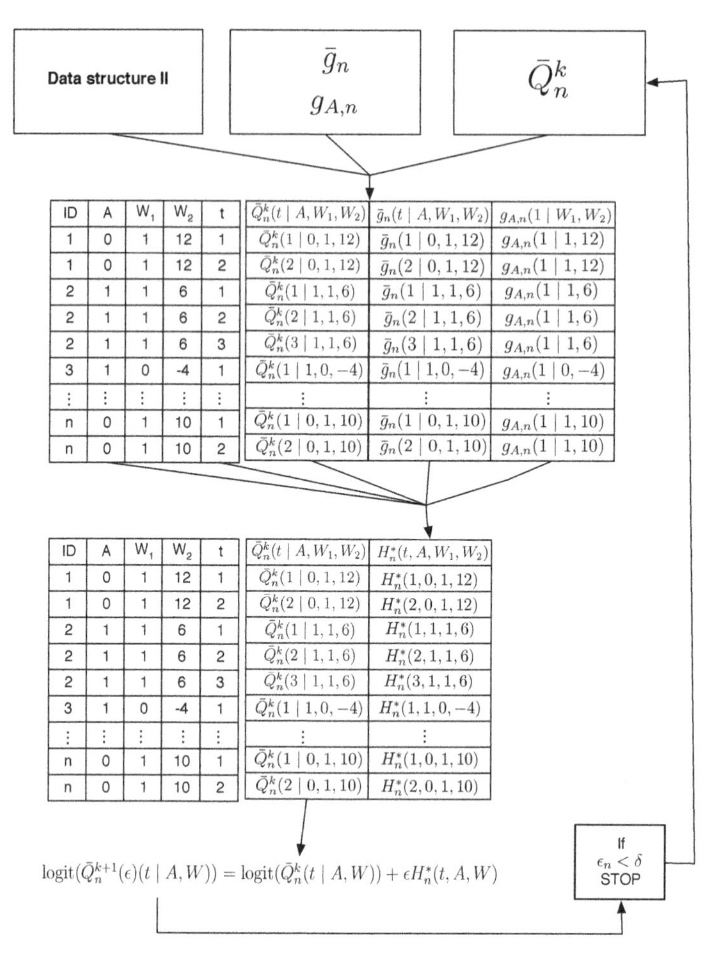

Fig. 18.4 One iteration of the TMLE algorithm

$$\Psi_{av}(Q_n^*)(t_k) = \frac{1}{n}\sum_{i=1}^{n} S_n^*(t_k \mid A = a, V = v, W_i),$$

where S_n^* is now the TMLE of the treatment-specific survival probability at $A = a$ and $V = v$.

The TMLE of $S_{0,a|v}(t_k)$ needed for constructing the parameter estimates of target parameters (18.7) and (18.8) may be constructed in the same way as for one treatment variable A but done separately for each level of V. So the TMLE of $S_{0,a|v}(t_k)$ is the same as the TMLE for $\Psi_a(P_0)(t_k)$ just estimated on a data set that only includes individuals with $V = v$.

There are a few clear advantages of TMLE for time-to-event analysis that are a consequence of the double robustness and local efficiency of the method. First, if the censoring is independent and treatment is randomized, then the estimator of the parameter of interest is guaranteed to be unbiased since the treatment mechanism $g_{A,0}(A \mid W)$ is known, and the required survivor function corresponding with the censoring mechanism $\bar{g}_0(t \mid A, W) = \bar{g}_0(t)$ can be consistently estimated with the Kaplan–Meier estimator. However, it has also been shown that by estimating these mechanisms, even when they are known, one can improve the efficiency of the estimates by adjusting for empirical confounding. This is done by positing a model for these mechanisms that contains the truth so that the estimates will converge to the truth. For a general account of how estimating the treatment and censoring mechanism can improve efficiency see van der Laan and Robins (2003, Sect. 2.3.7). Second, with informative censoring or observational treatment the double robustness allows one to reduce bias due to the initial estimate of $\bar{Q}_0(t \mid A, W)$ by estimating the treatment mechanism, $g_{A,0}(A, W)$, and censoring mechanism, $\bar{g}_0(t \mid A, W)$, as well as possible.

The TMLE also improves on estimating equation-based techniques, in which case ψ_0 is estimated with the closed-form solution of the efficient influence curve estimating equation $P_n D^*(Q_n^0, g_n^0, \psi) = 0$. This is due to the fact that TMLE is a substitution estimator that obeys the proper bounds of a survival probability. Estimating-equation-based results do not obey these bounds and may even result in estimates of probabilities that don't fall between zero and one. In cases where the treatment mechanism gets very close to zero, or the censoring hazard approximates 1, corresponding with practical violations of the positivity assumption stated above, the estimating-equation-based methods tend to become very unstable. When violations in the positivity assumption are a problem, the estimating-equation-based approaches may not only return estimates that are not a probability, but also suffer drastically in efficiency and not approach the semiparametric efficiency bound. However, the TMLE in such situations is more stable and may still achieve the semiparametric efficiency bound. For more details on how the TMLE compares to estimating-equation-based approaches see Stitelman and van der Laan (2010) and Chap. 20.

Confidence intervals may be constructed by relying on the fact that the TMLE solves the efficient influence curve estimating equation $0 = \sum_{i=1}^{n} D^*(Q_n^*, g_n)(O_i)$, where $D^*(Q_0, g_0) = D^*(Q_0, g_0, \Psi(Q_0))$ is the efficient influence curve for a particular parameter of interest. One can also state that $\Psi(Q_n^*)$ solves the estimating equation in ψ_0: $0 = \sum_i D^*(Q_n^*, g_n, \Psi(Q_n^*))(O_i)$, as defined by this efficient influence curve equation. Under regularity conditions, it can be shown that $\Psi(Q_n^*)$ is asymptotically linear with an influence curve $D^*(Q, g_0, \psi_0) + D_1$ for the case where Q_n^* possibly converges to a misspecified Q, and g_n converges to the true g_0 (van der Laan and Robins 2003, Sect. 2.3.7). If $Q_n = Q_0$, or $g_n = g_0$, then $D_1 = 0$. In addition, if g_n is an ML-based estimator of g_0, then ignoring contribution D_1 results in an asymptotically conservative influence curve and variance estimator. So the asymptotic variance of $n^{1/2}(\psi_{n,a}^* - \Psi_a(P_0))$ may be estimated by $\sigma_n^2 = \frac{1}{n}\sum_{i=1}^{n} D_a^{*2}(P_n^*)(O_i)$, where P_n^* is the TMLE of P_0 and $D_a^*(P_n^*)(O_i)$ the efficient influence curves for the treatment-specific survival curve above evaluated at P_n^*. Now 95% confidence intervals for the treatment-specific survival curve at a particular time point may be constructed as $\psi^*_{n,a} \pm 1.96(\sigma_n/\sqrt{n})$.

Variance estimates for the parameters of interests above that combine $\Psi_1(P_0)(t_k)$ and $\Psi_0(P_0)(t_k)$ may be estimated through the use of the delta method. The resulting efficient influence curves for the parameters of interest presented in Sect. 18.3 are

$$D^*_{RD}(P^*_n)(t_k) = D^*_1(P^*_n)(t_k) - D^*_0(P^*_n)(t_k),$$

$$D^*_{RR}(P^*_n)(t_k) = -\frac{1}{1-\psi^*_{n,1}(t_k)} D^*_1(P^*_n)(t_k) + \frac{1}{1-\psi^*_{n,0}(t_k)} D^*_0(P^*_n)(t_k),$$

$$D^*_{RH}(P^*_n)(t_k) = -\frac{1}{\psi^*_{n,1}(t_k)\log(\hat{\psi}^*_1)} D^*_1(P^*_n)(t_k) + \frac{1}{\psi^*_{n,0}(t_k)\log(\psi^*_{n,0})} D^*_0(P^*_n)(t_k).$$

Confidence intervals may now be constructed for these parameters at a particular time point using the above estimates of the corresponding efficient influence curve. Furthermore, the estimated influence curve for estimates that are means of these parameters may be constructed by taking means of the estimated efficient influence curves over the desired time points.

Appendix A presents an asymptotic linearity result generalized to hold for TMLE when Q^*_n converges to a possibly misspecified Q, and g_n converges to a true conditional censoring/treatment mechanism that adjusts for covariates that predict the residual bias between Q and Q_0. In particular, if either Q^*_n converges to Q_0 or g_n converges to g_0, then, under appropriate regularity conditions, we have that ψ^*_n is asymptotically linear with an influence curve $D(P_0)$:

$$n^{1/2}(\psi^*_n - \Psi(P_0)) = n^{-1/2}\sum_{i=1}^{n} D(P_0)(O_i) + o_p(1),$$

so that, by the central limit theorem,

$$n^{1/2}(\psi^*_n - \Psi(P_0)) \xrightarrow{D} N(0, E(D^2(P_0)(O)),$$

as sample size n converges to infinity.

18.6 Data Application: Tshepo Study

The Tshepo study is a 3-year randomized study using a $3 \times 2 \times 2$ factorial design comparing efficacy and tolerability among different drug regimens. For the purpose of this analysis we focus on the randomization to two NNRTI-based cART therapies: EFV and NVP. The Tshepo study is the first clinical trial evaluating the long-term efficacy and tolerability of EFV- vs. NVP-based cART among adults in Botswana. The study consists of 650 adults ranging in age from 20 to 64. Table 18.1

Table 18.1 Baseline characteristics of Tshepo study

Characteristic		NVP $n = 325$	EFV $n = 325$	Total $n = 650$
Age	Median [IQR]	33.2 [29.0, 38.3]	33.7 [28.8, 39.1]	33.3 [28.9, 38.7]
Male	Count (%)	95 (29.2%)	104 (32.0%)	199 (30.6%)
Weight	Median [IQR]	57.50 [51, 66]	57.0 [50.25, 65.50]	57.0 [51, 66]
BMI	Median [IQR]	21.2 [19.2, 24.3]	21.4 [19.2, 24.1]	21.3 [19.2, 24.3]
HIV-1 RNA (1,000s)	Median [IQR]	183 [63, 466]	204 [85, 499]	195 [70, 477]
CD4+ cell count	Median [IQR]	199 [138, 243]	199 [131, 260]	199 [136, 252]
WHO Clinical Stage 1	Count (%)	90 (27.7%)	108 (33.2%)	198 (30.5%)
WHO Clinical Stage 2	Count (%)	84 (25.8%)	77 (23.7%)	161 (24.8%)
WHO Clinical Stage 3	Count (%)	117 (36.0%)	99 (30.5%)	216 (33.2%)
WHO Clinical Stage 4	Count (%)	25 (7.7%)	33 (10.2%)	58 (8.9%)
Pulmonary TB	Count (%)	27 (8.3%)	32 (9.8%)	59 (9.1%)

displays summary statistics of the baseline characteristics, W, that were collected in the Tshepo study. The outcome of interest is the time to loss of virological response (TLOVR). The only censoring event for this outcome of interest is the end of study, and thus assuming independent censoring is appropriate. The following three questions will be addressed: (1) Is there a causal effect of NNRTI-based cART therapy? (2) Is the effect of NNRTI-based cART therapy modified by gender? (3) Is the effect of NNRTI-based cART therapy modified by baseline CD4 count?

18.6.1 Causal Effect of NNRTI

Table 18.2 presents estimates of the causal effect of taking EFV vs. NVP. The Cox proportional hazards estimate in the first column is the standard analysis performed in assessing the effect of a randomized control trial on a time to event outcome. We present two TMLEs for estimating the mean marginal additive difference in the probability of survival and the mean marginal log relative hazard. This second parameter is an extension of the Cox proportional hazards parameter. The mean is taken over the first 34 months after randomization and the weights are based on the variance of the influence curve. The marginal difference of survival at the final time point, 34 months, is also presented. A positive mean log relative hazard and a negative risk difference corresponds with longer times until the specified outcome for the individuals treated with EFV compared to NVP.

For TLOVR, which includes treatment modification, there is a highly significant causal effect of taking EFV vs. NVP. The TMLE estimates for this outcome are known to be unbiased since treatment is randomized and there is independent censoring (the only censoring event is end of study). Furthermore, the results are consistent with the results presented by Wester et al. (2010), where they concluded

Table 18.2 Causal effect of NNRTI

	Parametric	TMLE		
	Cox PH	Mean RH	Mean RD	RD at t = 34
Estimate	0.358	0.451	−0.072	−0.060
SE	0.156	0.165	0.025	0.034
p-value	0.022	0.006	0.003	0.072

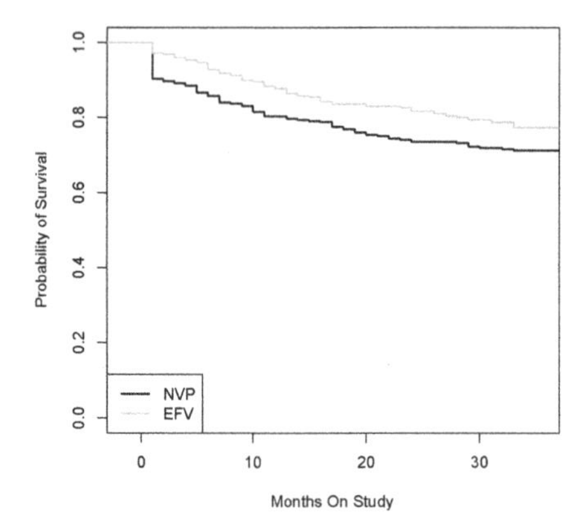

Fig. 18.5 EFV and NVP specific survival curves

that individuals treated with NVP tended to modify treatment sooner than individuals treated with EFV due to the toxicity of NVP.

Figure 18.5 presents the TMLE estimates of the treatment-specific survival curves for TLOVR. Examining the parameter estimates in conjunction with Fig. 18.5 reveals the difficulty in interpreting the Cox proportional hazards parameter (and our TMLE analog) compared to the marginal additive difference in the probability of survival. The mean additive difference is −0.072, which may be interpreted as: on average the EFV specific survival probability is 7.2% higher than the NVP-specific survival probability. A quick examination of Fig. 18.5 verifies this difference in the survival curves. The Cox proportional hazards estimate is 0.358 and would approximate the mean of $\Psi_{RH}(P_0)(t_k)$ over all time points according to the Cox proportional hazards model. This value has no easily interpretable meaning since it is the average of the log of the ratio of log survival probabilities. Alternatively, one could interpret it as an average of the log relative hazards, which requires the user to fully understand the definition of a conditional hazard (like a density). It is clear that when it is positive, the EFV-specific survival curve is larger. However, there is no intuitive meaning gained from the size of the value. In addition, we can see that the TMLE estimates are more statistically significant than the Cox proportional hazards estimates. Efficiency theory specific to the TMLE and simulation results suggest that this gain in significance is due to a reduction in bias from implementing TMLE (van der Laan and Rubin 2006; Moore and van der Laan 2009a). However, it is impossible to validate this claim for TMLE or any other method based on one sample of the data.

18.6.2 Causal Effect Modification by Baseline CD4

Table 18.3 presents the estimates that address whether or not there is a causal effect modification due to CD4 level (high/low) on the effect of cART treatment. The first column is the estimate from the Cox proportional hazards model. All main terms for W were included in the model as well as the interaction term EFV/NVP and the effect modifier CD4 level. The estimate presented is the estimate β_n in front of the cross term, $A \times V$, in the Cox proportional hazards model. The TMLEs presented are the parameters (18.5) and (18.6). The mean is taken over the first 34 months after

Table 18.3 Causal effect modification due to baseline CD4 level

	Parametric	TMLE		
	Cox PH	Mean RH	Mean RD	RD at $t = 34$
Estimate	0.675	0.829	−0.115	−0.144
SE	0.317	0.356	0.051	0.071
p-value	0.033	0.020	0.023	0.043

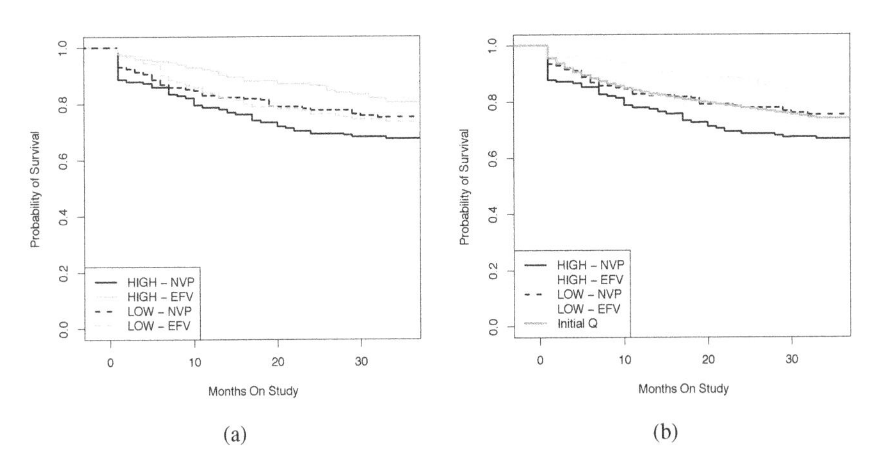

Fig. 18.6 Survival curves for time until viral failure, death, or treatment modification setting NNRTI and CD4. (a) Super learner. (b) Misspecified

randomization, and the weights are based on the variance of the influence curve. The difference in the risk difference at the final time point, 34 months, is also presented. A positive marginal difference in the log relative hazard (18.6), and a negative difference in the risk difference (18.5), indicates that EFV has a larger beneficial causal effect in the high CD4 group than in the low CD4 group.

Causal effect modification by CD4 is significant for all the parameter estimates presented. The Cox proportional hazards estimate is statistically significant; however, as was seen above, the p-value for the TMLE is more significant. These results are consistent with a decrease in bias or increase in efficiency due to using TMLE. Figure 18.6(b) shows the survival curves for TLOVR setting individuals to CD4 level and treatment group. The figure depicts the significant effect modification seen in Table 18.3. Not only is the effect of treatment among setting the individuals to high CD4 different than the effect when setting individuals to low CD4, but the effects are in opposite directions.

Figure 18.6(a) presents the TMLE survival curves where the survival probability at each time point is targeted and the initial estimate of the event hazard is estimated using the super learner. Figure 18.6(b) shows the targeted survival curves when the initial hazard is intentionally misspecified. In fact, the initial estimates for each of the four groups of differing CD4 level and treatment level are not different at all and a main terms logistic model that only accounts for t and t^2 was used. The bolded gray solid line in Fig. 18.6(b) shows the initial estimate of all four survival curves. Super learner was then used to estimate the treatment distribution, and since the only censoring event is the end of study, censoring is known to be independent of the baseline covariates, and Kaplan–Meier was used to estimate the censoring process. Figure 18.6(b) demonstrates that by using TMLE with a completely misspecified initial hazard, the effect modification is recovered, depicted by the separation of the four survival curves. This exemplifies the value of the double robustness of TMLE.

18.6.3 Causal Effect Modification Due to Gender

Table 18.4 present effect modification due to gender on the effect of cART treatment. Main terms were included for A and V, and $A \times V$ was included as well in the Cox proportional hazards model. The estimate is the β_n in front of $A \times V$. The targeted maximum likelihood estimates presented are the stratified effect modification parameters (18.7) and (18.8). The mean is taken over the first 34 months after randomization, and weighting is based on the estimated variance of the influence curve. The difference in the risk difference at the final time point, 34 months, is also presented. A negative marginal difference in the log relative hazard (18.8), and a positive difference in the risk difference (18.7), indicates that EFV has a larger beneficial causal effect for females. The treatment effect modification by gender on TLOVR is statistically significant for all three TMLE estimates and the Cox proportional hazards estimate. In fact, it is highly significant for the mean difference in

Table 18.4 Effect modification due to gender

	Parametric	TMLE		
	Cox-PH	Mean RH	Mean RD	RD at $t = 34$
Estimate	−0.952	−0.816	0.116	0.193
SE	0.353	0.329	0.035	0.054
p-value	0.007	0.013	0.001	0.000

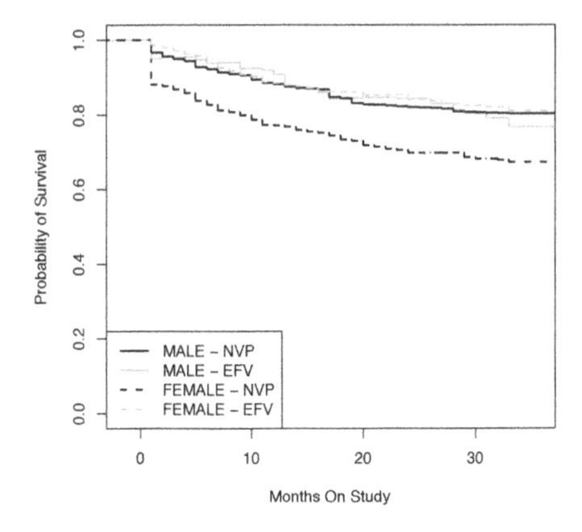

Fig. 18.7 Survival curves for time to viral failure, death, or treatment modification setting NNRTI and gender

the marginal log hazard of survival, and the difference in the marginal log hazard of survival at $t_k = 34$. Figure 18.7 shows the survival curves for the TLOVR outcome.

18.7 Discussion

The three statistical questions of interest presented in the introduction of this chapter may now be answered based on the TMLE methods and results presented above:

1. *Is there a causal effect of EFV vs. NVP on time to viral failure, death, or treatment modification?* There appears to be a causal effect of EFV vs. NVP on TLOVR. This suggests that viral failure, death, treatment modification or a combination of the three differs between individuals treated with EFV vs. NVP. The average risk difference in survival probability over the first 34 months after randomization is −7.2%.
2. *Does baseline CD4 level modify the effect of EFV vs. NVP on time to viral failure, death, or treatment modification?* Baseline CD4 level does modify the effect of EFV vs. NVP on time until TLOVR. EFV tends to be favorable compared to NVP for individuals at high CD4 levels. At low CD4 levels there is not much

of a difference in the treatment-specific survival curves (Fig. 6(a)). For TLOVR, the average risk difference between the effect in the high CD4 group vs. the low CD4 group is 12% (p-value = 0.023). One possible explanation for this is that the side effects associated with taking NVP were considered more acceptable for people with lower CD4 level so treatment was not modified. Healthier people would modify treatment because the advantages of treatment do not offset the risk of the side effects.

3. *Does the effect of EFV vs. NVP on time to viral failure, death, or treatment modification or some combination of the three differ by sex?* Gender does modify the effect of EFV vs. NVP on the time until TLOVR. Women tend to have more favorable outcomes using EFV, while males tend to have more favorable outcomes with NVP. For TLOVR, the average causal risk difference between the effect in the males vs. the females is 12% (p-value = 0.001). A possible reason for this result is that female NVP users tend to modify their treatment at a higher rate than the other groups. Based on Fig. 18.7, the major difference in the modification rate tends to occur right after starting the NVP therapy.

In addition to answering these statistical questions, the results illustrate the advantages of using TMLE over Cox proportional hazards regression for causal effects. The parameters estimated using TMLE are much easier to interpret than the parameter estimated using Cox regression. Furthermore, TMLE is double robust and locally efficient resulting in advantages over Cox regression in both producing unbiased estimates and gaining efficiency. The double robustness was illustrated by Fig. 6(b), where the effect modification due to CD4 level was regained after starting with an initial estimate of the four CD4/treatment-specific survival curves that was the same for all four combinations of CD4/treatment. The overall efficiency gains and bias reductions may not be directly exhibited through a single data analysis, as done here, but previous theoretical results and simulations have exhibited these advantages. Since TMLE targets the parameter of interest and, rather than relying on an a priori specified model to estimate the conditional hazard, it produces consistent estimates of a specified parameter of interest under very unrestrictive model assumptions, whereas the Cox proportional hazards estimate is only consistent if the Cox proportional hazards model and its restrictive parametric assumptions are true. For these reasons, the parameter estimates and significance levels produced by the TMLE should be considered more reliable than those produced using Cox proportional hazards.

Appendix

TMLE incorporating time-dependent covariates. In the Tshepo study, time-dependent measurements on viral load and CD4 count over time until end of follow-up were collected. The analysis presented in this chapter ignored these measurements. A general roadmap and algorithm for constructing TMLE based on general longitudinal data structures has been developed in van der Laan (2010a,b), is also presented in Appendix A, and demonstrated in Part VIII. This type of TMLE, with an enhanced implementation maximizing computational speed, has been fully implemented and evaluated in an upcoming article by Stitelman and van der Laan (forthcoming, 2011). The implementation can be easily adapted to handle general longitudinal data structures and target parameters, such as the causal effect of a dynamic treatment regimen on survival. In this upcoming article and corresponding technical report (forthcoming, 2011), full simulations and data analysis of the Tshepo study will be presented. It provides a TMLE of the causal effect of treatment on the survival function utilizing both the baseline covariates and the measured time-dependent covariates to improve efficiency as well as remove bias due to informative dropout. In this chapter appendix, we present preliminary results from this upcoming article, demonstrating the additional gains obtained by using a TMLE that incorporates the time-dependent covariates, and demonstrating the gain of TMLE relative to current practice in terms of IPCW estimation for dealing with time-dependent covariates.

We present the results of simulation studies that compare the bias and efficiency of six different estimators of the treatment specific survival curve $S_1(t_0)$: baseline TMLE, baseline IPCW, baseline A-IPCW, time-dependent TMLE, time-dependent IPCW, and time-dependent EE. Baseline refers to the data structure that excludes the time-dependent covariates, and EE is an an abbreviation for an estimating equation based estimator we developed for the complete longitudinal data structure [it can be viewed as an A-IPCW of the type presented in van der Laan and Robins (2003), but it is based on the representation of the efficient influence curve as used in the TMLE].

The EE involves representing the efficient influence curve for the longitudinal data structure as an estimating function in the target parameter ψ_0 and defining the estimator as the solution of the corresponding estimating equation, estimating the nuisance parameters with the initial estimators as used in the TMLE. No similar estimating equation based estimators have gained traction in the literature due to the computational difficulties of constructing such an estimate when there are many time points and intermediate variables. The algorithm proposed in the forthcoming article by Stitelman and van der Laan make the estimation of such an estimator computationally feasible. The EE is like the TMLE in that it is a double robust locally efficient estimator, but the TMLE is also a substitution estimator, while the EE is not. The time-dependent IPCW is defined as the empirical mean of

$$D_{IPCW}(O) = \frac{I(T > t_0, A = 1, C > t_0)}{\bar{G}_n(t_0- \mid X, A = 1)g_n(A \mid W)},$$

where g_n is an estimator of the treatment mechanism g_0, conditional on baseline covariates, $\bar{G}_n(t- \mid X, A = 1) = \prod_{t<t_0}(1 - \lambda_n(t \mid X, A = 1)$ is the estimator of the survivor function of censoring, conditional on baseline treatment, baseline covariates, and time-dependent covariates, and $\lambda_n(t \mid X, A = 1)$ is the conditional hazard of censoring at time t, adjusting for the observed past up to time $t-$.

The goal of the first set of simulations was to illustrate the bias reduction that occurs when one adjusts for time-dependent covariates that impact dropout beyond the effect of the baseline covariates on time to dropout. The second set of simulations show that if censoring is noninformative, a TMLE and EE incorporating the available time-dependent covariates improve efficiency relative to an estimator that ignores the time-dependent covariates, even though in this independent censoring scenario the latter is still a valid asymptotically linear estimator. Furthermore, our simulations also demonstrate that a locally efficient double-robust substitution estimator (time dependent TMLE) performs better in finite samples than both a locally efficient double-robust nonsubstitution estimator (time-dependent EE) and the current standard for accounting for time-dependent covariates (time-dependent IPCW). In fact, the simulations suggest that the benefit of targeted learning increases quickly, and dramatically, when the complexity (e.g., dimension of data structure) of the estimation problems increases.

In our simulations we simulated a longitudinal data structure

$$O = (W(0), A(0), N(1), W_4(1), W_5(1), A(1)..., N(K), W_4(K), W_5(K), A(K), N(K+1)),$$

for $t = 1, ..., K+1$. Here $W(0) = (W_1(0), W_2(0), W_3(0), W_4(0), W_5(0))$ are the baseline covariates, $A(0)$ is the binary baseline treatment randomized with probability 0.5, $N(t)$ is the indicator of observing a failure time event at time t, $A(t)$ is the indicator of observing a censoring event at time t, and $W_4(t)$ and $W_5(t)$ are the continuous time-dependent covariates. In each simulation, 100 simulated data sets with sample size $n = 500$ were generated, the treatment specific survival curve $S_1(t_0)$ at time point $t_0 = 3$ was estimated using each of the six different estimators, and estimates of bias and MSE were recorded. The true treatment specific survival $S_1(t_0)$ for each simulation equals 0.469. All six estimators were supplied consistent estimators of the hazards of censoring and failure, while the conditional distributions of the time-dependent covariates were estimated inconsistently by discretizing the continuous covariates $(W_4(t), W_5(t))$, coding the discretized covariates with binary indicators, and estimating the conditional distribution of the binary indicators with logistic parametric regression. Each estimator was evaluated using the same estimators Q_n and g_n (for each simulation) so that any difference in their performance may not be attributed to how Q_0 and g_0 were estimated.

Simulations with informative censoring. The precise data-generating mechanism is described as follows.

(1) Drawing baseline covariates $W(0)$ involved first generating from a mean-zero multivariate normal and truncating any component from above by 2 and from below by -2. The covariance matrix was defined as 1 on the diagonal and 0.2 off the diagonal.
(2) The two time-dependent covariates $W_4(t)$ and $W_5(t)$ were generated as follows:

$$W_4(t) = 0.2A(0) + 0.5W_1(0) - 0.4W_2(0) - 0.4W_3(0) + 2W_4(t-1) + 2W_5(t-1) + U_4$$
$$W_5(t) = 0.1A(0) + 0.1W_1(0) + 0.1W_2(0) - 0.4W_3(0) + 2W_4(t) + 2W_5(t-1) + U_5,$$

Table 18.5 Simulation results for low and highly informative censoring

	Time-dependent			Baseline		
	TMLE	EE	IPCW	TMLE	A-IPCW	IPCW
Low informative						
Mean of Estimates	0.471	0.471	0.451	0.469	0.469	0.469
MSE	0.00070	0.00073	0.00127	0.00082	0.00081	0.00093
Highly informative						
Mean of Estimates	0.472	0.472	0.172	0.436	0.437	0.394
MSE	0.00066	0.00067	0.08864	0.00215	0.00210	0.00773

where U_4 and U_5 are i.i.d. $N(0, \sigma = 0.4)$.

(3) The event indicators, $N(t)$, were generated as Bernoulli indicators with probability defined by the following conditional hazard of time to failure T:

$$\lambda_T(t) = \text{expit}(-3+0.3A(0)+0.3W_1(0)-0.3W_2(0)-0.3W_3(0)+2W_4(t-1)+2W_5(t-1)).$$

(4) The censoring indicators, $A(t)$, were generated as Bernoulli indicators with probability defined by the following conditional hazard for censoring for the low and highly informative censoring case, respectively:

$$\begin{aligned}\lambda_C(t) &= \text{expit}(-4 + 0.8A(0) + 0.3W_1(0) \\ &\qquad -0.3W_2(0) - 0.3W_3(0) - 0.01W_4(t) - 0.01W_5(t-1)), \\ \lambda_C(t) &= \text{expit}(-4 + 0.8A(0) + 0.3W_1(0) \\ &\qquad -0.3W_2(0) - 0.3W_3(0) - 0.1W_4(t) - 0.1W_5(t-1)).\end{aligned}$$

Table (18.5) presents the results for this simulation. The incorporation of the time-dependent covariates results in an important bias reduction (and MSE) for the TMLE and EE estimators. In the low informative censoring simulation, the time-dependent IPCW estimator has an MSE that is 1.8 times larger than the MSE of the time-dependent TMLE and EE estimator. In the highly informative censoring scenario, the MSE of the time-dependent IPCW estimator is 134 (!) times larger than the MSE of the time-dependent TMLE and EE estimator. The latter demonstrates a complete breakdown of the IPCW estimator, reflecting that it is simply a very unreliable estimator, even though it represents current practice.

Simulations with independent censoring. The data-generating distribution was the same as above, except the censoring mechanism was modified. The hazard of censoring was only a function of time, such that censoring was independent of the evolving processes, but three different hazards were considered, representing different levels of independent censoring: no censoring, medium censoring, and high censoring. In the first scenario, each individual was left uncensored. In the second and third scenario each subject was censored with either 20% probability (medium) or 60% probability (high).

Table 18.6 Simulation results for independent censoring

	Time-dependent			Baseline		
	TMLE	EE	IPCW	TMLE	A-IPCW	IPCW
No censoring						
Mean of Estimates	0.469	0.469	0.469	0.468	0.468	0.469
MSE	0.00047	0.00047	0.00054	0.00048	0.00048	0.00054
Medium censoring						
Mean of Estimates	0.467	0.467	0.470	0.469	0.469	0.468
MSE	0.00063	0.00086	0.00203	0.00093	0.00093	0.00169
High censoring						
Mean of Estimates	0.476	0.477	0.477	0.464	0.464	0.466
MSE	0.00111	0.00315	0.00566	0.00180	0.00181	0.00417

The results are presented in Table 18.6. We know that under independent censoring all six estimators are consistent. Indeed, the results demonstrate that all estimators are unbiased across the three simulations, so that the estimators only differ in their efficiency (i.e., variance). Under no censoring, all estimators behave similarly, with the exception of the IPCW estimators that are somewhat inefficient. Gains in efficiency due to incorporation of the time-dependent covariates can only be expected if a significant proportion of the subjects are right censored, since an efficient estimator treats a censored subject that is very sick at the censoring time differently than a censored subject that was relatively healthy at the censoring time. Indeed, the table shows that as the amount of independent censoring increases, the IPCW estimators become increasingly inefficient relative to the efficient TMLE and EE estimators.

It is also of interest to note that, under high censoring, the time-dependent TMLE is 1.6 times more efficient than the baseline TMLE. This demonstrates the substantial gain in efficiency one can obtain by utilizing time-dependent covariates. Furthermore, under high censoring, the locally efficient double-robust nonsubstitution estimator (time-dependent EE) has an MSE of almost three (!) times the MSE of the locally efficient double-robust substitution estimator (time-dependent TMLE). This demonstrates the enormous importance of being a substitution estimator. This gain is most likely due to estimated censoring probabilities that are empirically imbalanced across strata of the covariates, so that the estimators behave similarly, as in a highly informative censoring simulation. We repeatedly observed the problem with nonsubstitution estimators when there is strong confounding in a variety of situations. Finally, it is noteworthy that the time-dependent IPCW estimator has an MSE that is 5 times larger than the MSE of the time-dependent TMLE.

Part VI
C-TMLE

Chapter 19
C-TMLE of an Additive Point Treatment Effect

Susan Gruber, Mark J. van der Laan

C-TMLE is an extension of TMLE that pursues an optimal strategy for estimation of the nuisance parameter required in the targeting step. This latter step involves maximizing an empirical criterion over a parametric working model indexed by a nuisance parameter. For the sake of introduction and demonstration, we will focus on C-TMLE of a causal effect:

$$\Psi(P_0) = E_0[E_0(Y \mid A = 1, W) - E_0(Y \mid A = 0, W)],$$

based on n i.i.d. observations on the random variable $O = (W, A, Y) \sim P_0$, with nonparametric statistical model $\mathcal{M}$ for P_0. This target parameter depends on P_0 through the marginal distribution $Q_{W,0}$ of W and the conditional mean $\bar{Q}_0(A, W) = E_0(Y \mid A, W)$, such that we can also write $\Psi(Q_0)$, where $Q_0 = (Q_{W,0}, \bar{Q}_0)$. We denote the treatment mechanism $P_0(A = a \mid W)$ with $g_0(a \mid W)$, $a \in \{0, 1\}$, which plays the role of the nuisance parameter in TMLE and C-TMLE. This simple target parameter and data structure is sufficiently rich to convey the essential elements of this general estimation procedure C-TMLE.

As with other double robust estimators, TMLE relies on external estimation (using, for example, log-likelihood-based super learning) of the treatment mechanism $g_0(1 \mid W) = P_0(A = 1 \mid W)$ based on the log-likelihood loss function of a candidate g. TMLE uses the estimator g_n of g_0 in order to make the bias of the TMLE $\Psi(Q_n^1)$ of $\psi_0 = \Psi(Q_0)$ smaller than the bias of the initial substitution estimator $\Psi(Q_n^0)$ based on an initial estimator $Q_n^0 = (Q_{W,n}, \bar{Q}_n^0)$ of Q_0. Here $Q_{W,0}$ is estimated with the empirical distribution and is not updated by the TMLE. For example, if we use the squared error loss function for $\bar{Q}_0$, then we have that $\bar{Q}_n^1 = \bar{Q}_n^0 + \epsilon_n H(g_n)$, and the TMLE is defined as the substitution estimator $\Psi(Q_n^1)$, where $H(g_n)(W, A) = A/g_n(A \mid W) - (1 - A)/g_n(A \mid W)$ is the clever covariate used to define the parametric fluctuation working model, and ϵ_n is the corresponding least-squares regression estimator.

The choice of estimator g_n of g_0 can seriously affect the amount of bias reduction achieved by the TMLE $\Psi(Q_n^1)$ relative to the bias of the initial estimator $\Psi(Q_n^0)$. The likelihood for g is the only available guide for estimation of g_0, yet not all predictors of treatment are necessarily also predictive of the outcome and thus should be included in the estimator of the treatment mechanism. In addition, a covariate that is heavily predictive of the outcome, but mildly predictive of treatment, might be a more important covariate to include in the estimator of the treatment mechanism than a covariate that is mildly predictive of the outcome and strongly predictive of the treatment, but the log-likelihood of the treatment mechanism would heavily favor the latter nonimportant covariate. As a consequence, maximum-likelihood-based estimation of g_0, though fully effective for estimation of g_0 itself, is inherently limited for the purpose of TMLE by its inability to identify true confounders of the treatment effect.

Theory advanced in van der Laan and Gruber (2010) provides the key insight that the TMLE step achieves full bias reduction as long as it uses a true conditional distribution of treatment treatment that adjusts for the covariates that are predictive of the residual bias/error $\bar{Q}_n^0(a, W) - \bar{Q}_0(a, W)$, $a \in \{0, 1\}$, of the initial estimator of the true outcome-regression $\bar{Q}_0$. This result is intuitively a natural consequence of the fact that the clever covariate can only reduce bias if it is predictive of the outcome after taking into account the initial estimator. This theoretical collaborative double-robustness result provides the motivation and theoretical underpinning of the C-TMLE described in this chapter. This chapter is adapted from Gruber and van der Laan (2010a).

The C-TMLE and TMLE are both substitution estimators of the form $\Psi(Q_n^*)$, where Q_n^* is an update of Q_n^0. However, they differ in the subsequent targeted bias-reduction step applied to Q_n^0, and thereby the resulting update Q_n^*, and corresponding substitution estimator $\Psi(Q_n^*)$. The TMLE applies one TMLE step to Q_n^0 using a fully adjusted estimator g_n of the treatment mechanism. On the other hand, the C-TMLE builds iteratively a sequence of candidate TMLEs $Q_{n,k}^*$ that use a $g_{n,k}$, indexed by $k = 1, \ldots, K$, for which the empirical fit of both $Q_{n,k}^*$ and $g_{n,k}$ is increasing in k, and it uses cross-validation *based on the loss function for* Q_0 to select the best TMLE among these candidates. The final estimator $g_{n,K}$ in this sequence is as nonparametric as the g_n used by the TMLE and is supposed to be a consistent estimator of g_0. The rationale of the asymptotic consistency of C-TMLE can be phrased as follows. If, given a current running initial estimator of $\bar{Q}_0$, such as a TMLE using $g_{n,k}$, a next TMLE update of this initial estimator using an enlarged adjustment set in $g_{n,k+1}$, results in zero improvement in true fit (as meaured by cross-validation) of $\bar{Q}_0$, then the additional covariates added to the treatment mechanism cannot further reduce bias for ψ_0 either.

Specifically, such a sequence of candidate TMLEs and corresponding C-TMLE may be built as follows. Recall that we estimate the marginal distribution of W with the empirical distribution, so that we only need to describe the C-TMLE of $\bar{Q}_0$. For simplicity, the following algorithm is presented with a set of main terms extracted from W. One starts with the initial estimator $\bar{Q}_n^0$. The first candidate is defined as the TMLE that fluctuates the initial estimator $\bar{Q}_n^0$, using a logistic regression model fit for the treatment mechanism that only includes the intercept. Next consider a TMLE that fluctuates $\bar{Q}_n^0$ with a logistic regression model fit of the treatment mechanism that includes a main term (beyond the intercept). There are several such fits, each of which leads to a different TMLE. Focus on the TMLE that gives the best empirical fit to the data. If this TMLE indeed improves the $\bar{Q}_0$ empirical fit relative to the previous TMLE (in the sequence) using the intercept model for g_0, then this TMLE is the second candidate in the sequence of TMLEs we are building. If, on the other hand, this TMLE does not improve the empirical fit of $\bar{Q}_0$, then we do not accept this TMLE as our second candidate in the sequence of TMLEs. Instead we replace the initial estimator by the previous TMLE and we start over. We now consider a TMLE that fluctuates this new initial estimator with a logistic regression estimator of the treatment mechanism that includes the main term (beyond the intercept) that gives the best fit of the corresponding TMLE of $\bar{Q}_0$.

Since this TMLE is a fluctuation of the previous TMLE in the sequence, it will now always improve the $\bar{Q}_0$ empirical fit relative to the previous TMLE in the sequence we have built so far. Therefore, we select this TMLE as our second TMLE in the sequence. This process is iterated and results in a sequence of TMLEs $\bar{Q}^*_{n,k}$ with a corresponding estimator $g_{n,k}$ of the treatment mechanism, for which the empirical fits of both $\bar{Q}^*_{n,k}$ and $g_{n,k}$ improve in k. The estimator $g_{n,k}$ corresponds with a logistic regression fit with an intercept and $k-1$ main terms. Given these candidate estimators $\bar{Q}^*_{n,k}$, we select k with cross-validation selector k_n based on the loss function for $\bar{Q}_0$, the same loss function that was used in the TMLE step. The C-TMLE of $\bar{Q}_0$ is now defined as the corresponding $\bar{Q}^*_n = \bar{Q}^*_{n,k_n}$, and the C-TMLE of ψ_0 is the corresponding substitution estimator $\Psi(\bar{Q}^*_n)$. Note that this sequence of TMLEs puts in an increasing effort in targeted bias reduction (because the fit of $g_{n,k}$ is increasing in k), resulting in an improved empirical fit of $\bar{Q}_0$ (because the fit of $\bar{Q}^*_{n,k}$ is increasing in k), and cross-validation selects the largest k for which the observed increase in $\bar{Q}_0$ empirical fit is still reflective of an improvement in real fit of $\bar{Q}_0$.

A common misconception is that C-TMLE might not adjust for confounders as much as the TMLE. In fact, by careful selection of covariates in the treatment mechanism, the C-TMLE typically carries out a more effective bias reduction, and thereby delivers as much or more bias reduction than TMLE, at the cost of a smaller increase in finite sample variance. In the context of sparsity, the C-TMLE may strongly outperform the TMLE. That said, in settings in which the initial estimator is poor, and a thorough understanding on what covariates to include in the treatment mechanism estimator is available, a C-TMLE that builds many candidate TMLEs to select from may perform worse than the less adaptive TMLE.

19.1 Linear Fluctuation and Squared Error Loss

One first needs to define a valid loss function for $\bar{Q}_0$, such as the squared error loss function $L(\bar{Q})(O) = (Y - \bar{Q}(A, W))^2$, and a fluctuation working model, so that, given an initial estimator of $\bar{Q}_0$, an estimator of the treatment mechanism g_0, a corresponding TMLE is well defined. Given such a definition of the TMLE, the C-TMLE algorithm can be described as follows:

C-TMLE Algorithm

Step 1. Construct an initial estimator $\bar{Q}_n^0$ of $\bar{Q}_0(A, W) = E_0(Y \mid A, W)$, such as the super learner based on the squared error loss function.

Step 2. Create candidate TMLEs $\bar{Q}_{n,k}^*$, using a treatment mechanism estimator $g_{n,k}$, such that the empirical fits of $\bar{Q}_{n,k}^*$ (based on the loss function for $\bar{Q}_0$) and $g_{n,k}$ are increasing in k. This can be carried out with a forward greedy selection algorithm, described below.

Step 3. Select the best candidate, $\bar{Q}_n^* = \bar{Q}_{n,k_n}^*$, using loss-based cross-validation using the loss function for $\bar{Q}_0$ used in the TMLE.

Step 4. Evaluate its parameter value, $\psi_n = \Psi(Q_n^*)$, based on substitution of $\bar{Q}_n^*$ and the empirical distribution $Q_{W,n}$ as estimator of the marginal distribution of W.

Theory requires that the sequence $(g_{n,k} : k)$ of estimators grow toward and arrive at a consistent estimator of the true g_0. Building nested candidate estimators $g_{n,k}$ is one particular approach that satisfies this requirement, and ensures that for all $m < k$, $g_{n,k}$ is a better empirical fit for the treatment mechanism than $g_{n,m}$. At each step k in the iterative forward selection algorithm described below, it has a current initial estimator of $\bar{Q}_0$ and a current $g_{n,k}$ as a starting point. At this step k, it considers all the TMLE updates of the current initial estimator of $\bar{Q}_0$ using a $g_{n,k+1}$ that augments the current main term model $g_{n,k}$ with a single additional covariate W_k, among the remaining main terms to consider. It selects the main term that maximizes the TMLE fit of $\bar{Q}_0$. In this manner, for each $k = 1, 2, \ldots$, the k step in this iterative algorithm aims to improve the fit for g_0 in a way that maximally increases the corresponding TMLE fit of $\bar{Q}_0$.

Let's be specific. We define a TMLE in terms of the squared error loss function and linear fluctuation model. One begins with the intercept model for g_0 to construct a first clever covariate, $H^*(g_{n,1})$, used to create the first targeted maximum likelihood candidate, $\bar{Q}_{n,1}^* = \bar{Q}_n^0 + \epsilon_1 H^*(g_{n,1})$, where

$$g_{n,1}(a \mid W) = P_n(A = a), \ a \in \{0, 1\},$$
$$H^*(g_{n,1}) = \left(\frac{I(A = 1)}{g_{n,1}(1 \mid W)} - \frac{I(A = 0)}{g_{n,1}(0 \mid W)} \right),$$

and ϵ_1 is fitted by least-squares regression of Y on $H^*(g_{n,1})$ with offset $\bar{Q}_n^0$. The second candidate TMLE will be based on an updated model for g_0 that contains the intercept and one term. The best main term is selected based on an empirical fit of the TMLE of $\bar{Q}_0$. This empirical fit is defined as the empirical sum of squared residuals at the resulting $\bar{Q}_0$ fit.

Example. Consider the following example, illustrating the process of choosing the best term to add to the intercept model for g, given $W = (W_1, W_2, W_3)$.

C-TMLE Algorithm Example with $W = (W_1, W_2, W_3)$

- Construct tentative candidate estimators for $g_{n,2}$:
  - g_n^{2a}: regress A on W_1,
  - g_n^{2b}: regress A on W_2,
  - g_n^{2c}: regress A on W_3.
- Obtain each corresponding tentative candidate TMLE: $\bar{Q}_n^{2x} = \bar{Q}_n^0 + \epsilon_{2x} H^*_{g_n^{2x}}$, $x \in \{a, b, c\}$.
- Select the x that minimizes the negative log-likelihood $l(\bar{Q}_n^{2x})$.
- The best TMLE is given by $\bar{Q}_n^{2b}$, and note that $l(\bar{Q}_n^{2b}) < l(\bar{Q}_n^1)$, so that we accept this choice as our next $\bar{Q}_n^2$ in the sequence of TMLEs, with corresponding $g_{n,2} = g_n^{2b}$. We now have $\bar{Q}_n^1, \bar{Q}_n^2$ and corresponding $g_{n,1}, g_{n,2}$.

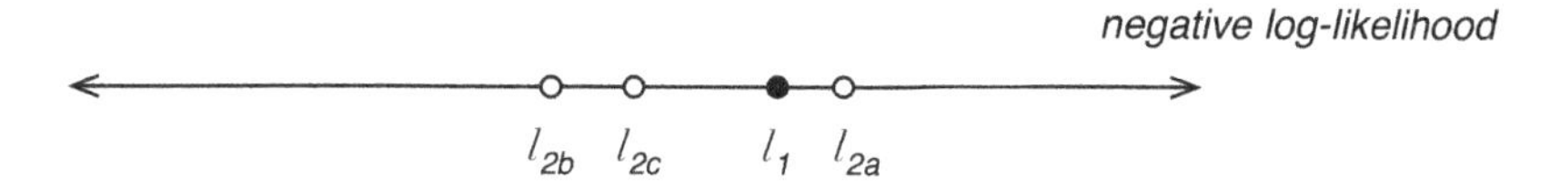

- Construct tentative candidate estimators for $g_{n,3}$:
  - g_n^{3a}: regress A on W_2, W_1,
  - g_n^{3b}: regress A on W_2, W_3.
- Obtain each corresponding tentative candidate TMLE: $\bar{Q}_n^{3x} = \bar{Q}_n^0 + \epsilon_{3x} H^*_{g_n^{3x}}$, $x \in \{a, b\}$.
- Select the x that minimizes the negative log-likelihood $l(\bar{Q}_n^{3x})$.
- The best TMLE is given by $\bar{Q}_n^{3a}$, but note that $l(\bar{Q}_n^{3a} > l(\bar{Q}_n^2)$. Therefore, we do not accept this best TMLE as our next TMLE $\bar{Q}_n^3$ in the sequence of TMLEs.

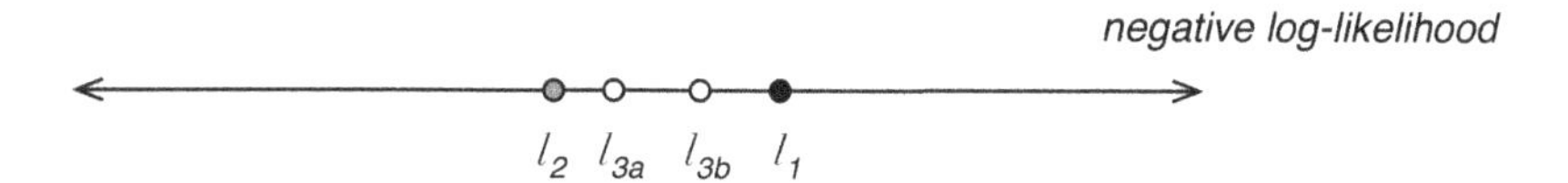

- Instead, we update the initial in our tentative candidate TMLEs by replacing the initial $\bar{Q}_n^0$ by $\bar{Q}_n^2$, and repeat our search for Q_n^3 with this new initial, as follows.
- Construct tentative candidate estimators for $g_{n,3}$:
  - g_n^{3c}: regress A on W_2, W_1,
  - g_n^{3d}: regress A on W_2, W_3.
- Obtain each corresponding tentative candidate TMLE: $\bar{Q}_n^{3x} = \bar{Q}_n^{2*} + \epsilon_{3x} H^*_{g_n^{3x}}$, $x \in \{c, d\}$.

- Select the x that minimizes the negative log-likelihood $l(\bar{Q}_n^{3x})$.
- The best TMLE is given by $\bar{Q}_n^{3c}$, and, note $l(\bar{Q}_n^{3c}) < l(\bar{Q}_n^2)$ (as it should), so that we accept this choice as our next $\bar{Q}_n^3$ in the sequence of TMLEs, with corresponding $g_{n,3} = g_n^{3c}$. We now have $\bar{Q}_n^1, \bar{Q}_n^2, \bar{Q}_n^3$ and corresponding $g_{n,1}, g_{n,2}, g_{n,3}$.

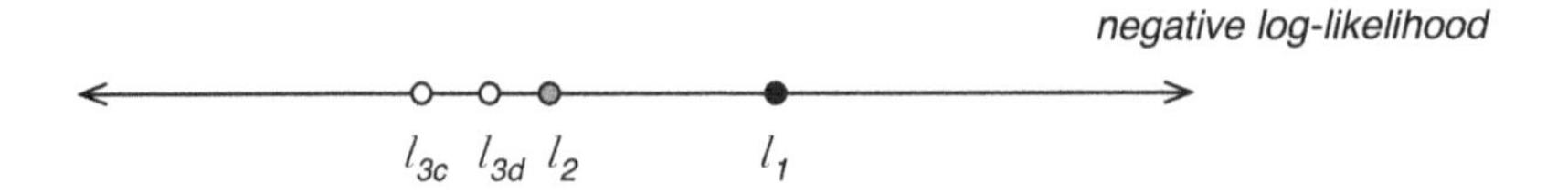

- Construct tentative candidate estimators for $g_{n,4}$:
  - g_n^{4a}: regress A on W_2, W_1, W_3.
- Obtain each corresponding tentative candidate TMLE:
  $\bar{Q}_n^{4a} = \bar{Q}_n^{2*} + \epsilon_{4a} H^*_{g_n^{4a}}$ (only one choice).
- Select the x that minimizes the negative log-likelihood $l(\bar{Q}_n^{4x})$: $x = a$.
- The best TMLE is given by $\bar{Q}_n^{4a}$, and, note $l(\bar{Q}_n^{3a}) < l(\bar{Q}_n^3)$, so that we accept this choice as our next $\bar{Q}_n^4$ in the sequence of TMLEs, with corresponding $g_{n,4} = g_n^{4a}$. The final sequence is thus given by: $\bar{Q}_n^1, \bar{Q}_n^2, \bar{Q}_n^3, \bar{Q}_n^4$, and we also have corresponding $g_{n,1}, g_{n,2}, g_{n,3}, g_{n,4}$.

A penalized RSS to make the empirical fit of $\bar{Q}_0$ more targeted. We have proposed to make the empirical fit of a candidate TMLE of $\bar{Q}_0$ more targeted than the empirical risk of the squared error loss function (i.e., the RSS) by adding to the RSS a penalty term proportional to the estimated variance of this candidate TMLE of the target parameter. Since this penalty is asymptotically negligible relative to RSS, this penalized RSS for a candidate TMLE of $\bar{Q}_0$ is still asymptotically minimized at the true $\bar{Q}_0$ and thereby represents a valid loss function. The variance of the candidate TMLE of the target parameter may be estimated using the empirical variance of the estimated efficient influence curve D^*.

Specifically, a penalized cross-validated sum of squared residuals, and the corresponding cross-validation selector of k can be defined as follows. The cross-validation selector is defined as

$$k_n = \underset{k}{\operatorname{argmin}}\ \text{cvRSS}_k + \text{cvVar}_k + n \times \text{cvBias}_k^2,$$

where these terms are given by

$$\text{cvRSS}_k = \sum_{v=1}^{V} \sum_{i \in Val(v)} (Y_i - \hat{\bar{Q}}_k^*(P_{nv}^0)(W_i, A_i))^2,$$

$$\text{cvVar}_k = \sum_{v=1}^{V} \sum_{i \in Val(v)} D^{*2}(\hat{\bar{Q}}_k^*(P_{nv}^0), \hat{g}^k(P_n), \hat{\Psi}(\hat{Q}_k^*(P_{nv}^0)))(O_i),$$

$$\text{cvBias}_k = \frac{1}{V} \sum_{v=1}^{V} \Psi(\hat{Q}_k^*(P_{nv}^0)) - \Psi(\hat{Q}_k^*(P_n)).$$

Here v indexes the validation set $Val(v)$ of size np and empirical distribution $P_{n,v}^0$ of the training sample of size $n(1-p)$ for the vth fold, $v = 1, \ldots, V$, and $p = 1/V$. For any Q, g, $D^*(Q, g, \Psi(Q))$ denotes the efficient influence curve of our target parameter at (Q, g):

$$D^*(Q, g, \Psi(Q))(O) = \frac{I(A=1) - I(A=0)}{g(A \mid W)}(Y - \bar{Q}(A, W)) + \bar{Q}(1, W) - \bar{Q}(0, W) - \Psi(Q).$$

Note that the logistic regression models for g_0 used by $g_{n,k}$ are not restricted to the univariate components of W only. For example, variables can be created that correspond to higher-order terms, such as interactions of the components of W. In addition, a categorical or continuous univariate covariate can be split into many binary covariates, thereby allowing for more nonparametric modeling of the effect of a single covariate. In addition, most importantly, a series of increasingly nonparametric propensity score estimates using super learning can be obtained based on different covariate sets. These super learner fits of the propensity score would then be used as the main terms in the algorithm described above. When there are many covariates, it might be desirable in practice to terminate the procedure before all covariates have been incorporated into the model for g_0, though care must be taken to ensure that none of the candidates thereby excluded from the subsequent selection process potentially maximizes the empirical criterion. In this manner the total number of candidates K is controlled without loss of practical performance of the resulting C-TMLE.

19.1.1 Simulations: Estimator Comparison

Three simulation studies illustrate the performance of the C-TMLE under different data-generating scenarios and are designed to provide insight into estimator performance under confounding of the relationship between treatment and outcome, complex underlying data-generating distributions, and practical violations of the positivity assumption. Other estimators commonly used to assess causal effects are also evaluated. A comparison of these estimators highlights the differences in their behavior and illustrates the importance of statistical properties such as double robustness, asymptotic efficiency, and robustness in the context of sparsity.

The unadjusted estimator is defined as

$$\psi_n^{unadj} = \frac{1}{n}\sum_{i=1}^{n}(2A_i - 1)Y_i.$$

If the covariates confound the relationship between treatment and outcome, the unadjusted estimator will be biased. Given an ML-based estimator $\bar{Q}_n^0$ of $\bar{Q}_0$, the MLE of ψ_0 is defined as

$$\psi_n^{MLE} = \frac{1}{n}\sum_{i=1}^{n}(\bar{Q}_n^0(1, W_i) - \bar{Q}_n^0(0, W_i)).$$

This estimator is consistent if $\bar{Q}_n^0$ is a consistent estimator of $\bar{Q}_0$. The IPTW estimator is defined as

$$\psi_n^{IPTW} = \frac{1}{n}\sum_{i=1}^{n}(I(A_i = 1) - I(A_i = 0))\frac{Y_i}{g_n(A_i \mid W_i)}.$$

Large weights, practical or theoretical violation of the positivity assumption $0 < g_0(1 \mid W) < 1$, is known to make this estimator variable and biased (Freedman and Berk 2008). The A-IPTW estimator is defined as

$$\psi_n^{A-IPTW} = \frac{1}{n}\sum_{i=1}^{n}\frac{I(A_i = 1) - I(A_i = 0)}{g_n(A_i \mid W_i)}(Y_i - \bar{Q}_n^0(A_i, W_i)) + \frac{1}{n}\sum_{i=1}^{n}(\bar{Q}_n^0(1, W_i) - \bar{Q}_n^0(0, W_i)),$$

and is asymptotically unbiased and efficient when both g_n and $\bar{Q}_n^0$ are asymptotically consistent estimators of g_0 and $\bar{Q}_0$, respectively. This estimator remains unbiased if at least one of these estimators is asymptotically consistent. Unlike C-TMLE, A-IPTW relies on external estimation of g_0, and may therefore include covariates that are predictive only of treatment, tending to increase both bias and variance.

The propensity score (pscore) estimator (Rosenbaum and Rubin 1983) that calculates the marginal treatment effect as the mean across strata defined by the conditional probability of receiving treatment is given by

$$\psi_n^{pscore} = \frac{1}{n}\sum_{i=1}^{n}(\bar{Q}_n^0(1, s_i) - \bar{Q}_n^0(0, s_i)),$$

where $\bar{Q}_n^0(a, s)$ is an estimator of the true conditional mean $E(Y \mid A = a, S = s)$, and s_i indicates a stratum of the pscore of covariate vector W_i. The pscore estimator is asymptotically consistent if g_n is a consistent estimator of g_0 and if one lets the number of strata converge to infinity as sample size increases. This will typically require a data-adaptive method for selection of the strata and the number of strata. Contrary to a nonparametric MLE based on the reduced-data structure $(g_n(1 \mid W), A, Y)$, it is commonly recommended in the literature to ignore the outcome data in the construction of these strata, even though this may heavily harm the performance of this estimator. Estimates can suffer even when overall match quality based on the pscore is high if only a small subset of the covariates are true confounders and these are unevenly distributed between treatment and control groups. Like most estimators, these are known to perform poorly when there are positivity violations (Sekhon 2008a). Because this estimator ignores covariate information and outcome data, it is known to not be asymptotically inefficient.

The matching estimator (Sekhon 2008a), an extension of pscore estimators that matches observations in treatment and control groups based on minimizing a distance between the covariates W of a treated and untreated unit, is defined as

$$\psi_n^{matching} = \frac{1}{n}\sum_{i=1}^{n}(\bar{Q}_n^0(1, m_i) - \bar{Q}_n^0(0, m_i)),$$

where $\bar{Q}_n^0(a, m)$ is a nonparametric estimator of the conditional mean $E(Y \mid A = a, M = m)$, and m_i indicates a set of matched observations to which subject i is assigned. The matching algorithm this estimator relies upon carefully matches observations in the treatment and control groups an effort to evenly distribute potential confounders. The matching procedure relies on the genetic algorithm (Holland and Reitman 1977) to achieve this goal. Candidate sets of matches are evaluated based on a loss function and a distance metric between covariate vectors, specified at run time, and are used to generate successive sets of candidates that achieve good balance (Sekhon 2008a). The matching estimator can be provided with a pscore estimator as one of the covariates. The marginal treatment effect is the average of the empirical effects across the strata defined by the sets of matches. As with the pscore estimator, this one also ignores the outcome in the construction of the strata.

The C-TMLE is defined as

$$\psi_n^{C-TMLE} = \frac{1}{n}\sum_{i=1}^{n}(\bar{Q}_n^*(1, W_i) - \bar{Q}_n^*(0, W_i)),$$

where $\bar{Q}_n^*$ refers to an update of an initial estimator $\bar{Q}_n^0$, as described previously. Note that the unadjusted estimator, the pscore estimator, the matching estimator, the TMLE, and the C-TMLE are all substitution estimators based on plugging in an estimator of $\bar{Q}_0$, so that these estimators only differ in the manner in which $\bar{Q}_0$ is estimated.

Covariates $W_1, \ldots W_5$ are generated as independent normal random variables, while W_6 is a binary variable. Specifically,

$$W_1, W_2, W_3, W_4, W_5 \sim N(0, 1),$$
$$P_0(W_6 = 1 \mid W_1, W_2, W_3, W_4, W_5) = \text{expit}(0.3W_1 + 0.2W_2 - 3W_3).$$

We use the following two treatment mechanisms:

$$g_{1,0}(1 \mid W) = \text{expit}(0.3W_1 + 0.2W_2 - 3W_3)$$
$$g_{2,0}(1 \mid W) = \text{expit}(0.15 \times (0.3W_1 + 0.2W_2 - 3W_3)).$$

We also use two conditional distributions of the outcome Y specified as follows:

$$Y = \bar{Q}_{i,0}(A, W) + \epsilon, \ \epsilon \sim N(0, 1),$$

with corresponding true outcome regressions:

$$\bar{Q}_{1,0}(A, W) = A + 0.5W_1 - 8W_2 + 9W_3 - 2W_5$$
$$\bar{Q}_{2,0}(A, W) = A + 0.5W_1 - 8W_2 + W_3 + 8W_3^2 - 2W_5.$$

We use three different data-generating distributions: $(\bar{Q}_{1,0}, g_{1,0})$ in simulation 1, $(\bar{Q}_{2,0}, g_{1,0})$ in simulation 2, and $(\bar{Q}_{2,0}, g_{2,0})$ in simulation 3.

Note that W_6 is strongly correlated with treatment A in simulations 1 and 2 (corr = 0.54) but is not an actual confounder of the relationship between A and Y. The true confounders are W_1, W_2, and W_3. The linear nature of the confounding due to W_3 in simulation 1 differs from that in simulations 2 and 3, where the true functional form is quadratic. In this way simulations 2 and 3 try to mimic realistic data analysis scenarios in which the unknown underlying functional form is seldom entirely captured by the regression model used in the analysis. Finally, the treatment mechanism in simulations 1 and 2 leads to positivity violations. Specifically, $P(A = 1 \mid W)$ ranges between 9×10^{-7} and 0.9999978, and approximately one-third of the probabilities are outside the range (0.05, 0.95). In simulation 3 there are no ETA violations since $0.11 < P(A = 1 \mid W) < 0.88$. In each simulation the true value of the parameter of interest equals 1: $\psi_0 = 1$.

One thousand samples of size $n = 1000$ were drawn from each data generating distribution. A main effects model fit for $\bar{Q}_n^0$ was obtained using the data-adaptive DSA algorithm restricted to main terms only for the MLE and A-IPTW estimators. A main terms logistic regression model fit for the treatment mechanism g_n was also selected by DSA, using the logistic link and restricted to main terms only, and provided as input into the IPTW, A-IPTW, pscore, and matching estimators. The pscore method was implemented by dividing observations into strata based on the five quintiles of the predicted conditional treatment probabilities. Any weights that were greater than 10 were set to 10 for the IPTW estimator.

Mean estimates of the treatment effect and standard errors for each simulation are shown in Table 19.1 and Fig. 19.1 illustrates each estimator's behavior. As expected, the estimators relying on consistent estimation of $\bar{Q}_0$ are unbiased in simulation 1, while those relying on consistent estimation of g_0 are unbiased in simulation 3. The unadjusted estimator yields biased results in all three simulations due to its failure to adjust for confounders. The ML-based estimator performs well in simulation 1 when the DSA estimator consistently estimates $\bar{Q}_0$. We understand that misspecification of $\bar{Q}_n^0$ (simulations 2 and 3) will often, though not always, lead to

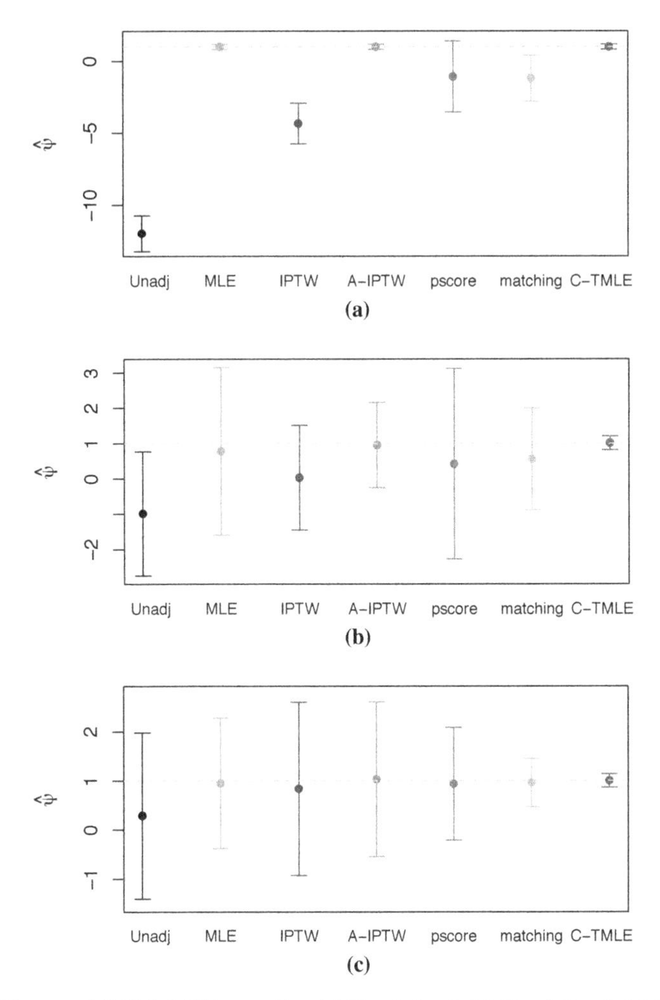

Fig. 19.1 Means and (0.025, 0.975) quantiles. (a) Simulation 1. (b) Simulation 2. (c) Simulation 3

Table 19.1 Means and standard errors for each estimator, 1000 iterations, n = 1000, ψ_0 = 1

	Simulation 1		Simulation 2		Simulation 3	
	ψ_n	SE	ψ_n	SE	ψ_n	SE
Unadj	−11.97	0.64	−0.98	0.91	0.29	0.86
MLE	0.99	0.09	0.76	1.22	0.95	0.68
IPTW	−4.36	0.72	0.03	0.76	0.83	0.90
A-IPTW	0.99	0.09	0.94	0.62	1.03	0.80
pscore	−1.09	1.27	0.42	1.38	0.93	0.59
matching	−1.22	0.82	0.54	0.73	0.96	0.25
C-TMLE	0.99	0.09	1.00	0.10	1.00	0.07

bias in the estimates. However, the plots highlight another phenomenon that is easy to overlook. The inability of the misspecified regression fit to explain the variance in the outcome often leads to large variance of the estimator of the treatment effect ψ_0. Truncation bias due to positivity violations causes the IPTW estimator using truncated weights to fail in simulations 1 and 2. The estimate is not biased in simulation 3, but the variance is so large that even in this setting where we'd expect IPTW to be reliable it fails to produce a significant result. A-IPTW estimates are unbiased and have low variance when the DSA algorithm selects the right model fit of $\bar{Q}_0$ (simulation 1). However, the variance of the A-IPTW estimator is large in simulations 2 and 3 because, despite not being a confounder, W_6, a strong predictor of A, is always included in the estimate of the treatment mechanism, thus needlessly increasing the variance.

The pscore has poor performance in simulations 1 and 2 when there are positivity violations. Without using information about the outcome the fit of the pscore can be based on the predictive power of the fit, but not on the potential bias reduction. The pscore method does a reasonable job in simulation 3. The matching estimator performs quite well; however, it is quite inefficient in simulation 1.

These simulation studies demonstrate the collaborative double robustness and efficiency of C-TMLE methodology, which allows for consistent efficient estimation in situations where other estimators can fail to perform adequately. In practice these failures may lead to biased estimates and to confidence intervals that fail to attain the correct coverage, as suggested by the IPTW results in simulations 1 and 2, where weights depend on a variable highly predictive of treatment that is not a true confounder of the relationship between Y and A.

As simulations 2 and 3 demonstrate, a misspecified parametric model not only results in biased estimates, but can also easily fail to adequately explain the variance in the outcome. Therefore maximum likelihood estimates of the parameter of interest based on such misspecified parametric models may have a larger variance than the semiparametric information bound achieved by an efficient estimator, such as a C-TMLE.

Estimators that rely on ML-based estimators of the treatment mechanism (IPTW, A-IPTW, TMLE, pscore) break down when there are positivity violations, failing to reduce bias, or even increasing bias, while incurring high variance that renders estimates meaningless (no statistical significance). An effort to reduce variance through truncation introduces bias into the estimate, and requires a careful tradeoff. C-TMLE addresses these issues, in the sense that it is able to utilize the covariates for effective bias reduction, avoiding harmful bias reduction efforts, reflected by the inclusion of W_6 in the treatment mechanism estimator.

To summarize, the collaborative nature of the estimation of the treatment mechanism in the C-TMLE confers three advantages:

1. The treatment mechanism model will exclude covariates that are highly predictive of treatment but do not truly confound the relationship between treatment and outcome.
2. The treatment mechanism model will strongly favor inclusion of covariates that help adjust for residual bias remaining after the initial estimator.
3. By employing the penalized RSS in the C-TMLE algorithm, the procedure will not select a treatment mechanism model that includes a term that leads to strong violations of the positivity assumption and thereby large variance of the corresponding TMLE without the benefit of a meaningful bias reduction.

19.1.2 Simulations: Comparison of C-TMLE and TMLE

The double robust property of TMLE minimizes the need for accurate estimation of both $\bar{Q}_0$ and g_0 since correct specification of either one leads to consistent estimates of the parameter of interest. However, accurate estimates of both are needed to achieve the Cramer–Rao efficiency bound. Implementations of the standard TMLE therefore strive for ideal estimates of both $\bar{Q}_0$ and g_0.

In contrast, the collaborative nature of the second stage of the C-TMLE algorithm leads to selection of an estimator, g_n, that targets that portion of the treatment mechanism needed to reduce bias not already adequately addressed by the initial estimator $\bar{Q}_n^0$ of $\bar{Q}_0$. For example, covariates included in the model fit $\bar{Q}_n^0$ might not be selected into the model fit for g_0 because they do not decrease the penalized RSS. At the same time, confounders that are not adequately adjusted for in the initial estimator $\bar{Q}_n^0$ are quickly added to model for g_0 unless the gain in bias reduction is offset by too great an increase in variance. When the initial estimate $\bar{Q}_n^0$ is a very good fit of $\bar{Q}_0$, the TMLE and C-TMLE have similar performance with respect to bias, but the C-TMLE may have a smaller finite sample variance by selecting a g_n that targets a non-fully-adjusted true conditional distribution of treatment, resulting in a possibly super efficient estimator. When the initial fit is less good, C-TMLE makes informed choices regarding inclusion of covariates in the treatment mechanism. As predicted by theory, again, this might lead to lower finite sample variances and more effective bias reduction.

The following simulation 4 illustrates these phenomena and shows the breakdown of the TMLE using the squared error loss function and linear fluctuation in the presence sparsity. The covariates W_1, W_2, and W_3 are generated as independent random uniform variables over the interval [0, 1], while W_4 and W_5 are independent normally distributed random variables. Specifically,

$$W_1, W_2, W_3 \sim U(0,1),$$
$$W_4, W_5 \sim N(0,1).$$

The treatment mechanism g_0 is designed so that W_3 is highly predictive of treatment:

$$g_0 = P_0(A = 1 \mid W) = \text{expit}(2W_1 + W_2 - 5W_3 + W_5).$$

The observed outcome Y is generated as:

$$Y = A + 4W_1 - 5W_2 + 5W_4 W_5 + \epsilon,\ \epsilon \sim N(0, 1).$$

The true causal effect ψ_0 equals 1.

C-TMLE and TMLE of ψ_0 were obtained for 1000 samples of size $n = 1000$ drawn from data-generating distribution implied by (Q_0, g_0). For this study we deliberately selected a misspecified main-terms-only model for $\bar{Q}_0$ by running the DSA algorithm restricted to main terms only. The propensity score $P(A = 1 \mid W)$ ranges from 0.004 to 0.996. Approximately 17% of the propensity scores are smaller than 0.05, indicating that practical positivity violations in finite samples cause the TMLE to be unstable.

We expect that the initial estimator of ψ_0 based on the misspecified $\bar{Q}_n^0$ (that excludes the interaction term) is biased. The targeting step for both targeted estimators are supposed to reduce this bias. The treatment mechanism g_0 is estimated with the DSA algorithm, allowing for quadratic terms and two-way interactions. The covariates that were candidates for inclusion in the model for g_n in the C-TMLE algorithm include $(W_1, \ldots, W_5, W_1^2, \ldots, W_5^2)$ and all two-way interaction terms $(W_i \times W_j)$ with $i \neq j$.

Results of the simulation are shown in Table 19.2. A small number of aberrant realizations of the TMLE were major contributors to the variance of that estimator. The three highest TMLEs of the treatment effect were 771.91, 37.22, and 9.52. It is likely that these high values arise from atypical samples containing observations that presented unusually strong positivity issues. In contrast, all C-TMLEs calculated from the same samples range from 0.307 to 1.698. Both estimators' average treatment effect estimates are not far from the true value, $\psi_0 = 1$. As expected, the variance of the TMLE is many times larger than that of the C-TMLE.

Not surprisingly, W_3, the strong predictor of treatment that is not a true confounder of the relationship between treatment and outcome, is included in every one of the 1000 models for g_n selected by the DSA algorithm, but it is included in only 35 of the models constructed in the estimator g_n selected by the C-TMLE

Table 19.2 Means and variance for each estimator, 1000 iterations, $n = 1000$, $\psi_0 = 1$

	Truncation level	# Obs truncated	ψ_n	Variance
C-TMLE	∞	0	0.98	0.04
TMLE	∞	0	1.73	597.52
	40	1	1.36	162.38
	10	2	0.94	1.99
	5	9	0.92	1.68

algorithm. At the same time, the interaction term $W_4 \times W_5$ is included in only two out of 1000 model fits for g_0 selected by DSA but is present in 576, more than half, of the estimators g_n selected by the C-TMLE.

This demonstrates the differences between the reliance of TMLE on an external estimate of g_0 and the collaborative approach to estimating the treatment mechanism used by C-TMLE. However, we note that the lack of robustness of the TMLE performance under sparsity is due to the unboundedness of the fluctuation function, and can be mitigated by employing the logistic fluctuation function (Chap. 7) that respects known bounds. These results were previously demonstrated for the TMLE and will also be demonstrated for the C-TMLE in a later section of this chapter.

19.1.3 Data Analysis

We apply the C-TMLE to an observational data set previously analyzed with the goal of identifying HIV mutations that affect response to the antiretroviral drug lopinavir (Bembom et al. 2008, 2009). For each analysis, which aims to assess the effect of one mutation A among the 26 mutations, the data structure on one subject can be represented as $O = (W, A, Y)$, where the outcome, Y, is the change in $\log_{10}$ viral load measured at baseline and at follow-up after treatment has been initiated, and W denotes the other 25 mutations and other summary measures of the history of the patient at baseline. If follow-up viral load was beneath the limit of detection, then Y was set to the maximal change seen in the population. Here $A \in \{0, 1\}$ is an indicator of the presence or absence of the mutation of interest. The covariate vector W consists of 51 covariates including treatment history, baseline characteristics, and indicators of the presence of additional HIV mutations. Practical positivity violations stemming from low probabilities of observing a given mutation of interest, given the other covariates, make it difficult to obtain a stable low variance estimate of the additive effect of A on the mean of Y, defined as $E_0[\bar{Q}_0(1, W) - \bar{Q}_0(0, W)]$.

Bembom et al. used a TMLE approach incorporating data-adaptive selection of an adjustment set (subset of W). Covariates whose inclusion in the adjustment set introduces an unacceptable amount of estimated bias were not selected. That study found substantial agreement with Stanford HIVdb mutation scores, values on a scale of 0 to 20 (http://hivdb.stanford.edu, as of September 2007, subsequently modified), where 20 indicates evidence exists that the mutation strongly inhibits response to drug treatment and 0 signifies that the mutation confers no resistance. Because the C-TMLE method includes covariates in the treatment mechanism only if they improve the targeting of the parameter of interest without having too much of an adverse effect on the MSE, we expect similar performance without having to specify an acceptable maximum amount of estimated bias.

The data set consists of 401 observations on 372 subjects. A C-TMLE of the additive effect of the mutation on change in viral load was carried out for each mutation. In each, a regression estimator $\bar{Q}_n^0$, was obtained using the DSA algorithm restricted to addition moves only, main terms only, and a maximum of 20 terms, where candidate terms in W include precomputed interactions detailed in Bembom et al. The mutation itself, A, was forced into the model fit of the DSA. Influence-curve-based variance estimates incorporating the contribution from estimating g_0 were used to construct 95% confidence intervals as detailed in Gruber and van der Laan (2010a).

Table 19.3 lists the Stanford mutation score associated with each of the HIV mutations under consideration, as well as the C-TMLE of the adjusted effect of mutation on lopinavir resistance. Confidence intervals entirely above zero indicate a mutation increases resistance to lopinavir. Eight of the twelve mutations having a mutation score of 10 or greater fall into this category. Point estimates for the remaining four mutations were positive, but the variance was too large to produce a significant result. Only one of the six mutations thought to confer slight resistance to lopinavir was flagged by the procedure, though, with the exception of p10FIRVY, point estimates were positive. Stanford mutation scores of 0 for four of the five mutations found to have a significantly negative effect on drug resistance support the conclusion that these mutations do not increase resistance, but are not designed to

Table 19.3 Stanford score (2007), C-TMLE estimate, and 95% confidence interval for each mutation. Starred confidence intervals do not include 0

Mutation	Score	Estimate	95% CI
p50V	20	1.703	(0.760, 2.645)*
p82AFST	20	0.389	(0.091, 0.688)*
p54VA	11	0.505	(0.241, 0.770)*
p54LMST	11	0.369	(0.002, 0.735)*
p84AV	11	0.099	(−0.139, 0.337)
p46ILV	11	0.046	(−0.222, 0.315)
p82MLC	10	1.610	(1.377, 1.843)*
p47V	10	0.805	(0.282, 1.328)*
p84C	10	0.602	(0.471, 0.734)*
p32I	10	0.544	(0.325, 0.763)*
p48VM	10	0.306	(−0.162, 0.774)
p90M	10	0.209	(−0.063, 0.481)
p33F	5	0.300	(−0.070, 0.669)
p53LY	3	0.214	(−0.266, 0.695)
p73CSTA	2	0.635	(0.278, 0.992)*
p24IF	2	0.229	(−0.215, 0.674)
p10FIRVY	2	−0.266	(−0.545, 0.012)
p71TVI	2	0.019	(−0.243, 0.281)
p23I	0	0.822	(−0.014, 1.658)
p36ILVTA	0	0.272	(−0.001, 0.544)
p16E	0	0.239	(−0.156, 0.633)
p20IMRTVL	0	0.178	(−0.111, 0.467)
p63P	0	−0.131	(−0.417, 0.156)
p88DTG	0	−0.426	(−0.842,−0.010)*
p30N	0	−0.440	(−0.853,−0.028)*
p88S	0	−0.474	(−0.781,−0.167)*

offer confirmation that a mutation can decrease drug resistance. However, Bembom et al. report that there is some clinical evidence that two of these mutations, 30N and 88S, do indeed decrease lopinavir resistance. These findings are consistent with the Stanford mutation scores and with the results from the previous analysis using the data-adaptively selected adjustment set TMLE approach.

19.2 Logistic Fluctuation for Bounded Continuous Outcomes

Chapter 7 described the importance of using a fluctuation working model in the TMLE procedure that respects the global constraints of the model. We introduced a logistic fluctuation procedure that ensures the TMLE of $\bar{Q}_0(A, W)$ remain within the bounds of the semiparametric model. This is especially relevant in sparse data situations, when outlying values for Y or $\bar{Q}_0(A, W)$ or extreme conditional treatment assignment probabilities inflate the variance of the efficient influence curve of the parameter of interest. An analysis of simulated data illustrates that employing a logistic fluctuation of $\bar{Q}_n^0$ in the targeting steps of the C-TMLE procedure further robustifies the C-TMLE under sparsity relative to the C-TMLE using the linear fluctuation function.

The targeting step of the TMLE procedure for a binary outcome uses logistic regression of Y on $H^*(A, W)$ with offset $\text{logit}(\bar{Q}_n^0)$ to fit its regression parameter ϵ, a parameter that dictates the magnitude of the fluctuation of the initial estimate. This naturally constrains the updated estimate, $\bar{Q}_n^1(A, W) = \text{expit}(\text{logit}(\bar{Q}_n^0(A, W)) + \epsilon H^*(A, W))$, to be between 0 and 1. If, instead, Y represents a continuous outcome known to be bounded between (0,1), for example, a proportion, then it is equally true that this same logistic regression updating algorithm, ignoring that Y is not binary, yields fitted values for Y that fall between 0 and 1.

Now suppose there is instead a continuous outcome Y known to be bounded by (a, b), with $a < b$. Ideally, an estimate of the conditional mean of Y given A and W should remain within $[a, b]$. We've just seen that this is easily arranged when $(a, b) = (0, 1)$. For arbitrary (a, b), $Y \in [a, b]$ can be mapped to $Y^* = (Y - a)/(b - a) \in [0, 1]$. We can then define the causal effect of treatment on the bounded outcome Y^* as $\Psi^*(P_0) = E_0[E_0(Y^* \mid A = 1, W) - E_0(Y^* \mid A = 0, W)]$. The same C-TMLE procedure outlined in Sect. 19.1 is applied to the data structure $O^* = (W, A, Y^*)$ to obtain an estimate ψ_n^*, but now using the logistic fluctuation (instead of linear) and the (possibly penalized) log-likelihood of a binary Y^*, given (W, A), as loss function for $\bar{Q}_0$ (instead of squared error loss function). This C-TMLE ψ_n^* immediately maps to a ψ_n of the causal effect on the original scale, using the relation $\Psi(P_0) = (b - a)\Psi^*(P_0)$. A confidence interval for ψ_0 can be obtained by multiplying the bounds on the confidence interval for $\Psi^*(P_0)$ by $(b - a)$. Similarly, the estimated variance $\hat{\sigma}^2$ of ψ_n is obtained by multiplying the estimated variance $\hat{\sigma}^{2*}$ of ψ_n^* with$(b - a)^2$.

19.2.1 Simulations: Logistic vs. Linear Fluctuation

The random variables were generated as follows:

$$W_1, W_2, W_3 \sim N(\mu_1, \mu_2, \mu_3, \Sigma),\ \mu_1 = \mu_2 = \mu_3 = 0,\ \ \Sigma = \begin{bmatrix} 2 & 1 & 0 \\ 1 & 1 & 0.2 \\ 0 & 0.2 & 1 \end{bmatrix},$$

$$W_4 \sim Bernoulli(0.2),$$
$$W_5 \sim Bernoulli(0.6),$$
$$W_6 \sim Bernoulli(0.7).$$

The treatment mechanism g_0 is given by $g_0 = P_0(A = 1 \mid W) = \text{expit}(2W_1 + 0.25W_2 - 0.5W_3 + W_4)$. The observed outcome Y is generated as $Y = A + 2A \times W_5 + W_1 + W_2 - W_3 \times W_5 + \epsilon$, $\epsilon \sim N(0, 1)$. Notice that the covariates (W_1, W_2, W_3, W_4) are causally related to treatment. The covariates W_1, W_2, and W_3 are also causally related to the outcome, and therefore confound the relationship between treatment and the outcome. Covariate W_6 was measured at baseline, but has no association with either the treatment or the outcome. Covariate W_5 is an effect modifier. The effect of treatment is larger for subjects having $W_5 = 1$ than for subjects having $W_5 = 0$. Though approximately one-half of the subjects receive treatment [$P_0(A = 1) = 0.53$ marginally], true treatment assignment probabilities vary between (0.0002, 0.9999), and for approx. 9% of observations the conditional probability of receiving treatment given the measured covariates is outside (0.05, 0.95). We drew 1000 samples of size $n = 1000$ from this data-generating distribution. Observed values for Y and fitted values $\bar{Q}_n^0$ of the conditional mean $\bar{Q}_0$ were truncated at the (0.01, 0.99)-quantiles of the marginal distribution of Y, given by (−5.83, 8.48). The true value of the marginal additive treatment effect on the bounded outcome Y is $\psi_0 = 2.192$.

Two C-TMLEs were applied to estimate the additive causal effect: C-TMLE$_{log}$, using a logistic fluctuation, and C-TMLE$_{lin}$, using a linear fluctuation. In order to demonstrate the impact the targeting step has on reducing bias, $\bar{Q}_n^0$ was obtained in

Table 19.4 Comparison of C-TMLE$_{log}$ and C-TMLE$_{lin}$, $\psi_0 = 2.192$

	$\bar{Q}$ correctly specified				$\bar{Q}$ misspecified			
	ψ_n	Bias	Var	MSE	ψ_n	Bias	Var	MSE
g_n bound = 0								
C-TMLE$_{log}$	2.222	0.030	0.008	0.009	2.154	−0.038	0.033	0.034
C-TMLE$_{lin}$	2.221	0.029	0.008	0.009	1.992	−0.200	0.349	0.389
g_n bound = 0.01								
C-TMLE$_{log}$	2.222	0.030	0.008	0.009	2.151	−0.041	0.032	0.034
C-TMLE$_{lin}$	2.221	0.029	0.008	0.009	2.057	−0.135	0.297	0.315
g_n bound = 0.025								
C-TMLE$_{log}$	2.222	0.030	0.008	0.009	2.146	−0.046	0.027	0.029
C-TMLE$_{lin}$	2.221	0.029	0.008	0.009	2.116	−0.076	0.054	0.060

two ways: (1) using the correct parametric regression model and (2) using a misspecified parametric regression model that assumes a univariate regression of Y on A only. Results in Table 19.4 illustrate that, as expected, when the model for $\bar{Q}_n^0$ is correctly specified, there is little difference between fluctuating on the logistic or linear scale.

Differences emerge when the model for $\bar{Q}_n^0$ is misspecified. At each level of bound on g_n, the linear fluctuation yields estimates that are much more biased and have higher variance than the logistic fluctuation-based estimates. Increasing the bound on g_n from 0 to 0.025 reduces both bias and variance for the linear fluctuation estimates, but imposes a bias–variance tradeoff on the logistic fluctuation estimates. In this simulation the MSE is smaller when g_n is bounded at (0.025,0.975) than when the bounds are closer to (0,1), but this is not always the case.

19.2.2 Simulations: Estimator Comparison

We implemented the estimators discussed in Sect. 19.1.1, the TMLE, and C-TMLE, both using the logistic fluctuation, of the additive treatment effect under the data-generating distribution scheme for the simulation given in Sect. 19.2.1. The treatment mechanism $g_n(A \mid W)$ was bounded from below at $\{0, 0.01, 0.025\}$. Table 19.5 displays the results.

These results indicate that when the parametric model for $\bar{Q}_0$ is correctly specified, estimators that rely on consistent estimation of $\bar{Q}_0$ perform very well. However, estimators that rely only on consistent estimation of g_0 and fail to exploit the information from estimation of $\bar{Q}_0$ (i.e., IPTW, pscore, and matching) are less efficient, in spite of being given the correct model for g_0. Misspecifying the model for $\bar{Q}_0$ does not harm these estimators, but in situations like the one in this simulation, they are still less efficient than TMLE and C-TMLE.

The unadjusted estimate is biased due to confounding by covariates W_1, W_2, W_3. The MLE has the smallest mean squared error when the ML-based estimator of $\bar{Q}_0$ is correctly specified, but it is not robust to misspecification. The IPTW estimator, A-IPTW estimator, matching estimator, TMLE, and C-TMLE, all of which rely on an estimator g_n, show improvements in MSE as the bounds on g_n increase from 0 to 0.025 due to a decrease in the variance at the cost of increasing bias. The IPTW estimator is consistent but very inefficient. The A-IPTW estimator has lower bias than IPTW but pays a high price in variance when $\bar{Q}_n^0$ is heavily misspecified. The pscore estimator is quite stable across all truncation levels for g_n; however, its lack of data adaptiveness yields an estimate that is quite biased in comparison with the other methods. The matching estimator is less biased than pscore and also quite stable with respect to changes in the bounds on g_n. The MSE of the matching estimator is slightly smaller than the MSE of TMLE when $\bar{Q}_n^0$ is inconsistent and approximately the same as the MSE of the C-TMLE, but the matching estimate is more biased than either TMLE or C-TMLE. Both the TMLE and C-TMLE are able to exploit information that is unavailable to the matching algorithm when $\bar{Q}_n^0$

Table 19.5 Comparison of all estimators, $\psi_0 = 2.192$

	$\bar{Q}$ correctly specified					$\bar{Q}$ misspecified				
	ψ_n	Bias	Var	MSE	RE	ψ_n	Bias	Var	MSE	RE
g_n bound = 0										
Unadj	4.590	2.398	0.021	5.771	–	4.590	2.398	0.021	5.771	–
MLE	2.222	0.031	0.007	0.008	0.001	4.590	2.398	0.021	5.771	1.000
IPTW	2.210	0.018	0.090	0.090	0.016	2.210	0.018	0.090	0.090	0.016
A-IPTW	2.186	−0.006	0.011	0.011	0.002	2.193	0.001	0.157	0.157	0.027
pscore	2.454	0.262	0.014	0.083	0.014	2.454	0.262	0.014	0.083	0.014
matching	2.316	0.124	0.018	0.033	0.006	2.316	0.124	0.018	0.033	0.006
TMLE	2.185	−0.007	0.011	0.011	0.002	2.174	−0.018	0.049	0.049	0.008
C-TMLE	2.222	0.030	0.008	0.009	0.002	2.154	−0.038	0.033	0.034	0.006
g_n bound = 0.01										
Unadj	4.590	2.398	0.021	5.771	–	4.590	2.398	0.021	5.771	–
MLE	2.222	0.031	0.007	0.008	0.001	4.590	2.398	0.021	5.771	1.000
IPTW	2.225	0.033	0.063	0.064	0.011	2.225	0.033	0.063	0.064	0.011
A-IPTW	2.187	−0.005	0.011	0.011	0.002	2.216	0.024	0.092	0.093	0.016
pscore	2.454	0.262	0.014	0.083	0.014	2.454	0.262	0.014	0.083	0.014
matching	2.317	0.125	0.018	0.033	0.006	2.317	0.125	0.018	0.033	0.006
TMLE	2.185	−0.006	0.011	0.011	0.002	2.168	−0.024	0.044	0.044	0.008
C-TMLE	2.222	0.030	0.008	0.009	0.002	2.151	−0.041	0.032	0.034	0.006
g_n bound = 0.025										
Unadj	4.590	2.398	0.021	5.771	–	4.590	2.398	0.021	5.771	–
MLE	2.222	0.031	0.007	0.008	0.001	4.590	2.398	0.021	5.771	1.000
IPTW	2.277	0.085	0.041	0.049	0.008	2.277	0.085	0.041	0.049	0.008
A-IPTW	2.188	−0.004	0.010	0.010	0.002	2.285	0.093	0.055	0.064	0.011
pscore	2.454	0.262	0.014	0.083	0.014	2.454	0.262	0.014	0.083	0.014
matching	2.319	0.127	0.018	0.034	0.006	2.319	0.127	0.018	0.034	0.006
TMLE	2.187	−0.005	0.010	0.010	0.002	2.152	−0.040	0.031	0.032	0.006
C-TMLE	2.222	0.030	0.008	0.009	0.002	2.146	−0.046	0.027	0.029	0.005

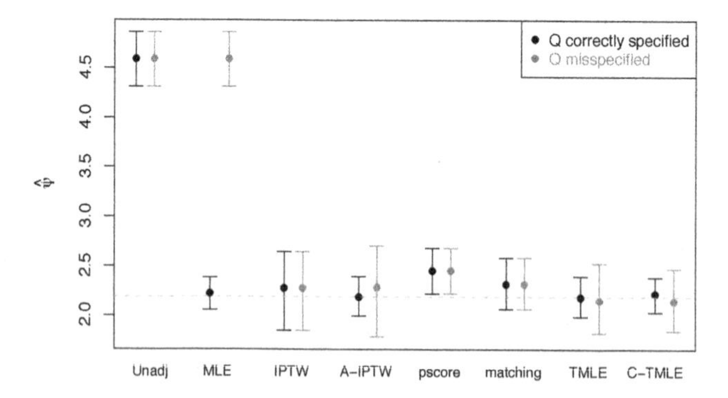

Fig. 19.2 Means and (0.025, 0.975)-quantiles, with $g_n(1 \mid W)$ bounded at (0.025, 0.975), and the parametric model for $\bar{Q}_0$ correctly specified (*left*) and misspecified (*right*)

is consistent, and thus have lower bias and variance than the matching estimator. These results also indicate that C-TMLE may trade off a small increase in bias for a larger reduction in variance, relative to TMLE, thereby minimizing overall MSE.

The MSE provides only one of several points of comparison for estimators. Minimizing MSE is an important goal, and, as we just observed, C-TMLE can make a beneficial data-adaptive tradeoff between bias and variance, but Fig. 19.2 illustrates that an estimator with a significant bias relative to the standard error, but good MSE, such as the pscore estimator, can be problematic. The plot in Fig. 19.2 shows the mean and (0.025, 0.975)-quantiles of the estimates obtained from the 1000 generated samples. 91% of the pscore estimates were larger than ψ_0. This suggests that, though an estimate far from the null with a tight confidence interval may look convincing, it might in fact be misleading, and that confidence intervals for the pscore estimator might fail to achieve the nominal coverage rate under circumstances resembling those found in this simulation. This is in marked contrast to the TMLE and C-TMLE, double robust efficient substitution estimators that have desirable properties across a range of data-generating distributions.

19.3 Discussion

The sparsity in the data with respect to the target parameter of interest, as often induced by the high dimension of covariate profiles and lack of firm knowledge about the data-generating distribution, demands estimators that carry out a very careful bias–variance tradeoff when making decisions. Estimators that are asymptotically efficient under regularity conditions may still show a very different practical performance under sparsity. For that purpose, it is important that an efficient estimator also be a substitution estimator, based on substituting an estimator that respects the global bounds on the statistical model. In addition, the estimator of the nuisance parameter used by such an efficient estimator will need to be evaluated by its effectiveness in achieving bias reduction at the cost of a reasonable increase in variance. Using an estimator of the nuisance parameter that is blinded from this benchmark will generally not result in good estimators of the target parameter under sparsity. C-TMLE using the logistic fluctuation is an asymptotically efficient substitution estimator that also targets fitting of the nuisance parameter toward its goal. Simulations demonstrate that, under sparsity, the C-TMLE indeed outperforms other efficient estimators that either ignore global bounds or contraints or use blinded estimators of the nuisance parameter.

Chapter 20
C-TMLE for Time-to-Event Outcomes

Ori M. Stitelman, Mark J. van der Laan

In this chapter, the C-TMLE for the treatment-specific survival curve based on right-censored data will be presented. It is common that one wishes to assess the effect of a treatment or exposure on the time it takes for an event to occur based on an observational database. Chapters 17 and 18 discussed the treatment-specific survival curve in RCTs. The TMLE presented there improves upon common methods for analyzing time-to-event data in robustness, efficiency, and interpretability of parameter estimates. Observational data differ from RCTs in that the exposure/treatment is not set according to a known mechanism. Moreover, in situations where there is dependent censoring the censoring mechanism is also unknown. As a consequence, in observational studies, the TMLE needs to estimate the treatment and censoring mechanism, and this needs to be done in such a way that the resulting targeted bias reduction carried out by the TMLE is fully effective.

The C-TMLE, introduced in the previous chapter, is an extension of TMLE specific to situations where treatment is not randomized or censoring is informative. The C-TMLE is often more efficient for finite samples and in observational data than a standard TMLE and all other available estimators. In fact, in some instances, the C-TMLE is asymptotically super efficient in the sense that its asymptotic variance improves on the semiparametric efficiency bound for regular estimators. Furthermore, the C-TMLE is a well-behaved estimator in situations where the parameter of interest is borderline identifiable.

When exposure is not randomized there may be strata defined by baseline characteristics that never experience a particular level of exposure. This phenomenon, discussed throughout this text and in detail in Chap. 10, is a violation of the positivity assumption. Violations of the positivity assumption render the parameters of interest as presented in Chaps. 17 and 18 unidentifiable. However, many times, in finite samples, certain parameters are weakly identifiable due to practical violations of the positivity assumption. Practical violations occur when a certain value of baseline covariates are almost completely predictive of a certain treatment within the sample. C-TMLE addresses this issue and represents a stable estimator of borderline identifiable parameters. Thus, the C-TMLE methodology may be applied in the time-to-event setting to gain efficiency as well as produce estimators of weakly identifiable parameters of interest. Readers will benefit from reading Chaps. 17–19, in addition to Part I before tackling this chapter, which is adapted from Stitelman and van der Laan (2010).

20.1 Estimating Parameters Based on Coarsened Data

We briefly introduce the parameter estimation problem for a general coarsened data structure. Coarsened data structures are data structures where the full data are not observed. Right-censored data structures are an example of a coarsened data structure since the full data absent right censoring are not observed. Collaborative targeted methods for estimating parameters with this data structure will be introduced.

Suppose one observes a censored data structure $O = \Phi(C, X)$ of the full data X and censoring variable C, where O has a probability distribution P_0. Let $\mathcal{M}$ be a semiparametric model for the probability distribution P_0. To minimize notation, we will assume O is discrete so that $P_0(o) = P_0(O = o)$ denotes a probability density. By assuming that the conditional distribution of O, given X, satisfies the CAR assumption, the density factorizes as $P_0(O) = Q_0(O)g_0(O \mid X)$, where Q_0 is the part of the density associated with the full data X and g_0 is the conditional distribution of the observed data O given the full data X. Here C may encode both treatment and censoring variables, so that g_0 includes both the censoring and treatment mechanisms, both of which act to coarsen the full data. The factorization of the probability density P_0 implies that the model $\mathcal{M}$ for P_0 may be partitioned into a model $\mathcal{Q}$ for Q_0 and model $\mathcal{G}$ for g_0. The probability distribution, P_0, may be indexed in the following way: P_{Q_0,g_0}. One is typically interested in estimating a parameter, $\Psi(P_0)$, which is a function of the true data-generating distribution. More specifically, the parameter of interest is often a function of the true full-data-generating distribution absent coarsening, and can thus be represented as $\Psi(Q_0)$.

Many methods have been developed to estimate $\Psi(Q_0)$. The MLE approach has been discussed throughout this text, and its use in time-to-event data structures is presented in Chap. 18. An alternative method for estimating $\Psi(Q_0)$ is the IPCW-based approach, originally proposed by Koul et al. (1981) and Keiding et al. (1989). IPCW estimators solve an estimating equation in order to yield estimates, ψ_n^{IPCW}, of the parameter of interest, and ψ_n^{IPCW} is a consistent estimator of $\Psi(Q_0)$ if the estimator of the g_0-factor is consistent. However, an IPCW estimator is ad hoc and unstable because (1) it does not solve the efficient influence curve estimating equation and is therefore generally inefficient and (2) it is not a substitution estimator and therefore does not respect the global restraints of the observed data model. As a result, an IPCW estimator is highly variable, very sensitive to the choice of estimator of g_0, and may act erratically in finite samples.

Another method for estimating $\Psi(Q_0)$ is an A-IPCW estimator. As discussed earlier in this text, Robins and Rotnitzky (1992) proposed this general estimating-equation-based approach, which constructs estimators ψ_n^{A-IPCW} that solve the efficient influence curve estimating equation. An A-IPCW estimator is double robust because it is consistent when either Q_0 or g_0 is estimated consistently. Furthermore, an A-IPCW estimator also improves on the standard IPCW estimator in terms of efficiency since it solves the efficient influence curve estimating equation. Thus, under appropriate regularity conditions, the A-IPCW estimator is locally asymptotically efficient. However, like the IPCW estimator, the A-IPCW estimator is not a substitution estimator and may also be unstable.

20.2 C-TMLEs

The collaboratively double robustness property states that a TMLE Q^*_{n,g_n} of Q_0 is consistent if the estimator g_n of g_0 correctly adjusts for the variables that explain the additive residual bias of the initial estimator Q_n with respect to Q_0. Thus the collaborative double robustness of TMLE teaches us that consistency of the TMLE does not require that either the estimator of Q_0 or the estimator of g_0 is consistent, but rather, one should be concerned with reducing the distance between, Q^*_{n,g_n} and Q_0, and, g_n and g_0, such that the resulting estimator $\Psi(Q^*_{n,g_n})$ is close to $\Psi(Q_0)$. If Q_n does a very good job estimating Q_0, very little adjustment is necessary through the estimate of g_0; on the other hand, if Q_n is a poor estimator of Q_0, the estimator g_n will have to do a better job of approximating g_0.

C-TMLE is an extension of TMLE that takes advantage of the collaborative double robustness property of those estimators by constructing g_n in collaboration with Q_n. C-TMLE uses the log-likelihood or another loss function for Q_0 to choose from a sequence of K targeted maximum likelihood estimates Q_n^{k*} indexed by initial estimates of Q_0 and g_0. Recall the procedure:

1. Create Q_n, an initial estimator of Q_0.
2. Generate a sequence of estimates of g_0: $g_n^0, g_n^1, \ldots, g_n^{K-1}, g_n^K$, where g_n^0 is the least data-adaptive estimate and g_n^K is the most data-adaptive estimate of g_0.
3. Generate the initial TMLE estimate, Q_n^{0*}, indexed by Q_n and g_n^0.
4. Generate a sequence of TMLE estimates: $Q_n^{0*}, Q_n^{1*} \ldots, Q_n^{K-1*}, Q_n^{K*}$, indexed by corresponding estimators $g_n^0, \ldots, g_n^K$, where each TMLE in this sequence has a larger log-likelihood than the previous TMLE. This monotonicity is ensured by defining the next TMLE as the TMLE that uses the previous TMLE in the sequence as initial estimator, each time the log-likelihood of the TMLE does not increase with the same initial estimator just by virtue of using the more data-adaptive estimate of g_0.
5. Finally, choose among the sequence of TMLEs using loss-based cross-validation with log-likelihood loss.

One adjustment to the above methodology, discussed in the previous chapter, is to use a penalized loss function when parameters are borderline identifiable. This is an important consideration in observational studies and the issue of choosing an appropriate penalty is addressed in Sect. 20.5.

The C-TMLE has two distinct advantages over the TMLE methodology:

1. C-TMLE may be used to produce stable estimators of borderline identifiable parameters while TMLE may breakdown in these situations (the estimating equation methods discussed above are even more susceptible than TMLE to breaking down). The reason many parameters are not identifiable, or are borderline identifiable, is due to violations of ETA or the more general positivity assumption, where a certain level of a covariate or group of covariates is completely predictive of treatment/exposure/censoring. In these situations, where sparsity of the data with respect to the target parameter is an issue, C-TMLE is able to weight the bias–variance tradeoff of adjusting for certain covariates in estimating these weakly identifiable parameters. C-TMLE only adjusts for covariates in estimating g_0 when they appear to be beneficial to the estimate of the parameter of interest and selects against adjusting for covariates which are detrimental to the estimate of $\Psi(Q_0)$, weighing both bias and variance. All other methods that rely on an estimate of g_0 use a loss function that measures the fit of g_0 itself, or a priori specify a parametric model, and thereby ignore the effect adjusting for certain covariates has on the final estimate of the parameter of interest.
2. The C-TMLE is often more efficient in finite samples than the TMLE. In fact, in some rare situations, the C-TMLE is super efficient by having an asymptotic variance smaller than the semiparametric efficiency bound. For example, if the initial estimator Q_n is an MLE for a correctly specified parametric model. The finite sample and asymptotic super-efficient behavior is a consequence of the collaborative double robustness exploited by the C-TMLE. In situations where the initial estimate Q_n is a very good estimate of Q_0 in the targeted sense, little adjustment is needed from the estimate of g_0. The more one adjusts for covariates in the estimator of g_0, the larger the variance of the final estimator of the parameter of interest. In fact, it can be shown that once the estimator of g_0 adjusts for all covariates that explain the residual bias of the initial estimator as an estimator of Q_0, then a TMLE update of this latter TMLE will (asymptotically) estimate zero fluctuation. In other words, the theory teaches us that more aggressive efforts for bias reduction are fitting noise! Thus not adjusting much in g_n when one doesn't have to provides estimators with smaller variance.

The C-TMLE exhibits all of the advantages of the TMLE discussed in previous chapters, as well as these two major advantages. The advantages of the C-TMLE are particularly useful in observational studies, where practical violations of the positivity assumption are a concern. However, in studies where treatment is randomized, C-TMLEs are also appropriate for two distinct reasons. First, informative censoring may be an issue, and practical violations of the ETA assumption may be attributed to this censoring. Second, one may adjust for covariates in the treatment mechanism g_0 in order to gain efficiency since C-TMLEs address the bias–variance tradeoff of adjusting for particular variables. Thus, implementation of the C-TMLE in RCTs will help ensure that one does not adjust in g_n for the covariates in a way that hinders the estimate of the parameter of interest.

20.3 Data, Model, and Parameters of Interest

The time-to-event data structure presented in Sect. 18.1 is the data structure of interest here. However, since we are now interested in observational data, there is an additional arrow from W to A in the causal graph. This new data structure suggests the following orthogonal factorization of the likelihood of the observed data structure O under a probability distribution P:

$$\mathcal{L}(O \mid P) = \overbrace{P(W)}^{Q_W}\overbrace{P(A \mid W)}^{g_A}\prod_{t=1}^{K}\overbrace{P(dN(t) \mid \bar{N}(t-1), \bar{A}(t-1), A, W)}^{Q_{dN(t)}}$$
$$\underbrace{P(dA(t) \mid \bar{N}(t), \bar{A}(t-1), A, W)}_{g_{A(t)}}.$$

Thus, the likelihood of O factorizes, just as the general censored data structure presented in Sect. 20.1, into a portion corresponding to the full-data distribution Q_0 and a portion corresponding to the censoring and treatment mechanism g_0. Q_0 is composed of the baseline covariate distribution $Q_{W,0}(W)$ and $\bar{Q}_0(t \mid A, W) \equiv E_0(dN(t) \mid \bar{N}(t-1) = 0, \bar{A}(t-1) = 0, A, W)$, the intensity of the event-counting process given A and W, conditioning on "no event yet." We further factorize g_0 into the treatment mechanism $g_{A,0}$ and censoring mechanism intensity $\bar{g}_0(t \mid A, W) \equiv E_0(dA(t) \mid \bar{N}(t) = 0, \bar{A}(t-1) = 0, A, W)$, which is the intensity of the censoring process given A and W, conditioning on "no event yet." Let's also define $S_0(t_k \mid A, W) = P_0(T > t_k \mid A, W)$, which is the conditional survival function of the event of interest and can be expressed in terms of the intensity of the event process $\bar{Q}_0$ under the CAR assumption:

$$S_0(t_k \mid A, W) = \prod_{t=1}^{t_k}\left[1 - \bar{Q}_0(t \mid A, W)\right].$$

Note that $\bar{Q}_0(t \mid A, W)$ is the conditional hazard of T at t, given A, W, under CAR, which holds if T and C are conditionally independent, given A, W (which is implied by our causal graph). The parameters of interest depicted in Sect. 18.3, when A is randomized, are the same parameters of interest now that we have moved to the observational setting. Moreover, the methods in Sect. 18.5 for estimating the TMLE of these parameters are exactly the same for the observational setting.

20.4 Estimators of the Treatment-Specific Survival Function

In this section we will briefly discuss the MLE, IPCW estimator, and A-IPCW estimator for the treatment-specific survival curve. These three methods will then be compared to the TMLE/C-TMLE in a simulation study. MLEs are one class of estimators for estimating the treatment-specific survival function, discussed in

Chap. 18, and we show in Sect. 18.3 how to map $\bar{Q}_n$ into $\psi_n^{MLE} = \Psi_a(Q_n)(t_k)$, the MLE of the treatment-specific survival curve $\Psi_a(Q_0)(t_k)$ at time t_k. The IPCW method for estimating the treatment-specific survival curve only relies on an estimator of g_0. This estimating-equation-based estimator may take the following form:

$$\psi_{n,a}^{IPCW} = \frac{1}{n} \sum_{i=1}^{n} \frac{I(T_i > t_k)I(C_i > t_k)I(A_i = a)}{g_{n,A}(a|W_i) \prod_{s=1}^{t-} (1 - \bar{g}_n(s \mid A_i, W_i))}.$$

The A-IPCW estimator is a double robust estimator that solves the efficient-influence-curve-based estimating equation. Thus, this estimator requires estimates of Q_0 and g_0. The efficient influence curve for the treatment-specific survival curve at time t_k for the observed data structure is

$$D_a^*(P_0) = \sum_{t \le t_k} H_{0,a}^*(t \mid A, W) \left[I(\tilde{T} = t, \Delta = 1) - I(\tilde{T} \ge t)\bar{Q}_0(t \mid A = a, W) \right]$$
$$+ S_0(t_k \mid A = 1, W) - \Psi_a(P_0)(t_k),$$

where

$$H_{0,a}^*(t \mid A, W) = -\frac{I(A = a)}{g_{A,0}(A = a \mid W) \prod_{i=1}^{t-} (1 - \bar{g}_0(i \mid A, W))} \frac{S_0(t_k \mid A, W)}{S_0(t \mid A, W)} I(t \le t_k).$$

Recall that $H_{0,a}^*(t \mid A, W)$ is the time-dependent clever covariate used to define the TMLE of the treatment-specific survival function $S_{0,a}(t_k) = P_0(T_a > t_k)$, and, by the δ-method, it forms the building block of the time-dependent clever covariate of any desired causal contrast in terms of such treatment-specific survival functions. Hubbard et al. (1999) develop the one-step A-IPCW estimator that solves the efficient influence curve estimating equation. The resulting A-IPCW estimate is given by

$$\psi_{n,a}^{A-IPCW} = \frac{1}{n} \sum_{i=1}^{n} \sum_{t \le t_k} H_{n,a}^*(t, A_i, W_i) \left[I(\tilde{T}_i = t, \Delta_i = 1) \right.$$
$$\left. - I(\tilde{T}_i \ge t)\bar{Q}_n(N_1(t) = 1 \mid A = a, W_i) \right] + S_n(t_k \mid A = a, W_i),$$

where $H_{n,a}^*(t \mid A, W)$ is $H_a(t \mid A, W)$ with estimates $g_{n,A}$, $\bar{g}_n$, and S_n substituted for $g_{A,0}$, $\bar{g}_0$, and S_0. It is important to note that $\psi_{n,a}^{IPCW}$ and $\psi_{n,a}^{A-IPCW}$ might not be written as a substitution estimator $\Psi_a(Q_n)$ for a particular Q_n.

20.5 C-TMLE of the Treatment-Specific Survival Function

There are two requirements for extending the TMLE to a C-TMLE. First, a sequence of estimates of g_0 and corresponding sequence of TMLEs of Q_0 must be generated. Second, the TMLE from that sequence of TMLEs that has the minimum cross-validated risk based on the initial loss function (or a loss function that is asymptotically equivalent with that loss function) for Q_0 is chosen. Thus, in order to implement the C-TMLE, one must choose a method for sequencing the estimates of g_0, and a loss function for Q_0 that is asymptotically equivalent to the log-likelihood loss function used by the TMLE.

Since g_0 factorizes into both a treatment mechanism $g_{A,0}$ and censoring intensity $\bar{g}_0$, the sequence of estimates of g_0 must be a sequence of estimates of both the treatment and censoring mechanisms. Therefore, we propose a sequence of estimates where, for each element in the sequence, either the censoring or treatment mechanism is more nonparametric than it was in the previous step. Since main terms that are data-adaptive fits of the covariate profile may be constructed, using main terms regressions for these estimates is reasonable and lends itself nicely to defining a sequence of estimates of g_0. We describe the process below for main terms, which are simply the observed covariates.

Suppose one observes A, and K baseline covariates $W_1 \ldots W_K$, and τ is the last time point observed for any subject. First, an initial estimate $\bar{Q}_n$ of the conditional hazard $\bar{Q}_0$ is constructed using super learner based on the log-likelihood loss function. This estimate $\bar{Q}_n$ is held fixed. Next, we present an iterative algorithm that generates a sequence of J moves $M_0, \ldots, M_J$, where $J = 2 \times K + 1$. For each move, there is a corresponding TMLE: $(\bar{Q}_n^{0*}, g_n^0), \ldots, (\bar{Q}_n^{J*}, g_n^{J*})$. Note, that the superscript now denotes the number of moves that index the TMLE. There should be no confusion with the superscript before, which denoted the iteration number since the * indicates a TMLE that is fully iterated. Each move M_j corresponds with two main terms regression models: a main terms logistic regression model for $g_{A,0}$, and a main terms logistic regression model for $\bar{g}_0$. M_0 is the logistic intercept model for $g_{A,0}$, and a logistic regression fitting time nonparametrically for $\bar{g}_0$:

$$M_0 = \begin{cases} \text{logit}\,[P(A = 1|W_1, \ldots, W_K)] = \beta_0, \\ \text{logit}\,[P(A(t) = 1|A(t-1) = 0, N(t) = 0, A, W_1, \ldots, W_K)] \\ \qquad\qquad = \alpha_0 + \alpha_1 I(t = 2) +, \ldots, +\alpha_L I(t = L). \end{cases}$$

The next step M_1 in the sequence consists of g_{A,M_1} and $\bar{g}_{M_1}$, which are constructed by adding a main term to either g_{A,M_0} or $\bar{g}_{M_0}$. So the set of possible g_{A,M_1} is constructed by adding a main term from the set $\{W_1, \ldots, W_K\}$ to g_{A,M_0} and the set of possible $\bar{g}_{M_1}$ are constructed by adding a main term from the set $\{A, W_1, \ldots, W_K\}$ to $\bar{g}_{M_0}$. The TMLE corresponding with such a candidate estimator of g_0, and using $\bar{Q}_n$ as initial estimator of the hazard, is evaluated at each possible M_1, and the main term that maximizes the increase in the penalized log-likelihood of the TMLE is the next move in the sequence. The estimate for which a main term is not added remains the same as in the previous step in the sequence. The variable that is added is then removed from the possible set of moves in the next step for that particular component of g_0 (i.e., the treatment mechanism or the censoring mechanism). This process is continued until none of the possible steps for augmenting the fit of g_0 increases the penalized log-likelihood of the corresponding TMLE. At this point, the construction of the clever covariate H_1 is complete, and the corresponding TMLE becomes the initial estimator for the next TMLE in the sequence. The TMLE estimate based on M_j, where j is the last completed step in the sequence, becomes the new initial $\bar{Q}_n$ for the TMLE algorithm and a new clever covariate H_2 is constructed. The estimates of g_0 in M_{j+1} are now chosen based on adding a main term to the previous fit of g_0 implied by M_j as before. Thus, given this choice M_j, the g_{A,M_j}, $\bar{g}_{M_j}$, and jth TMLE $\bar{Q}_n^{j*}$ are used to construct the next TMLE, $\bar{Q}_n^{(j+1)*}$, in the sequence. This process is continued until all $2 \times K + 1$ possible moves are completed, updating the initial estimator of $\bar{Q}_0$ each time, and building a new clever covariate when necessary. The number of moves completed indexes the different candidate TMLEs, and the optimal number of moves should be chosen by using V-fold (possibly penalized) log-likelihood-based cross-validation.

Figure 20.1 presents a diagram of the sequencing algorithm for an example data set with two baseline covariates. The top displays how an initial estimate $\bar{Q}_n$ and the first move M_0, resulting in two fits g_{A,M_0} and $\bar{g}_{M_0}$, map into the first TMLE of the conditional hazard in the sequence, $\bar{Q}_n^{0*}$. Furthermore, that TMLE has a particular penalized log-likelihood fit. In the example, the penalized log-likelihood of $\bar{Q}_n^{0*}$ associated with M_0 is −3,364. The remainder of the diagram shows how the moves are constructed by building on M_0. Each box includes, in the upper left hand corner the main terms that are available to construct the possible moves, in the upper right hand corner the initial estimate of $\bar{Q}_0$ for that move, and in the bottom right hand corner the possible moves that may be made. In the box for M_1, the move that maximizes the penalized log-likelihood is the one that adds W_2 to g_{A,M_0} (penalized log-likelihood of −3,349). This move is chosen and added to the list of chosen moves as M_1 and $\bar{g}_{M_1}$ is set to $\bar{g}_{M_0}$. Subsequently, the variable that was chosen is removed from the table of available moves in the next step (W_2 is crossed out in the table of available moves for $\bar{g}_{M_2}$ in the next box). This process is continued until none of the moves increases the penalized log-likelihood from the preceding step. This occurs at M_3. Then, the initial estimate of $\bar{Q}_0$ is set to the previous TMLE in the sequence, $\bar{Q}_n^{2*}$, and the process is continued. The rest of sequence of chosen moves is populated in this fashion.

An extension of the above sequencing procedure that uses data-adaptive methods to estimate g_0 is also possible. One may incorporate more data-adaptive techniques by allowing the main terms to be super learning fits of both the treatment and censoring mechanisms based on a growing set of explanatory variables. Furthermore, the suggested sequencing algorithm presented here is one of many possible ways to construct a sequence of increasingly nonparametric estimates of g_0; in practice, alternative sequencing methods may be implemented.

Chapter 19 discusses a penalty to robustify the estimation procedure in the context of sparsity, specifically, in situations where the efficient influence curve has large values for good fits of g_0. The penalty term should make the criterion more targeted toward the parameter of interest while preserving the log-likelihood as the dominant term in situations where identifiability is not in jeopardy, as it is when there is no practical violation of the positivity assumption. Thus, the penalty term should be asymptotically negligible but of importance in a sparse data setting. For this reason we choose an estimator of the variance of the $\bar{Q}_0$-component of the efficient influence curve as our penalty, where the $\bar{Q}_0$-component is the sum over time

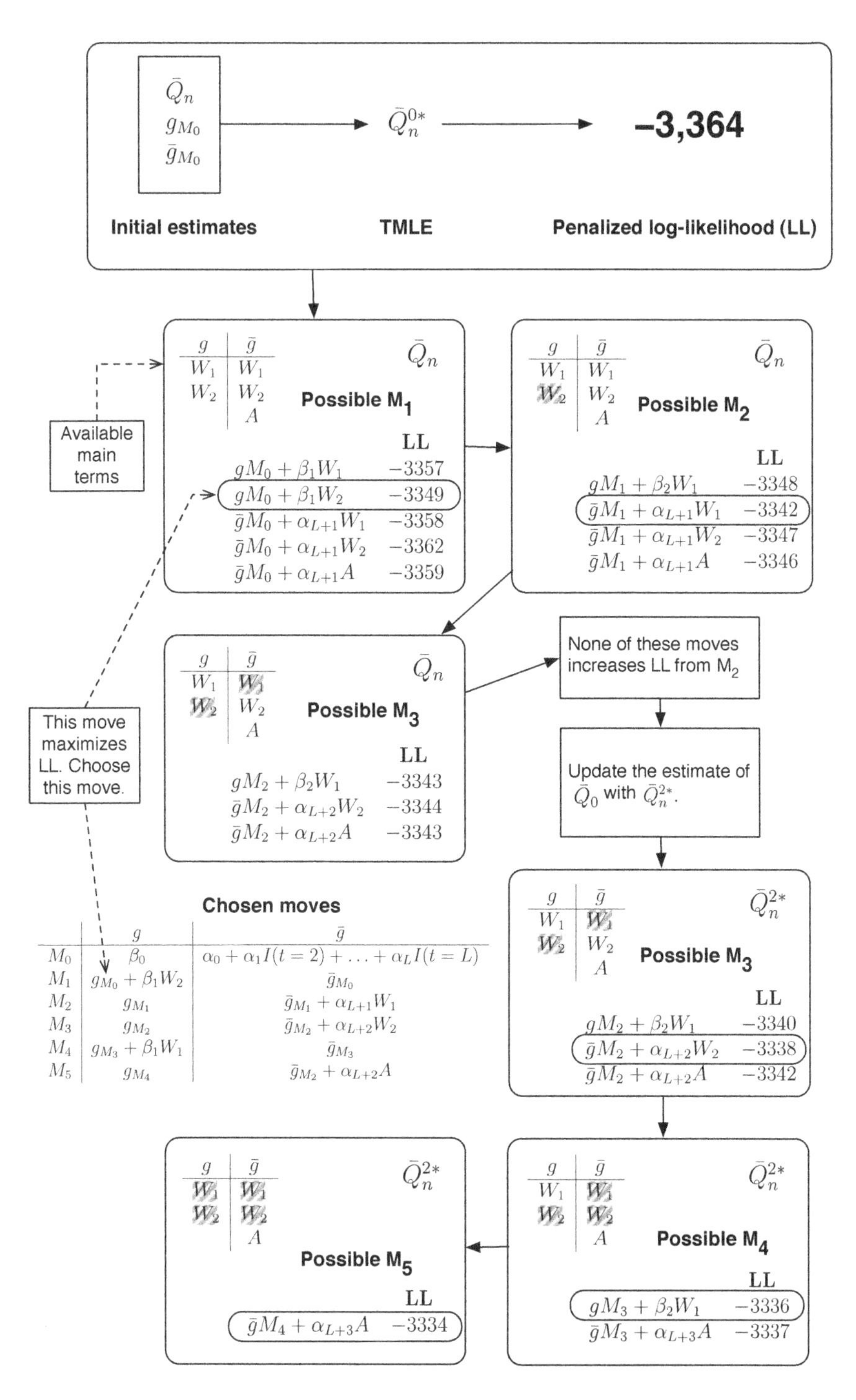

Fig. 20.1 Example of sequencing algorithm for data set with two baseline covariates

of the the time-specific clever covariate multiplied by the counting process residual. The variance of the efficient influence curve is asymptotically negligible relative to the log-likelihood, and in situations where there is a violation of the positivity assumption, as in the case when $g_{n,A}$ or $\prod_{i=1}^{t-} (1 - \bar{g}_n(i \mid A, W))$ is very close to zero for a given subject, it will severely penalize the log-likelihood. Using a standard method for estimating the variance of a martingale, we obtain the following variance term:

$$\frac{1}{n}\sum_{i}^{n}\sum_{t}^{t_k}\frac{1}{g_{n,A}(a \mid W)\prod_{i=1}^{t-}(1 - \bar{g}_n(i \mid a, W))}\frac{S_n(t_k \mid a, W)}{S_n(t \mid a, W)}I(t \leq t_k)\bar{Q}_n(1 - \bar{Q}_n)(t \mid a, W).$$

This penalty becomes large when the probability $A = a$ is small, even for values of W for which $A = a$ is not observed in the data. Thus, this penalty is sensitive to lack of identifiability, including theoretical nonidentifiability.

Now that a sequence of fits of g_0 and a penalized loss function for $\bar{Q}_0$ have been defined, the C-TMLE algorithm can be implemented:

1. Estimate $Q_{W,0}$ with the empirical probability distribution.
2. Generate $\bar{Q}_n$, an estimate of the discrete failure time hazard $\bar{Q}_0$, using super learner based on the log-likelihood loss function (step 1 in Fig. 20.2).
3. Use V-fold cross-validation with the log-likelihood loss function penalized by the variance term above to choose among the TMLE algorithms indexed by the number of moves (steps 2–6 in Fig. 20.2).
4. Implement the sequencing algorithm on the full data set for the chosen number of moves.
5. The resulting $\bar{Q}_n^*$ from the TMLE indexed by the chosen number of moves is the C-TMLE of the conditional hazard.
6. Construct the substitution estimator $\Psi(Q_n^*)$ with $Q_n^* = (Q_{W,n}, \bar{Q}_n^*)$, which is the C-TMLE of the parameter of interest.

Several variations of this sequencing algorithm and penalized likelihood can also be explored to see if they produce more robust estimators in sparse data situations.

Trimming. Observations that led to identifiability problems are removed from fitting g_0. This is done in order to obtain estimates that are not as influenced by outlying values in W and were highly predictive of treatment/censoring.

Truncation. Observations that led to identifiability problems are set to a minimum probability. All subjects who have a treatment mechanism that predicted treatment less than $p\%$ of the time, where p is small, are set to $p\%$.

Using binary covariates. Transform the continuous variables into binary variables that are indicators of the quantiles of the original variable. This allows the C-TMLE algorithm to adjust for only the regions that do not cause positivity violations, as opposed to the entire variable. Thus, the larger the number of binary variables constructed from an initial covariate, the more flexibility the C-TMLE algorithm has. However, too many binary variables for a single continuous covariate may contribute to loss of signal and a large increase in the computation time of the algorithm.

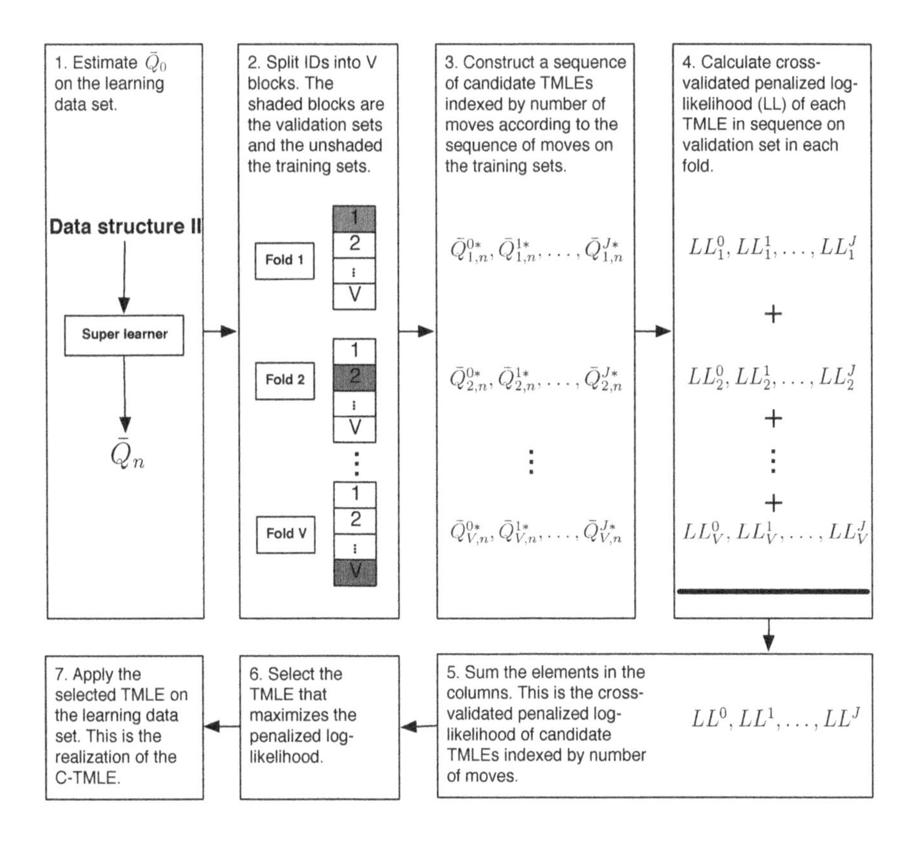

Fig. 20.2 Cross-validation using penalized log-likelihood to choose among a sequence of TMLEs

Using binary covariates had the largest positive effect on producing robust estimates in our simulations, and trimming and truncation had little effect on the results in the simulations presented below. Furthermore, a dimension-reduction step in between the initial fit of $\bar{Q}_0$ and the C-TMLE sequencing step improved computation time tremendously. This was done by removing all variables from the sequencing step that fell below a certain cutoff in terms of association with the outcome of interest after accounting for the initial fit. Univariate regression was performed with the initial estimate as an offset and all variables that fell below a 0.10-FDR-adjusted p-value were no longer considered in the sequencing step. All C-TMLEs presented in the remainder of this chapter include the dimension-reduction step, and use binary covariates for the secondary sequencing step.

C-TMLEs and corresponding estimates g_n solve the efficient influence curve equation, just like the TMLE. This provides the basis for the generally applicable asymptotic linearity theorem for C-TMLE as presented in Chap. 19 and Appendix A. Thus, confidence intervals may be constructed for C-TMLE in the same way as they are constructed for TMLE in Chap. 18.

20.6 Simulations

The simulations consist of data sets generated under three scenarios: no ETA violation, medium ETA violation, and high ETA violation. Within each scenario, estimates are presented for each of the methods using a correct parametric model for the conditional hazard and a purposely misspecified parametric model. The simulated data were generated as follows:

1. Baseline covariates $W = \{W_1, W_2, W_3, W_4, W_5\}$ were generated from a multivariate normal with mean 0, variance 1, and covariance 0.2. If any W was greater than 2 or less than -2, it was set to 2 or -2, respectively, to ensure that the treatment and censoring mechanisms were appropriately bounded.
2. Treatment A was generated as a binomial:
$$P_0(A = 1 \mid W) = \text{expit}\,(0.4 + 0.4W_1 + 0.4W_2 - 0.5W_3 + \log(\text{ETA}_{OR}) \times W_4),$$
where ETA_{OR} is the odds ratio implied by the coefficient of W_4, and W_4 is the baseline covariate responsible for violations in the ETA assumption in the simulated data sets. ETA_{OR} equals 1 for the scenario under no ETA violation, 10 for medium ETA violation, and 15 for high ETA violation.
3. The event process was generated using the following hazard at each t:
$$P_0(T = t \mid T \geq t, A, W) = \text{expit}\,(0.25 - 0.6W_1 - 0.6W_2 - 0.6W_3 - A).$$
4. The censoring process was generated using the following hazard at each t:
$$P_0(C = t \mid C \geq t, A, W) = \text{expit}\,(-3 - 0.1W_1 - 0.1W_2 - 0.1W_3 - 0.1A).$$

Under each level of ETA violation, 500 data sets of 500 observations were generated. The following estimators were used to estimate the parameter of interest, which is the treatment-specific survival curve for $A = 1$ at time 2: IPCW estimator $\psi_{n,1}^{IPCW}(2)$, MLE $\psi_{n,1}^{MLE}(2)$, A-IPCW estimator $\psi_{n,1}^{A-IPCW}(2)$, TMLE $\psi_{n,1}^{TMLE}(2)$, A-IPCW estimator without W_4, TMLE without W_4, and C-TMLE $\psi_{n,1}^{C-TMLE}(2)$ as described in Sect. 20.5 with dimension reduction, penalized log-likelihood loss function, and binary baseline covariates split at the 33rd and 66th precentile. Each of these methods was implemented twice for each data set: once using the correct parametric model for $\bar{Q}_0$ and once using a purposely misspecified parametric model for $\bar{Q}_0$ that only included A and W_5 as main terms in the logistic hazard regression. Note that W_5 is just a noise variable and does not play a role in the outcome process, censoring process, or treatment mechanism. For estimators requiring an estimate of $g_{A,0}$ and $\bar{g}_0$, they were estimated based on the correctly specified parametric model.

The A-IPCW estimator without W_4 and TMLE without W_4 are not estimators one could implement based on a real data set, but were evaluated to compare the C-TMLE algorithm to methods where the irrelevant variable causing identifiability problems was known and removed. Furthermore, all of the estimation methods except for C-TMLE were given the true parametric model for g_0, an advantage they would not have when analyzing real data. In a real data analysis, model selection that uses a loss function for fitting the treatment and censoring mechanisms would be implemented.

The problem variable may be a confounder in some scenarios. In order to evaluate the methods under this situation, we reran the high ETA violation scenario with a minor change. The treatment was generated as a binomial as $P_0(A = 1 \times W) = \text{expit}(0.4 + log(15) \times W_1 + 0.4W_2 - 0.5W_3)$. Instead of varying the odds ratio for W_4, we set the odds ratio for W_1, one of the variables that affects the hazard of the event of interest, to 15.

20.6.1 Results: Point Estimates

Tables 20.1–20.3 display the simulation results where the variable causing identifiability concerns is not a confounder. The true value of the parameter being estimated is 0.462. Table 20.1 shows that all estimators of the parameter of interest are unbiased when the initial model for $\bar{Q}_0$ is specified correctly (Q_C). However, when the initial model for $\bar{Q}_0$ is misspecified (Q_M), the MLE is biased. The IPCW estimate is the same for the misspecified and correctly specified model for $\bar{Q}_0$ since this estimate does not depend on an estimate of the conditional hazard of T.

The fact that all of the methods produce unbiased estimators of the parameter of interest, even for the moderate sample sizes examined here, suggests that bias should not be the standard by which these estimators are judged. Assessing the methods in terms of MSE begins to distinguish the methods from one another. Table 20.2 presents the root mean square error, relative efficiency (on the variance scale), and the efficiency bound for each scenario. Again, in the no ETA scenario, all estimators have essentially the same MSE. However, as the ETA becomes larger, some of the methods begin to demonstrate their advantages while others lose all stability.

1. The IPCW estimator is highly unstable with increasing ETA. In fact, the C-TMLE is six times more efficient when the conditional failure time hazard $\bar{Q}_0$ is estimated consistently and almost 3.5 times more efficient when $\bar{Q}_0$ is misspecified with medium ETA. For the high ETA case, the C-TMLE is 15.5 times more efficient for a consistently estimated $\bar{Q}_0$ and eight times more efficient when the parametric model for $\bar{Q}_0$ is misspecified. The C-TMLE is 3.5 more times efficient than the A-IPCW estimator for a consistently estimated $\bar{Q}_0$, and 2.6 times more efficient for a misspecified parametric model for $\bar{Q}_0$ with medium ETA. For high ETA, the C-TMLE is 6.5 and 4.5 times more efficient for the respective ways of estimating $\bar{Q}_0$.
2. The TMLE, regardless of ETA, tends to have an MSE that approaches the efficiency bound, unlike the IPCW or A-IPCW estimator.
3. The C-TMLE shows super efficient behavior, and even as the ETA violation increases, the MSE remains close to the level it was under no ETA violation. This is true whether $\bar{Q}_0$ is fit well or misspecified. The MSE is lower when $\bar{Q}_0$ is es-

Table 20.1 Mean estimates ($\psi_0 = 0.462$); variable causing violation in ETA is not a confounder

Method	No ETA		Medium ETA		High ETA	
	Q_C	Q_M	Q_C	Q_M	Q_C	Q_M
TMLE	0.460	0.460	0.463	0.460	0.465	0.458
MLE	0.461	0.473	0.461	0.499	0.461	0.501
IPCW	0.460	0.460	0.461	0.461	0.460	0.460
A-IPCW	0.460	0.460	0.463	0.464	0.464	0.466
A-IPCW w/o W_4	0.460	0.460	0.460	0.455	0.460	0.455
TMLE w/o W_4	0.460	0.460	0.460	0.455	0.460	0.455
C-TMLE	0.460	0.463	0.460	0.460	0.461	0.463

Table 20.2 RMSE and relative efficiency; variable causing violation in ETA is not a confounder

Method	No ETA		Medium ETA		High ETA	
	Q_C	Q_M	Q_C	Q_M	Q_C	Q_M
Efficiency bound	0.028		0.046		0.060	
RMSE						
TMLE	0.029	0.029	0.051	0.056	0.062	0.065
MLE	0.027	0.030	0.028	0.047	0.028	0.049
IPCW	0.029	0.029	0.071	0.071	0.106	0.106
A-IPCW	0.029	0.029	0.054	0.061	0.070	0.081
A-IPCW w/o W_4	0.029	0.029	0.030	0.031	0.029	0.031
TMLE w/o W_4	0.029	0.029	0.030	0.031	0.029	0.030
C-TMLE	0.028	0.031	0.029	0.037	0.029	0.040
Relative efficiency						
TMLE	1.0	1.1	1.2	1.5	1.0	1.2
MLE	0.9	1.1	0.4	1.0	0.2	0.7
IPCW	1.0	1.0	2.4	2.4	3.1	3.1
A-IPCW	1.0	1.1	1.4	1.8	1.3	1.8
A-IPCW w/o W_4	1.0	1.1	0.4	0.5	0.2	0.3
TMLE w/o W_4	1.0	1.1	0.4	0.4	0.2	0.3
C-TMLE	1.0	1.2	0.4	0.7	0.2	0.4

Table 20.3 Characteristics of C-TMLE; variable causing violation in ETA is not a confounder

Method	No ETA		Medium ETA		High ETA	
	Q_C	Q_M	Q_C	Q_M	Q_C	Q_M
Mean # of moves	0.1	13.4	0.1	10.5	0.1	10.1
% of time C-TMLE algorithm chose:						
Zero Moves	0.98	0.00	0.98	0.06	0.99	0.08
W_1	0.00	0.99	0.00	0.93	0.00	0.89
W_2	0.00	0.99	0.00	0.91	0.00	0.89
W_3	0.00	0.99	0.00	0.81	0.00	0.81
W_4 (ETA Variable)	0.01	0.84	0.00	0.47	0.00	0.41
W_5	0.01	0.00	0.01	0.00	0.01	0.00

timated consistently; however, it still outperforms any of the other estimators in terms of efficiency when the parametric model for $\bar{Q}_0$ is misspecified.

Of note, for high ETA, the A-IPCW estimates range from 17.5 to 103%, the estimates generated by the TMLE range from 30.3 to 63.8%, and the C-TMLE produces estimates ranging from 35.6 to 59.2%. Thus, it becomes immediately clear that the A-IPCW estimator does not respect the global constraints of the model by producing an estimate that is not a probability (one of the estimates is greater than 100%). In addition, the A-IPCW estimator is an empirical mean of an unbounded function of the data; thus when the estimates of g_0 are close to zero, the contribution from one observation may be too large or even infinite. On the other hand, the estimates generated by TMLE and C-TMLE are empirical means of probabilities. Since they are substitution estimators, each observation's contribution is bounded and may be no larger than 1. The advantage of substitution estimators is directly observed in the simulation results by the smaller RMSE for TMLE than A-IPCW.

Table 20.3 presents characteristics of the C-TMLE algorithm. When $\bar{Q}_0$ is consistently estimated, the C-TMLE algorithm makes very few moves and, in almost all cases, it makes zero moves relying on the intercept models for g_0. However, when $\bar{Q}_0$ is misspecified, the C-TMLE algorithm selects more moves and attempts to adjust in the estimator of g_0 for the variables that were not adjusted for in the initial estimate of $\bar{Q}_0$. Also, the algorithm resists choosing the region of the variable that causes the ETA violations illustrated by the fact that W_4 is selected fewer times as ETA increases.

Tables 20.4–20.6 display the results where confounder W_1 is also the variable causing identifiability problems. The "No ETA" columns are the same as in the previous tables. As before, when $\bar{Q}_0$ is consistently estimated, all of the estimators are unbiased. However, when the parametric model for $\bar{Q}_0$ is misspecified, the TMLE, IPCW estimator, and A-IPCW estimator remain unbiased, the MLE is highly biased, and the C-TMLE is slightly biased. The bias in the C-TMLE is due to the fact that it is not fully adjusting for W_1 when regions of that variable contribute to nonidentifiability of the parameter of interest. This bias is compensated for by the small variance, as the C-TMLE does as well as any of the other methods in terms of RMSE. Furthermore, the A-IPCW estimator fails to achieve the efficiency bound and performs twice as poorly as the C-TMLE in terms of RMSE, as seen in Table 20.5. Though the IPCW estimator behaved reasonably in terms of bias and MSE, its potential to generate highly unstable estimates was displayed in the previous simulations.

Table 20.6 displays the characteristics of the C-TMLE algorithm. Again, when $\bar{Q}_0$ is consistently estimated, very few moves are made, and when it is misspecified, the algorithm adjusts by choosing a fuller model for g_0. As expected, the C-TMLE algorithm has a difficult time choosing what variables to adjust for now that the ETA variable is a confounder. This can be seen by the fact that the algorithm continues to adjust for W_1 more often than it did for W_4 in Table 20.3. The algorithm uses the penalized loss function to weight whether it is better to adjust for a variable that is associated with the outcome or remove it since it causes identifiability problems. In this case, the algorithm has chosen to adjust for at least some region of the variable

Table 20.4 Mean estimates ($\psi_0 = 0.462$); variable causing violation in ETA is a confounder

	No ETA		High ETA	
Method	Q_C	Q_M	Q_C	Q_M
TMLE	0.460	0.460	0.468	0.459
MLE	0.461	0.473	0.462	0.552
IPCW	0.460	0.460	0.461	0.461
A-IPCW	0.460	0.460	0.462	0.466
A-IPCW w/o W_1	0.460	0.460	0.462	0.533
TMLE w/o W_1	0.460	0.460	0.462	0.533
C-TMLE	0.460	0.463	0.462	0.482

Table 20.5 RMSE and relative efficiency; variable causing violation in ETA is a confounder

	No ETA		High ETA	
Method	Q_C	Q_M	Q_C	Q_M
Efficiency bound	0.028		0.054	
RMSE				
TMLE	0.029	0.029	0.053	0.050
MLE	0.027	0.030	0.029	0.094
IPCW	0.029	0.029	0.058	0.058
A-IPCW	0.029	0.029	0.052	0.077
A-IPCW w/o W_1	0.029	0.029	0.032	0.076
TMLE w/o W_1	0.029	0.029	0.031	0.076
C-TMLE	0.028	0.031	0.031	0.055
Relative efficiency				
TMLE	1.0	1.1	1.0	0.9
MLE	0.9	1.1	0.3	3.0
IPCW	1.0	1.0	1.2	1.2
A-IPCW	1.0	1.1	0.9	2.0
AIPW w/o W_1	1.0	1.1	0.3	2.0
TMLE w/o W_1	1.0	1.1	0.3	2.0
C-TMLE	1.0	1.2	0.3	1.1

Table 20.6 Characteristics of C-TMLE; variable causing violation in ETA is a confounder

	No ETA		High ETA	
Method	Q_C	Q_M	Q_C	Q_M
Mean # of moves	0.103	13.389	0.134	8.448
% of time C-TMLE algorithm chose:				
Zero Moves	0.98	0.00	0.97	0.12
W_1 (ETA Variable)	0.00	0.99	0.00	0.88
W_2	0.00	0.99	0.00	0.80
W_3	0.00	0.99	0.00	0.59
W_4	0.01	0.84	0.01	0.48
W_5	0.01	0.00	0.02	0.00

a large percentage of the time. Had the algorithm decided to remove the variable completely from the adjustments, the estimator would have been more biased, and the RMSE would be very large, like those seen for the TMLE without W_1 estimator. This difference in RMSE illustrates the value of generating binary variables for the C-TMLE.

20.6.2 Results: Inference

Table 20.7 presents the coverage probabilities where the ETA variable is not a confounder. Ideally, a well-behaved method would produce confidence intervals that include the truth 95% of the time. Since each scenario was only simulated 500 times, some variation from 95% is not unexpected. (The confidence intervals for the MLE are not reported as that would require an application of a δ-method to compute the correct influence curve based on the assumed parametric model, and no theory is available when MLE is based on a machine learning algorithm.) The A-IPCW estimator is the only method that has 95% confidence intervals over all scenarios (excluding the estimator that doesn't adjust for the ETA variable since that estimator is not feasible in a real data setting). The influence-curve-based confidence intervals for the TMLE begin to deteriorate with increasing ETA. The C-TMLE coverage probability also decreases with increasing ETA but not as quickly as for the TMLE, and only when Q_0 is misspecified. Table 20.8 displays the 95% coverage probabilities when the ETA variable is a confounder. Again, the TMLE and C-TMLE coverage probabilities are less than 95% when Q_0 is misspecified. Thus, we can conclude that the theoretically valid asymptotic influence-curve-based confidence intervals are not producing proper coverage in finite samples when lack of identifiability is an issue. Furthermore, as the parameter becomes more nonidentifiable, the coverage probabilities further deteriorate.

Tables 20.7 and 20.8 also present the mean width of the influence-curve-based confidence intervals for each estimator. While the A-IPCW estimator provides confidence intervals with proper coverage, the width of these intervals are larger than the intervals of both the TMLE and C-TMLE. In fact, in Table 20.7, the average A-IPCW confidence-interval width for high ETA with inconsistent initial estimator of Q_0 is almost twice as large as the C-TMLE interval width. When the ETA variable is a confounder, under high ETA and misspecified Q_0, the A-IPCW intervals are 67% larger on average than the C-TMLE intervals.

Although the A-IPCW intervals include the truth 95% of the time, in many cases they are extremely large, rendering these estimates useless. The data sets where A-IPCW estimates have large intervals are not the ones where TMLE/C-TMLE have difficulty with coverage. In fact, for high ETA, the TMLE/C-TMLE influence-curve-based confidence intervals include the truth for almost all data sets where the AIPW estimate is below 0.35 or above 0.60. The TMLE/C-TMLE intervals that do not include the truth are very close to including it. This suggests that a small adjustment

Table 20.7 Coverage probabilities and mean width of confidence intervals; variable causing violation in ETA is not a confounder

Method	No ETA Q_C	No ETA Q_M	Medium ETA Q_C	Medium ETA Q_M	High ETA Q_C	High ETA Q_M
Coverage probabilities						
TMLE	0.94	0.96	0.86	0.85	0.80	0.83
IPCW	0.98	0.98	0.92	0.92	0.88	0.88
A-IPCW	0.94	0.95	0.95	0.95	0.94	0.94
A-IPCW w/o W_4	0.94	0.95	0.95	0.96	0.95	0.96
TMLE w/o W_4	0.94	0.96	0.96	0.95	0.95	0.96
C-TMLE	0.94	0.94	0.95	0.92	0.94	0.89
Mean width of confidence intervals						
TMLE	0.11	0.12	0.19	0.21	0.21	0.24
IPCW	0.14	0.14	0.24	0.24	0.27	0.27
A-IPCW	0.11	0.12	0.18	0.22	0.20	0.25
A-IPCW w/o W_4	0.11	0.12	0.11	0.12	0.11	0.12
TMLE w/o W_4	0.11	0.12	0.11	0.12	0.11	0.12
C-TMLE	0.11	0.12	0.11	0.13	0.11	0.13

Table 20.8 Coverage probabilities and mean width of confidence intervals; variable causing violation in ETA is a confounder

Method	No ETA Q_C	No ETA Q_M	High ETA Q_C	High ETA Q_M
Coverage probabilities				
TMLE	0.94	0.96	0.87	0.93
IPCW	0.98	0.98	0.94	0.94
A-IPCW	0.94	0.95	0.94	0.92
A-IPCW w/o W_1	0.94	0.95	0.94	0.38
TMLE w/o W_1	0.94	0.96	0.94	0.38
C-TMLE	0.94	0.94	0.94	0.82
Mean width of confidence intervals				
TMLE	0.11	0.12	0.18	0.20
IPCW	0.14	0.14	0.21	0.21
A-IPCW	0.11	0.12	0.17	0.25
A-IPCW w/o W_1	0.11	0.12	0.12	0.12
TMLE w/o W_1	0.11	0.12	0.12	0.12
C-TMLE	0.11	0.12	0.11	0.15

to the TMLE/C-TMLE influence-curve-based confidence intervals would cause the TMLE/C-TMLE intervals to include the truth.

For high ETA, the A-IPCW confidence intervals tend to be larger than the TMLE confidence intervals in the region of standard errors that produce useful confidence intervals; however, in the region where the confidence intervals are not useful, the reverse is true. The average length of the A-IPCW confidence interval is 0.255 compared to 0.237 for the TMLE and 0.132 for the C-TMLE. Even though the A-IPCW estimator produces confidence intervals with proper coverage, they are larger than the TMLE intervals and almost twice as large as the C-TMLE intervals, which have only slightly less coverage. The standard errors are almost always larger for the A-IPCW estimator vs. the C-TMLE for this simulation. In fact, none of the standard errors for C-TMLE exceeds 0.1, while 5.4% of the A-IPCW standard errors exceed 0.15. Thus, the difference in coverage probabilities (0.94 vs. 0.89) is compensated for by the fact that a large percent of A-IPCW confidence intervals are too large to be practically useful.

Adjustment for targeted methods. The TMLE and C-TMLE confidence intervals would include the truth if the intervals were slightly shifted to the left or the right. We hypothesize that this departure from normality is the result of a distribution of estimates that is slightly skewed in finite samples. This suggests that bootstrap methods, which use the 0.025 and 0.975 bootstrap quantiles to construct confidence intervals, would produce valid 95% confidence intervals. In order to test this hypothesis, 500 additional data sets were generated according to the original simulation high ETA scenario and bootstrap confidence intervals, both based on quantiles and estimated standard error, as well as influence-curve-based confidence intervals were compared for the TMLE. We note this was not done for the C-TMLE due to the prohibitive amount of time it would take to run the bootstrap for 500 data sets; however, for one data set it is a feasible method for inference, and the bootstrap results for the TMLE intervals should hold for C-TMLE. These results are presented in Table 20.9. The resulting coverage probability was 94% using quantile-based-bootstrap intervals, compared to 88% for bootstrap intervals based on the estimated standard error, and 87% using influence-curve-based confidence intervals. Furthermore, the average length of the confidence intervals was 0.21, 0.22, and 0.26, respectively. This suggests that the quantile-based bootstrap, which naturally accounts for the skewness in finite samples, is able to produce valid 95% confidence intervals. The lack of coverage for the standard-error-based bootstrap confidence intervals confirms that the skewness of the distribution of the estimates in finite samples contributes to the poor influence curve based confidence intervals. This is due to the fact that both of these methods depend on the standard normal quantiles to generate confidence intervals. Not only do the quantile-based bootstrap confidence intervals produce the proper coverage, but they also are 20% smaller than the influence-curve-based intervals. Thus, the quantile-based bootstrap intervals should be the preferred method for constructing TMLE and C-TMLE confidence intervals in the presence of sparsity.

Table 20.9 Bootstrap vs. influence-curve-based 95% confidence intervals for TMLE

	Coverage probabilities	Mean CI width
Quantile bootstrap	0.94	0.21
Wald bootstrap	0.88	0.22
Wald influence curve	0.87	0.26

20.7 Discussion

Ultimately, a choice must be made to implement an estimator that behaves the best across the largest number of possible scenarios. The simulations presented here illustrate the advantages of the C-TMLE methodology for estimating causal parameters when analyzing time-to-event outcomes. The results show that the C-TMLE does at least as well as the best estimator under every scenario and, in many of the more realistic scenarios, behaves much better than the next best estimator in terms of both bias and variance. Unlike other estimators that rely on an external estimator of nuisance parameters, the C-TMLE algorithm estimates the nuisance parameters with consideration for the parameter of interest. The C-TMLE is an entirely a priori specified method that accounts for the fact that there are identifiability concerns in observational data and addresses these issues uniformly, rather than handling them on a case-by-case basis, or ignoring them completely. The C-TMLE algorithm accomplishes this by using a targeted (penalized) loss function to make smart choices in determining what variables to adjust for in the estimate of g_0 and only adjusts for variables that have not been fully adjusted for in the initial estimate of Q_0. This allows the C-TMLE estimates to exhibit super efficiency and behave almost as well as the MLE when the model for Q is specified correctly. In addition, when the initial estimator of Q_0 is not specified correctly, the C-TMLE adjusts in the secondary step only for the variables that improve the estimate of the parameter of interest by considering the bias–variance tradeoff for each adjustment. These decisions are always made with respect to how they affect the estimate of the parameter of interest and are not dependent on a loss function designed for the prediction of the treatment/censoring mechanism itself, as it is in the other methods presented. By ignoring the effect of each adjustment on the estimate of the parameter of interest, the other methods have been shown to be highly unstable in finite samples. Furthermore, the TMLE and C-TMLE are substitution estimators and obey the proper bounds of the true model contributing to their overall stability. Lastly, the bootstrap provides a method to construct valid 95% confidence intervals for the C-TMLE that are tighter than the intervals produced by other methods when estimating weakly identifiable parameters.

Chapter 21
Propensity-Score-Based Estimators and C-TMLE

Jasjeet S. Sekhon, Susan Gruber, Kristin E. Porter, Mark J. van der Laan

In order to estimate the average treatment effect $E_0[E_0(Y \mid A = 1, W) - E_0(Y \mid A = 0, W)]$ of a single time-point treatment A based on observing n i.i.d. copies of $O = (W, A, Y)$, one might use inverse probability of treatment (i.e., propensity score) weighting of an estimator of the conditional mean of the outcome (i.e., response surface) as a function of the pretreatment covariates. Alternatively, one might use a TMLE defined by a choice of initial estimator, a parametric submodel that codes fluctuations of the initial estimator, and a loss function used to determine the amount of fluctuation, where either the choice of submodel or the loss function will involve inverse probability of treatment weighting. Asymptotically, such double robust estimators may have appealing properties. They can be constructed such that if either the model of the response surface or the model of the probability of treatment assignment is correct, the estimatosr will provide a consistent estimator of the average treatment effect. And if both models are correct, the weighted estimator will be asymptotically efficient. Such estimators are called double robust and locally efficient (Robins et al. 1994, 1995; Robins and Rotnitzky 1995; van der Laan and Robins 2003).

By factorization of the likelihood of O into a factor that identifies the average treatment effect, and the conditional probability of treatment, given the covariates W (i.e, the treatment mechanism), estimation of the propensity score $g_0(1 \mid W) = P_0(A = 1 \mid W)$ should be based solely on the log-likelihood of the treatment mechanism. In particular, estimation of g_0 should not involve examining the data on the final outcome Y. The double robust estimators exhibit a particularly interesting and useful type of asymptotics with respect to the choice of estimator of the propensity score. Due to this factorization of the likelihood, if one uses a maximum likelihood estimator of g_0 according to a particular model for g_0, then the influence curve of the double robust estimator equals the influence curve it would have had if g_0 were known and not estimated, minus a projection term whose size is implied by the size of the model for g_0 (van der Laan and Robins 2003). As a consequence of this result, the larger the model for g_0, the more efficient the double robust estimator will be. In addition, an estimator of the variance of the double robust estimator that ignores the fact that g_0 was estimated is asymptotically conservative, and thus provides valid conservative confidence intervals and tests. In the special case that the estimator of the response surface is consistent, it follows that the influence curve of the double robust estimator is not affected at all by the choice of estimator of g_0 (the above-mentioned projection term equals zero): under this assumption, even estimators that rely on sequential learning based on the log-likelihood of g_0, will not affect the statistical inference. Of course, such statements are not warranted if the choice of model for g_0 is based on examining the data on the final outcomes Y.

In finite samples, however, double robust estimators can increase variance and bias for the average treatment effect, relative to the estimator of the average treatment effect based on the unweighted estimator of the outcome, especially when some observations have an extreme probability of assignment to treatment, corresponding with practical or theoretical violations of the positivity assumption. Recall, that the positivity assumption states that the conditional probability of treatment assignment is bounded away from 0 and 1 for all covariate values. As a result, Kang and Schafer (2007) and Freedman and Berk (2008) warn against the routine use of estimators that rely on IPCW, including double robust estimators. This is in agreement with the past and ongoing literature defining and analyzing this issue (Robins 1986, 1987a, 2000; Robins and Wang 2000; van der Laan and Robins 2003), simulations demonstrating the extreme sparsity bias of IPCW estimators (e.g., Neugebauer and van der Laan 2005), diagnosing violations of the positivity assumptions in response to this concern (Kish 1992; Wang et al. 2006; Cole and Hernan 2008; Bembom and van der Laan 2008; Moore et al. 2009; Petersen et al. 2010), data-adaptive selection of the truncation constant to control the influence of weighting (Bembom and van der Laan 2008), and selecting parameters that rely on realistic assumptions (van der Laan and Petersen 2007a; Petersen et al. 2010).

One problem with reliance on the propensity score is that it may condition on variables that are either unrelated to the outcome of interest or only weakly related. Adding a pretreatment variable that is unrelated to the outcome but related to treatment (i.e., an instrument) to a propensity score model may increase bias. If the relationships between the variables are linear, bias will always be increased (Bhattacharya and Vogt 2007; Wooldridge 2009). In the nonparametric case, the direction of the bias is less straightforward, but increasing bias is a real possibility and expected (Pearl 2010a). This type of bias implied by such bias-amplifying variables has been termed Z-bias. In the nonparametric case, bias may result even when there are no unobserved confounders.

Including variables in a propensity score model that are unrelated to the outcomes of interest also exacerbates the problem of small or large estimated probabilities of treatment assignment. Such probabilities make inverse probability of treatment-weighted estimators unstable, and may, in finite samples, appear to cause violations of the positivity assumption. But these violations may be innocuous because the variable causing the violation may be unrelated to the outcome, and, therefore, one need not condition on it.

Even ignoring concerns about Z-bias, another consideration may lead one to want to examine the outcomes in order to decide on the fit of the propensity score: It is often impossible to balance all of the theoretically plausible confounders in a given sample. In such cases, one cannot estimate the treatment effect without making functional form assumptions outside the support of the data. However, if the pretreatment variables that we cannot balance are unrelated to the outcomes, it may be possible to make progress. Of course, it would be preferable if a priori our scientific beliefs were sufficient to exclude the problematic pretreatment variables, but that is often unrealistic.

The foregoing paragraphs present us with a conundrum. For effective bias reduction based on the propensity score, we need to examine outcomes to include covariates in the propensity score fit that are meaningful confounders, but that contradicts the goal of fitting a propensity score, conditional on all the available covariates, and, as a consequence, it will alter the statistical understanding of the estimator, and its inference in a fundamental way. If we go the route of modeling the propensity score and the response surface together, then it is essential that the stability problems created by weighting be resolved. In addition, this will need to be done with an a priori specified algorithm.

C-TMLEs have desirable features that help to mitigate many of the concerns regarding the use of double robust estimators. First, the estimation of the response surface is automated by an a priori specified machine learning algorithm, such as the super learner. Second, the whole procedure for selecting the propensity score fit is automated. That is, the C-TMLE is an a priori specified estimator of the average treatment effect. Instead of giving the designer the freedom to select a fit of the propensity score based on the orthogonal log-likelihood of the propensity score before committing to an estimator of the average treatment effect that will use this fit of the propensity score, the C-TMLE lets an a priori specified machine determine this choice based on all the available data. It is important to note that choices that define the manner in which the C-TMLE fits the propensity score may still be based on inspection of the ancillary log-likelihood of the propensity score (i.e., not examining final outcome data).

Third, C-TMLE, by construction, only aims to include the variables in the propensity score that are related to the outcome of interest. More precisely, C-TMLE only includes variables in the propensity score if they are inadequately adjusted for by the fit of the response surface. Thus, concerns about Z-bias are reduced. Fourth, the estimated probabilities of treatment assignment are less likely to be extreme because typically fewer variables and fewer problematic variables will be included in the propensity score model by C-TMLE than by noncollaborative methods. The theory of collaborative double robustness provides the theoretical underpinning of the C-TMLE algorithm, showing that full bias reduction is achieved by using a propensity score that only adjusts for the covariates that explain the residual bias between the initial estimator of the response surface and the true response surface (Appendix A). Finally, as outlined in Chap. 7, both TMLE and C-TMLE can make use of a logistic fluctuation to make sure that the fit of the response surface either respects a priori known bounds of the continuous outcome or enforces the bounds implied by the range of the continuous outcome observed in the data. With a logistic fluctuation, the TMLE and C-TMLE will have the predicted outcome bounded to its observed range even in finite samples. This bounding stabilizes the estimator because the influence function of the estimator is bounded, even in finite samples, and this controls the instability in the context of sparsity.

To summarize, Z-bias and the inability to balance all of the a priori plausible confounders suggests that one may want to use an a priori defined estimator that views fitting the propensity score as a task that needs to be carried out in collaboration with fitting the response surface. C-TMLEs have a number of desirable advantages relative to other double robust estimators that view fitting the propensity score as an external task based on the orthogonal log-likelihood of the propensity score that ignores the outcome data.

Chapter Summary

Above, we made a compelling case for the C-TMLE. Statistical properties of estimators, and thereby the comparison between different estimation procedures, are not affected by the choice of causal model, only by the statistical target parameter and the statistical model. Nonetheless, causal models represent an intrinsic component of our road map for targeted learning of causal effects. Chapter 2 was devoted to the SCM, and this causal model was repeatedly invoked in this book. In this causal model, counterfactuals, and thereby the causal quantities of interest, were derived from the SCM. An important and popular alternative causal model directly states the existence of counterfactuals of scientific interest as the main assumption (often defined in words in terms of an experiment), which avoids the representation of assumptions in terms of structural equations. This is called the Neyman–Rubin model and is presented in the next section. The debate over which estimator to select for estimation of a causal effect should not be concerned with the choice of causal model.

We then reexamine prominent Monte Carlo simulations by implementing the C-TMLE and TMLE. These estimators may overcome the more detailed, but in some sense second-order, concerns regarding the instability of double robust estimators under sparseness. Specifically, we reanalyze and extend the simulations of Kang and Schafer (2007), which were designed to highlight the limitations of double robust estimators. The outcome is a linear function of the covariates, and the error term is small relative to the size of the coefficients. In addition, the missingness mechanism results in many positivity violations in finite samples. For the double robust estimators Kang and Schafer considered, the double robust weighted least squares and A-IPTW result in volatile estimates due to the high-leverage data points generated by large weights. We also examine the simulations of Freedman and Berk (2008). These simulations were originally designed to demonstrate how weighting by the propensity score can result in highly unstable estimates in conditions that are less extreme than those of Kang and Schafer. In both simulation studies, we show that the TMLEs, and, in particular, the C-TMLEs, perform well.

21.1 Neyman–Rubin Causal Model and Potential Outcomes

The Neyman–Rubin causal model consists of more than simply the notation for potential outcomes that was originated by Neyman (1923). Rubin and others, such as Cochran, Holland, and Rosenbaum, have developed a general framework that helps to clarify some important issues of inference and design. Beginning with Rubin (1974), the model began to unify how one thinks about observational and experimental studies, and it gives a central place to the treatment assignment mechanism.

The Neyman–Rubin framework has become increasingly popular in many fields, including statistics (Holland 1986; Rubin 1974, 2006; Rosenbaum 2002), medicine (Rubin 1997; Christakis and Iwashyna 2003), economics (Dehejia and Wahba 1999, 2002; Galiani et al. 2005; Abadie and Imbens 2006), political science (Herron and Wand 2007; Imai 2005; Sekhon 2008b), sociology (Morgan and Harding 2006; Diprete and Engelhardt 2004; Winship and Morgan 1999; Smith 1997), and even law (Rubin 2002).The framework originated with Neyman's model, which is non-parametric for a finite number of treatments. In the case of one treatment and one control condition, each unit has two potential outcomes, one if the unit is treated and the other if untreated. A causal effect is defined as the difference between the two potential outcomes, but only one of the two potential outcomes is observed. Rubin (1974, 2006) developed the model into a general framework for causal inference with implications for observational research. Holland (1986) wrote an influential review article that highlighted some of the philosophical implications of the framework. Consequently, instead of the "Neyman–Rubin model," the model is often simply called the Rubin causal model (e.g., Holland 1986) or sometimes the Neyman–Rubin–Holland model (e.g., Brady 2008) or the Neyman–Holland–Rubin model (e.g., Freedman 2006).

The intellectual history of the Neyman–Rubin model is the subject of some controversy (e.g., Freedman 2006; Rubin 1990; Speed 1990). Neyman's 1923 article never mentions the random assignment of treatments. Instead, the original motivation was an urn model, and the explicit suggestion to use the urn model to physically assign treatments is absent from the paper (Speed 1990). It was left to R. A. Fisher in the 1920s and 1930s to note the importance of the physical act of randomization in experiments. Fisher first did this in the context of experimental design in his 1925 book, expanded on the issue in a 1926 article for agricultural researchers, and developed it more fully and for a broader audience in his 1935 book *The Design of Experiments*.

This gap between Neyman and Fisher points to the fact that there was something absent from the Neyman mathematical formulation, which was added later, even though the symbolic formulation was complete in 1923. What those symbols *meant* changed. And in these changes lies what is causal about the Neyman–Rubin model—i.e., a focus on the mechanism by which treatment is assigned. The Neyman–Rubin model is more than just the math of the original Neyman model. Obviously, it relies not on an urn model motivation for the observed potential outcomes but, for experiments, a motivation based on the random assignment of treatment. And for observational studies, one relies on the assumption that the assignment of treatment can be treated as if it were random. In either case, the mechanism by which treatment is assigned is of central importance. And the realization that the primacy of the assignment mechanism holds true for observational data no less than for experimental, is due to Rubin (1974).

The basic setup of the Neyman model is simple. Let A_i be a treatment indicator: 1 when i is in the treatment regime and 0 otherwise. But an additional assumption must be made to link potential outcomes to observed outcomes. The most common assumption used is the one of "no interference between units" (Cox 1958, Sect. 2.4). With this assumption, one can assume that the observed outcome for observation i is

$$Y_i = A_i Y_{1,i} + (1 - A_i) Y_{0,i}, \tag{21.1}$$

where $Y_{1,i}$ denotes the potential outcome for unit i if the unit receives treatment and $Y_{0,i}$ denotes the potential outcome for unit i in the control regime. The treatment effect for observation i is defined by $\tau_i = Y_{1,i} - Y_{0,i}$. Causal inference is a missing-data problem because $Y_{1,i}$ and $Y_{0,i}$ are never both observed.

The "no interference between units" is often called the stable unit treatment value assumption (SUTVA). SUTVA implies that the potential outcomes for a given unit do not vary with the treatments assigned to any other unit, and that there are not different versions of treatment (Rubin 1978). The mapping from potential outcomes to observed outcomes is not a primitive in the potential-outcomes framework. This point is often missed. Equation (21.1) only follows because of the no interference assumption. Otherwise, Y_i may depend on A_j, $Y_{0,j}$, and $Y_{1,j}$, where $j \neq i$. Therefore, one may argue that there is a structural model embedded in the Neyman model as commonly used, although a simple one with clear behavioral implications.

The next key part of the Neyman–Rubin model is the assignment mechanism. It is the process by which the potential outcomes are missing. The treatment assignment mechanism may satisfy the no unmeasured confounding assumption:

$$P(A \mid W, Y_0, Y_1) = P(A \mid W), \tag{21.2}$$

where W are some confounders. If the randomization is not conditional on W, then $P(A \mid W, Y_0, Y_1) = P(A \mid W) = P(A)$. Beyond randomization, one wishes that

$$0 < P(A_i = 1 \mid W_i) < 1. \tag{21.3}$$

Equation (21.3) is also referred to as the positivity assumption, as discussed in detail in Chaps. 2 and 10. It is a common support condition.

Equations (21.2) and (21.3) make clear that randomized experiments are free of any dependence between the treatment *and* potential outcomes, conditional on observables that were used to define the randomization probabilities. Before Rubin (1975), the potential-outcomes framework was used by various authors to formalize randomized experiments, but never observational studies. Freedman (2006), Rubin (2008), and Sekhon (2010) review some of the relevant history.

It was unprecedented when Rosenbaum and Rubin (1983) used Eqs. (21.2) (ignorability) and (21.3) (common support) to define "strong ignorability." Ignorability dates from Rubin (1976). Importantly, these concepts were applied, for the first time, to observational data and not just experimental data. This gave a formal language to the tradition of thinking of observational studies as broken experiments, where many of the lessons of experimental design are maintained. This tradition goes back to at least Cochran (1965) – also see Cochran and Rubin (1973) and Cochran (1983). Rubin and his various co-authors formalized and extended it to become a way of thinking about causality. There are no observed outcomes in Eqs. (21.2) and (21.3), but they define an assumption by which the average treatment effect may be identified: selection on observables.

If the principle of defining an estimator in terms of an a priori fitted propensity score, in which the fitting process can be flexible but is ignorant of the outcomes, is a valid one, then the statistical properties of double robust estimators (such as the TMLE with an externally fitted treatment mechanism) that live by this principle should be fully competitive with a (double robust) C-TMLE that ignores this principle and lives by the principle of targeted learning that views the goal of the fit of the propensity score as an ingredient to obtain a best estimator of the target quantity.

Three questions arise that we wish to address. First, can an automated estimation strategy be used effectively? Second, can the TMLE and the C-TMLE overcome the demonstrated instability problems of other double robust estimators? Third, overall, which one wins, the TMLE, which lives by the principle of using an externally fitted propensity score, or the C-TMLE, which fits the propensity score as an ingredient for targeted fitting of the response surface?

21.2 Kang and Schafer Censored-Data Simulations

In this section, motivated by Kang and Schafer (2007) (hereafter, KS) and a response by Robins et al. (2007b), we compare the performance of TMLEs to that of estimating-equation-based double robust estimators, in the context of sparsity. This set of simulations was originally designed by KS to highlight the stability problems of double robust estimators. We will demonstrate that TMLEs can perform well in these simulations. The KS simulations focus on the problem of estimating a population mean from censored data. The data are CAR but not completely at random. We explore the relative performance of the estimators under the original KS simulation and a number of alternative data-generating distributions that involve different and stronger types of violations of the positivity assumption. These new simulation settings were designed to provide more diverse and challenging test cases for evaluating robustness and thereby finite sample performance of the different estimators.

Original Kang and Schafer simulation. KS considered n i.i.d. units of $O = (W, \Delta, \Delta Y) \sim P_0$, where W is a vector of four baseline covariates and Δ is an indicator of whether the continuous outcome, Y, is observed. KS were interested in estimating $\mu(P_0) = E_0(Y) = E_0[E_0(Y \mid \Delta = 1, W)]$. Let $(Z_1, \ldots, Z_4)$ be independent normally distributed random variables with mean zero and variance one.

The covariates W we actually observe were generated as follows: $W_1 = \exp(Z_1/2)$, $W_2 = Z_2/(1+\exp(Z_1)) + 10$, $W_3 = (Z_1Z_3/25+0.6)^3$, and $W_4 = (Z_2+Z_4+20)^2$. The outcome Y was generated as $Y = 210+27.4Z_1+13.7Z_2+13.7Z_3+13.7Z_4+N(0,1)$. From this one can determine that the conditional mean $\bar{Q}_0$ of Y, given W, which equals the same linear regression in $Z_1(W),\ldots,Z_4(W)$, where $Z_j(W)$, $j = 1,\ldots,4$, are the unique solutions of the four equations above in terms of $W = (W_1,\ldots,W_4)$. Formally, $\bar{Q}_0(W) = E_0[E_0(Y \mid Z) \mid W]$. Thus, if the data analyst had been provided the functions $Z_j(W)$, then the true regression function was linear in these functions, but the data analyst is measuring the terms W_j instead.

The other complication of the data-generating distribution is that Y is subject to missingness, and the true censoring mechanism, denoted by $g_0(1 \mid W) = P_0(\Delta = 1 \mid W)$, is given by $g_0(1 \mid W) = \text{expit}(-Z_1(W) + 0.5Z_2(W) - 0.25Z_3(W) - 0.1Z_4(W))$. With this data-generating mechanism, the average response rate is 0.50. Also, the true population mean is 210, while the mean among respondents is 200. These values indicate a small selection bias.

In these simulations, a linear main term model in the main terms $(W_1,\ldots,W_4)$ for either the outcome-regression or missingness mechanism is misspecified, while a linear main term model in the main terms $(Z_1(W),\ldots,Z_4(W))$ would be correctly specified. Note that there are finite sample violations of the positivity assumption given in Eq. (21.3). Specifically, we find $g_0(\Delta = 1 \mid W) \in [0.01, 0.98]$, and the estimated missingness probabilities $g_n(\Delta = 1 \mid W)$ were observed to fall in the range $[4 \times 10^{-6}, 0.97]$.

Modified Kang and Schafer simulation 1. In the KS simulation, when $\bar{Q}_0$ or g_0 is misspecified, the misspecifications are small. The selection bias is also small. Therefore, we modified the KS simulation in order to increase the degree of misspecification and to increase the selection bias. This creates a greater challenge for estimators and better highlights their relative performance. As before, let Z_j be i.i.d. $N(0,1)$. The outcome Y was generated as $Y = 210 + 50Z_1 + 25Z_2 + 25Z_3 + 25Z_4 + N(0,1)$. The covariates actually observed by the data analyst are now given by the following functions of $(Z_1,\ldots,Z_4)$: $W_1 = \exp(Z_1^2/2)$, $W_2 = 0.5Z_2/(1+\exp(Z_1^2)) + 3$, $W_3 = (Z_1^2 Z_3/25+0.6)^3 + 2$, and $W_4 = (Z_2+0.6Z_4)^2 + 2$. From this, one can determine the true regression function $\bar{Q}_0(W) = E_0(E_0(Y \mid Z) \mid W)$. The missingness indicator was generated as follows: $g_0(1 \mid W) = \text{expit}(-2Z_1 + Z_2 - 0.5Z_3 - 0.2Z_4)$. A misspecified fit is now obtained by fitting a linear or logistic main term regression in $W_1,\ldots,W_4$, while a correct fit is obtained by providing the user with the terms $Z_1,\ldots,Z_4$, and fitting a linear or logistic main term regression in $Z_1,\ldots,Z_4$. With these modifications, the population mean is again 210, but the mean among respondents is 184.4. With these modifications, we have a higher degree of practical violation of the positivity assumption: $g_0(\Delta = 1 \mid W) \in [1.1 \times 10^{-5}, 0.99]$ while the estimated probabilities, $g_n(\Delta = 1 \mid W)$, were observed to fall in the range $[2.2 \times 10^{-16}, 0.87]$.

Modified Kang and Schafer simulation 2. Here we made one additional change to the modified simulation 1: We set the coefficient in front of Z_4 in the true regression of Y on Z equal to zero. Therefore, while Z_4 is still associated with missingness, it is not associated with the outcome, and is thus not a confounder. Given $(W_1, \ldots, W_3)$, W_4 is not associated with the outcome either, and therefore as misspecified regression model of $\bar{Q}_0$ we use a main term linear regression in (W_1, W_2, W_3). This modification to the KS simulation enables us to take the debate on the relative performance of double robust estimators one step further, by addressing a second key challenge of the estimators: They often include nonconfounders in the censoring mechanism estimator. This unnecessary inclusion could unnecessarily introduce positivity violations. Moreover, this can itself introduce substantial bias and inflated variance, sometimes referred to as Z-bias. While this problem is not presented in the Kang and Schafer paper and responses, it is highlighted in the literature, including Bhattacharya and Vogt (2007), Wooldridge (2009), and Pearl (2010a). As discussed earlier, the C-TMLE provides an innovative approach for estimating the censoring mechanism, preferring covariates that are associated with the outcome and censoring, without "data snooping."

21.2.1 Estimators

As illustrated in KS and Robins et al. (2007b), semiparametric efficient double robust estimators typically rely on IPCW. These weights will be very large when there are violations of the positivity assumption. As a benchmark, KS compare all estimators in their article to the ordinary least squares estimator:

$$\mu_{OLS,n} = \frac{1}{n} \sum_{i=1}^{n} \bar{Q}_n(W_i),$$

where $\bar{Q}_n$ is the least squares estimator of $\bar{Q}_0$ according to a main term linear regression model $m_\beta(W) = \beta W^\top$, only using the observations with $\Delta_i = 1$.

Kang and Schafer present comparisons of several double robust (and nondouble robust) estimators. We focus on the weighted least squares (WLS) estimator and the A-IPCW estimator. The WLS estimator is defined as

$$\mu_{WLS,n} = \frac{1}{n} \sum_{i=1}^{n} m_{\beta_n}(W_i),$$

where m_β is a linear regression model for $\bar{Q}_0$ and β_n is an IPCW linear regression estimator given by

$$\beta_n = \arg\min_\beta \sum_{i=1}^{n} \frac{\Delta_i}{g_n(1 \mid W_i)} (Y_i - m_\beta(W_i))^2.$$

The A-IPCW estimator is defined as

$$\mu_{A-IPCW,n} = \frac{1}{n} \sum_i \frac{\Delta_i}{g_n(1 \mid W_i)} (Y_i - \bar{Q}_n(W_i)) + \bar{Q}_n(W_i).$$

We compare these estimators with the TMLE and the C-TMLE with logistic fluctuation for a continuous outcome (Chap. 7). These estimators are guaranteed to stay within the global bounds of the model, which is essential when $g_0(1 \mid W)$ has values close to 0. The logistic fluctuation TMLE for continuous $Y \in (a, b)$ involves defining a normalized outcome $Y^* = (Y - a)/(b - a) \in (0, 1)$, computing the TMLE of $E_0(Y^*)$, and transforming back this TMLE into a TMLE of $E_0(Y) = (b - a)E_0(Y^*) + a$. The TMLE with logistic fluctuation requires setting a range $[a, b]$ for the outcomes Y. If such knowledge is available, one simply uses the known values. If Y is not subject to missingness, then one would use the minimum and maximum of the empirical sample, which represents a very accurate estimator of the range. In these simulations, Y is subject to informative missingness such that the minimum or maximum of the biased sample represents a biased estimate of the range, resulting in a small unnecessary bias in the TMLE (negligible relative to MSE). We enlarged the range of the complete observation by a factor of 1.1, which seemed to remove most of the unnecessary bias. We expect that some improvements can be obtained by incorporating a valid estimator of the range that takes into account the informative missingness, but such second order improvements are outside the scope of this chapter. The TMLE of $E_0(Y^*)$ involves obtaining an initial estimator of $E_0(Y^* \mid W, \Delta = 1)$, representing it as a logistic function, and subsequently fluctuating it according to the logistic fluctuation function. Let $\bar{Q}_n^0 \in (0, 1)$ be an initial estimator of $E_0(Y^* \mid \Delta = 1, W)$ obtained by regressing Y^* onto W among the observations with $\Delta_i = 1$. Consider the logistic fluctuation working model

$$\text{logit}\bar{Q}_n^0(\epsilon)(W) = \text{logit}\bar{Q}_n^0(W) + \epsilon H^*_{g_n}(W),$$

where $H^*_{g,n}(1, W) = 1/g_n(1 \mid W)$. One estimates the amount of fluctuation ϵ with maximum likelihood estimation using logistic regression software for binary outcomes. One can use standard software for this fluctuation, ignoring that Y^* is not binary. (See Chap. 7 for the proof that the binary outcome log-likelihood loss function is the correct loss function in this case.) This now defines the first-step TMLE $\bar{Q}_n^1 = \bar{Q}_n^0(\epsilon_n)$, which is also the TMLE of $\bar{Q}_0$. The TMLE of $E_0(Y^*)$ is now given by the corresponding substitution estimator $\mu^*_{TMLE,n} = \frac{1}{n} \sum_i \bar{Q}_n^*(W_i)$. The latter estimator maps into the desired TMLE $\mu_{TMLE,n} = (b - a)\mu^*_{TMLE,n} + a$ of $\mu_0 = E_0(Y)$.

The C-TMLE $\mu_{C-TMLE,n}$ is defined in Chap. 20 for the mean outcome $E_0 Y_1$ based on $O = (W, A, Y)$, but now treating $A = \Delta$. The C-TMLE differs from the standard TMLE above in its estimation procedures for $\bar{Q}_0$ and g_0. The TMLE fluctuates an initial estimator of $\bar{Q}_0$ using an external estimate of g_0, while the C-TMLE estimate considers a sequence of subsequent TMLE updates of this initial estimator indexed by increasingly nonparametric estimators of g_0 and, based on the "log-likelihood" for $\bar{Q}_0$ of these candidate TMLEs, data-adaptively determines the desired TMLE and, in particular, the desired fit of g_0. The C-TMLE involves building an estimator of the distribution of Δ as a function of a set of covariates that are still predictive of Y, after taking into account the initial estimator. That is, the C-TMLE relies on a collaboratively estimated g_n that at times only targets a true conditional distribution of Δ, given a *reduction* of W, yet delivers full bias reduction.

21.2.2 Results

For the three simulations described above, the OLS, WLS, A-IPCW, TMLE, and C-TMLE were used to estimate $\mu(P_0)$ from 250 samples of size 1000. We evaluated the performance of the estimators by their bias, variance, and MSE. We compared the estimators of $\mu(P_0)$ using different specifications of the estimators of $\bar{Q}_0$ and g_0. In the tables below, CC indicates that the estimators of both were specified correctly; CM indicates that the estimator of $\bar{Q}_0$ was correct, but the estimator for g_0 was misspecified; MC indicates that the estimator for $\bar{Q}_0$ was misspecified, but the estimator for g_0 was correct; and MM indicates both estimators were misspecified.

For all estimators, we compared results with $g_n(1 \mid W) \in [0, 1]$ by also truncating $g_n(1 \mid W)$ from below at three different levels: 0.010, 0.025, and 0.050. We note that neither KS nor Robins et al. (2007b) included bounding $g_n(1 \mid W)$ from below when applying their estimators. In any given application, it is difficult to determine which bounds to use, but the theory teaches us that double robust estimators can only be consistent if $g_n(1 \mid W)$ stays bounded away from zero, even if the true g_0 is

Table 21.1 Simulation results, 250 samples of size 1000. (a) Kang and Schafer simulation. (b) Modified simulation 1. (c) Modified simulation 2

	CC			*CM*			*MC*			*MM*		
(a)	Bias	Var	MSE	Bias	Var	MSE	Bias	Var	MSE	Bias	Var	MSE
OLS	−0.09	1.4	1.4	−0.09	1.4	1.4	−0.93	2.0	2.8	−0.93	2.0	2.8
WLS	−0.09	1.4	1.4	−0.09	1.4	1.4	0.10	1.8	1.8	−3.0	2.1	11
A-IPCW	−0.09	1.4	1.4	−0.10	1.4	1.5	0.04	2.5	2.5	−8.8	2e+2	3e+2
TMLE	−0.10	1.4	1.4	−0.11	1.4	1.4	−0.09	2.1	2.1	−4.6	3.6	25
C-TMLE	−0.10	1.4	1.4	−0.11	1.4	1.4	0.09	1.8	1.8	−1.5	2.8	5.0
(b)												
OLS	−0.17	4.7	4.7	−0.17	4.7	4.7	−36	17	1e+3	−36	17	1e+3
WLS	−0.16	4.7	4.7	−0.16	4.7	4.7	−4.4	42	61	−35	16	1e+3
A-IPCW	−0.16	4.7	4.8	−0.16	4.7	4.7	−1.8	2e+2	2e+3	−35	17	1e+3
TMLE	−0.22	4.7	4.7	−0.23	4.7	4.7	−0.04	89	89	−34	6.5	1e+3
C-TMLE	−0.26	4.7	4.7	−0.22	4.7	4.7	−0.64	16	16	−34	6.6	1e+3
(c)												
OLS	−0.06	3.9	3.9	−0.06	3.9	3.9	−34	15	1e+3	−34	15	1e+3
WLS	−0.06	4.0	3.9	−0.06	3.9	3.9	−3.6	40	53	−33	15	1e+3
A-IPCW	−0.05	4.0	4.0	−0.06	3.9	3.9	−1.1	2e+2	2e+3	−33	16	1e+3
TMLE	−0.10	3.9	3.9	−0.11	3.9	3.9	0.15	76	76	−32	5.6	1e+3
C-TMLE	−0.14	3.9	3.9	−0.11	3.9	3.9	−0.88	11	11	−33	5.8	1e+3

Table 21.2 Kang and Schafer simulation results by truncation level of g_n, 250 samples of size 1000

Bound on g_n	*CC*			*CM*			*MC*			*MM*		
by estimator	Bias	Var	MSE	Bias	Var	MSE	Bias	Var	MSE	Bias	Var	MSE
OLS	−0.09	1.4	1.4	−0.09	1.4	1.4	−0.93	2.0	2.8	−0.9	2.0	2.8
WLS												
None	−0.09	1.4	1.4	−0.09	1.4	1.4	0.10	1.8	1.8	−3.0	2.1	11
0.010	−0.09	1.4	1.4	−0.09	1.4	1.4	0.10	1.8	1.8	−3.0	2.0	11
0.025	−0.09	1.4	1.4	−0.09	1.4	1.4	0.10	1.8	1.8	−2.9	2.0	11
0.050	−0.09	1.4	1.4	−0.09	1.4	1.4	0.11	1.8	1.8	−2.7	1.9	9.4
A-IPCW												
None	−0.09	1.4	1.4	−0.10	1.4	1.5	0.04	2.5	2.5	−8.8	2e+2	3e+2
0.010	−0.09	1.4	1.4	−0.09	1.4	1.4	0.04	2.5	2.5	−6.1	18	56
0.025	−0.09	1.4	1.4	−0.09	1.4	1.4	0.04	2.4	2.4	−4.9	6.1	30
0.050	−0.09	1.4	1.4	−0.09	1.4	1.4	0.08	2.3	2.3	−3.8	3.2	18
TMLE												
None	−0.10	1.4	1.4	−0.11	1.4	1.4	−0.09	2.1	2.1	−4.6	3.6	25
0.010	−0.10	1.4	1.4	−0.10	1.4	1.4	−0.09	2.1	2.1	−4.4	4.2	24
0.025	−0.10	1.4	1.4	−0.10	1.4	1.4	−0.09	2.1	2.1	−4.1	3.1	20
0.050	−0.10	1.4	1.4	−0.10	1.4	1.4	−0.06	2.0	2.0	−3.6	2.4	15
C-TMLE												
None	−0.10	1.4	1.4	−0.11	1.4	1.4	0.09	1.8	1.8	−1.5	2.8	5.0
0.010	−0.10	1.4	1.4	−0.10	1.4	1.4	0.09	1.7	1.7	−1.3	2.2	4.0
0.025	−0.10	1.4	1.4	−0.10	1.4	1.4	0.11	1.7	1.7	−1.4	2.3	4.2
0.050	−0.10	1.4	1.4	−0.10	1.4	1.4	0.10	1.8	1.8	−1.3	2.1	3.8

not bounded away from zero (e.g., van der Laan and Robins 2003). Therefore, only presenting the (interesting) results for not bounding at all (but $g_n(1 \mid W) \in [0,1]$) provides insight about an estimator that should never be used in practice. Ideally, the choice of bounding $g_n(1 \mid W)$ should depend on, among other things, the data-generating process and the sample size, so that one desires an estimator adaptively determines the truncation level (such as particular implementations of C-TMLE).

Table 21.1 presents the simulation results without any bounding of g_n.The tables show that in all three simulations, the TMLE and C-TMLE with a logistic fluctuation achieve comparable or better MSE than the other estimators. When $\bar{Q}_n$ is misspecified, TMLE performs well and C-TMLE stands out with a much lower MSE. Together, the results from modified simulation 1 and modified simulation 2 show that the C-TMLEs have similar or superior performance relative to estimating-equation-based double robust estimators when not all covariates are associated with Y. At the same time, even in cases in which *all* covariates are associated with Y, the C-TMLE still performs well. Tables 21.2 and 21.3 compare results for each estimator when bounding g_n at different levels. We see that bounding g_n can improve the bias and variability of the estimators, often substantially. However, we also see that bounding can easily increase bias. The effect of bounding and the desired level

Table 21.3 Simulation results by truncation level of g_n, 250 samples of size 1000. (a) Modified Kang and Schafer simulation 1. (b) Modified Kang and Schafer simulation 2

	CC			*CM*			*MC*			*MM*		
(a)	Bias	Var	MSE	Bias	Var	MSE	Bias	Var	MSE	Bias	Var	MSE
OLS	−0.17	4.7	4.7	−0.17	4.7	4.7	−36	17	1e+3	−36	17	1e+3
WLS												
None	−0.16	4.7	4.7	−0.16	4.7	4.7	−4.4	42	61	−35	16	1e+3
0.010	−0.16	4.7	4.7	−0.16	4.7	4.7	−4.6	39	60	−35	16	1e+3
0.025	−0.17	4.7	4.7	−0.16	4.7	4.7	−5.5	32	62	−35	16	1e+3
0.050	−0.17	4.7	4.7	−0.16	4.7	4.7	−7.3	25	78	−35	16	1e+3
A-IPCW												
None	−0.16	4.7	4.8	−0.16	4.7	4.7	−1.8	2e+2	2e+3	−35	17	1e+3
0.010	−0.16	4.7	4.7	−0.16	4.7	4.7	−3.7	74	88	−35	17	1e+3
0.025	−0.17	4.7	4.7	−0.16	4.7	4.7	−5.9	43	77	−35	17	1e+3
0.050	−0.17	4.7	4.7	−0.16	4.7	4.7	−8.8	28	1e+2	−35	17	1e+3
TMLE												
None	−0.22	4.7	4.7	−0.23	4.7	4.7	−0.04	89	89	−34	6.5	1e+3
0.010	−0.22	4.7	4.7	−0.22	4.7	4.7	0.71	53	54	−34	6.5	1e+3
0.025	−0.22	4.7	4.7	−0.22	4.7	4.7	1.0	22	23	−34	6.5	1e+3
0.050	−0.22	4.7	4.7	−0.22	4.7	4.7	−0.49	11	11	−34	6.5	1e+3
C-TMLE												
None	−0.26	4.7	4.7	−0.22	4.7	4.7	−0.64	16	16	−34	6.7	1e+3
0.010	−0.24	4.7	4.8	−0.22	4.7	4.7	−0.84	22	22	−34	6.7	1e+3
0.025	−0.24	4.7	4.7	−0.22	4.7	4.7	−1.5	12	14	−34	6.8	1e+3
0.050	−0.23	4.7	4.7	−0.22	4.7	4.7	−2.6	8.7	15	−34	6.8	1e+3

(b)												
OLS	−0.06	3.9	3.9	−0.06	3.9	3.9	−34	15	1e+3	−34	15	1e+3
WLS												
None	−0.06	4.0	3.9	−0.06	3.9	3.9	−3.6	40	53	−33	15	1e+3
0.010	−0.06	4.0	3.9	−0.06	3.9	3.9	−4.0	35	51	−33	15	1e+3
0.025	−0.06	4.0	3.9	−0.06	3.9	3.9	−4.9	29	53	−33	15	1e+3
0.050	−0.06	4.0	3.9	−0.06	3.9	3.9	−6.7	23	68	−33	15	1e+3
A-IPCW												
None	−0.05	4.0	4.0	−0.06	3.9	3.9	−1.1	2e+2	2e+2	−33	16	1e+3
0.010	−0.06	4.0	4.0	−0.06	3.9	3.9	−3.1	70	80	−33	16	1.e+3
0.025	−0.06	4.0	3.9	−0.06	3.9	3.9	−5.4	39	68	−33	16	1e+3
0.050	−0.06	3.9	3.9	−0.06	3.9	3.9	−8.3	26	94	−33	16	1e+3
TMLE												
None	−0.10	3.9	3.9	−0.11	3.9	3.9	0.15	76	76	−32	5.6	1e+3
0.010	−0.10	3.9	3.9	−0.10	3.9	3.9	0.95	43	44	−32	5.6	1e+3
0.025	−0.10	3.9	3.9	−0.10	3.9	3.9	1.3	18	19	−32	5.6	1e+3
0.050	−0.10	3.9	3.9	−0.10	3.9	3.9	−0.20	8.5	8.5	−32	5.6	1e+3
C-TMLE												
None	−0.14	3.9	3.9	−0.11	3.9	3.9	−0.88	11	11	−33	5.8	1e+3
0.010	−0.13	3.9	3.9	−0.10	3.9	3.9	−0.91	12	12	−33	6.1	1e+3
0.025	−0.12	3.9	3.9	−0.10	3.9	3.9	−1.4	8.5	10	−33	6.1	1e+3
0.050	−0.12	3.9	3.9	−0.10	3.9	3.9	−2.5	6.4	12	−33	6.0	1e+3

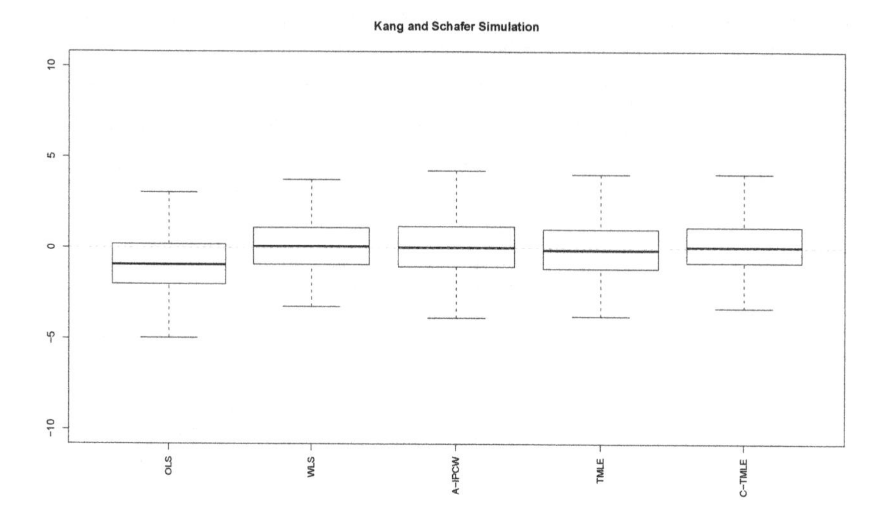

Fig. 21.1 Kang and Schafer simulation, MC, truncation level 0.025

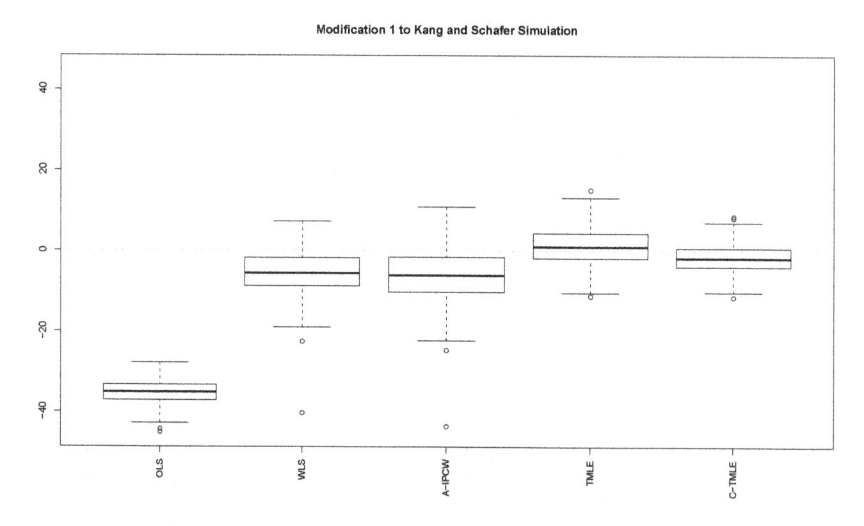

Fig. 21.2 Modified Kang and Schafer simulation 1, MC, truncation level 0.025

of bounding varies by estimator. It is important to note C-TMLE and TMLE are always well behaved. In no simulation do they show marked instability. C-TMLE performs particularly well. Results from the KS simulation, modified simulation 1, and modified simulation 2 are presented visually for MC with $g_n(1 \mid W)$ truncated from below at 0.025 in Figs. 21.1–21.3.

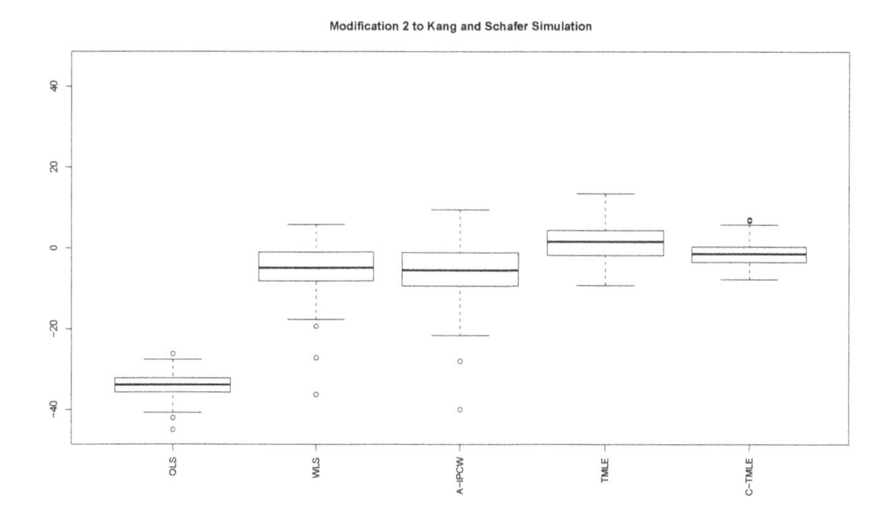

Fig. 21.3 Modified Kang and Schafer simulation 2, MC, truncation level 0.025

21.2.3 Super Learning and the Kang and Schafer Simulations

The misspecified formulation in KS can illustrate the benefits of coupling data-adaptive (super) learning with the TMLE. Results for the case that both $\bar{Q}_0$ and g_0 are inconsistently estimated indicate that the C-TMLE, constrained to use a main term regression model with misspecified covariates (W_1, W_2, W_3, W_4), has smaller variance than $\hat{\mu}_{OLS}$ but is more biased. The MSE of the TMLE is larger than the MSE of C-TMLE, with increased bias and variance. How would the estimation process be affected if we chose to act, based on the widespread understanding that models are seldom correctly specified and main term regressions generally fail to adequately capture the true relationships between predictors and an outcome, by turning to data-adaptive machine learning?

We coupled super learning with TMLE and C-TMLE to estimate both $\bar{Q}_0$ and g_0. For C-TMLE, four missingness-mechanism-score-based covariates were created based on different truncation levels of the propensity score estimate $g_n(1 \mid W)$: no truncation, and truncation from below at the 0.01, 0.025, and 0.05 percentile. These four scores were supplied along with the misspecified main terms $W_1, \ldots, W_4$ to the targeted forward selection algorithm in the C-TMLE used to build a series of candidate nested logistic regression estimators of the missingness mechanism and corresponding candidate TMLEs. The C-TMLE algorithm used 5-fold cross-validation to select the best estimate from the eight candidate TMLEs. This allows the C-TMLE algorithm to build a logistic regression fit of g_0 that selects among the misspecified main-terms and super-learning fits of the missingness mechanism score $g_n(1 \mid W)$ at different truncation levels.

Table 21.4 Super learning simulation results, MM, $g_n(1 \mid W)$ truncated at 0.025

	Bias	Var	MSE
TMLE+ SL	−0.771	1.51	2.10
C-TMLE+ SL	−1.047	1.54	2.64

An important aspect of super learning is to ensure that the collection of prediction algorithms includes a variety of approaches for fitting the true function $\bar{Q}_0$ and g_0. For example, it is sensible to include a main terms regression algorithm in the super learner library. Should that algorithm happen to be correct, the super learner will behave as the main terms regression algorithm. It is also recommended to include algorithms that search over a space of higher-order polynomials, nonlinear models, and, for example, cubic splines. For binary outcome regression, as required for fitting g_0, classification algorithms such as classification and regression trees, support vector machines (Cortes and Vapnik 1995), and k-nearest-neighbor algorithms (Friedman 1994) could be added to the collection of algorithms. Super learning relies on the oracle property of V-fold cross-validation to asymptotically select the optimal convex combination of estimates obtained (Chap. 3).

Consider the misspecified scenario proposed by KS. The truth for both the outcome regression and the propensity for missingness regression is captured by a main terms linear regression of the outcome on Z_1, Z_2, Z_3, Z_4. This simple truth is virtually impossible to discover through the usual model selection approaches when the observed data consist of misspecified covariates $O = (W_1, W_2, W_3, W_4, \Delta, \Delta Y)$, given that $Z_1 = 2\log(W_1)$, $Z_2 = (W_2 - 10)(1 + 2W_1)$, $Z_3 = (25 \times (W_3 - 0.6))/(2\log(W_1))$, and $Z_4 = \sqrt[3]{W_4} - 20 - (W_2 - 10)(1 + 2W_1)$. This complexity illustrates the importance of including prediction algorithms that attack the estimation problem from a variety of directions. The collection of algorithms employed included glm, step, ipredbagg, DSA, earth, loess, nnet, svm, and k-nearest-neighbors. (We note that k-nearest-neighbors is only for binary outcomes, and it was used to estimate g only.)

In Table 21.4 we report the results for TMLE and C-TMLE based on 250 samples of size 1000, with predicted values for $g_n(1 \mid W)$ truncated from below at 0.025. The MSE for both estimators is smaller than the MSE of $\hat{\mu}_{OLS}$. The C-TMLE bias is slightly higher than the $\hat{\mu}_{OLS}$ bias, and TMLE is slightly better with respect to both bias and variance. More importantly, data-adaptive estimation improved efficiency of TMLE by a factor of 8.5. C-TMLE efficiency improved by a factor of 1.5.

21.3 Freedman and Berk Simulations

Freedman and Berk (2008) (hereafter, FB) compared weighted and unweighted regression approaches to estimating coefficients in parametric causal models. They demonstrated that propensity score weighting can increase the bias and variance of the estimators relative to unweighted regression, even when the true propensity score model is known. FB were concerned with how applied researchers were using double robust estimators: to perform structural estimation using parametric models. FB noted that this was far from the original intention of Robins and his collaborators for double robust estimators. Robins et al. were estimating treatment effects (contrasts) and using semiparametric model to perform the estimation. We use the FB simulations to engage exactly that setting: we are estimating treatment effects and we compare the performance of two semiparametric estimators, the TMLE and C-TMLE, relative to alternative estimators. We replicated the original FB simulation study and offer additional simulations based on modifications of their setup. We should note up front that our intention is not to question the take-home point of the FB article: Using double robust estimators to perform structural estimation is fraught with difficulties. We explore different questions, including that of whether nonparametric double robust estimators can be used to estimate treatment effects without the observed instability of the usual estimators relying on the inverse probability of treatment weighting.

We examine the behavior of TMLE, C-TMLE, and A-IPTW, in addition to the WLS and OLS estimators FB consider. The additive treatment effect in the FB simulations is defined nonparametrically as $\Psi(P) = E_P[E_P(Y \mid A = 1, W) - E_P(Y \mid A = 0, W)]$, where n i.i.d. copies of $O = (W, A, Y) \sim P_0$ represents the observed data, with outcome Y, binary treatment assignment A, and covariates W.

FB simulation 1 presents weighted and unweighted linear regression results based on the correct model and two misspecified parametric models, using a data-generating distribution that has conditional treatment assignment probabilities that come close to 0 and 1. We present results from applying each estimator discussed below to FB simulation 1 as well as additional results using modified data-generating distributions that provide additional insight into estimator performance.

21.3.1 Estimators

Given a linear regression model for $E_0(Y \mid A, W)$, the unweighted linear regression (OLS) estimator is obtained with least squares regression, while the weighted linear regression (WLS) estimator is obtained with weighted least squares regression assigning weight $w_i = 1/g_n(A_i \mid W_i)$ to observation $O_i = (W_i, A_i, Y_i)$. The A-IPTW estimator is given by

$$\psi_{A-IPTW,n} = \frac{1}{n}\sum_{i=1}^{n} \frac{I(A_i = 1) - I(A_i = 0)}{g_n(A_i \mid W_i)}(Y_i - \bar{Q}_n^0(A_i, W_i)) + \bar{Q}_n^0(1, W_i) - \bar{Q}_n^0(0, W_i),$$

where $\bar{Q}_n^0(A, W)$ is a least squares regression estimator of $\bar{Q}_0$, the true conditional mean of Y, given (A, W). The TMLE is a substitution estimator:

$$\psi_{TMLE,n} = \frac{1}{n}\sum_{i=1}^{n}(\bar{Q}_n^*(1, W_i) - \bar{Q}_n^*(0, W_i)),$$

where $\bar{Q}_n^*$ is a targeted estimate of the true regression $\bar{Q}_0(A, W) = E_0(Y \mid A, W)$, obtained by fluctuating the initial estimate, $\bar{Q}_n^0$, in a manner designed to reduce bias in the estimate of the parameter of interest. A logistic fluctuation working model was employed, guaranteeing that the TMLE $\bar{Q}_n^*$ would remain within the bounds $[a, b]$ for the outcome Y, set by design, by the user, or based on the observed outcomes. Since Y is generated from a normal distribution, the bounds were arbitrarily chosen to be the $[0.01, 0.99]$ quantiles of the observed values for Y in each simulated data set, and Y was truncated by these quantiles. The truncated data set can now be viewed as (W, A, Y), with $Y \in [a, b]$ for known bounds $[a, b]$. The TMLE procedure maps $Y \in [a, b]$ into $Y^* = (Y - a)/(b - a) \in [0, 1]$, then regresses Y^* onto A, W to obtain an initial estimator of $E_0(Y^* \mid A, W)$. Since the TMLE involves fluctuating the logit of this initial estimator, the values of the initial estimator were bounded away from 0 and 1 by truncating them from above and below at $\alpha = [0.005, 0.995]$. Recall that a TMLE is defined by a choice of submodel and loss function. Two TMLEs were implemented. In the first TMLE, we used the logistic regression submodel with clever covariate $(2A - 1)/g_n(A \mid W)$ and the quasi-log-likelihood loss function. This TMLE of the additive effect was described in Chap. 7. The second TMLE used the logistic regression submodel with clever covariate $(2A - 1)$, and the weighted quasi-log-likelihood loss function, where the weights are $1/g_n(A_i \mid W_i)$, $i = 1, \ldots, n$. We will denote this latter TMLE with TMLE$_w$. The latter TMLE is a less aggressive in weighting, and might therefore be more robust under violations of the positivity assumption.

The C-TMLE is also a substitution estimator:

$$\psi_{C-TMLE,n} = \frac{1}{n} \sum_{i=1}^{n} (\bar{Q}_n^*(1, W_i) - \bar{Q}_n^*(0, W_i)).$$

The C-TMLE is described in Chap. 19 and involves building a main term logistic regression estimator of a conditional distribution of A in terms of a set of covariates that are still predictive of Y, after taking into account the initial estimator. Two sets of C-TMLE results were obtained. For the first, labeled C-TMLE in Tables 21.5–21.6, the covariate set W used to create the series of treatment mechanism estimators is restricted to main term covariates. In the second set, labeled C-TMLE(augW), the set of main terms is augmented with four terms corresponding to the propensity score estimate supplied to all other estimators and truncated propensity scores, truncated at level $(p, 1 - p)$, with p set to $(0.10, 0.25, 0.50)$.

21.3.2 Simulations

Two data-generating distributions are defined. For each one, 250 samples of size $n = 1000$ are drawn from the given data-generating distribution. The propensity score g_0 is estimated using the correct probit model for treatment, and the estimator is denoted by g_n. The correct linear regression statistical model includes A, W_1, and

W_2 as main terms. Two increasingly misspecified models are defined, one with A and W_1 as main terms and one with only A as a main term. Estimates of the marginal additive treatment effect are obtained based on an MLE fit of $\bar{Q}_0$ according to these parametric models paired with the MLE g_n of g_0.

Freedman and Berk simulation 1. This simulation replicates FB simulation 1. Both covariates, W_1 and W_2, confound the relationship between treatment and the outcome, so one expects OLS to be biased when the regression model for $\bar{Q}_0$ is misspecified. Incorporating estimated propensity scores should allow the remaining estimators to be unbiased, at the cost of higher variance. Specifically, the data-generating distribution is defined as follows:

$$\begin{aligned}
&Y = 1 + A + W_1 + 2W_2 + U,\ U \sim N(0,1),\\
&P_0(A = 1 \mid W) = \Phi(0.5 + 0.25W_1 + 0.75W_2),\\
&(W_1, W_2) \text{ is bivariate normal, } N(\mu, \Sigma),\\
&\text{with } \mu_1 = 0.5, \quad \mu_2 = 1, \quad \Sigma = \begin{bmatrix} 2 & 1 \\ 1 & 1 \end{bmatrix},
\end{aligned}$$

where Φ is the CDF of the standard normal distribution, so that the treatment mechanism conforms to a probit model. These settings lead to finite sample violations of the positivity assumption: conditional treatment probabilities $g_0(1 \mid W) = P_0(A = 1 \mid W)$ range from 0.03 to 0.99995.

Freedman and Berk simulation 2. This simulation was designed to demonstrate that weighting can introduce bias in the estimate of the additive treatment effect, even when the correct propensity score model is known. In this simulation, $P_0(A = 1 \mid W)$ is between 0.0003 and 0.9997. The linear form of the relationships between the covariates and the outcome is unchanged, but the strengths of those relationships are altered to weaken the association between W_1 and W_2, and between W_2 and A, but strengthen the relationships between W_1 and Y and W_2 and Y. As in simulation 2, W_3 is associated with A, but not with the outcome Y. Specifically, the data-generating distribution is defined as follows:

$$\begin{aligned}
&Y = 1 + A + 5W_1 + 10W_2 + U,\ U \sim N(0,1),\\
&P_0(A = 1 \mid W) = \Phi(0.25W_1 + 0.001W_2 + W_3),\\
&(W_1, W_2) \text{ is bivariate normal, } N(\mu, \Sigma), \text{with } \mu_1 = 0.5, \quad \mu_2 = 2, \quad \Sigma = \begin{bmatrix} 0.1 & 1 \\ 1 & 1 \end{bmatrix}.
\end{aligned}$$

21.3.3 Results

OLS, WLS, A-IPTW, TMLE, and C-TMLE were applied to each simulated data set. In all simulations, when the model for the true conditional mean $\bar{Q}_0$ was correctly specified, OLS, the unweighted parametric estimator, had the smallest MSE, but when $\bar{Q}_0$ was misspecified, all other estimators outperformed OLS with respect to both MSE and bias. Simulation 1 results suggest that TMLE and C-TMLE are more robust than WLS and A-IPTW to practical violations of the positivity assumption. C-TMLE results in simulation 2 demonstrate that performance improves under lack of positivity by using a procedure that estimates only the necessary portion of the treatment mechanism. C-TMLEs' MSE and variance are superior to those of the other estimators that incorporate propensity score estimates. Under extreme misspecification (misspecified model 2) bias is almost entirely removed. Additionally, augmenting the covariate set with truncated propensity scores improves the performance of the C-TMLE. This augmentation confers the greatest benefit when the parametric model for $\bar{Q}_0$ is most severely misspecified. The results for the two simulations are presented in Tables 21.5 and 21.6. It is also of interest to note that for the truncated g_n setting, the TMLE that incorporates g_n in the clever covariate performs better than the TMLE that moves g_n into the weight, while the opposite is true for the unbounded g_n. Since it is theoretically sound to use some bounding, this particular simulation seems to favor the first type of TMLE.

Table 21.5 Freedman and Berk simulation 1, 250 samples of size 1000

	g_n unbounded				g_n bound = (0.025, 0.975)			
	Bias	Var	MSE	RE*	Bias	Var	MSE	RE
Unadj	4.061	0.046	16.538	–	4.061	0.046	16.538	–
Correct model								
OLS	0.010	0.009	0.010	1.000	–	–	–	–
WLS	0.012	0.039	0.039	4.144	0.016	0.024	0.024	2.526
A-IPTW	0.019	0.058	0.059	6.153	0.014	0.017	0.017	1.766
TMLE	0.190	0.475	0.509	53.460	0.019	0.027	0.027	2.834
TMLE_w	0.016	0.047	0.048	4.994	0.015	0.018	0.018	1.909
C-TMLE	0.004	0.014	0.014	1.449	0.013	0.013	0.013	1.410
C-TMLE(augW)	0.011	0.010	0.010	1.092	0.014	0.014	0.014	1.501
Misspecified model 1								
OLS	1.138	0.020	1.314	1.000	–	–	–	–
WLS	0.133	0.115	0.133	0.101	0.295	0.040	0.127	0.096
A-IPTW	0.120	0.344	0.357	0.272	0.433	0.033	0.220	0.167
TMLE	−0.588	0.380	0.724	0.551	−0.001	0.048	0.048	0.037
TMLE_w	0.134	0.177	0.194	0.148	0.359	0.032	0.161	0.123
C-TMLE	0.262	1.516	1.579	1.202	−0.412	0.098	0.267	0.203
C-TMLE(augW)	−0.242	1.068	1.122	0.854	−0.077	0.054	0.060	0.046
Misspecified model 2								
OLS	4.061	0.046	16.538	1.000	–	–	–	–
WLS	0.431	0.660	0.843	0.051	1.070	0.091	1.234	0.075
A-IPTW	0.381	3.039	3.172	0.192	1.507	0.130	2.402	0.145
TMLE	−0.451	1.392	1.590	0.096	−0.132	0.120	0.137	0.008
TMLE_w	0.430	1.226	1.406	0.085	1.260	0.105	1.693	0.102
C-TMLE	1.885	5.358	8.889	0.537	0.456	0.276	0.482	0.029
C-TMLE(augW)	−0.046	0.158	0.160	0.010	0.011	0.063	0.063	0.004

*Relative to OLS estimator using the same model specification

Table 21.6 Freedman and Berk simulation 2, 250 samples of size 1000

	g_n unbounded				g_n bound = (0.025, 0.975)			
	Bias	Var	MSE	RE	Bias	Var	MSE	RE
Unadj	3.022	0.688	9.816	–	3.022	0.688	9.816	–
Correct model								
OLS	0.002	0.004	0.004	1.000	–	–	–	–
WLS	0.002	0.012	0.012	3.175	0.004	0.009	0.009	2.476
A-IPTW	0.004	0.018	0.018	4.694	0.004	0.009	0.009	2.470
TMLE	0.001	0.067	0.067	17.676	0.002	0.011	0.011	3.003
TMLE_w	0.002	0.015	0.015	4.027	0.003	0.009	0.009	2.490
C-TMLE	0.002	0.004	0.004	0.991	0.002	0.004	0.004	0.989
C-TMLE(augW)	0.001	0.004	0.004	1.044	0.001	0.004	0.004	1.059
Misspecified model 1								
OLS	0.024	0.447	0.446	1.000	–	–	–	–
WLS	−0.108	0.500	0.510	1.143	−0.037	0.223	0.224	0.501
A-IPTW	−0.144	0.830	0.847	1.898	−0.037	0.223	0.224	0.502
TMLE	−0.127	1.077	1.089	2.440	−0.053	0.291	0.293	0.656
TMLE_w	−0.134	0.678	0.693	1.553	−0.039	0.227	0.228	0.511
C-TMLE	−0.077	0.050	0.056	0.125	−0.077	0.047	0.053	0.118
C-TMLE(augW)	−0.091	0.042	0.050	0.112	−0.094	0.045	0.054	0.120
Misspecified model 2								
OLS	3.022	0.688	9.816	1.000	–	–	–	–
WLS	−0.077	1.686	1.685	0.172	0.186	0.392	0.425	0.043
A-IPTW	−0.167	3.727	3.740	0.381	0.232	0.406	0.459	0.047
TMLE	−0.940	1.357	2.235	0.228	−0.294	0.555	0.639	0.065
TMLE_w	−0.120	2.181	2.187	0.223	0.180	0.400	0.430	0.044
C-TMLE	0.002	0.073	0.073	0.007	−0.005	0.021	0.021	0.002
C-TMLE(augW)	−0.049	0.073	0.075	0.008	−0.033	0.045	0.046	0.005

The C-TMLE outperforms all of the other estimators except for when the correct OLS model is used. And the performance of the C-TMLE is never poor in any simulation. The usual instability problems of weighted estimators has been minimized. The combination of properties in the C-TMLE proved especially robust in these Monte Carlos: it is a double robust (asymptotically efficient) substitution estimator that respects global constraints, makes use of a logistic fluctuation to respect the bounds even in finite samples, and performs internal collaborative estimation for g_0.

Domain knowledge can be incorporated into both stages of the TMLE and C-TMLE procedures. One example is the use of the augmented covariate set when the true treatment assignment mechanism is known. The strength of this approach is most clearly illustrated in simulation 2 with $\bar{Q}_0$ modeled with misspecified model 2, where the right thing to do is adjust for all covariates, yet that causes strong positivity violations. In this case, the inclusion of truncated propensity scores in W offered a more refined choice beyond simply including or excluding an entire covariate. These additional terms can be helpful in situations where including a particular covariate causes an positivity violation, but in fact, experimentation is lacking in only some portion of the covariate values.

21.4 Discussion

Researchers spend too little time on design and too much time on analysis in an attempt to overcome design defects. Sometimes – and in some fields, such as the social sciences, often – the correct answer is that the data at hand cannot answer the research question. Often new data must be gathered with a better design, ideally a design in which the researcher exploits natural or intentional variation to mitigate confounding instead of having to make a selection on observables assumption.

An essential goal of a scientific study is objectivity. Relying on an estimation strategy where one adjusts the model specification or estimator after one has observed estimated treatment effects cannot be considered objective. However, this objectivity is fully addressed by any estimator of the target parameter that is a priori specified, or at most influenced by ancillary statistics, so that the pursuit of objectivity itself should not limit the choice of estimators. The utilization of an a priori specified machine (and, specifically, super) learning algorithm to perform the modeling helps to mitigate the data-snooping concerns: the estimation procedure is fully specified before the analyst observes any final outcome data or estimated treatment effects. Having resolved the concern for objectivity, the remaining concern then centers on the instability of most double robust estimators when the data are sparse. C-TMLE is more stable than the other estimators considered here, and the TMLE and C-TMLE with logistic fluctuations perform well in these simulations.

The TMLE and C-TMLE and their accompanying technology, such as the super learner, are powerful and promising tools that overcome some of the common objections to double robust estimators. Demonstrating that the TMLE and C-TMLE perform well in general when the positivity assumption is violated is difficult because sparsity is a finite sample concern, and the efficiency and double robustness of TMLE and C-TMLE are asymptotic statistical properties, but the fact that these estimators are also *substitution* estimators (i.e., obtained by plugging an estimator of the data-generating distribution into the statistical model) explains the observed robustness. In particular, a substitution estimator puts bounds on the influence of one observation fully implied by the statistical model and the target parameter as a mapping on that statistical model. We hope that by showing that these estimators perform well in simulations created by *other* researchers for the purposes of showing the weaknesses of double robust estimators, we provide probative evidence in support of TMLE and C-TMLE. Indeed, we also extended the original simulations to make the estimation problems more challenging. Of course, much can happen in finite samples, and we look forward to exploring how these estimators perform in other settings. Of particular interest are applications of this technology to applied problems.

Part VII
Genomics

Chapter 22
Targeted Methods for Biomarker Discovery

Catherine Tuglus, Mark J. van der Laan

The use of biomarkers in disease diagnosis and treatment has grown rapidly in recent years, as microarray and sequencing technologies capable of detecting biological signatures have become more effective research tools. In an attempt to create a level of quality assurance with respect to biological and more specifically biomarker research, the FDA has called for the development of a standard protocol for biomarker qualification (Food and Drug Administration 2006). Such a protocol would define "evidentiary" standards for biomarker usage in areas of drug development and disease treatment and provide a standardized assessment of a biomarker's significance and biological interpretation. This is especially relevant for RCTs, where the protocol would prohibit the use of unauthenticated biomarkers to determine treatment regime, resulting in safer and more reliable treatment decisions (Food and Drug Administration 2006). Consequentially, identifying accurate and flexible analysis tools to assess biomarker importance is essential. In this chapter, we present a measure of variable importance based on a flexible semiparametric model as a standardized measure for biomarker importance. We estimate this measure with the TMLE.

Many biomarker discovery methods only measure the association between the marker and the biological outcome. However, a significant association is often difficult to interpret and does not guarantee that the biomarker will be a suitable and reliable drug candidate or diagnostic surrogate. This is especially true with genomic data, where genes are often present in multiple pathways and can be highly correlated amongst themselves. Applying association-based methods to these data will often lead to a long and ambiguous listing of biomarkers, which can be expensive to analyze.

Ideally, biomarker discovery analyses should identify markers that systematically affect the outcome through a biological pathway or mechanism, in other words, markers causally related to the outcome of interest. Once these markers are identified, they can be further analyzed and eventually applied as potential drug targets or prognostic markers. Due to the complex nature of the human genome, this is not a straightforward task, and certain assumptions are required to identify a causal effect.

In general, causal effects are often difficult if not impossible to estimate correctly, especially based on high-dimensional and highly correlated genomic data structures. The required identifiability assumptions such as the time-ordering assumption, the randomization assumption, and the positivity assumption are often only fully realized in RCTs, making their utility in a standard protocol limited. However, measures that are causally interpretable in RCTs can still be biologically interpretable based on observational data as measures of importance.

Here, we present the typical representation of a causal effect as a potential measure of importance for a biomarker A:

$$\Psi(P_0)(a) = E_0[E_0(Y \mid A = a, W) - E_0(Y \mid A = 0, W)].$$

Given the observed data structure $O = (W, A, Y) \sim P_0$, this measure corresponds to the effect of a biomarker (A) on the outcome (Y), adjusting for confounders (W). Here, A can represent a single biomarker or set of biomarkers. This chapter will focus on the univariate case. This measure can be estimated in semiparametric models for P_0, and with formal inference, using the TMLE.

In this chapter, we present the TMLE of the variable importance measure (VIM) above under a semiparametric regression model, which can accommodate continuous treatment or exposure variables often seen in biomarker analyses. We will primarily focus on its application to biomarker discovery. However, this method also has important applications to clinical trial data when the treatment is binary or continuous, and when one wishes to test for possible effect modification by baseline variables, for instance, treatment modified by biomarkers measured at baseline.

We demonstrate the efficacy and functionality of this VIM and its TMLE in a simulation study. The simulations provide a performance assessment of our estimated measure under increasing levels of correlation of A with W. We show the accuracy with which the TMLE of the VIM can detect "true" variables from amongst increasingly correlated "decoy" variables. Additionally, we also evaluate the accuracy of three commonly used methods for biomarker discovery under the same conditions: univariate linear regression, lasso regression (Efron et al. 2004), and random forest (Breiman 1999, 2001a). We also apply the method in an application to a leukemia data set (Golub et al. 1999).

22.1 Semiparametric-Model-Based Variable Importance

Previous chapters have focused on the TMLE of the above VIM in a nonparametric model for variables A that are discrete; for instance, A might be an indicator for receiving a particular treatment or exposure. However, particularly in the worlds of genomics and epidemiology, the variable of interest is often continuous. In this chapter, we present a semiparametric-regression-model-based measure of variable importance that is flexible enough to accommodate the typical data structures in genomics, epidemiology, and medical studies.

This VIM was proposed in van der Laan (2006) and estimated with the TMLE in van der Laan and Rubin (2006). These semiparametric regression models have been considered in Robins et al. (1992), Robins and Rotnitzky (2001), and Yu and van der Laan (2003). Under the semiparametric regression model, only the effect of A on the mean outcome of Y needs to be modeled with a parametric form, while the remainder of the conditional mean of the outcome Y remains unspecified. The semiparametric nature can accommodate both continuous and binary variables of interest as well as incorporate effect modification by W in a straightforward and interpretable manner.

We assume

$$E_0(Y \mid A, W) = m(A, V|\beta_0) + r(W),$$

for a specified parametric model $\{m(A, V \mid \beta) : \beta\}$ that satisfies $m(0, V \mid \beta) = 0$ for all β, and unspecified function $r(W)$. Here V is a user-supplied set of effect modifiers contained in the covariate vector W. This is equivalent to assuming $E_0(Y \mid A = a, W) - E_0(Y \mid A = 0, W) = m(a, V \mid \beta_0)$. For our purposes, we assume a linear form for $m(A, V \mid \beta_0)$, which puts this model in the class of partial linear regression models. Given this semiparametric form with user-supplied $m(.)$, the marginal variable importance of a particular A is defined generally as

$$\mu_0(a) = E_{W,0}(m(a, V \mid \beta_0)).$$

However, it is important to remember that the maximum likelihood estimator is developed under the assumption that $m()$ is correct.

Given an estimator β_n of β_0, an estimate of this parameter of interest at a particular $A = a$ is defined as

$$\mu_n(a) = \frac{1}{n}\sum_{i=1}^{n}(m(a, V_i \mid \beta_n)).$$

If we assume a linear model $m(A, V \mid \beta) = A\beta^{\top}V$, the variable importance can be represented as a linear curve at the level a for the biomarker given by $E_{W,0}(m(A = a, V \mid \beta_0)) = a\beta_0^{\top}E_0V$. Thus, given this linear model, the VIM is identified by a simple linear combination (i.e., $\beta_0^{\top}E_0V$), and formal statistical inference is obtained with a straightforward application of the delta method. Further details are provided in Tuglus and van der Laan (2008). Here, we focus on the simplest linear case $m(A, V \mid \beta) = A\beta$, where the marginal importance of A can be represented by single coefficient value β.

22.2 The TMLE

The data structure is $O = (W, A, Y) \sim P_0$ and the statistical model $\mathcal{M}$ consists of all probability distributions P for which $\bar{Q}(P)(A, W) = E_P(Y \mid A, W)$ is of the form $A\beta + E_P(Y \mid A = 0, W)$ for some β. The target parameter $\Psi : \mathcal{M} \to \mathbb{R}$ is defined as $\Psi(P) = \beta(P)$, the β-coefficient in front of A. This target parameter has an efficient influence curve at P that is given by $D^*(P)(O) = 1/\sigma^2(A, W)H^*(g(P))(A, W)(Y - \bar{Q}(P)(A, W))$, where

$$H^*(g(P))(A, W) = \frac{d}{d\beta}m(A, V \mid \beta) - \frac{E_P(\frac{d}{d\beta}m(A, V \mid \beta)/\sigma^2(A, W) \mid W)}{E_P(1/\sigma^2(A, W) \mid W)},$$

$g(P)(A \mid W) = P(A \mid W)$, and $\sigma^2(A, W)$ is the conditional variance of Y, given (A, W). It is of interest to note that σ^2 cancels out in the efficient influence curve *if* $\sigma^2(A, W) = \sigma^2(W)$ is only a function of W.

The TMLE requires selecting a loss function for $\bar{Q}$, $L(\bar{Q})$, and a submodel $\{\bar{Q}_g(\epsilon) : \epsilon\} \subset \mathcal{M}$ through $\bar{Q}$ at $\epsilon = 0$, so that the linear span of $d/d\epsilon\, L(\bar{Q}_g(\epsilon))$ at $\epsilon = 0$ includes this efficient influence curve $1/\sigma^2 H^*(g)(Y - \bar{Q}(A, W))$. We select the squared error loss function, $L(\bar{Q})(O) = (Y - \bar{Q}(A, W))^2/\sigma^2(A, W)$, and the univariate linear regression submodel, $\bar{Q}_g(\epsilon) = \bar{Q} + \epsilon H^*(g)$ with "clever covariate" $H^*(g)$. The TMLE is now defined as usual and the iterative TMLE algorithm converges in a single step.

For the sake of implementation, we restrict ourselves to the choice $\sigma^2 = 1$ (that is, we are estimating the nuisance parameter σ^2 with the trivial constant 1). For this choice $\sigma^2 = 1$, we have that the clever covariate $H^*(g) = (A - E_g(A \mid W))$ only depends on g through the conditional mean of A, given W. The consistency of the TMLE does not rely on σ^2 since the efficient influence curve is an unbiased estimating function in β for each choice of σ^2: the TMLE is consistent if either $\bar{Q}_0$ or g_0 is estimated consistently. However, as a consequence of not estimating σ^2, even if both $\bar{Q}_0$ and g_0 are consistently estimated, the TMLE will only be efficient if $\sigma_0^2(A, W)$ is only a function of W.

Implementation. In biomarker discovery analyses, one is interested in assessing the VIM for a whole collection of biomarkers. For each biomarker, one defines a corresponding adjustment set (e.g., all other biomarkers). We outline the TMLE implementation below for a single biomarker A and corresponding adjustment set W. There are three initial components necessary for applying TMLE to estimate the parameter of interest.

1. A model $m(A, V \mid \beta)$ satisfying $m(0, V \mid \beta) = 0$ for all β and V. In this case, it is defined as $m(A, V \mid \beta) = \beta A$.
2. An initial regression estimate of $\bar{Q}_0(A, W) = E_0(Y \mid A, W)$ of the form $\bar{Q}_n^0(A, W) = m(A, V \mid \beta_n^0) + r_n^0(W)$. The initial regression estimate of the

proper form may be obtained from semiparametric regression methods such as those of Hastie and Tibshirani (1990), among others, or by using methods like DSA, which allow the user to fix a portion of the regression model. However, we recommend a more flexible approach that allows one to use a wider range of data-adaptive software. This approach is outlined as follows. (i) Obtain an initial regression estimate of $\bar{Q}_0(A,W)$ of general form using data-adaptive machine learning algorithms such as the super learner, (ii) evaluate $r_n^0(W) = \bar{Q}_n^0(A=0,W)$, and (iii) determine the least squares regression estimate β_n^0 for the linear regression working model $\bar{Q}_n^0(A,W) = m(A,W \mid \beta) + \alpha\bar{Q}_n^0(A=0,W) + \text{error}$, treating $\bar{Q}_n^0(A=0,W)$ as a covariate, and α and β as unknown coefficients.
3. An estimate of the conditional mean $\bar{g}_0(W) = E_0(A \mid W)$.

Given the obtained initial estimator $\bar{Q}_n^0$ of the correct form, the TMLE is now obtained as follows:

1. Estimate the "clever covariate" that will allow us to update the initial regression in a direction that targets the parameter of interest. In this case, the clever covariate is defined as

$$H^*(A,W) = \frac{d}{d\beta}m(A,V \mid \beta) - E\left(\frac{d}{d\beta}m(A,V \mid \beta)|W\right),$$

which for this particular form $m(A,V \mid \beta) = \beta A$ simplifies to $H^*(\bar{g})(A,W) = A - \bar{g}(W)$, where $\bar{g}(W) = E_g(A \mid W)$. Let $\bar{g}_n$ be the estimator of the true conditonal mean $\bar{g}_0$ of A, given W.
2. Use least squares regression to regress the outcome Y onto the clever covariate $H^*(\bar{g}_n)(A,W)$ using $\bar{Q}_n^0(A,W)$ as offset, and define the resulting coefficient in front of the clever covariate as ϵ_n.
3. Update the initial estimate $\beta_n^1 = \beta_n^0 + \epsilon_n$, $r_n^1 = r_n^0 - \epsilon_n\bar{g}_n$, and thereby the corresponding regression $\bar{Q}_n^1(A,W) = \bar{Q}_n^0(A,W) + \epsilon_n H^*(\bar{g}_n)(A,W)$. Iteration of this updating procedure does not result in further updates of $\bar{Q}_n^1$. As a consequence, the TMLE of $\bar{Q}_0$ is given by $\bar{Q}_n^* = \bar{Q}_n^1$.

Statistical inference. The TMLE $\bar{Q}_n^* = (\beta_n^*, r_n^*)$ solves the estimating equation $0 = P_n D^*(\bar{Q}_n^*, \bar{g}_n)$, where $D^*(\bar{Q}_n^*, \bar{g}_n)(W,A,Y) = H^*(\bar{g}_n)(W,A)(Y - m(A,V \mid \beta_n^*) - r_n^*(W))$. We can represent the efficient influence curve $D^*(\bar{Q}_n^*, \bar{g}_n) = D(\beta_n^*, r_n^*, \bar{g}_n)$ as an estimating function for β. As a consequence, if one is willing to assume that $\bar{g}_n$ is consistent, then statistical inference can be based on the conservative influence curve $IC(O) = -c^{-1}D(\beta_0, r^*, \bar{g}_0)$ with scale factor $c = E_0\left(d/d\beta_0\, D(\beta_0, r^*, \bar{g}_0)\right)$, and r^* represents the possibly misspecified limit of r_n^*.

The asymptotic covariance of $\sqrt{n}(\beta_n^* - \beta_0)$ can be estimated with the empirical estimate of the covariance matrix of this influence curve: $\Sigma_n = \frac{1}{n}\sum_{i=1}^{n} IC_n(O_i)IC_n(O_i)^\top$. For the sake of statistical inference we can use as working model $\sqrt{n}(\beta_n^* - \beta_0) \sim N(0, \Sigma_n)$. For example, one may test the null hypothesis $H_0 : \beta_0(j) = 0$, using a standard test statistic $T_n = (\sqrt{n}\beta_n^*(j))/\sqrt{\Sigma_n(j,j)}$, which is asymptotically $N(0,1)$ under the null hypothesis. Similarly, a multiple testing methodology can be applied based on the influence curves of the biomarker-specific variable importance estimator across a large collection of biomarkers. Statistical inference can also be based on the bootstrap, but in high-dimensional biomarker analyses it is important to have a computational friendly method available as well.

22.3 Variable Importance Methods

In this section we compare TMLE to three other methods commonly used for determining variable importance in biomarker discovery analyses: univariate linear regression, lasso regression with cross-validation-based model selection (Efron et al. 2004) using R package lars (Efron and Hastie 2007), and random forest (Breiman 1999, 2001a) using R package randomForest (Liaw and Wiener 2002).

For each component of the covariate vector, using each of the methods, we assess the variable importance of this component, controlling for all other variables. For the univariate regression and TMLE methods that report p-values we may adjust for multiple testing using Benjamini–Hochberg step-up FDR-controlling procedure (Benjamini and Hochberg 1995) implemented with the mt.rawp2adjp() R function in package multtest (Ge and Dudoit 2002), and thereby classify the biomarkers as important or not accordingly. However, since the lasso method and random forest method do not allow for cutoffs based on valid p-values, we will focus on comparing the method-specific ranked lists, ranked by VIM or p-value when available.

Univariate linear regression (lm). Marginal variable importance is represented by the coefficient and p-value resulting from the univariate linear regression fit, $E_n(Y \mid A) = \beta_n A$. P-values are calculated using a standard t-test. This method does not account for any confounding and will often misclassify biomarkers correlated with the "true" biomarkers as significant.

Penalized regression (lasso). Marginal variable importance is represented by the coefficient of A in a lasso regression main term fit of $\bar{Q}_0(A, W_s) = E_0(Y \mid A, W_s)$, with $W_s \subset W$ representing the subset of W found significant according to their univariate regression on Y at p-value cutoff $\alpha = 0.05$. Lasso does not provide any formal statistical inference, therefore, p-values are not recorded. Lasso does attempt to account for confounding, but will only allow for main term linear regression fits with maximally $n-1$ nonzero coefficient values, making its applicability to high-dimensional data limited (Tibshirani 1996). Lasso is also a maximum likelihood method that focuses on estimating the overall regression $E_0(Y \mid A, W)$, and not the parameter of interest.

TMLE. The VIM is obtained by applying a TMLE to the initial regression estimator provided by the lasso fit of $\bar{Q}_0(A, W_s)$. We estimate $\bar{g}_0(W) = E_0(A \mid W)$ using lasso regression as well. P-values are calculated using a standard t-test.

Random forest (RF1, RF2). Random forest is a tree-based algorithm commonly used in biomarker discovery analyses, though it does not estimate the same measure as lm, lasso, or TMLE. Due to the nature of random forest, there is no guarantee that all biomarkers will receive a measure of importance. Also, as with lasso, no formal statistical inference is available. Two measures of importance, RF1 and RF2, are provided by the R function randomForest(), and we used the default setting with 500 trees. Random forest provides two measures of importance based on the perturbing effect the variable of interest has on overall classification error and node splits. The first, denoted RF1, is based on an"out-of-bag" error rate, and the second, RF2, is based on the accuracy of the node split (both with no p-values provided) (Breiman 1999, 2001a; Liaw and Wiener 2002).

22.4 Simulations

We simulate data to compare the four approaches for variable importance analysis under increasing correlation levels among the biomarkers, using a diagonal block correlation structure. The structure of the simulated data allows us to study the effects that both correlated and uncorrelated variables have on the reported importance of the true variables. For each approach, the biomarkers will be ranked by the resulting importance measure and p-value (when available). The sensitivity and specificity of methods will be compared based on both p-value and rank-based cutoff values, and will be summarized using ROC plots. We will also determine the ability of each approach to identify the true variables and each variables true importance rank by comparing the length of list required to label all true variables as "important."

The data structure is defined as $O = (W^*, Y) \sim P_0$, with a 100-dimensional covariate vector W^* and univariate outcome Y. The sample size is set at $n = 300$. The covariate vector W^* is simulated from a multivariate normal distribution with block diagonal correlation structure and mean vector created by randomly sampling mean values from $\{0.1, 0.2, ..., 9.9, 10.0, 10.1, ..., 50\}$, resulting in $K = 10$ independent clusters of 10 variables, each variable having unit variance, and any pair of variables within the cluster has correlation ρ_{TRUE}. The outcome Y is simulated from a main effect linear model using one variable from each of the K clusters. These K variables are designated as "true variables." The importance of a variable is determined by its coefficient value in the linear regression of Y. Two sets of values are used: a constant value $\{\beta_k = 4 : k = 1, ..., 10\}$ and an increasing set $\{\beta_k = k : k = 1, ..., 10\}$. A normal error with mean zero and variance σ_Y^2 is added as noise. Simulations are run for $\rho_{TRUE} = 0, 0.1, 0.2, 0.3, 0.4, 0.5, 0.6, 0.7, 0.8, 0.9$, and $\sigma_Y^2 = 10$, using both sets of coefficient values.

For each setting of $\{\rho, \sigma_Y\}$ we simulated 100 data sets of size $n = 300$. The recorded importance measures and p-values are translated into a list of ranks, and the ranks are averaged over the 100 iterations. A rank of one is the largest importance value or smallest p-value. Sensitivity and specificity calculations for each simulation are also determined for each simulated data set and averaged across the 100 simulated data sets to produce the final estimates. Simulation results are summarized here in terms of area under the curve (AUC) and length of list.

AUC. The overall performance of a ranked list is often summarized in terms of the AUC, the area under the curve derived from the basic ROC curve, which plots the true positive rate (sensitivity) by the false positive rate (1-specificity) as a function of the cutoff for the list.Under pure noise conditions the AUC= 0.5, indicating that at any threshold the false positive and true positive rates are equal (random classifier). The more convex the curve becomes, the higher the AUC, and the better the ranked list, and a perfect ranked list will have AUC = 1. The calculated AUC values are plotted vs. correlation for each of the five methods using importance measure importance rank and p-values when available for correlations, $\rho_{TRUE} \in \{0, 0.1, 0.2, 0.3, 0.4, 0.5, 0.6, 0.7, 0.8, 0.9\}$. From Fig. 22.1 we can see that

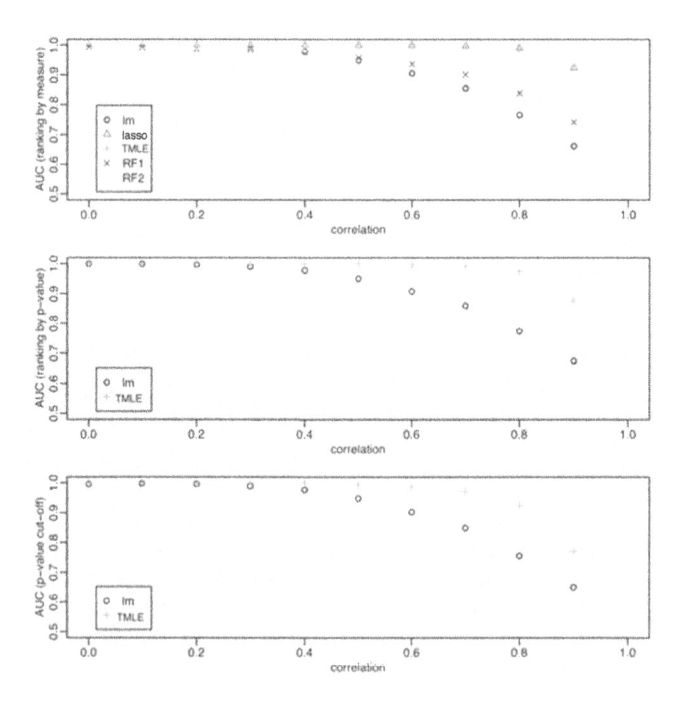

Fig. 22.1 AUC value from ROC curves by pairwise correlation $\rho = 0, ..., .9$, completed for ranking by measure (top), ranking by p-value (middle), and ranking by p-value using p-value cutoff, where $\sigma_Y = 10$, $n = 300$. Plots are shown for constant $\beta = 4$, but results are comparable when $\beta = \{1, ..., 10\}$

the TMLE performs well up to $\rho = 0.6$, performing only marginally better than lasso for $\rho > 0.2$, but with AUC visibly greater than random forest and lm as the correlation increases. As expected, lm is most susceptible to increases in correlation, performing perfectly when the correlation between biomarkers equals zero but failing consistently as the correlation increases, reaching below 0.8 by $\rho = 0.5$.

Average length of list. We can also compare the method-specific ranked lists of biomarkers based on the average cutoff for the list required to capture all "true" variables. Having a short cutoff allows the biologist to spend money analyzing the top genes with confidence, knowing that the most important genes are at the top of the list. The average required list length to find all ten "true" variables is plotted vs. correlation for all five measures and two p-value average ranked lists. These plots are shown for both constants $\beta_{true} = 4$ and $\beta_{true} = \{1 \ldots 10\}$. More detailed required length of lists for capturing the top k true variables, $k = 1, ..., 10$, for each available ranked list (rank by measure, rank by p-value) at each correlation level, as well as plots of the average rank and importance value, can be found in Tuglus and van der Laan (2008).

Length of list is a direct reflection of the type I error or false discovery rate associated with different cutoffs for the ranked lists of variables. Overall, the TMLE performs well up to correlations of 0.9, though the improvement over lasso is less clear when β_{TRUE} is constant (Figs. 22.2(a) and 22.2(b)). In the case where $\beta_{TRUE} = \{1, ..., 10\}$, (Figs.22. 2(c) and 22.2(d)), the improvement of TMLE over lasso is more pronounced, but detection of the first variable (with the lowest β value) is difficult for all methods. When ranking by measure or p-value, all methods have their lowest list length around 20 variables. In contrast, when β was constant at 4, the lowest list length was near its minimum at 10. The shift in list length is due to the importance value for the variable associated with $\beta = 1$. At such a high noise level ($\sigma_Y = 10$), the lower importance values are more difficult to distinguish from the noise. This is apparent by comparing the average importance rank and average importance value for the variable with $\beta = 1$ (Tuglus and van der Laan 2008). The rank is much higher than 10, but the value is close to one as it should be. In general, the TMLE has the shortest list and is less affected by increases in correlation between the biomarkers than any other methods.

Though TMLE performs better than the three other methods, it is still sensitive to more extreme correlations (0.7–0.9). Our simulations show a small increase in bias for the measure of the true variables at higher correlations (see Tuglus and van der Laan 2008). However, in practice, high correlation can adversely affect the TMLE estimate due to violation of the positivity assumption. The increased length of the variable list when ranked by importance measure at correlations 0.8 and 0.9 indicates that the TMLE cannot distinguish the true variable from among a group of variables when the correlation is very high. Positivity violations or strong pairwise correlations can often be avoided if the "problem" variables (the variables highly correlated with the biomarker of interest A) are removed from the set of confounders (W). One simple method is to apply a correlation cutoff, where all W whose corre-

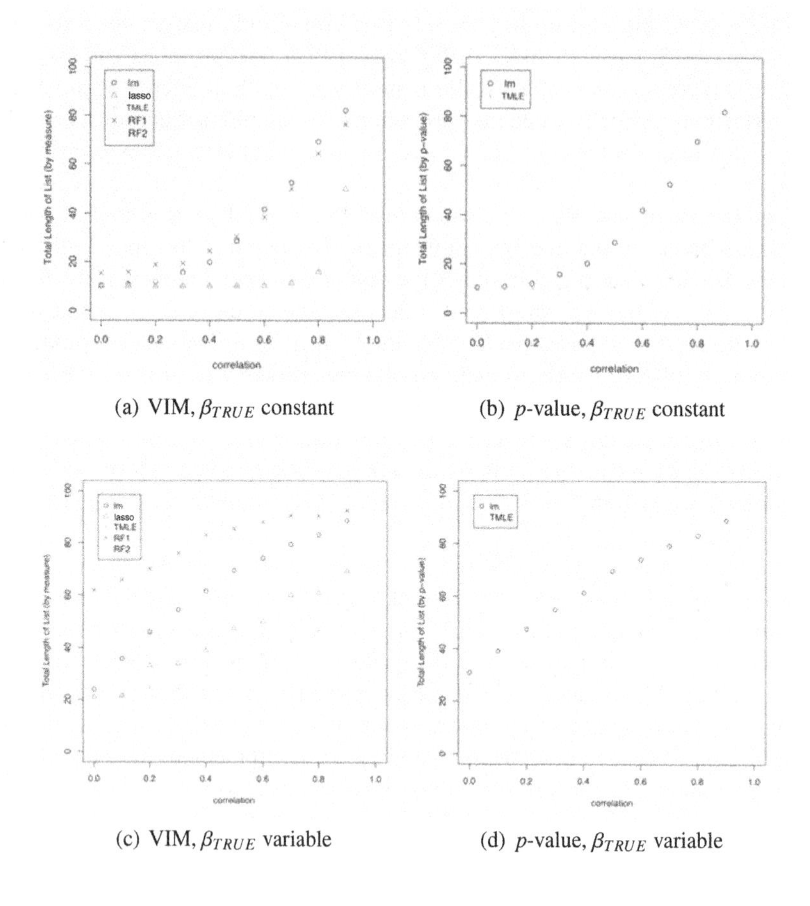

(a) VIM, β_{TRUE} constant (b) p-value, β_{TRUE} constant

(c) VIM, β_{TRUE} variable (d) p-value, β_{TRUE} variable

Fig. 22.2 Total length of list required to have all ten true variables in the list by $\rho = 0, ..., 0.9$ $\sigma_Y = 10$, $\beta_{TRUE} = 4$, (a) ranking by importance measure and (b) ranking by p-value. Then β_{TRUE} set at $\{1, ..., 10\}$ and plotted (c) ranking by importance measure and (d) ranking by p-value

lation with A is greater than a particular correlation (ρ_δ) are removed from the set of possible confounders for variable A prior to the application of the TMLE method.

The restriction of ρ_δ results in the algorithm's identifying all true variables as well as variables whose correlation with the true variables is higher than ρ_δ. Once we select ρ_δ, we are conceding that variables with correlations greater than ρ_δ cannot be teased apart to determine the true underlying (important) variable. By applying the correlation cutoff we are redefining our parameter. It is no longer the singular effect of A. Instead, we admit that, given the data, the true important variable cannot be targeted when the data are highly correlated and redefine our measure as a W_δ-adjusted importance where W_δ is a newly defined subset of W based on the correlation cutoff. Given this new definition of the parameter, important variables according to the W_δ-adjusted method include all important variables as well as all variables whose correlation to an important variable is greater than a particular delta cutoff.

In the next section, we apply the correlation cutoff ($\rho_\delta = \{0.5, 0.75\}$) to a leukemia application, where the truth is unknown and the data are noisy. In practice, it is reasonable to label all potentially relevant variables as important when their effects cannot be disentangled. Setting a correlation cutoff explicitly specifies and acknowledges the method's threshold to detect the important variables among highly correlated confounders. We recommend that future applications use a larger set of ρ_δ values and provide importance measures and rankings for all variables given each ρ_δ, or data-adaptively select ρ_δ using the methods outlined in Bembom et al. (2008).

22.5 Leukemia Data Application

Biomarker data are generally high-dimensional and highly correlated; therefore, certain prescreening is necessary prior to performing a biomarker analysis. We are primarily concerned with screening the potential covariate set W. Reducing this set to relevant biomarkers can not only decrease computation time but, also result in better estimates from data-adaptive algorithms.

We want to reduce this set of covariates to include only potential confounders. Potential confounders for a given A are any W that are related to both Y and A. However, it can be time consuming to screen the confounder set for every A separately. We recommend screening only in terms of the association of the biomarkers with Y. This can be accomplished by discounting any components of W that are not significantly associated with Y based on simple univariate or bivariate (e.g., including A) regression, or a combination of results from multiple methods (e.g., all variables significant according to at least one of the following methods: linear regression, random forest, or lasso).

The above screening can also serve to reduce the number of variables for which we estimate variable importance (i.e., variables A). Removing these variables presumes they have insignificant importance. If the data are reduced based on the outcome Y, this reduction must be accounted for in any subsequent multiple testing procedures. An easy way to accomplish this is, after estimating the importance measure and calculating the associated p-values for a subset of the full variable set, automatically assign all prescreened variables (i.e., variables with no estimate) a p-value of one. Then apply the Benjamini–Hochberg step-up FDR-controlling multiple testing procedure (Benjamini and Hochberg 1995) to the full set of p-values as usual. This two-stage FDR multiple testing procedure still controls the FDR, and, if the prescreening has only discounted variables that would have had p-values greater than the cutoff, the procedure will also retain the type II control of the Benjamini–Hochberg step-up FDR-controlling procedure. See Tuglus and van der Laan (2009) for more details on the reasoning behind and performance of this procedure.

The data set from Golub et al. (1999) has been used in many papers for methodological comparison due to its relevance, limited gene set, and biological interpretability. One goal in the original study was to identify differentially expressed genes in patients with acute lymphoblastic leukemia (ALL) and acute myeloid leukemia (AML). Gene expression levels were measured using Affymetrix oligonucleotide arrays with 6,817 human genes for $n = 38$ patients (27 ALL, 11 AML). The gene expression set was preprocessed and reduced to 3,051 genes according to methods described in Dudoit et al. (2002).

This analysis mirrors the procedure implemented in the previous simulations. We first apply univariate linear regression to all genes and control for multiple testing using Benjamini–Hochberg step-up FDR controlling procedure. This resulting set contains 876 genes. To minimize bias due to positivity violations, a simple correlation cutoff of $\rho_c = \{0.5, 0.75\}$ is applied.

As in the simulation, we model the importance as $m(A, V \mid \beta) = \beta A$ for all A. For the initial $\bar{Q}_n^0(A, W)$ and $\bar{g}_n(W_s)$ we use a polynomial spline fit. We recommend using a data-adaptive algorithm such as super learner over lars/lasso in application, since in reality the structure of $E_0(Y \mid A, W)$ and $E_0(A \mid W)$ may have more than just additive main effects.

In this application, the outcome is binary, ALL ($Y = 0$) vs. AML ($Y = 1$); therefore we can interpret $\beta_0 a$ as the excess risk $P_0(Y = 1 \mid A = a) - P_0(Y = 1 \mid A = 0)$. The TMLE update presented in this chapter uses a linear regression working model, thereby not respecting the known probability bounds. For the sake of discovery, this limitation might not be that important. However, it is of interest to develop VIMs and the corresponding TMLE specifically designed for binary and bounded continuous outcomes.

The TMLEs of the VIMs and corresponding p-values are recorded and adjusted for multiple testing using Benjamini–Hochberg step-up FDR-controlling procedure. We selected all genes with adjusted p-values less than or equal to 0.05 and then ranked the selected set of genes by their absolute importance measures. The same method is used to rank genes according to the univariate regression measures, and p-values. RF1 and RF2 importance measures are simply ranked.

Using a p-value cutoff of 0.05, TMLE results in 272 significant genes at $\rho_c = 0.5$ and 225 significant genes at $\rho_c = 0.75$, while univariate regression identifies 681 significant genes. It is difficult to determine which list is better, especially when the lists include hundreds of genes. In this analysis, we compare the top then of each list in an effort to compare their biological relevance. In any given list, we include the top ten genes of the particular method along with their ranks for all other methods. For many of the genes, these ranks vary greatly over the different methods. By consulting the literature, we hope to gain insight on the biologically validity of each list. The top ten genes according to their importance ranking for lm, RF1, RF2, and TMLE ($\rho_c = \{0.5, 0.75\}$) are shown in Tables 22.1–22.5.

Among the top ten genes according to the univariate regression results, CSTA, CD33, MYB, and ELA2 have all been associated with various types of cancer in the literature in previous quantitative analyses. CSTA has been proposed as a diagnostic and prognostic biomarker for cancer (Kos and Lah 1998). CD33 antigen has been shown in vitro to induce apoptosis in AML cells (Vitale et al. 2001). MYB is the homolog of an avian viral oncogene (Clappier et al. 2007), and ELA2 has been related to acute promyelocytic leukemia (Lane and Ley 2003).

Among the top 10 genes according to RF1 and RF2, all genes in RF1 were also in the top 10 for RF2, except CBX1 was replaced by CSTA in the list for RF1. CSTA was also in the top 10 of lm. Out of the top 10 the following genes have been associated with various cancers: TCF3, TOP2B, CCND3, and CSTA. Chromosomal abnormalities in TCF3 have been linked to T-cell and B-cell ALL (Hunger 1996). TOP2B is a current drug target having been linked to drug resistant cancers (Nebral et al. 2005; Kaufmann et al. 1998a). CCND3 is a cyclin D. In the absence of cyclin Ds, cells have shown increased resistance to oncogenic transformation in mouse models (Kozar et al. 2004).

There are marked differences and similarities between the TMLE-based results using a correlation cutoff of 0.5 and 0.75. There are five genes that are common between the two lists, four of which have some cancer-related association: TOP2B, CHRNA7, BCL3, and TCF7. Directional relationships remain consistent between the two lists, but the magnitudes shift due to the different covariate sets. TOP2B, a current drug target (Nebral et al. 2005; Kaufmann et al. 1998a), was also identified by random forest. BCL3 is a proto-oncogene biologically associated with B-cell ALL (Martin-Subero et al. 2007). TCF7 is a known biomarker for T-cell ALL, and is rarely expressed in AML cancer cells (Palomero et al. 2006). CHRNA7 was recently found to inform the role of nicotine in colon cancer (Wong et al. 2007). It is also important to note that CHRNA7 is highly correlated with CD33. Cancer-relevant genes found only in Table 22.4 ($\rho_c = 0.5$) are PTTG1IP, MCL1, PI3K, and CAMK2G. PTTG1IP has been consistently found overly expressed in human tumors (Ramaswamy et al. 2003; Puri et al. 2001; Fujii et al. 2006; Zhu et al. 2006). MCL1 is related to BCL2 and is a negative regulator of apoptosis (Kaufmann et al. 1998b). PI3K is activated by cellular agents known to stimulate B and T cells (Fruman et al. 1999). CAMK2G has an active role in cell growth control and has tumor-cell-specific variants (Tombes and Krystal 1997). Cancer-relevant genes found only in Table 22.5 ($\rho_c = 0.75$) are CAT and E2F4. CAT regulates BCL-2 and is often underexpressed in ALL tissues (Senturker et al. 1997; Komuro et al. 2005). E2F4 has an essential role in cell proliferation and cell fate decisions (Balciunaite et al. 2005) as well as activation of tumor suppressor proteins (Leone et al. 2001).

Using simple univariate linear regression, 681 genes were significant at the 0.05 level after adjusting for multiple testing. However, we know from general knowledge and our simulations that lm is highly sensitive to correlation among the variables, leading to large increases in type I error rate. Given this and a set of 681 genes, attempting to further analyze the lists to identify and biologically verify the relevant genes seems a nearly impossible and very expensive task. Attempting to control type I error by adding additional covariates requires model selection methods that are geared toward prediction.

Random forest is a prediction and classification method, and the importance measures it provides are difficult to interpret. Given an importance value of 0.612, the relationship between the variable and the outcome is unclear – is it highly expressed in AML or ALL? We only know that the variable is more "important" than a vari-

Table 22.1 Top ten ranked genes according to absolute importance measures among significant genes according to a p-value cutoff of 0.05 using lm

Gene name/symbol	Mapped IDs	**lm**	**lm** rankp	**TMLE** rankp (0.75)	**TMLE** rankp (0.5)	**RF1** rank	**RF2** rank
CST3	M27891	0.258	1	13	17	6	3
CSTA	D88422	0.341	2	521	466	12	8
Zyxin	X95735	0.345	3	287	534	2	2
Macmarcks	HG1612-HT1612	−0.619	4	1041	1768	9	9
CD33	M23197	0.517	5	906	28	26	22
C-MYB	U22376.cds2.s	−0.403	6	69	99	40	28
ELA2	M27783.s	0.334	7	104	1970	15	14
DF	M84526	0.262	8	175	145	96	149
P48	X74262	−0.431	9	291	266	57	31
LTC4S	U50136.rna1	0.725	10	146	2110	38	60

Table 22.2 Top ten ranked genes according to their importance measures using RF1

Gene name/symbol	Mapped IDs	**RF1**	**RF1** rank	**RF2** rank	**TMLE** rankp (0.75)	**TMLE** rankp (0.5)	**lm** rankp
FAH	M55150	0.953	1	1	588	234	52
Zyxin	X95735	0.823	2	2	287	534	3
TCF3	M31523	0.718	3	6	155	400	12
ADM	D14874	0.693	4	5	329	2136	57
PTX3	M31166	0.691	5	33	33	201	28
CST3	M27891	0.682	6	3	13	17	1
TOP2B	Z15115	0.654	7	4	1	2	33
CCND3	M92287	0.621	8	10	481	924	19
Macmarcks	HG1612-HT1612	0.613	9	9	1041	1768	4
APLP2	L09209.s	0.610	10	7	160	408	25

Table 22.3 Top ten ranked genes according to their importance measures using RF2

Gene name/symbol	Mapped IDs	**RF2**	**RF2** rank	**RF1** rank	**TMLE** rankp (0.75)	**TMLE** rankp (0.5)	**lm** rankp
FAH	M55150	0.426	1	1	588	234	52
Zyxin	X95735	0.282	2	2	287	534	3
CST3	M27891	0.218	3	6	13	17	1
TOP2B	Z15115	0.208	4	7	1	2	33
ADM	D14874	0.200	5	4	329	2136	57
TCF3	M31523	0.186	6	3	155	400	12
APLP2	L09209.s	0.183	7	10	160	408	25
CSTA	D88422	0.171	8	12	521	466	2
Macmarcks	HG1612-HT1612	0.164	9	9	1041	1768	4
CCND3	M92287	0.159	10	8	481	924	19

Table 22.4 Top ten ranked genes according to absolute importance measures among significant genes according to a p-value cutoff of 0.05 using TMLE with correlation cutoff $\rho_c = 0.5$

Gene name/symbol	Mapped IDs	TMLE	TMLE rankp (0.5)	TMLE rankp (0.75)	lm rankp	RF1 rank	RF2 rank
TOP2B	Z15115	−0.973	1	2	33	7	4
CHRNA7	X70297	0.839	2	1	48	69	61
corneodesmosin	L20815	0.338	3	3	1875	1846	2004
BCL3	U05681.s	0.314	4	4	477	558	821
KTN1	Z22551	−0.311	5	18	373	2967	118
CaM	U81554	0.272	6	81	367	476	749
TCF7	X59871	−0.159	7	6	569	635	887
PTTG1IP	Z50022	0.310	8	5	2753	2674	483
MCL1	L08246	0.293	9	2406	61	75	65
PI3K	Z46973	−0.172	10	113	734	772	1009

Table 22.5 Top ten ranked genes according to absolute importance measures among significant genes according to a p-value cutoff of 0.05 using TMLE with correlation cutoff $\rho_c = 0.75$

Gene name/symbol	Mapped IDs	TMLE	TMLE rankp (0.75)	TMLE rankp (0.5)	lm rankp	RF1 rank	RF2 rank
CHRNA7	X70297	1.260	1	2	48	69	61
TOP2B	Z15115	−0.946	2	1	33	7	4
corneodesmosin	L20815	0.327	3	3	1875	315	621
BCL3	U05681.s	0.181	4	4	477	316	622
Surface glycoprotein	Z50022	0.310	5	8	2753	317	474
TCF7	X59871	−0.175	6	7	569	318	623
CAT	X04085.rna1	0.163	7	21	92	56	59
E2F4	U18422	−0.256	8	42	1752	319	624
UGP2	U27460	−0.244	9	14	155	186	303
SELL	M15395	0.183	10	43	340	84	316

able with a value of 0.611. Also, out of the top ten lists for RF1 and RF2 (12 genes total), only four genes were found to be biologically associated with cancer, and only one specifically relating to ALL/AML distinction, TCF3. Why TCF3 is rated second for RF1 and sixth for RF2 is unclear. In comparison, lm found four related to cancer, two of which specifically related to AML/ALL.

The TMLE measure provides directionality and is less sensitive to increases in correlation (Sect. 22.3). Given an importance measure of −0.175, we can conclude that this particular gene is up-regulated in ALL patients when compared to AML patients. This particular measure is for TCF7 using a correlation cutoff of 0.75. TCF7 is rarely expressed in AML and often highly expressed in ALL patients (especially T-cell related). Out of the six cancer-related genes in the top ten list for 0.75 cutoff, three are biologically related to the AML/ALL distinction. When the cutoff is 0.5, there are eight cancer-related genes, three related to the AML/ALL distinction. For all three AML/ALL-related genes, the directionality of the relationship is biologically correct.

The TMLE results do have a greater number of cancer-related genes and a greater number of specifically AML/ALL-related genes. However, the increase over lm is small, and the comparison only includes the top ten genes. Further support for TMLE is gained from the previous simulations where we demonstrated its resistance to increases in correlation and its control of type I error, while still being an interpretable and meaningful measure of importance.

22.6 Discussion

Variable importance results vary widely, leading to long lists and confusion. In this chapter, we proposed using the statistical analogs of causal effects as VIMs and using TMLE to statistically assess these effect measures. In simulation, this proved resilient to increases in correlation while controlling the type I error. It also provides an interpretable and meaningful measure of importance, which, given an appropriate study design, is interpretable as a causal effect. In comparison, the commonly employed univariate linear regression is highly susceptible to increases in type I error due to increased correlation between the biomarkers. The utilization of machine learning algorithms, such as lasso/lars, to estimate these same target parameters is incomplete without the targeting carried out by the TMLE update, which removes bias and allows for statistical inference in terms of p-values, multiple testing, and confidence intervals.

Chapter 23
Finding Quantitative Trait Loci Genes

Hui Wang, Sherri Rose, Mark J. van der Laan

The goal of quantitative trait loci (QTL) mapping is to identify genes underlying an observed trait in the genome using genetic markers. In experimental organisms, the QTL mapping experiment usually involves crossing two inbred lines with substantial differences in a trait, and then scoring the trait in the segregating progeny. A series of markers along the genome is genotyped in the segregating progeny, and associations between the trait and the QTL can be evaluated using the marker information. Of primary interest are the positions and effect sizes of QTL genes.

Early literature (Sax 1923; Thoday 1960) focused on directly analyzing a single marker using analysis of variance (ANOVA). The biggest disadvantage of such marker-based analysis is its inability to assess QTL genes between markers. In 1989, Lander and Botstein proposed the interval mapping (IM) method (Lander and Botstein 1989). With IM, the genotypic value of a QTL follows a multinomial distribution, determined by the distance of the QTL to its flanking markers and the genotypes of the flanking markers. The trait value is modeled as a Gaussian mixture with the mixing proportions being the multinomial probabilities of the QTL genotype. The significance of the QTL effect is then assessed using likelihood ratio test. By testing positions at small increments along the genome, a whole-genome finely scaled test statistic profile can be constructed. IM has greatly increased the accuracy of estimating QTL parameters, and it has gained wide popularity in the genetic mapping community. Later, Haley and Knott developed a regression method to approximate IM (Haley and Knott 1992). This method imputes the unobserved genotypic value of a putative QTL with its expected value.

IM methods unrealistically assume there is only one gene underlying the observed trait in the entire genome, represented as testing each potential position separately (Lander and Botstein 1989) or computing the univariate association between the expected genotypic value and the phenotypic trait in Haley–Kott regression. In other words, IM only considers the current QTL; all other QTL genes are ignored. When this assumption is violated, the effects of other QTL genes are contained within the residual variance, affecting the assessment of QTL parameters.

To handle multiple QTL genes, Jansen (1993) and Zeng (1994) developed a composite interval mapping (CIM) approach. In CIM, background markers are added to a standard IM statistical model to reduce noise and increase the precision of QTL effect estimates. Thus, the CIM approach estimates QTL effects adjusted for confounding markers and can substantially improve the performance of IM when the background markers are properly chosen. Multiple interval mapping (MIM) was also developed to simultaneously estimate effects and positions of multiple QTL genes (Kao et al. 1999). MIM enjoys greater power but is computationally difficult. It also has a long-standing estimator selection problem: Which QTL genes are to be included? Bayesian approaches have also been studied and applied in QTL mapping (Satagopan et al. 1996; Heath 1997; Sillanpaa and Arjas 1998).

In recent years, with finely scaled single nucleotide polymorphism (SNP) markers replacing the traditional widely spaced microsatellite markers, identifying QTL genes between markers has become less concerning. Due to the high-dimensional nature of SNP data, the univariate marker-trait regression is widely used for its simplicity and computational feasibility despite its noisy results. Machine learning algorithms, such as random forests (Breiman 2001b), are also used to map QTL genes (Lee et al. 2008).

Most of these QTL methods are fully parametric and typically assume a Gaussian distribution for the phenotypic trait, as well as require specification of a parametric regression model. The estimation of QTL effects often relies on the method of maximum likelihood estimation. Maximum likelihood estimation based on such parametric regression models is widely used and well studied, with software available in many platforms. However, quite often, these parametric models represent an over-simplified description of the underlying genetic mechanism and leads to biased estimates. In addition, if the parametric model is data-adaptively selected among a set of candidate parametric regression models, then the reported standard errors and the p-values are not interpretable.

In this chapter, we address the QTL mapping problem through the use of a semiparametric regression model and the TMLE. The only assumption of the semiparametric regression model is that the phenotypic trait changes linearly with the QTL gene. We also define the C-TMLE, which is a particularly appealing estimator for the high-dimensional genomic data structures. Portions of this chapter were adapted from Wang et al. (2010).

23.1 Semiparametric Regression Model and TMLE

Suppose the observed data are i.i.d. realizations of $O_i = (Y_i, M_i) \sim P_0, i = 1, \ldots, n$, where Y represents the phenotypic trait value, M represents the marker genotypic values, and i indexes the ith subject. Let A be the genotypic value of the putative QTL under consideration. When A lies on a marker, A is observed. When A lies between markers, it is unobserved. In this case, we impute A with its expected value from a multinomial distribution computed from the genotypes and the relative locations of its flanking markers. This is the same strategy used in Haley–Knott regression (Haley and Knott 1992), and we will thus only be estimating the effect of an imputed A. The semiparametric regression model for the effect of A at value $A = a$ relative to $A = 0$, adjusted for a user-supplied set of other markers M^-, is given by

$$E_0(Y \mid A = a, M^-) - E_0(Y \mid A = 0, M^-) = \beta_0 a.$$

Other parametric forms, such as $a \sum_{j=1}^{J} \beta_j V_j$ incorporating effect modification by other markers V_j, can be incorporated as well. We view β_0 as our parameter of interest, which also corresponds with a marginal average effect obtained by averaging this conditional effect over the distribution of M^-.

The TMLE of β_0 was presented in the previous chapter and involves an initial machine learning (e.g., super learner) fit of $E_0(Y \mid M)$, which yields a fit of $E_0(Y \mid A = 0, M^-)$, mapping the latter into an initial estimator of β_0 and thereby of $E_0(Y \mid A, M^-)$ in the semiparametric regression model. After obtaining this initial estimator of $E_0(Y \mid A, M^-)$ of the semiparametric form as enforced by the semiparametric regression model, we carry out a single targeted update step by adding an estimate of the clever covariate $A - E_0(A \mid M^-)$, and fitting the coefficient ϵ in front of this clever covariate with univariate regression, using the initial estimator of $E_0(Y \mid A, M^-)$ as offset. Note that the TMLE of β_0 is now simply $\beta_n^0 + \epsilon_n$.

The estimation of the clever covariate requires an estimator of $E_0(A \mid M^-)$. The latter can be carried out with a machine learning algorithm regressing A on M^-. In particular, one could decide to fit this regression of the marker of interest on two flanking markers, thereby dramatically simplifying the estimation problem, while potentially capturing most of the confounding by the total marker set M^-. The choice of how great the distance between the flanking markers will be is a delicate issue. If one selects the flanking markers right next to the marker of interest, the data might not allow the separation of the effect of interest from the effect of the flanking markers. That is, one is aiming to adjust for confounders that are too predictive of the marker of interest. On the other hand, if one selects the flanking markers too far away from the marker of interest, the flanking markers will not adjust well for the markers that are in between the marker of interest and the flanking markers. Simulations in the previous chapter suggest that the TMLE shows no sign of deterioration for correlations smaller than 0.7 between the marker of interest and the confounders. This could be used to set the window width defined by the two flanking markers. Subject matter considerations, such as that the scientist would be satisfied with a claim that the targeted effect of the marker can be due to other markers in a window of a particular size, could also be used to set this window width of the flanking markers.

An alternative approach is to let the data decide what other markers to include in the model for $E_0(A \mid M^-)$. For that purpose, we can employ the C-TMLE (using a linear regression working model for fluctuation of initial estimator), first presented in Chap. 19 for estimation of an additive effect $E_0(E_0(Y \mid A = 1, W) - E_0(Y \mid A = 0, W))$ for the observed data structure $O = (W, A, Y)$ and nonparametric model for the probability distribution P_0 of O. This C-TMLE has also been implemented for this estimation problem, but, obviously, now in terms of TMLEs in this semiparametric regression model. Thus, this algorithm involves using forward selection of main terms to build a main term linear regression fit for $E_0(A \mid M^-)$, based on the sum of squared residuals (i.e., MSE) of the corresponding TMLE of $E_0(Y \mid A, M^-)$ that uses this main term regression fit of $E_0(A \mid M^-)$ in the clever covariate. Cross-validation is used to select the number of main terms (i.e., the number of forward selection steps that the algorithm carries out) that will actually be included in the fit of $E_0(A \mid M^-)$. The candidate main terms can include fits of $E_0(A \mid M^-)$ such as one based on two flanking markers defined by a choice of window width, across a number of possible window widths. In this manner the C-TMLE algorithm can data-adaptively decide how aggressive the targeting step should be in its effort to reduce bias due to residual confounding.

As in Chap. 19, the C-TMLE implementation may also involve the selection of a penalty to be added to the MSE in order to make the procedure more robust in the context of having to adjust for highly correlated markers: for details we refer to the technical report (Wang et al. 2011). C-TMLE allows one to data-adaptively determine the markers to include in the fit of $E_0(A \mid W)$. For example, one may wish to only adjust for the two closest markers that are farther than δ-apart from the marker A, and one can use C-TMLE to data-adaptively select this choice δ based on the log-likelihood of the TMLE of the semiparametric regression fit. In our simulations and data analysis we have implemented both TMLEs as well as C-TMLEs.

23.2 The C-TMLE

Let $Q_n^0 = m(A, V \mid \beta_n^0) + r(M^-)$ be the initial estimate of Q_0 contained in the same semiparametric regression model that we also used in the TMLE. The C-TMLE is concerned with iteratively updating this initial estimate of Q_0. Firstly, we compute a set of K univariate covariates $W_1, \ldots, W_K$ from M^-, which we will refer to as main terms, even though a term could be an interaction term or a super learning fit of the regression of A on a subset of the components of M^-. Let's refer to M^- by $W = (W_1, \ldots, W_K)$. In this subsection we will suppress in the notation for estimates of Q_0 and g_0 their dependence on the sample size n. Let $\Omega = \{W_1, \ldots, W_K\}$ be the full collection of main terms. A linear regression model fit g^K of $g_0(W) = E_0(A \mid W)$ using all main terms in Ω is viewed as the most nonparametric estimate of g_0. For a given subset of main terms $\mathcal{S} \subset \Omega$, let $\mathcal{S}^c$ be its complement within Ω. For a given subset $\mathcal{S}^k$, we will define g^k as the least squares fit of the linear regression model for $E_0(A \mid W)$ that includes as main terms all the terms in $\mathcal{S}^k$. In the C-TMLE algorithm we use a forward selection algorithm that augments a given set $\mathcal{S}^k$ into a next set $\mathcal{S}^{k+1}$ obtained by adding the best main term among all main terms in the complement $\mathcal{S}^{k,c}$ of $\mathcal{S}^k$. In other words, the algorithm iteratively updates a current estimate g^k into a new estimate g^{k+1}, but the criterion for g does not measure how well g fits g_0; it measures how well the TMLE using this g fits Q_0.

Let $L(Q)(O) = (Y - Q(A, W))^2$ be the squared error loss function for the true regression function $Q_0 = E_0(Y \mid A, W) = \beta_0 A + E_0(Y \mid A = 0, W)$. For a given initial estimate Q, let $Q_g(\epsilon) = Q + \epsilon(A - g(W))$ be the parametric working fluctuation model used in the TMLE of Q_0 defined in the previous section. For a given estimate g of g_0 and initial Q of Q_0, the corresponding TMLE (as defined in the previous section) of Q_0 is given by $Q_g(\epsilon_n)$, where $\epsilon_n = \arg\min_\epsilon P_n L(Q_g(\epsilon))$ is the univariate least squares estimator of ϵ using the initial estimate Q as offset, and P_n denotes the empirical probability distribution of $O_1, \ldots, O_n$. Here we used the notation $Pf \equiv \int f(o)dP(o)$. That is, an initial estimate Q, an estimate g, and the data $O_1, \ldots, O_n$ are mapped into a new targeted maximum likelihood estimate $Q^* = Q_g(\epsilon_n)$. Let's refer to this mapping as $Q^* = \text{TMLE}(Q, g)$, suppressing its dependence on P_n.

The C-TMLE algorithm defined below generates a sequence $(Q^k, \mathcal{S}^k)$ and corresponding TMLEs Q^{k*}, $k = 0, \ldots, K$, where Q^k represents an initial estimate, $\mathcal{S}^k$ a subset of main terms that defines g^k, and Q^{k*} the corresponding TMLE that updates Q^k using g^k. These TMLEs Q^{k*} represent subsequent updates of the initial estimator Q_n^0, and the corresponding main term set $\mathcal{S}^k$, as used to define g^k in this k-specific TMLE, increases in k, one unit at a time: $\mathcal{S}^0$ is empty, $\mid \mathcal{S}^{k+1} \mid = \mid \mathcal{S}^k \mid +1$, $\mathcal{S}^K = \Omega$. The C-TMLE uses cross-validation to select k, and thereby to select the TMLE Q^{k*} that yields the best fit of Q_0 among the $K + 1$ k-specific TMLEs that are increasingly aggressive in their bias-reduction effort. This C-TMLE algorithm is defined as follows:

Initiate algorithm: Set initial TMLE. Let $k = 0$. $Q^k = Q_n^0$ is the initial estimate of Q_0, and $\mathcal{S}^k$ is the empty set so that g^k is the empirical mean of A. Thus, Q^{k*} is the TMLE updating this initial estimate Q^k using as clever covariate $A - g^k$.

Determine next TMLE. Determine the next best main term to add to the linear regression working model for $g_0(W) = E_0(A \mid W)$:

$$\mathcal{S}^{k+1,cand} = \arg \min_{\mathcal{S}^k \cup W_j : W_j \in \mathcal{S}^{k,c}} P_n L(\text{TMLE}(Q^k, \mathcal{S}^k \cup W_j)).$$

If

$$P_n L(\text{TMLE}(Q^k, \mathcal{S}^{k+1,cand})) \leq P_n L(\text{TMLE}(Q^{k*})),$$

then $(\mathcal{S}^{k+1} = \mathcal{S}^{k+1,cand}, Q^{k+1} = Q^k)$, else $Q^{k+1} = Q^{k*}$, and

$$\mathcal{S}^{k+1} = \arg \min_{\mathcal{S}^k \cup W_j : W_j \in \mathcal{S}^{k,c}} P_n L(\text{TMLE}(Q^{k*}, \mathcal{S}^k \cup W_j)).$$

[In words: If the next best main term added to the fit of $E_0(A \mid W)$ yields a TMLE of $E_0(Y \mid A, W)$ that improves upon the previous TMLE Q^{k*}, then we accept this best main term, and we have our next TMLE Q^{k+1*}, g^{k+1} (which still uses the same initial estimate as Q^{k*} uses). Otherwise, reject this best main term, update the initial estimate in the candidate TMLEs to the previous TMLE Q^{k*} of $E_0(Y \mid A, W)$, and determine the best main term to add again. This best main term will now always result in an improved fit of the corresponding TMLE of Q_0, so that we now have our next TMLE Q^{k+1*}, g^{k+1} (which now uses a different initial estimate than Q^{k*} used).]

Iterate. Run this from $k = 1$ to K at which point $\mathcal{S}^K = \Omega$. This yields a sequence (Q^k, g^k) and corresponding TMLE Q^{k*}, $k = 0, \ldots, K$.

This sequence of candidate TMLEs Q^{k*} of Q_0 has the following property: the estimates g^k are increasingly nonparametric in k and $P_n L(Q^{k*})$ is decreasing in k, $k = 0, \ldots, K$. It remains to select k. For that purpose we use V-fold cross-validation. That is, for each of the V splits of the sample in a training and validation sample, we apply the above algorithm for generating a sequence of candidate estimates $(Q^{k*} : k)$ to a training sample, and we evaluate the empirical mean of the loss function at the resulting Q^{k*} over the validation sample, for each $k = 0, \ldots, K$. For each k we take the average over the V-splits of the k-specific performance measure over the validation sample, which is called the cross-validated risk of the k-specific TMLE. We select the k that has the best cross-validated risk, which we denote with k_n. Our final C-TMLE of Q_0 is now defined as Q^{k_n*}, and the corresponding updated regression coefficient is our TMLE β_n^* of β_0.

Remark. The candidate main terms can also include fits of $E_0(A \mid M^-)$ such as one based on two flanking markers defined by a choice of window width, across a number of possible window widths. In this manner, the above C-TMLE algorithm data-adaptively decides which window width yields effective bias reduction. C-TMLE implementation in the following data analysis involved a penalized mean squared error as a measure of fit instead of the mean squared error, where the penalty is defined as a variance estimator of the corresponding TMLE of β_0.

Statistical Properties of the C-TMLE

To understand the appeal of the C-TMLE, we make the following remarks. Including a main term in the fit of the clever covariate that has no effect on the outcome will only harm the TMLE of β_0 both with respect to bias and mean squared error. If one uses the log-likelihood (i.e., MSE) of the regression of A on M^- as a criterion for selection of the main terms, then one will easily select main terms that have a weak effect on the outcome, while truly important main terms are not included. Therefore, it is crucial to use a main term selection criterion for $E_0(A \mid M^-)$ that actually measures the fit of the resulting TMLE of the outcome regression. In addition, one can formally prove that the TMLE achieves the full bias reduction with respect to β_0 if the clever covariate uses a true regression, $E_0(A \mid M^s)$, with M^s being a reduction of M^- that is rich enough so that $E_0(Y \mid A = 0, M^-)$ is captured. In fact, the result is stronger, since M^s only needs to capture the function of M^- that is obtained by taking the difference between the true $E_0(Y \mid A = 0, M^-)$ and its initial estimator $E_n(Y \mid A = 0, M^-)$ (van der Laan and Gruber 2010). Thus, theory indeed fully supports that we should be selecting main terms in the clever covariate that are predictive of residual bias of the initial estimator of $E_0(Y \mid A = 0, M^-)$, and the C-TMLE algorithm presented above indeed targets such main terms.

23.3 Simulation

A single chromosome of 100 markers was simulated on 600 backcross subjects. Markers were evenly spaced at 2 centimorgan (cM). A single QTL main effect was generated at marker position 100 cM, denoted by $M_{(100)}$. Here, the number in the subscript of M indicates the position of the marker. There were also four epistatic effects on markers $M_{(60)}$, $M_{(90)}$, $M_{(120)}$, and $M_{(150)}$. Phenotypic values were generated from the data-generating distribution: $Y = 5 + 1.2M_{(100)} - 0.8M_{(60)}M_{(90)} - 0.8M_{(90)}M_{(120)} - 0.8M_{(120)}M_{(150)} - 0.8M_{(150)}M_{(60)} + U$, where U is the error term drawn from an exponential distribution scaled to have a variance of 10. We generated 500 simulated data sets of this type.

In this simulation, the density of markers is fairly high, the phenotypic outcome follows a nonnormal distribution, and there are strong counteracting epistatic effects in linked markers. A univariate regression effect estimate of the effect of, for example, $M_{(100)}$ will be biased due to the lack of adjustment for the effect of the highly correlated markers. Indeed, the CIM estimate for the effect of $M_{(100)}$ is negative, far away from the true value 1.2. On the other hand, taking the CIM prediction function as the initial estimator $\bar{Q}_n^{(0)}$, TMLE was then able to recover some of the signal and hence improved on the CIM estimates. In TMLE, the true regression of A on the other 99 markers, M^-, was estimated with a main terms linear regression including two flanking markers with a prespecified distance to A. We used two distances, 20 cM and 40 cM, and denote the estimators by $\text{TMLE}_{(20)}$ and $\text{TMLE}_{(40)}$. The CIM analysis was carried out using QTL Cartographer (Basten et al. 2001), with default settings. We analyzed markers without considering positions between them. For CIM, the mean effect estimate for $M_{(100)}$ is −0.2731 and is dominated by the epistatic effects from its nearby markers. $\text{TMLE}_{(40)}$ is able to correct some of the bias, and its effect estimate is 0.5365. $\text{TMLE}_{(20)}$ utilizes an estimator of $E_0(A \mid M^-)$ with more predictive power than $\text{TMLE}_{(40)}$ and produced an estimate closest to the truth. We list the averages of the effect estimates for $M_{(100)}$ across 500 simulations in Table 23.1 along with their standard errors for CIM, $\text{TMLE}_{(20)}$, and $\text{TMLE}_{(40)}$.

We also used a univariate regression (UR) fit for $\bar{Q}_n^{(0)}$ within TMLE, and these results can be found in Table 23.1. The UR initial estimate was even more biased than that of CIM. $\text{TMLE}_{(20)}$, using UR as $\bar{Q}_n^{(0)}$, produced very similar estimates to $\text{TMLE}_{(20)}$ using CIM as initial estimator. On the other hand, $\text{TMLE}_{(40)}$ using the CIM as initial estimator produced a better estimator than $\text{TMLE}_{(40)}$ using the

Table 23.1 Mean effect estimates of $M_{(100)}$ over 500 simulations

	$\bar{Q}_n^{(0)}$=CIM		$\bar{Q}_n^{(0)}$=UR	
	Estimate	SE	Estimate	SE
Initial Estimate	−0.2731	0.3273	−0.6248	0.2684
$\text{TMLE}_{(40)}$	0.5365	0.4538	0.2705	0.3135
$\text{TMLE}_{(20)}$	0.8478	0.4508	0.8093	0.4079

univariate regression as initial estimator. This demonstrates the robustness of TMLE with respect to misspecification of the initial estimator, which predicts that the more predictive the regression of A on M^-, the more robust TMLE will be to the choice of its initial estimator. A closer look at Table 23.1 also reveals that compared to $\text{TMLE}_{(40)}$, the additional bias reduction of $\text{TMLE}_{(20)}$, using univariate regression as initial estimator, comes with an increase in standard error.

23.4 Wound-Healing Application

In this section, we analyze a data set published in Masinde et al. (2001). The original study was designed to identify QTL genes involved in the wound-healing process. A genomewide scan of 119 codominant markers was performed using 633 F2 (MRL/MP x SJL/J) mice. Each mouse was punctured with a 2-mm hole in its ear, and the phenotypic trait was the hole closure measurement at day 21. The marginal distribution of the phenotypic trait is bell-shaped.

We analyzed this data set with TMLE (results not shown; see Wang et al. 2011), C-TMLE, and CIM. Based on the evaluation of a discrete super learner (Chap. 3) that included both DSA and random forests, the DSA machine learning algorithm was selected as initial estimator of $E_0(Y \mid M)$, and subsequently mapped into the desired initial estimator for $E_0(Y \mid A, M^-)$ satisfying the semiparametric regression model. To lessen the computational load, we first screened additive and dominant effects of all markers with univariate regression and supplied to this machine learning algorithm the markers with a p-value less than 0.10. In the TMLE, the conditional mean of A, given M^- is fitted with a main terms linear regression model with main

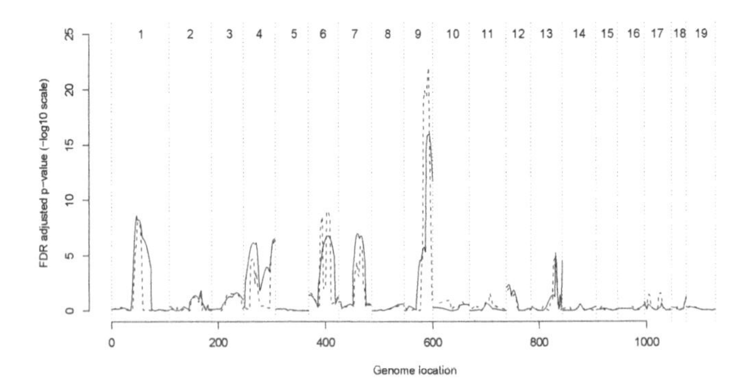

Fig. 23.1 —The genomewide FDR-adjusted p-value profile for the additive effects in the wound-healing data set. The *solid line* represents CIM, and the *dashed line* represents C-TMLE. Chromosome numbers are superimposed on top of the picture

terms A_c, W_1^a, W_1^d, W_2^a, W_2^d, where A_c denotes the dominant effect of A when A is additive and the additive effect of A when A is dominant, W_1 and W_2 are the closest flanking markers 20 cM away from A, and the superscript a denotes the additive effect and d the dominant effect.

Four hundred putative QTL positions were tested at 2-cM increments for both the additive and dominant effects. The p-values were adjusted using FDR. The TMLE and C-TMLE produced similar results, and we only present C-TMLE results in this chapter. Figure 23.1 displays the genomewide FDR-adjusted p-value profile for the additive effect at each tested position. The CIM p-values were computed from the asymptotic χ^2 distribution. No significant dominant effect was detected in this data set. The (C)-TMLE essentially identified the same QTL genes as CIM, albeit with an improved resolution. Many of these genes were also reported in Masinde et al. (2001). However, on chromosome 6, the (C-)TMLE suggests two linked QTL genes instead of one, as indicated by CIM.

23.5 Listeria Application

Boyartchuk et al. (2001) published a data set on the survival time of 116 age-matched female mice following infection with *Listeria monocytogenes*, a Gram-positive bacteria causing a wide range of diseases. The mice were an F2 intercross population derived from susceptible BALB/cByJ and resistant C57BL/6ByJ strains, and the goal of the study was to map genetic factors of susceptibility to *L. monocytogenes*. The phenotypic trait is the recorded time to death for each mouse upon infection with *L. monocytogenes*. One hundred and thirty-one codominant markers were genotyped on the autosomal chromosomes. When a mouse survived beyond 240 h, it was considered recovered. About 30% of the mice recovered, and we refer to them as survivors and the remaining mice as nonsurvivors. This creates a spike in the phenotypic trait distribution, violating the normality assumption in traditional approaches of QTL mapping.

The outcome Y was defined as the logarithm of the phenotypic trait. The first step of TMLE is to obtain an initial estimator of $E_0(Y \mid M)$, which can then be mapped into an initial estimator of $E_0(Y \mid A, M^-)$, satisfying the semiparametric regression model. Y can be decomposed into a binary trait of survival or nonsurvival and a continuous trait of survival time among nonsurvivors (Broman 2003). We denote this binary trait of survival by $Z = I(Y = \log 264)$. Then, the expected value of Y given the marker data M can be represented as

$$E_0(Y \mid M) = P_0(Z = 1 \mid M) \log 264 + P_0(Z = 0 \mid M) E_0(Y \mid Z = 0, M).$$

In the above formula, $P_0(Z = 1 \mid M)$ and $P_0(Z = 0 \mid M)$ are conditional probabilities of whether a mouse has survived ($Z = 1$) or died ($Z = 0$) given the marker data M. We fit this with a super learning algorithm for binary outcomes. $E_0(Y \mid Z = 0, M)$ is the conditional expectation of Y on M given that the mouse has died, which can

Table 23.2 Mean risk of candidate initial regressions in discrete super learner from the Listeria data set

	DSA	RF	SL	2-part SL
CV risk	0.2212	0.1581	0.1589	0.1463

be obtained by applying super learning on nonsurvivors. We refer to this machine learning algorithm as the 2-part super learner.

The collection of algorithms in the super learner included DSA and random forests. As before, the machine learning algorithms were only provided the additive and dominant markers that had a significant univariate effect based on a p-value threshold of 0.10. Since we wished to evaluate if this 2-part super learner provided a better fit than a regular super learner, we implemented a discrete super learner whose library consisted of a total of four algorithms for estimation of $E_0(Y \mid M)$: DSA, random forests, super learner, and a 2-part super learner. In Table 23.2, we report the honest cross-validated risk of DSA, random forests, super learner, and the 2-part super learner. In the super learning fits, more than 95% of the weight was put on random forests, thereby strongly favoring a fit that allows for complex interactions.

The 2-part super learner had the smallest honest cross-validated risk and was therefore selected as the estimator of $E_0(Y \mid M)$. In the TMLE, we fitted the conditional mean of A, given M^-, with a main term linear regression model including the main terms used A_c, W_1^a, W_1^d, W_2^a, W_2^d, where A_c denotes the dominant effect of A when A is additive and the additive effect of A when A is dominant, W_1 and W_2 are the closest flanking markers 20 cM away from A, and the superscript a denotes the additive effect and d the dominant effect.

When inspecting Fig. 23.2, TMLE displays much less noise than the parametric CIM. Three additive genes on chromosomes 1, 5, and 13 are clearly identified. Two additive effects on chromosomes 15 and 18 are borderline significant. In addition, TMLE also detected dominant effects on chromosomes 12, 13, and 15. The chromosome 15 QTL gene is identified as carrying both the additive and dominant effects. The literature suggests that the chromosome 1 QTL gene has an effect on how long a mouse can live given it will eventually die, the chromosome 5 gene has an effect on a mouse's chance of survival, and the genes on chromosomes 13 and 15 are involved in both (Boyartchuk et al. 2001; Broman 2003; Jin et al. 2007). We detected all of these genes and, in addition, an additive gene on chromosome 18 and a dominant gene on chromosome 12. CIM also identified those major genes, however, with less significance and many more suspicious positives. See Table 23.3. This data analysis was first published in Wang et al. (2010).

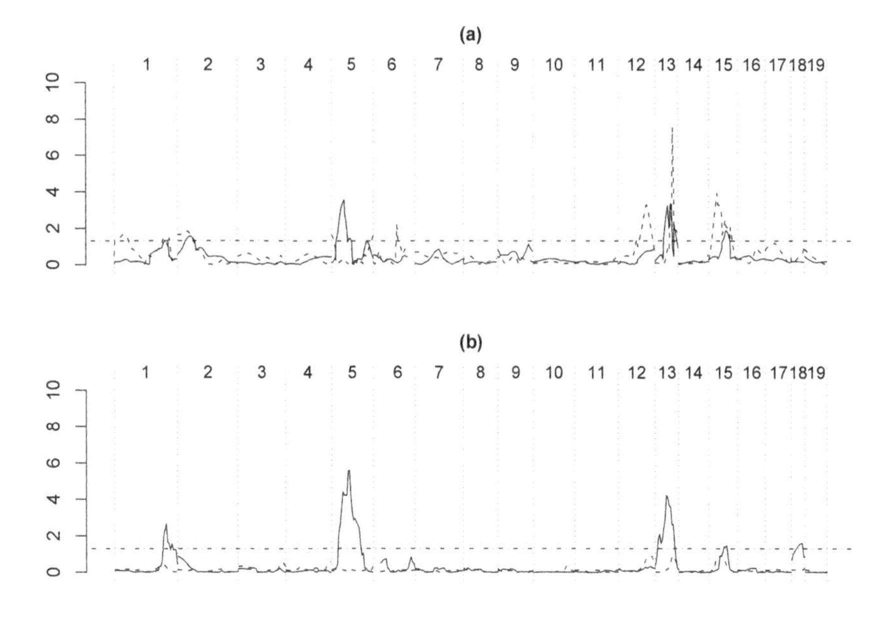

Fig. 23.2 The genomewide p-value profile for the additive and dominant effects in the Listeria data set. The p-values are FDR adjusted and on a negative log10 scale. (a) p-value profile from the CIM. (b) p-value profile from TMLE. In both panels, the *solid line* represents additive effects, and the *dashed line* represents dominant effect. The *dash-dot* line indicates the 0.05 p-value threshold. Chromosome numbers are superimposed on top of each panel

Table 23.3 The estimates of effect sizes and positions of QTL genes from CIM and TMLE in Listeria data set. QTL genes with FDR-adjusted p-values smaller than 0.05 are reported

		CIM			C-TMLE		
QTL ID	Type	Chr	cM	Effect size	Chr	cM	Effect size
1	dom	1	15.0	−0.2351	–	–	–
2	dom	1	72.8	0.1606	–	–	–
3	add	1	78.8	−0.1349	1	78.1	−0.1074
4	dom	2	14.0	−0.2623	–	–	–
5	add	2	18.0	−0.1744	–	–	–
6	dom	5	0.0	−0.1468	–	–	–
7	dom	5	61.0	−0.1693	–	–	–
8	add	5	18.1	0.2764	5	26.1	0.1960
9	dom	6	33.8	−0.1235	–	–	–
10	dom	12	41.8	−0.2352	12	40.1	−0.1372
11	add	13	22.7	−0.3409	13	14.4	−0.1668
12	dom	13	25.9	0.3525	13	26.4	0.1458
13	add	15	25.1	0.1540	15	22.1	0.0678
14	dom	15	12.0	0.2042	15	22.1	0.1438
15	add	18	–	–	18	14.1	−0.0692

23.6 Discussion

Current practice for assessing the effects of genes on a phenotype involves the utilization of parametric regression models. One of the advantages of parametric regression models is that they also provide a p-value, allowing one to rank the different estimated effects and assess their significance. However, both the effect estimates as well as the reported statistical significance are subject to bias due to model misspecification. On the other hand, machine learning algorithms such as random forests, are not sufficient when used alone since these algorithms are tailored for prediction, report generally poor effect estimates, and do not provide a measure of significance. TMLE allows us to incorporate the state of the art in machine learning, without significant computational burden (the targeting step is relatively trivial, although it needs to be carried out for each effect), while still providing an estimate tailored for the effect of interest and CLT-based statistical inference.

Part VIII
Longitudinal Data Structures

Chapter 24
Case Study: Longitudinal HIV Cohort Data

Maya L. Petersen, Mark J. van der Laan

In this chapter, we introduce a case study based on the treatment of HIV infection. A series of scientific questions concerning how best to detect and manage antiretroviral treatment failure in resource-limited settings are used to illustrate the general road map for targeted learning. We emphasize the translation of background knowledge into a formal causal and statistical model and the translation of scientific questions into target causal parameters and corresponding statistical parameters of the distribution of the observed data. Readers may be interested in first reading the longitudinal sections of Appendix A for a rigorous treatment of longitudinal TMLE and related topics.

HIV is a virus that damages the human immune system, resulting in a decline in CD4+ T lymphocytes and increased susceptibility to opportunistic infections. Antiretroviral drugs used in combination can suppress HIV replication to the point that HIV becomes undetectable in the blood stream, allowing CD4+ T-cell counts and immunologic function to recover. Unfortunately, HIV may develop resistance to the initial combination antiretroviral regimen used, allowing viral replication to rebound despite ongoing treatment. Failure to modify antiretroviral regimens once resistance and viral failure have occurred results in the evolution of additional resistance mutations and can compromise future treatment options. Delayed modification can also increase morbidity and mortality as a result of both CD4+ T cell depletion and inflammation-associated immune damage (Petersen et al. 2008; Rodger et al. 2009). In order to prevent these complications, the standard of care in resource-rich settings is to measure plasma HIV RNA levels (viral loads) regularly and modify a patient's antiretroviral regimen as soon as viral failure is detected (Hammer et al. 2008).

The majority of HIV-infected individuals, however, live in settings where resource and infrastructure limitations currently preclude regular viral load monitoring (Stringer et al. 2006). As a result, patients in much of the world may remain for extended periods on regimens that permit ongoing viral replication at detectable levels. The consequences of this limited monitoring capacity and resulting delays in regimen modification remain incompletely understood. Further, less resource-intensive modes of effectively detecting treatment failure remain to be identified. With this motivation, this chapter focuses on the following public health questions: What impact does delayed regimen modification following emergence of resistance have on long-term mortality? To what extent will use of less resource-intensive modification strategies, such as those based on CD4+ T cell measurements rather than viral loads, result in worse patient outcomes? How can CD4+ T cell measurements best be used to guide regimen modification? We illustrate how these questions can be approached using a formal causal inference framework and answers estimated using data drawn from observational HIV cohorts.

24.1 Data

Let baseline time $t = 0$ denote time of failing first-line antiretroviral therapy, where first-line therapy is defined as a combination antiretroviral (cART) regimen containing two nucleoside reverse transcriptase inhibitors (NRTIs) and one nonnucleoside reverse transcriptase inhibitor (NNRTI), and failure is defined as the second of two consecutive plasma HIV RNA levels greater than 500 copies/ml, measured at least 6 months after starting cART. We use a discrete time scale, with $t = 0, ..., \tau$. For simplicity, we refer to the time scale as days for the remainder of the chapter; however, time increments could also represent months, quarters, or longer intervals. The appropriate time scale will depend on the frequency with which treatment decisions and measurements are made. The target population is defined as adults who are antiretroviral-naive prior to initiating cART and who fail first-line cART a minimum of τ days prior to the calendar date at which the database is administratively closed.

We consider two types of treatment variables; $A_1(t)$ is defined as an indicator that jumps to zero if a subject interrupts first-line therapy, and $A_2(t)$ is defined as an indicator that jumps to zero if a subject modifies first-line therapy (or in other words, starts second-line therapy). Modification is defined as initiation of a protease inhibitor drug plus two new NRTIs. Interruption is defined as stopping all drugs for at least 2 weeks. All other changes to the antiretroviral regimen are assumed to represent substitutions due to patient preference, availability, or adverse effects and are not coded as treatment changes.

Subjects may also leave the cohort or be "lost to follow-up." We define a censoring time C as the time point at which a subject leaves the cohort and define $C(t) \equiv I(C \leq t)$ as the indicator that a subject is no longer in follow-up at time t. We treat censoring as an additional intervention variable because we are interested in the effect of treatment if all subjects remained in the cohort (and thus under observation) until time τ. All intervention variables by definition jump only once; changes in antiretroviral regimen after interruption or modification are not considered part of the treatment of interest, and a subject does not return to the cohort once he or she has been censored. Time-varying covariates can be considered under the following categories: laboratory measurements, diagnoses of new comorbidities, clinic visit dates, and vital status. The latter three categories, as well as the days on which laboratory measurements are updated, can be coded as counting processes.

The most recent laboratory covariate values at a given time t are coded as $W(t) = (W_1(t), ..., W_J(t))$. In clinical cohort data from resource-rich settings, $W(t)$ often includes the following J time-varying covariates: CD4+ T cell count, CD8+ T cell count, viral load, hepatitis C virus antibody, and hepatitis B virus surface antigen. In resource-limited settings such as Africa, $W(t)$ may be limited to CD4+ T cell count, complete blood count, or body mass index. Each time-dependent covariate may be measured at different and possibly irregular time points. We denote the process tracking when new laboratory measurements are made as $\Delta(t) = (\Delta_1(t), ..., \Delta_J(t))$, where $\Delta_j(t)$ denotes an indicator that covariate j is measured at time t. A covariate $W_j(t)$ is missing until $\Delta_j(t)$ first jumps; subsequently $W_j(t)$ is coded as the covariate's most recent value. New diagnoses made at time t are coded using a vector of counting processes $D(t) = (D_1(t), ..., D_K(t))$. These K counting processes include diagnosis of AIDS-defining illnesses and, in data from resource-rich settings, diagnosis of major non-AIDS comorbidities.

Clinic visits are coded as a separate counting process $M(t)$. Note that only when $dM(t) = 1$ (i.e., a patient visits the clinic) are any of the counting processes in $D(t)$ or the treatment process $A_2(t)$ at risk of jumping. In contrast, $\Delta(t)$, corresponding to updates of the laboratory covariates, can jump on any date, as can losses to follow-up and treatment interruptions. Finally, data are collected on vital status. Let T denote time of death and $\tilde{T} = \min(T, C, \tau)$ be the follow-up time. In addition, let $Y(t) = I(T \leq t)$ indicate whether a subject has died by time t, a counting process that can jump on any day.

In addition to the time-varying covariates above, the data include the following non-time varying-covariates: age at baseline, calendar year at baseline, sex, ethnicity, HIV risk group, nadir CD4 count prior to baseline, and peak viral load prior to baseline. We denote these non-time-varying covariates with B.

24.2 Causal Model

We separate variables into intervention variables $A(t) = (A_1(t), A_2(t), C(t))$, nonintervention variables $L(t) \equiv (M(t), D(t), \Delta(t), W(t))$, and the outcome $Y(t)$ and assume the following time ordering, as shown more explicitly below: $(Y(t), L(t), A(t))$. Baseline variables $L(0)$ include non-time-varying covariates and the baseline values of time-varying covariates $L(0) \equiv (B, M(0), D(0), \Delta(0), W(0))$. We use $\bar{X}(t) = (X(0), X(1), ..., X(t))$ to denote the history of any covariate X through time t. We define covariate values after death deterministically as their last observed value $L(t) \equiv L(T-1)$ and $A(t) \equiv A(T-1)$ for $t \geq T$. We also specify the following set of structural equations ($t = 1, ..., \tau$):

$$
\begin{aligned}
L(0) &= f_{L(0)}(U_0),\\
Y(t) &= f_{Y(t)}(Y(t-1), \bar{L}(t-1), \bar{A}(t-1), U_{Y(t)}),\\
M(t) &= f_{M(t)}(Y(t), \bar{L}(t-1), \bar{A}(t-1), U_{M(t)}),\\
D_k(t) &= f_{D_k(t)}(M(t), Y(t), \bar{L}(t-1), \bar{A}(t-1), U_{D_k(t)}); k = 1, ..., K,\\
\Delta_j(t) &= f_{\Delta_j(t)}(D(t), M(t), Y(t), \bar{L}(t-1), \bar{A}(t-1), U_{\Delta_j(t)}); j = 1, ..., J,\\
W_j(t) &= f_{W_j(t)}(\Delta(t), D(t), M(t), Y(t), \bar{L}(t-1), \bar{A}(t-1), U_{W_j(t)}); j = 1, ..., J,\\
A_1(t) &= f_{A_1(t)}(Y(t), \bar{L}(t), \bar{A}(t-1), U_{A_1(t)}),\\
A_2(t) &= f_{A_2(t)}(Y(t), A_1(t), \bar{L}(t), \bar{A}(t-1), U_{A_2(t)}),\\
C(t) &= f_{C(t)}(Y(t), A_1(t), A_2(t), \bar{L}(t), \bar{A}(t-1), U_{A_1(t)}).
\end{aligned}
$$

All subjects are assumed alive, on first-line therapy, and uncensored at baseline ($A_1(0) = A_2(0) = 1$, $Y(0) = C(0) = 0$). Specification of the causal model also involves specification of the joint distribution of the background factors or errors U:

$$
\begin{aligned}
U_0 &= (U_B, U_{M(0)}, U_{D(0)}, U_{W(0)}, U_{\Delta(0)}),\\
U &= (U_0, U_{Y(t)}, U_{M(t)}, U_{D_k(t)}, U_{\Delta_j(t)}, U_{W_j(t)}, U_{A_1(t)}, U_{A_2(t)}, U_{C(t)} : t, k, j),\\
U &\sim P_U.
\end{aligned}
$$

If it were known, for example, that the decision to modify therapy (among subjects who were alive and still on first-line therapy) was randomly assigned and perfectly complied with, this knowledge would justify an assumption that $U_{A_2(t)}$ is independent of all other errors [as well as an exclusion restriction on the structural equation model such that $A_2(t) = f_{A_2(t)}(Y(t), A_1(t), \bar{A}(t-1), U_{A_2(t)})$]. However, given the observational nature of the data, we avoid making any assumptions at this stage regarding the joint distribution P_U.

We denote the observed history of a covariate X as $\bar{X} \equiv \bar{X}(\tilde{T})$. The observed data consist of n i.i.d. copies of $O = \bar{O}(\tilde{T}) = (\bar{Y}, \bar{L}, \bar{A})$. These data are observed for a given individual until he or she either leaves the cohort (is lost to follow-up), dies, or time τ. We denote the distribution of O as P_0 and corresponding density p_0. We assume that the observed data correspond to n repeated draws from the SCM. In other words, for $i = 1, ..., n$, O_i is drawn by first drawing U_i from the distribution of background factors P_U (e.g., this might correspond to drawing a subject from a population), then generating each component of O sequentially for either τ time points or until $C(t)$ jumps to one. If $Y(t)$ jumps to one, covariate values for all subsequent time points are set equal to their last observed values.

24.3 Target Causal Parameters

In this section, we introduce a range of target causal parameters. For each, we begin with a scientific question and describe a hypothetical randomized trial that could be used to answer it. Each of these trials targets a distinct causal parameter. We illustrate how each target parameter in turn can be expressed in terms of counterfactuals, where the relevant counterfactuals are defined in terms of an intervention on the causal model.

24.3.1 Standard Marginal Structural Models

In assessing how changes in the availability of viral load monitoring will impact patient outcomes, the first question is whether delayed regimen modification following viral failure increases patient mortality, and if so, by how much. Previous analyses documented an increased risk of mortality with delayed modification of virologically failing NNRTI-based regimens; however, these analyses were based on subjects treated in resource-rich settings and included patients exposed to antiretroviral therapy prior to initiating cART (Petersen et al. 2008). Understanding how mortality varies as a function of cumulative delay until modification, and whether any increased risk of mortality resulting from delayed modification persists after second-line therapy has been initiated, could further inform the design of alternative monitoring strategies. For example, if most of the harm of delayed modification accrues during the first 3 months of failure, use of a semiannual vs. annual viral load testing strategy may have a smaller benefit than if mortality increases linearly with cumulative time spent on failing therapy. In theory, these questions could be addressed by enrolling subjects at the time of viral failure and randomly assigning each subject to remain on first-line failing therapy until a fixed switching time, ranging from immediate switch to switch after some maximum delay. In such an ideal trial, subjects would be prevented from interrupting therapy or leaving the cohort. Survival could then be compared between subjects randomized to different modification times.

In order to translate this ideal trial into a target causal parameter, we define counterfactuals indexed by interventions on interruptions and modifications of first-line therapy and on losses to follow-up. We denote counterfactual covariate and outcome values (the values that covariates and outcome would have taken under a specific treatment history $\bar{a}$) as $\bar{L}_{\bar{a}}$ and $\bar{Y}_{\bar{a}}$. These counterfactuals are defined as the solutions to the corresponding structural equations under an intervention on the SCM in which the structural equations $f_{A(t)}$, for $t = 1, ..., \tau$, are replaced with the constant values implied by $\bar{a}$. Our outcome of interest is counterfactual survival $\bar{Y}_{\bar{a}}(\tau)$. We focus on counterfactuals indexed by interventions under which first-line therapy is not interrupted and is modified at a fixed time (ranging from immediate switch to no switch during follow-up) and where no loss to follow-up occurs. The set of counterfactual interventions of interest is thus

$$\mathcal{A} \equiv \left\{ \bar{c} = 0, \bar{a}_1 = 1, \bar{a}_2 : \sum_{t=1}^{\tau} a_2(t) \in \{0, \tau\} \right\}. \tag{24.1}$$

Let

$$X_{SM} = \left(\bar{Y}_{\bar{a}}(\tau) : \bar{a} \in \mathcal{A}\right)$$

denote the collection of counterfactual survival times under each possible treatment regimen and let $X_{SM} \sim F_{X_{SM}}$. If we believe that the SCM accurately represents the processes that generated our observed data, this distribution represents the distribution of survival times that would have been observed if we had intervened on the data-generating system to change the mechanism by which treatment decisions were made (i.e., by forcing all subjects, rather than a self-selected subgroup, to follow each regimen $\bar{a} \in \mathcal{A}$), without altering any of the remaining data-generating processes.

Multiple target parameters can be defined using the counterfactual outcomes $(\bar{Y}_{\bar{a}}(\tau) : \bar{a} \in \mathcal{A})$ and corresponding counterfactual survival times. For example, if the counterfactual (discrete) hazard under every possible delay time is of interest, one option is to smooth across time points and delay times using a marginal structural model (Robins 2000, 1998, 1999b), such as

$$\text{logit}\,(P(T_{\bar{a}} = t \mid T_{\bar{a}} \geq t)) = m_{SM}(t, \bar{a} \mid \beta)\,.$$

For example, one might specify the following model to investigate a linear summary of the relationship between counterfactual hazard at time t and and cumulative time spent on failing therapy up till time t:

$$m_{SM}(t, \bar{a} \mid \beta) = \beta_0 + \beta_1 \sum_{j=1}^{t-1} a_2(j) + \beta_2 t + \beta_3 \sum_{j=1}^{t-1} a_2(j) \times t. \tag{24.2}$$

For this particular specification, $\exp(\beta_1 + \beta_3 t)$ is the relative (discrete) odds of death at time t for each additional day spent on failing therapy. Alternatively, more flexible model specifications could be used, such as models in which splines allow for nonlinear changes in baseline hazard over time and nonlinear effects of delayed modification. We refer to model (24.2), indexed by an intervention beginning at a single time point and applied uniformly to all subjects in the population, as a "standard" marginal structural model, to contrast it with the history-adjusted and dynamic marginal structural models described in the following sections.

At this stage in the road map, we are aiming purely to define our target parameter and wish to avoid introducing new model assumptions. We thus define our target causal parameter as a projection of true counterfactual hazard under different possible values for $\bar{a}$ onto the model $m_{SM}(t, \bar{a} \mid \beta)$ using a marginal structural working model (Neugebauer and van der Laan 2007). For model (24.2), the target causal parameter is defined as

$$\beta_{SM} = \arg\max_{\beta} E_{F_{X_{SM}}}\left[\sum_{\bar{a}}\sum_{t} \log\left((\lambda_{SM,\beta})^{I(T_{\bar{a}}=t)}(1 - \lambda_{SM,\beta})^{I(T_{\bar{a}}>t)}\right)\right], \tag{24.3}$$

where to simplify notation we use $\lambda_{SM,\beta}$ to refer to $\text{expit}(m_{SM}(\bar{a}, t \mid \beta))$. In other words, β_{SM} is defined as the parameter value of β that minimizes the average of the

Kullback–Liebler divergence between the model $m_{SM}(t, \bar{a} \mid \beta)$ and the distribution $F_{X_{SM}}$ across time points and possible switching times. One way to understand this projection is to think of the target parameter as the parameter value that would have been obtained if the investigator had access to the true counterfactual survival times (or a perfectly executed randomized trial) for an infinite population under every possible modification time and regressed these counterfactual outcomes on modification time according to model $m(t, \bar{a} \mid \beta)$. In this manner, the causal parameter β_{SM} is explicitly defined as a function of the distribution of the counterfactual survival times:

$$\beta_{SM} = \Psi_{SM}(F_{X_{SM}}). \tag{24.4}$$

24.3.2 History-Adjusted Marginal Structural Models

Target parameters defined using standard marginal structural models can be used to estimate counterfactual survival if the entire population of patients failing antiretroviral therapy (or subgroups defined by baseline covariate values $V \subset L(0)$) were forced to delay regimen modification. In practice, however, such a uniform treatment pattern is unlikely to occur. When viral loads are not available, the World Health Organization (WHO) currently recommends the use of CD4+ T cell counts to guide regimen modification (World Health Organization 2006). Specifically, any of the following three immunologic criteria can be interpreted as evidence of regimen failure and used to trigger modification to second-line therapy: (1) decline of CD4+ T cell counts to pretherapy baseline or below, (2) $\geq$ 50% decline of CD4+ T cell counts from on-treatment peak value, or (3) persistent CD4+ T cell counts < 100 cells/μl. While requiring fewer resources to implement than viral-load-based monitoring, however, CD4-based monitoring of antiretroviral treatment is complicated by the fact that in some patients CD4 counts remain stable for weeks or months despite ongoing viral replication (Reynolds et al. 2009). As a result, immunologic criteria have poor sensitivity for detecting virologic failure, and if used exclusively to guide switching decisions would result in delayed regimen modification for many patients.

The findings that (1) delayed regimen modification enforced across the entire target population would result in lower expected survival and (2) use of CD4+ T cell counts would on average result in delayed regimen modification do not in themselves imply that use of CD4+ T cell counts to guide modification decisions would necessarily increase mortality. Specifically, if CD4+ T cell counts are used to trigger regimen modification, delays will be longest for those subjects who maintain elevated CD4 counts despite ongoing viral replication and will be shortest for those subjects whose CD4 counts are low at the time of or decline rapidly following viral failure. This suggests an additional scientific question: Among subjects with viral failure, is delayed modification less harmful for those subjects who maintain CD4 counts above WHO switching criteria than it is for subjects with low CD4 counts? A CD4-based monitoring strategy would have a substantially smaller impact on mortality if delayed modification resulted in increased mortality primarily among those subjects with low CD4 counts on failing therapy.

In order to address whether CD4 count during virologic failure modifies the effect of additional delays in regimen modification, a clinical trial could enroll subjects who had remained on virologically failing first-line regimens for varying durations, stratify them on the basis of their current CD4+ T cell count, and within each CD4 count stratum randomly assign each subject an additional fixed delay time. Such a trial would allow the effect of additional delay time on survival to be compared between subjects who did vs. did not meet WHO CD4 switching criteria in the context of viral failure. Importantly, however, the effect of delayed modification within CD4 count strata would be estimated among a selected subpopulation: those who remained alive and on first-line therapy. Petersen et al. (2007a), Robins et al. (2007a), van der Laan et al. (2007a), van der Laan and Petersen (2007b), and Petersen et al. (2007b) provide further discussion of this issue.

We define counterfactual outcomes indexed by a series of baseline time points: $r = 1, ..., \tau - m$. For each baseline time point r, the counterfactual outcome is defined as the probability of survival for at least m additional time points under an intervention on treatment decisions beginning at time r. Treatment decisions from time 0 through time $r - 1$ are left random and treatment decisions from time r until the outcome is measured at $r + m$ are intervened on. More formally, the counterfactuals of interest are $Y_{\bar{A}(r-1)\underline{a}(r)}(r + m)$ for $r = 1, ..., \tau - m$, where $\underline{a}(r) \equiv (a(r), a(r + 1), ..., a(r + m - 1)) \in \mathcal{A}_r$. We consider $\mathcal{A}_r$ (the set of possible treatment regimens beginning at time r) such that for each $\underline{a}(r) \in \mathcal{A}_r$ we have $(\bar{A}(r - 1), \underline{a}(r)) \in \mathcal{A}$, where $\mathcal{A}$ (the set of possible treatments from $t = 1, ..., \tau$) is defined as in (24.1) to include all possible modification times and no losses to follow-up or interruptions. To simplify notation, we use $Y_{\underline{a}(r)}(r + m)$ to refer to $Y_{\bar{A}(r-1)\underline{a}(r)}(r + m)$ and $T_{\underline{a}(r)}$ to refer to $T_{\bar{A}(r-1)\underline{a}(r)}$. Let $F_{X_{HM}}$ denote the distribution of

$$X_{HM} = \left(\left\{\bar{A}(r - 1), Y(r), \mathrm{CD4}(r), \left(Y_{\underline{a}(r)}(r + m) : \underline{a}(r) \in \mathcal{A}_r\right)\right\} : r = 1, ..., \tau - m\right).$$

Here $\mathrm{CD4}(r) \in W(r)$ denotes the most recent CD4 measurement available at time r.

We aim to estimate how the effect of additional time spent on a failing regimen differs depending on a subject's most recent CD4+ T cell count among those subjects who remain alive, in follow-up, and on first-line therapy. In order to define a target parameter that addresses this question, we could estimate counterfactual survival probability m days in the future as a function of additional time spent on failing therapy and current CD4+ T cell count using a series of standard marginal structural working models and treating each time point $0, ..., \tau - m - 1$ in turn as baseline. Alternatively, the use of history-adjusted marginal structural models (van der Laan et al. 2005; Petersen et al. 2007a) allows us to use a common working model and smooth across baseline time points:

$$\begin{aligned}&\mathrm{logit}\left(P\left(T_{\underline{a}(r)} \leq r + m \mid \bar{A}_1(r - 1) = \bar{A}_2(r - 1) = 1, C \geq r, T > r, \mathrm{CD4}(r)\right)\right)\\&\quad = m_{HM}(r, \underline{a}(r), \mathrm{CD4}(r) \mid \beta),\end{aligned}$$

for $r = 1, ..., \tau - m$. For example, we might define our target parameter using the following working model:

$$m_{HM}\left(r, \underline{a}(r), \text{CD4}(r)|\beta\right) = \beta_0 + \beta_1 \sum_{t=r}^{r+m-1} a_2(t) + \beta_2 I(\text{CD4}(r) > w*)$$
$$+\beta_3 \sum_{t=r}^{r+m-1} a_2(t) \times I(\text{CD4}(r) > w*), \tag{24.5}$$

where $w*$ is the CD4 modification threshold recommended by the WHO. Such a model provides a linear summary of the effect of additional delay until regimen modification ($\sum_{t=r}^{r+m-1} a_2(t)$) on probability of survival m time points in the future and allows this effect to differ depending on current CD4 count. An alternative model specification could also allow this effect to differ depending on duration of time already spent on failing therapy (r). For the particular working model specification (24.5), $\beta_3 = 0$ corresponds to the null hypothesis that the effect of additional delay until regimen modification is the same regardless of current CD4 count, and $\exp(\beta_1 + \beta_3)$ corresponds to the discrete hazard ratio associated with an incremental increase in delay until regimen modification for subjects with a CD4 count $> w*$. A finding that $\beta_1 > 0$ while $(\beta_3 + \beta_1) \leq 0$ would suggest that increased mortality resulting from delayed regimen modification was occurring primarily in those subjects with CD4 counts below the WHO-recommended modification threshold.

Again, rather than assuming that equality (24.5) holds for some value of β, the target parameter β_{HM} can be defined using a projection as

$$\beta_{HM} = \arg\max_{\beta} E_{F_{X_{HM}}}\left[\sum_{\underline{a}(r)}\sum_{r} \log\left((\lambda_{HM,\beta})^{I(T_{\underline{a}(r)} \leq r+m)}(1 - \lambda_{HM,\beta})^{I(T_{\underline{a}(r)} > r+m)}\right)\right], \tag{24.6}$$

where to simplify notation we use $\lambda_{HM,\beta}$ for $\text{expit}(m_{HM}(r, \underline{a}(r), \text{CD4}(r) \mid \beta))$. In this manner, the history-adjusted marginal structural model target causal parameter is explicitly defined as a function of the distribution of the counterfactual survival times indexed by interventions beginning at time r:

$$\beta_{HM} = \Psi_{HM}(F_{X_{HM}}). \tag{24.7}$$

24.3.3 Dynamic Marginal Structural Models

The target parameters defined using standard and history-adjusted marginal structural models address the scientific questions of whether delayed regimen modification following viral failure results in increased mortality, whether the effect of additional delay until regimen modification among subjects who remain on first-line therapy differs depending on current CD4+ T cell count, and whether delayed modification remains detrimental to those subjects with CD4 counts above the WHO-recommended modification threshold. The target parameters defined thus far do not, however, address the following questions: (1) How would patient outcomes have differed if a CD4-based rule *vs.* a viral load-based rule had been used to decide when to modify therapy? (2) Which CD4 -based rule would have resulted, on average, in optimal patient outcomes?

A clinical trial to address the latter two questions would enroll subjects at the time of cART initiation and randomly assign them to a strategy for deciding when to modify therapy. Random assignment of subjects to remain on failing therapy until they met a CD4-based switching criterion *vs.* a viral-load-based switching criterion would allow patient outcomes to be compared under these two strategies, while random assignment of subjects to a range of different CD4-based switching criteria would provide insight into the best choice of CD4-based rule. The randomized exposure in such hypothetical trials can be contrasted with the exposure in the hypothetical trials described in Sects. 24.3.1 and 24.3.2, in which subjects were randomly assigned a fixed delay time until modification rather than assigned a strategy for deciding when to modify.

The target parameters defined in Sects. 24.3.1 and 24.3.2 focused on subjects who were virologically failing cART. In order to focus on the larger population of subjects starting cART, we redefine our baseline time point in the current section such that $t = 0$ corresponds to time of cART initiation rather than the time of cART failure. We define counterfactuals indexed by dynamic treatment regimens, or rules that assign treatment decisions at each time point in response to patient characteristics. Our focus is on dynamic rules that assign subjects to switch to second-line therapy as soon as (and no sooner than) their CD4+ T cell count reaches a specified threshold, and that do not allow subjects to either interrupt first-line therapy or to leave the cohort. A similar approach could be used to define counterfactuals under viral-load-based rules.

Let $d_\theta(t, \overline{\mathrm{CD4}}(t), \bar{A}(t-1))$ denote a treatment rule that deterministically assigns values to the intervention variables $A(t) = (A_1(t), A_2(t), C(t))$ based on treatment history and CD4 count up till time t according to the following algorithm:

- Do not interrupt first-line therapy (set $A_1(t) = 1$ for all t).
- Remain in follow-up (set $C(t) = 0$ for all t).
- If most recent CD4+ T cell count is $< \theta$ and a subject is still on first-line therapy, switch to second-line therapy (set $A_2(t) = 0$ if $A_2(t-1) = 1$ and $\mathrm{CD4}(t) < \theta$).
- If most recent CD4+ T cell count is $\geq \theta$ and a subject is still on first-line therapy, do not switch to second-line therapy (set $A_2(t) = 1$ if $A_2(t-1) = 1$ and $\mathrm{CD4}(t) < \theta$).
- Once a subject has modified regimens, $A_2(t) = 0$ by definition.

We focus on counterfactual survival times $(\bar{Y}_{d_\theta}(\tau) : \theta \in \Theta)$ under an intervention on the SCM that assigns interruption, modification, and censoring according to the rule $d_\theta(t, \overline{\mathrm{CD4}}(t), \bar{A}(t-1))$, $t = 1, .., \tau$, where Θ is a set of CD4 switching thresholds of interest. In other words, $Y_{d_\theta}(t)$ is defined as the solution to the structural equation $f_{Y(t)}$ under an intervention on the system of equations in which $f_{A_1(t)}, f_{A_2(t)}$, and $f_{C(t)}$ are replaced with the treatment rule $d_\theta(t, \overline{\mathrm{CD4}}(t), \bar{A}(t-1))$. Let $F_{X_{DM}}$ denote the distribution of

$$X_{DM} = \left(\bar{Y}_{d_\theta}(\tau) : \theta \in \Theta\right).$$

We are interested in how the counterfactual survival distribution differs as a function of the CD4+ T cell count (or viral load) threshold θ used to trigger regimen modification. A dynamic marginal structural model can be used to summarize this relationship, smoothing over possible values of the threshold θ (Hernan et al. 2006; van der Laan and Petersen 2007a; Robins et al. 2008). For example, one could specify a working model for the discrete counterfactual hazard as a function of θ:

$$\text{logit}\left(P(T_{d_\theta} = t \mid T_{d_\theta} \geq t)\right) = m_{DM}(\theta, t \mid \beta).$$

For example, one might specify the following working model:

$$m_{DM}(t, \theta \mid \beta) = \beta_0 + \beta_1\theta + \beta_2\theta^2 + h(t), \tag{24.8}$$

where $h(t)$ is some user-specified function of t. For example, if $h(t)$ corresponds to an indicator variable for each time point t, (24.8) approximates a Cox proportional hazards model for fine enough time scale t. Alternative model specifications could allow the effect of the threshold θ on the discrete hazard to vary by time (or, in other words, relax the proportional hazards assumption). As with β_{SM} and β_{HM}, rather than assuming that equality (24.8) holds for some value θ, we define β_{DM} using a projection:

$$\beta_{DM} = \arg\max_{\beta} E_{F_{X_{DM}}}\left[\sum_{\theta}\sum_{t} \log\left((\lambda_{DM,\beta})^{I(T_{d_\theta}=t)}(1-\lambda_{DM,\beta})^{I(T_{d_\theta}>t)}\right)\right], \tag{24.9}$$

where to simplify notation we use $\lambda_{DM,\beta}$ to refer to $\text{expit}(m_{DM}(t, \theta \mid \beta))$. The dynamic marginal structural model parameter is now defined a a function of the distribution of the counterfactual survival times indexed by rules d_θ:

$$\beta_{DM} = \Psi_{DM}(F_{X_{DM}}). \tag{24.10}$$

24.4 Statistical Model and Identifiability Results

Recall that the observed data consist of n i.i.d. copies of $O \sim P_0$, while the target parameters are functions of the counterfactual distributions $F_{X_{SM}}$, $F_{X_{HM}}$, and $F_{X_{DM}}$. In order to estimate these target causal parameters, we must thus first be able to express $\Psi_{SM}(F_{X_{SM}})$, $\Psi_{HM}(F_{X_{HM}})$, and $\Psi_{DM}(F_{X_{DM}})$ as parameters of the observed data distribution P_0. The sequential randomization assumption is one sufficient assumption for β_{SM} and β_{HM} to be identified as parameters of the observed data distribution (Robins 1986, 1987a,b):

$$Y_{\bar{a}}(j) \coprod A_1(t) \mid \bar{L}(t) = \bar{l}(t), \bar{A}(t-1) = \bar{a}(t-1), \tag{24.11}$$
$$Y_{\bar{a}}(j) \coprod A_2(t) \mid \bar{L}(t) = \bar{l}(t), \bar{A}(t-1) = \bar{a}(t-1), A_1(t) = a_1(t),$$
$$Y_{\bar{a}}(j) \coprod C(t) \mid \bar{L}(t) = \bar{l}(t), \bar{A}(t-1) = \bar{a}(t-1), A_1(t) = a_1(t), A_2(t) = a_2(t),$$

for $t < j \leq \tau$.

For β_{DM} the corresponding assumption is

$$Y_{d_\theta}(j) \coprod A_1(t) \mid \bar{L}(t) = \bar{l}(t), \bar{A}(t-1) = \bar{a}(t-1), \tag{24.12}$$
$$Y_{d_\theta}(j) \coprod A_2(t) \mid \bar{L}(t) = \bar{l}(t), \bar{A}(t-1) = \bar{a}(t-1), A_1(t) = a_1(t),$$
$$Y_{d_\theta}(j) \coprod C(t) \mid \bar{L}(t) = \bar{l}(t), \bar{A}(t-1) = \bar{a}(t-1), A_1(t) = a_1(t), A_2(t) = a_2(t),$$

for $t < j \leq \tau$.

In words, modification, interruption, and loss to follow-up at each time point are assumed to be independent of counterfactual survival, given the observed past up till that time point. In terms of the causal model, these identifiability assumptions impose restrictions on the allowable joint distribution of the error terms P_U. We refer to the resulting SCM, corresponding to the model in Sect. 24.2 augmented with the restrictions on the joint distribution of the errors needed for identifiability, as the working SCM. We use the term "working" to refer to the SCM under which the target causal parameter is identified, which might include assumptions not fully supported by background knowledge and thus not part of the original SCM. We pursue estimation under the working model, while emphasizing that any interpretation of resulting estimates as causal effects is based on the plausibility of these working model assumptions. In the current example, neither the original SCM nor the working SCM imposes restrictions on the allowable joint distributions of the observed data. Thus for the purpose of estimation we commit to a nonparametric statistical model for each of the target parameters.

24.4.1 Likelihood

Let $Q_{L(0),0}(l(0)) \equiv P_0(L(0) = l(0))$ denote the conditional distribution of the baseline covariates and

$$Q_{L(t),0}(l(t) \mid Y(t), \bar{L}(t-1), \bar{A}(t-1)) \equiv P_0(L(t) = l(t) \mid Y(t), \bar{L}(t-1), \bar{A}(t-1))$$

denote the conditional distribution at time t of the nonintervention covariates (other than vital status), given past covariates, vital status, and treatment. Let

$$g_{A(t),0}(a(t) \mid Y(t), \bar{L}(t), \bar{A}(t-1)) \equiv P_0(A(t) = a(t) \mid Y(t), \bar{L}(t), \bar{A}(t-1))$$

denote the conditional distribution at time t of treatment and censoring given the past. Let

$$Q_{Y(t),0}(y(t) \mid Y(t-1), \bar{L}(t-1), \bar{A}(t-1)) \equiv P_0(Y(t) = y(t) \mid Y(t-1), \bar{L}(t-1), \bar{A}(t-1))$$

denote the conditional distribution of vital status at time t given past covariates and treatment, and

$$\bar{Q}_{Y(t),0}(Y(t-1), \bar{L}(t-1), \bar{A}(t-1)) \equiv P_0(Y(t) = 1 \mid Y(t-1), \bar{L}(t-1), \bar{A}(t-1)).$$

The likelihood can be factorized as follows:

$$P_0(O) = Q_{L_0,0}(L(0)) \prod_{t=1}^{\tilde{T}} \left\{ \begin{array}{l} \bar{Q}_{Y(t),0}(Y(t-1), \bar{L}(t-1), \bar{A}(t-1))^{Y(t)} \\ (1 - \bar{Q}_{Y(t),0}(Y(t-1), \bar{L}(t-1), \bar{A}(t-1)))^{1-Y(t)} \\ Q_{L(t),0}(L(t) \mid Y(t), \bar{L}(t-1), \bar{A}(t-1)) \\ g_{A(t),0}(A(t) \mid Y(t), \bar{L}(t), \bar{A}(t-1)) \end{array} \right\}.$$

The components of this likelihood $Q_{L(t),0}$ and $g_{A(t),0}$, $t = 1, ..., \tilde{T}$ can be further factorized into their respective components, where each factor represents the conditional distribution of a variable given its parents, those covariates on the right-hand side of the corresponding structural equation in the SCM presented in Sect. 24.2. For example,

$$\begin{aligned} g_{A(t),0}(A(t) \mid Y(t), \bar{L}(t), \bar{A}(t-1)) \equiv\ & g_{A_1(t),0}(A_1(t) \mid Y(t), \bar{L}(t), \bar{A}(t-1)) \\ & \times g_{A_2(t),0}(A_2(t) \mid A_1(t), Y(t), \bar{L}(t), \bar{A}(t-1)) \\ & \times g_{C(t),0}(C(t) \mid A_1(t), A_2(t), Y(t), \bar{L}(t), \bar{A}(t-1)). \end{aligned}$$

$Q_{L(t),0}$ can similarly be factorized into a series of conditional distributions, corresponding to $Q_{M(t),0}$, $Q_{D(t),0}$, $Q_{\Delta(t),0}$, and $Q_{W(t),0}$. Finally, the likelihood for the multidimensional variables $D(t)$, $W(t)$, and $\Delta(t)$ can be further factorized according to some arbitrary ordering. The data can be organized in long format, with a subject contributing a new line of data each time at least one of the counting processes jumps.

24.4.2 Target Parameters $\Psi(P_0)$

When (24.11) (or its graphical counterpart) holds, the target counterfactual parameters $\Psi(F_X)$ defined in Sect. 24.3 are identified (with slight abuse of notation) as parameters $\Psi(P_0)$ of the observed data distribution by the longitudinal g-computation formula (Robins 1986, 1987a,b; Pearl 2009). The g-computation formula for the marginal distribution of the counterfactual survival time indexed by a given intervention is derived by (1) intervening on the likelihood to remove those factors that correspond to the structural equations for the intervention variables, (2) evaluating the resulting truncated likelihood at the value of the intervention variables used to index the counterfactual, and (3) integrating with respect to the distribution of all nonintervention variables other than the outcome. The target parameters β_{SM} and β_{DM} are identified as the projections of these counterfactual survival times under each possible intervention ($\bar{a} \in \mathcal{A}$ and d_θ for $\theta \in \Theta$, respectively) onto the corresponding working model. The target parameter β_{HM} is identified as the projection of the joint distribution of the counterfactual survival times under each possible intervention $(Y_{\underline{a}}(r+m) : \underline{a}(r) \in \mathcal{A}_r)$ and $(\text{CD4}(r), Y(r), \bar{A}(r-1))$, for each baseline time point r, onto working model m_{HM}.

We provide the full identifiability result for the distribution of the counterfactual survival time $T_{\bar{a}}$ [and thus for $\beta_{SM} = \Psi_{SM}(F_{X_{SM}})$] as an illustration:

$$P(T_{\bar{a}} = t) \overset{24.11}{=}$$

$$\sum_{\bar{l}(t-1)} \left\{ \begin{array}{l} \bar{Q}_{Y(t),0}(T \geq t, \bar{L}(t-1) = \bar{l}(t-1), \bar{A}(t-1) = \bar{a}(t-1)) \times \\ \prod_{j=1}^{t-1}(1 - \bar{Q}_{Y(j),0}(T \geq j, \bar{L}(j-1) = \bar{l}(j-1), \bar{A}(j-1) = \bar{a}(j-1)) \times \\ \prod_{j=1}^{t-1} Q_{L(j),0}(l(j) \mid Y(j) = 0, \bar{L}(j-1) = \bar{l}(j-1), \bar{A}(j-1) = \bar{a}(j-1)) \\ Q_{L(0),0}(l(0)) \end{array} \right\},$$

where the right-hand side of this equation is a parameter of the observed data distribution P_0.

This identifiability result implies that the target parameter β_{SM} can be evaluated by drawing repeatedly from the truncated likelihood to generate the distribution of $Y_{\bar{a}}(t)$ for $t = 0, ..., \min(T, \tau)$ and $\bar{a} \in \mathcal{A}$. In other words, β_{SM} is evaluated using the following algorithm:

1. Draw $L(0)$ from the distribution $Q_{L(0),0}$ and draw $Y(1)$ from the conditional distribution $Q_{Y(1),0}$ given the draw of $L(0)$. If $Y(1) = 1$, skip to step 6.
2. Draw $L(1)$ from the conditional distribution $Q_{L(1),0}$ given $L(0)$ (noting that $Q_{L(1),0}$ is itself is composed of multiple conditional distributions and thus requires multiple sequential draws).
3. Draw $Y(2)$ from the conditional distribution $Q_{Y(2),0}$ given $\bar{L}(1)$ and setting $A(1) = a(1)$. If $Y(2)$=1, skip to step 6.
4. Draw $L(2)$ from the conditional distribution $Q_{L(2),0}$ given $\bar{L}(1)$ and setting $A(1) = a(1)$.
5. Repeat steps 3 and 4 to draw $Y(t)$ and $L(t)$ until $Y(t) = 1$ or $t = \tau$, whichever happens first.
6. Repeat steps 1–5 an infinite number of times for each treatment regimen $\bar{a} \in \mathcal{A}$
7. Evaluate β_{SM} by regressing the counterfactuals $Y_{\bar{a}}(t)$ simulated in steps 1–6 on treatment history $\bar{a}$ and t using pooled logistic regression model $m_{SM}(t, \bar{a}|\beta)$.

The parameter β_{DM} can be evaluated using a similar process, with the modifications that $A(t)$ in steps 3–5 is set by evaluating the function $d_\theta(t, \overline{\text{CD4}}(t), \bar{A}(t-1))$, steps 1–5 are repeated for each $\theta \in \Theta$, and in step 7 the simulated counterfactuals $Y_{d_\theta}(t)$ are regressed on θ and t using pooled logistic regression model $m_{DM}(t, \theta \mid \beta)$.

Evaluation of β_{HM} requires a modification of the algorithm such that a draw for a given time point r involves drawing from the nontruncated likelihood up till r

and the truncated likelihood after r. In other words, β_{HM} can be evaluated using the following algorithm:

1. Draw $(Y(r), \bar{L}(r), \bar{A}(r-1))$ by first drawing $L(0)$ from $Q_{L(0),0}$, then drawing $Y(j)$ from $Q_{Y(j),0}$, $L(j)$ from $Q_{L(j),0}$, and $A(j)$ from $g_{A(j),0}$ for $j = 1, ..., r-1$, and finally drawing $Y(r)$ from $Q_{Y(r),0}$ and $L(r)$ from $Q_{L(r),0}$. If $Y(r) = 1$, $C(r-1) = 1$, $A_1(r-1) = 0$ or $A_2(r-1) = 0$, skip to step 5.
2. Draw $Y(r+1)$ from the conditional distribution $Q_{Y(r+1),0}$ given draw $(\bar{L}(r), \bar{A}(r-1))$ and setting $A(r) = a(r)$. If $Y(r+1) = 1$, skip to step 5.
3. Draw $L(r+1)$ from the conditional distribution $Q_{L(r+1),0}$ given draw $(\bar{L}(r), \bar{A}(r-1))$ and setting $A(r) = a(r)$.
4. Repeat steps 2 and 3 to draw $Y(t)$ and $L(t)$ until $Y(t) = 1$ or $t = r + m$, whichever happens first.
5. Repeat steps 1–4 an infinite number of times for each $\underline{a}(r) \in \mathcal{A}_r$ and each $r = 1, ..., \tau - m$.
6. Evaluate β_{HM} by regressing the counterfactuals $Y_{\underline{a}}(r+m)$ simulated in steps 2–5 in those draws for which $Y(r) = C(r-1) = 0$ and $A_1(r-1) = A_2(r-1) = 1$ on $\underline{a}(r)$, CD4(r), and r using pooled logistic regression model $m_{HM}(r, \underline{a}(r), \text{CD4}(r) \mid \beta)$.

Each of these parameters $\beta = \Psi(P_0)$ can now be targeted for estimation, under the additional assumption of positivity needed to ensure that the relevant conditional probabilities are well defined (Chap. 10).

24.5 Estimation

We provide a succinct summary of MLE, IPCW estimation, TMLE, and IPCW reduced-data TMLE. Inference can be based on the nonparametric bootstrap or the influence curve; details are not provided in this chapter. We use the shorthand

$$Q_{\bar{L}(t),0} \equiv \prod_{j=0}^{t} Q_{L(j),0}(L(j) \mid Y(j), \bar{L}(j-1), \bar{A}(j-1)), \tag{24.13}$$

$$Q_{\bar{Y}(t),0} \equiv \prod_{j=1}^{t} Q_{Y(j),0}(Y(j) \mid Y(j-1), \bar{L}(j-1), \bar{A}(j-1)), \tag{24.14}$$

and $Q_0 \equiv Q_{\bar{L}(\tilde{T}),0} \times Q_{\bar{Y}(\tilde{T}),0}$ to refer to the L and Y components of P_0. We use

$$g_{\bar{A}(t),0} \equiv \prod_{j=1}^{t} g_{A(j),0}(A(j) \mid Y(j), \bar{L}(j), \bar{A}(j-1)) \tag{24.15}$$

and $g_0 \equiv g_{\bar{A}(\tilde{T}),0}$ to refer to the conditional distributions of the A components in $P_0 = Q_0 g_0$.

24.5.1 MLE

Above, each target parameter was expressed as a function of P_0 and algorithms were provided that described how each parameter could be evaluated given knowledge of the true data-generating distribution. A substitution estimator for each parameter is provided by plugging in an estimator of the data-generating distribution to these algorithms. The parameters β_{SM} and β_{DM} are only functions of Q_0; thus a substitution estimator of these parameters only requires an estimator Q_n of Q_0. In order to implement such an estimator, the conditional distribution of $L(t)$ can be factorized in terms of conditional distributions of the components of $L(t)$, where many of these components are binary indicators. The continuous or ordered discrete components of $L(t)$, such as the biomarkers CD4 count and viral load, can be discretized and coded accordingly in terms of binary indicators as well. These different conditional distributions can then be estimated based on the log-likelihood of the data $O_1, \ldots, O_n$, where, for each type of conditional distribution, we only have to work with the relevant factor of the likelihood that represents the particular conditional distribution we wish to estimate.

In estimating the t-specific conditional distribution of a given variable, one option is to pool across time or across different levels of an ordered discrete variable. For example, we could estimate the probability of a clinic visit at time t given the past by pooling across time points and including some function of time t as a covariate in a corresponding regression model. MLE according to parametric models for these conditional distributions can be carried out with standard multivariate logistic regression software. In addition, we can utilize machine learning algorithms such as log-likelihood-based super learning to construct data-adaptive estimators that avoid reliance on a priori specified parametric forms of these conditional distributions. This results in an initial estimator Q_n^0 of Q_0 (where we use the 0 superscript to differentiate this initial estimator of Q_0 from targeted estimators of Q_0 created by updating this initial fit when implementing TMLE in Sect. 24.5.3). An estimator Q_n^0 defines the maximum-likelihood-based substitution estimators $\Psi_{SM}(Q_n^0)$ and $\Psi_{DM}(Q_n^0)$ of the target parameters β_{SM} and β_{DM}.

The target parameter β_{HM} is a function of both Q_0 and g_0 (its evaluation according to the algorithm defined in Sect. 24.4.2 requires $g_{\bar{A}(r-1),0}$ in addition to $Q_{\bar{Y}(r+m),0}$ and $Q_{\bar{L}(r+m-1),0}$ for each time point r). Thus implementation of an MLE of β_{HM} according to this algorithm requires an estimator g_n of g_0. As with Q_0, g_0 can be factorized into a series of conditional distributions of binary variables, and these conditional distributions can be estimated using either parametric logistic regression models or with data-adaptive estimators. Rather than simulating data using Q_n^0 and g_n beginning at time $t = 0$, step 1 of the algorithm can alternatively be implemented by drawing from the empirical distribution of the observed data at time r $(\bar{L}(r), Y(r), \bar{A}(r-1))$. Consistency of the MLEs of β_{SM} and β_{DM} requires consistency of the estimator Q_0^n, consistency of the MLE of β_{HM} also requires consistent estimation of either $g_{\bar{A},0}(r-1)$ or the distribution of $(\bar{L}(r), Y(r), \bar{A}(r-1))$ for each time point r (which will be achieved if estimation of this distribution is based on sampling from the empirical distribution of the data at time r).

24.5.2 Inverse-Probability-Weighted Estimation

An alternative approach is to define an inverse probability of treatment and censoring-weighted estimating function for each of our target parameters as described in previous chapters.The following estimating functions are unbiased estimating functions for the target parameters β_{SM} and β_{DM}:

$$D^{SM}_{IPCW}(g_0,\beta_{SM}) = \sum_{t\leq\tilde{T}} \frac{I(A_1(t-1)=1)\frac{d}{d\beta}m_{SM}(t,\bar{A}(t-1)\mid\beta)}{g_{\bar{A}(t-1),0}}(Y(t)-\lambda_{SM,\beta}),$$

$$D^{DM}_{IPCW}(g_0,\beta_{DM}) = \sum_{\theta}\sum_{t\leq\tilde{T}} \frac{I(\bar{A}(t-1)=d_\theta(\bar{L}))\frac{d}{d\beta}m_{DM}(t,\theta\mid\beta)}{g_{\bar{A}(t-1),0}}(Y(t)-\lambda_{DM,\beta}).$$

The estimating function for β_{HM} involves a sum over those baseline time points r for which $Y(r)=C(r-1)=0, A_1(r-1)=A_2(r-1)=1$, and $r\leq\tau-m$. To facilitate definition of the estimating function, let $\mathcal{R}$ refer to this set. Further, let

$$\begin{aligned}&\mathcal{W}(C(r+m-1),A_1(r+m-1),m_{HM},g_0)\\ &\quad\equiv \frac{I(C(r+m-1)=0,A_1(r+m-1)=1)\frac{d}{d\beta}m_{HM}(r,\underline{A}(r),\text{CD4}(r)\mid\beta)}{\prod_{j=r}^{r+m-1} g_{A(j),0}(A(j)\mid\bar{L}(j),\bar{A}(j-1))}.\end{aligned}$$

The following is now an unbiased estimating function for β_{HM}:

$$D^{HM}_{IPCW}(g_0,\beta_{HM}) = \sum_{r\in\mathcal{R}}\mathcal{W}(C(r+m-1),A_1(r+m-1),m_{HM},g_0)(Y(r+m)-\lambda_{HM,\beta}).$$

Given an estimator g_n of g_0, an estimate β_n is then defined as the solution of $0=\sum_{i=1}^n D_{IPCW}(g_n,\beta_n)(O_i)$. These estimators can be implemented with weighted logistic regression software. For example, β_{SM} can be implemented by fitting a pooled weighted logistic regression of the observed outcomes $Y(t)$ on the observed modification times implied by $\bar{A}_2(t-1)$ among subjects that remain alive and uncensored and who have not interrupted therapy by time $t-1$, with weights corresponding to the inverse of the product of $g_{A(j),0}$ taken up to time $t-1$. Consistency of the IPCW estimators relies on consistency of the estimator g_n.

24.5.3 TMLE

In the interest of space, we focus on estimation of $\beta_{SM} = \Psi_{SM}(Q_0)$, with brief comments regarding estimation of β_{DM} and β_{HM}. The MLE of the parameter β_{SM} is implemented based on an initial estimator of the conditional distributions of binary nonintervention variables, where this estimator, Q_n^0, was represented as a series of logistic regression fits. The TMLE of β_{SM} involves adding a clever covariate to each of these logistic regression fits, using the current logistic regression fit as an offset, and fitting the coefficients ϵ in front of the clever covariate with parametric logistic regression (van der Laan 2010a,b). This TMLE corresponds with using the log-likelihood loss function $L(P) = -\log P$ and using these parametric logistic regression working models with parameter ϵ as the parametric submodel through the initial estimator that encodes the fluctuations of an initial estimator.

The clever covariate for the conditional distribution $Q_B(B \mid Pa(B))$ of a binary indicator B given its parents $Pa(B)$ (the variables on the right-hand side of the corresponding structural equation) is a function $H_B(Q_n^0, g_n)$ of the same dimension as the target parameter, and it can be evaluated for each observation O_i as a function of the parent set $Pa_i(B)$ for that observation. Specifically,

$$H_B(Q_n^0, g_n) = E_{Q_n^0, g_n}(D_{IPCW}^{SM}(g_n, \beta_n^0) \mid B = 1, Pa(B)) \\ -E_{Q_n^0, g_n}(D_{IPCW}^{SM}(g_n, \beta_n^0) \mid B = 0, Pa(B)),$$

where $D_{IPCW}^{SM}(g_n, \beta_n^0)$ is the inverse probability of treatment and censoring-weighted estimating function for the target parameter as presented above (formally, any gradient of the pathwise derivative of the target parameter can be selected). The resulting update of Q_n^0 is denoted by Q_n^1, and this process is iterated until convergence to Q_n^*, at which point the coefficients in front of the clever covariate (i.e., the fluctuation parameters ϵ) approximate zero. Current experience shows very fast convergence of this targeted maximum likelihood algorithm, with the majority of bias reduction achieved in the first step.

One can also use a separate ϵ for each factor of the likelihood, and carry out the updates Q_n^k of Q_n^0 sequentially, starting at the last factor of Q, each time using the clever covariate evaluated at the most recent update Q_n^k, and proceeding till the update of the first factor. The latter closed-form TMLE has been presented in van der Laan (2010a,b).

The TMLE for β_{SM} is defined as the substitution estimator $\Psi_{SM}(Q_n^*)$. Consistency of the TMLE relies on consistent estimation of Q_0 or consistent estimation of g_0 (as well as use of an estimator g_n that converges to a distribution that satisfies the positivity assumption). Efficiency of the TMLE requires the consistency of both estimators.

The TMLE for the target parameter $\beta_{DM} = \Psi_{DM}(Q_0)$ is implemented in the same fashion, with Q_n^* used to implement the substitution estimator $\Psi_{DM}(Q_n^*)$. A similar approach can be used for a history-adjusted target parameter that is defined by specifying a separate working model for each time point r. In this special case of history-adjusted parameters, the TMLE can be implemented using sequential applications of the TMLE standard marginal structural model algorithm to estimate the parameters of each r-specific working model, treating covariates up till time r (including $\bar{A}(r-1)$) as baseline nonintervention covariates. When the history-adjusted target parameter is defined by pooling over time points r, as with β_{HM}, the TMLE involves additional updates of g_n; however, details are beyond the scope of this chapter.

24.5.4 IPCW Reduced-Data TMLE

Implementation of the TMLE in Sect. 24.5.3 requires fitting all conditional distributions of the Q_0-factor of the likelihood and carrying out the TMLE update for each. The need to update the fit for each conditional distribution prior to simulating from Q_n^* can make the TMLE procedure quite computer intensive. Further, the initial estimation step requires estimation of a very high-dimensional Q_0-factor. Due to the curse of dimensionality, Q_n^0 may be a highly biased estimator of Q_0, resulting in a TMLE that is inefficient and relies heavily on the consistency of g_n for its consistency. We provide an overview of the IPCW reduced-data TMLE (IPCW-R-TMLE) as one response to these challenges (van der Laan 2008b). In order to simplify the discussion, we again focus on the target parameter β_{SM}, noting that a parallel approach could be used to estimate and β_{DM} while estimation of β_{HM} would require additional steps.

We motivate development of the estimator by considering a scenario in which the same SCM holds, but in which the observed data available to the analyst have been reduced such that the only time-varying covariates observed are the intervention variables (interruption, modification, and censoring), the outcome, and CD4+ T cell count. We denote the reduced covariate set by $L^r(t) \equiv \text{CD4}(t)$ and the corresponding reduced observed data $O^r \equiv \left(\bar{Y}, \bar{L}^r, \bar{A}\right)$. Parallel to the notation introduced for P_0, we use $P_0^r = Q_0^r g_0^r$ to denote the distribution of O^r, where $Q_{0L^r(t)}^r$, $Q_{0Y(t)}^r$ and $g_{0A(t)}^r$ are defined by replacing $L(t)$ with $L^r(t)$ in the conditional distributions (24.13), (24.14), and (24.15), and where $Q_0^r \equiv Q_{0\bar{L}^r(\tilde{T})}^r \times Q_{0\bar{Y}(\tilde{T})}^r$.

Identifiability of the target causal parameter based on this new reduced-data structure requires stronger assumptions; each conditional independence statement of (24.11) needs to hold conditional on $\bar{L}^r(t)$ rather than $\bar{L}(t)$. This stronger identifiability assumption would impose additional restrictions on the allowed distributions of the error terms P_U and thus imply a working SCM different from that defined in (24.4). We develop a TMLE for this reduced observed data structure, then consider how this reduced-data TMLE can be modified such that it remains a consistent estimator of the target causal parameter β_{SM} under the original SCM working model implied by the weaker identifiability assumption (24.11) (given consistency of g_n or Q_n^0 and convergence of g_n to an appropriate distribution).

Under the reduced-data identifiability assumption, the target causal parameter β_{SM} can be represented as a function of the distribution of the reduced observed data distribution $\Psi_{SM}^r(Q_0^r)$, where Q_0^r is much lower dimensional than Q_0. We can estimate this target parameter with TMLE as described in Sect. 24.5.3, now applied to the reduced-data structure O^r. Briefly, Q_0^r and g_0^r can be factorized into a series of conditional distributions of binary variables, and maximum likelihood methods, potentially combined with data-adaptive approaches, can be applied to provide an initial estimator Q_n^{r0} and an estimator g_n^r. Updating Q_n^{r0} until convergence provides an estimate Q_n^{r*} of Q_0^r.

The problem is that the stronger identifiability assumption with respect to the reduced-data structure O^r might not hold, and as a result the substitution estimator $\Psi^r_{SM}(Q^{r*}_n)$ may be an inconsistent estimator of $\beta_{SM} = \Psi_{SM}(Q_0)$, even when $\Psi^r_{SM}(Q^{r*}_n)$ is a consistent (and efficient) estimator of $\Psi_{SM}(Q^r_0)$. That is, conditioning on time-varying covariates in addition to CD4 count may be required for the counterfactual outcome to be independent of censoring, treatment modifications, and interruptions and thus for the causal parameter to be identified as a parameter of the distribution of the observed data. The reduced-data TMLE can be modified to adjust for any such residual confounding by observed time-varying covariates other than CD4 count by using an estimator g_n of the true g_0 (the conditional distribution of the intervention variables in the nonreduced observed data), and applying inverse weights g^r_n/g_n to each of the estimation steps in the reduced-data TMLE procedure.

Specifically, for maximum-likelihood-based estimation of a conditional distribution $Q_B(B \mid Pa(B))$, where $Pa(B)$ only depends on $\bar{A}$ through $\bar{A}(t)$, we use weights $g^r_{n\bar{A}(t)}/g_{n\bar{A}(t)}$ to obtain an IPCW-R-ML-based initial estimator Q^{r0}_n of Q^r_0, and an IPCW-R-ML estimator of the fluctuation parameter ϵ in the TMLE step. The resulting IPCW-R-TMLE $\Psi_{SM}(Q^{r*}_n)$ is now a consistent estimator of $\Psi_{SM}(Q_0)$ if the true treatment and censoring mechanism g_0 is estimated consistently, and, in the case where g^r_n/g_n converges to 1, then this estimator is double robust with respect to misspecification of estimators of Q^r_0 and $g^r_0 = g_0$. For further details we refer the interested reader to Appendix A and van der Laan (2008b).

24.6 Discussion

An additional issue complicates the link between an SCM and the observed data. Ideally, the exact date at which censoring occurred would be known. For example, a subject transferring care to an alternative clinic would report the date of the transfer. In practice, however, censoring time C must often be approximated using an operational definition. Any algorithm used to define C should be based on past covariates in order to respect the temporal ordering in the underlying causal model. A common approach is to define censoring time based on a minimum duration during which no counting process for a subject has jumped. In order to maintain the link between the observed data and the underlying SCM, any data that do become available on a subject subsequent to C should not be used. Even when this approach is employed, however, the link between the observed data and the SCM will remain imperfect. For some subjects a period will exist during which a subject's follow-up status is incorrectly classified (e.g., a subject already died before our definition of censoring, but we do not know), resulting in time-updated observed covariates and outcomes that fail to reflect the true underlying processes.

In summary, SCMs are a useful tool for translating background knowledge and scientific questions into statistical models and target parameters, and for informing the interpretation of resulting parameter estimates by providing transparency regarding the assumptions needed in order for these estimates to approximate causal effects. As our discussion makes clear, however, the steps of specifying an SCM and its link to the observed data, defining a target causal parameter that adequately addresses the scientific question of interest, and implementing estimators of this parameter can each increase dramatically in complexity when applied to real clinical cohort data. We have raised several examples of possible complications as illustrations, but many more remain. Issues not addressed include the fact that the subjects in a clinical cohort are rarely a random sample from a well-defined population, and that many covariates will have substantial measurement error and/or potentially informative reporting processes. Acknowledgement of these challenges is not intended as a disincentive to using observational data to target causal questions, but rather as encouragement to approach such analyses systematically, to use a road map that clearly delineates between true causal knowledge and working models, and to remain humble in the interpretation of resulting estimates.

Chapter 25
Probability of Success of an In Vitro Fertilization Program

Antoine Chambaz

About 9 to 15% of couples have difficulty in conceiving a child, i.e., do not conceive within 12 months of attempting pregnancy (Boivin et al. 2007). In response to subfertility, assisted reproductive technology has developed over the last 30 years, resulting in in vitro fertilization (IVF) techniques (the first "test-tube baby" was born in 1978). Nowadays, more than 40,000 IVF cycles are performed each year in France and more than 63,000 in the USA (Adamson et al. 2006). Yet, how to quantify the success in assisted reproduction still remains a matter of debate. One could, for instance, rely on the number of pregnancies or deliveries per IVF cycle. However, an IVF program often consists of several successive IVF cycles. So, instead of considering each IVF cycle separately, one could rather rely on an evaluation of the whole program. IVF programs are emotionally and physically burdensome. Providing the patients with the most adequate and accurate measure of success is therefore an important issue that we propose to address in this chapter.

25.1 The DAIFI Study

Our contribution is based on the French Devenir Après Interruption de la FIV (DAIFI) study (Soullier et al. 2008; de la Rochebrochard et al. 2008, 2009). In France, the four first IVF cycles are fully reimbursed by the national health insurance system. Therefore, as in the previous references, we conclude that the most adequate measure of success for French couples is the probability of delivery (resulting from embryo transfer) during the course of a program of at most four IVF cycles. We will refer to this quantity as the probability of success of a program of at most four IVF cycles, or even sometimes as the probability of success.

Data were provided by two French IVF units (Cochin in Paris and Clermont-Ferrand, a medium-sized city in central France). All women who followed their first IVF cycle in these units between 1998 and 2002 and who were under 42 at the start of the cycle were included. Women over 42 were not included, unless they had a normal ovarian reserve and a specific IVF indication. For every enrolled woman, the data were mainly the attended IVF unit and the woman's date of birth, and for each IVF cycle, its start date, number of oocytes harvested, number of embryos transferred or frozen, indicators of pregnancy, and successful delivery (for a comprehensive description, see de la Rochebrochard et al. 2009). Data collection was discontinued after the woman's fourth IVF cycle. Since the first four IVF cycles are fully reimbursed, it is reasonable to assume that economic factors do not play a role in the phenomenon of interest. Specifically, whether a couple will abandon the IVF program mid-course without a successful delivery or undergo the whole program does not depend on economic factors (on the contrary, if the IVF cycles were not fully reimbursed, then disadvantaged couples would likely abandon the program mid-course more easily). Furthermore, successive IVF cycles occur close together in time: hence, the sole age at the start of the first IVF cycle is a relevant summary of the successive ages at the start of each IVF cycle during the program. Likewise, we make the assumption that the number of embryos transferred or frozen during the first IVF cycle is a relevant summary of the successive number of harvested oocytes and transferred or frozen embryos associated to each IVF cycle (i.e., a relevant summary measure of the couple's fertility during the program). Relaxing this assumption will be considered in future work.

Estimating the probability of success of a program of at most four IVF cycles is not easy due to couples who abandon the IVF program mid-course without a successful delivery. Moreover, since those couples have a smaller probability of having a child than couples that undergo the whole program, it would be wrong to ignore the right censoring, and simply count the proportion of successes (Soullier et al. 2008), even if the decision to abandon the program is not informed by any relevant factors. In addition, it seems likely that some of the baseline factors, such as baseline fertility, might be predictive of the dropout time (measured on the discrete scale of number of IVF cycles): in statistical terms, we expect that the right-censoring mechanism will be informative.

Three approaches to estimating the probability of success of a program of at most four IVF cycles are considered in Soullier et al. (2008). The most naive approach estimates the probability of success as the ratio of the number of deliveries successive to the first IVF cycle to the total number of enrolled women, yielding a point estimate of 37% and a 95% confidence interval given by $(0.35, 0.38)$. This first approach obviously overlooks a lot of information in the data.

A second approach is a standard nonparametric survival analysis based on the Kaplan–Meier estimator. Specifically, Soullier et al. (2008) compute the Kaplan–Meier estimate S_n of the survival function $t \mapsto P(T \geq t)$, where T denotes the number of IVF cycles attempted after the first one till the first successful delivery. The observed data structure is represented as $(\min(T, C), I(T \leq C))$, with C the right-censoring time. The estimated probability of success is given by $1 - S_n(3)$. This method resulted in an estimated probability of success equal to 52% and a 95% confidence interval $(0.49, 0.55)$. This much more sensible approach still neglects the baseline covariates and thus assumes that a woman's decision to abandon the program is not informed by relevant factors that predict future success, such as those measured at baseline. One could argue that this method should provide an estimated upper bound on the probability of success.

Actually, formulating the problem of interest in terms of survival analysis is a sensible option, and indeed the methods in Part V for right-censored data can be employed to estimate the survival function of T. In Sect. 25.6, we discuss the equivalence between our approach presented here and the survival analysis approach.

In order to improve the estimate of the probability of success, Soullier et al. (2008) finally resort to the so-called multiple imputation methodology (Schafer 1997; Little and Rubin 2002). Based on iteratively estimating missing data using the past, this third approach leads to a point estimate equal to 46%, with a 95% confidence interval given by (0.44, 0.48).

The three methods that we summarized either answer only partially the question of interest (naive approach and nonparametric Kaplan–Meier analysis) or suffer from bias due to reliance on parametric models (multiple-imputation approach). We expose in the next sections how the TMLE methodology paves the way to solving this delicate problem with great consideration for theoretical validity.

25.2 Data, Model, and Parameter

The observed data structure is longitudinal:

$$O = (L_0, A_0, L_1, A_1, L_2, A_2, L_3 = Y),$$

where $L_0 = (L_{0,1}, L_{0,2}, L_{0,3}, L_{0,4})$ denote the baseline covariates and $L_{0,1}$ indicates the IVF center, $L_{0,2}$ indicates the age of the woman at the start of the first IVF cycle, $L_{0,3}$ indicates the number of embryos transferred or frozen at the first IVF cycle, and $L_{0,4}$ indicates whether the first IVF cycle is successful, i.e., yields a delivery, ($L_{0,4} = 1$) or not ($L_{0,4} = 0$). For each $1 \le j \le 3$, A_{j-1} indicates whether the woman completes her jth IVF cycle ($A_{j-1} = 1$) or not ($A_{j-1} = 0$) this also encodes for dropout, and L_j indicates whether the jth IVF cycle is successful ($L_j = 1$) or not ($L_j = 0$). The longitudinal data structure becomes degenerate after a time point t at which either the woman abandons the program ($A_t = 0$) or has a successful IVF cycle ($L_t = 1$ for some t). By encoding convention, the data structure O is constrained as follows. (1) If $A_{j-1} = 0$ for some $1 \le j < 3$, then $A_j = \ldots = A_2 = 0$ and $L_j = \ldots = L_3 = Y = 0$. (2) If $L_{0,4} = 1$, then $L_1 = \ldots = L_3 = Y = 1$ and $A_0 = \ldots = A_2 = 1$, and similarly if $L_j = 1$ for some $1 \le j < 3$, then $L_{j+1} = \ldots = L_3 = Y = 1$ and $A_j = \ldots = A_2 = 1$, too.

The true data generating distribution of O is denoted by P_0. We assume that the following positivity assumption holds: P_0–almost surely, for each $0 \le j \le 2$:

$$0 < P_0\left(A_j = 1 \mid L_{1:j} = 0_{1:j}, A_{0:j-1} = 1_{0:j-1}, L_{0,4} = 0, (L_{0,1}, L_{0,2}, L_{0,3})\right),$$

with notation $x_{i:j} = (x_i, \ldots, x_j) \in \mathbb{R}^{j-i+1}$ for $i \le j$, and the obvious convention $x_{1:0} = A_{1:0} = L_{1:0} = \emptyset$. This assumption states that, for each $0 \le j \le 2$, conditionally on observing a woman who already went through $(j+1)$ unsuccessful IVF cycles, it cannot be certain, based on past information $(L_{0:j}, A_{0:j-1})$, that a $(j+2)$-th IVF cycle will not be attempted. As discussed in Chap. 10, positivity can be tested from the data.

We see P_0 as an element of the statistical model $\mathcal{M}$ of all possible probability distributions of O (satisfying, in particular, the constraints imposed by the encoding convention and positivity assumption). Set $\mathcal{M}$ is large because a model should reflect only true knowledge and because we lack any meaningful knowledge about the true data-generating distribution P_0 that would allow us to enforce further restrictions.

The parameter mapping of interest, $\Psi(P)$, is the following explicit functional of a candidate data-generating distribution P:

$$\Psi(P) = E_P\Bigg(\sum_{\ell_{1:2}\in\{0,1\}^2} P(Y = 1 \mid A_{0:2} = 1_{0:2}, L_{1:2} = \ell_{1:2}, L_0) \\ \times P(L_2 = \ell_2 \mid A_{0:1} = 1_{0:1}, L_1 = \ell_1, L_0) \times P(L_1 = \ell_1 \mid A_0 = 1, L_0) \Bigg), \quad (25.1)$$

where, by convention, for each $2 \leq j \leq 3$,

$$P\Big(L_j = \ell_j \mid A_{0:j-1} = 1_{0:j-1}, L_{1:j-1} = \ell_{1:j-1}, L_{0,4} = \ell_{0,4}, (L_{0,1}, L_{0,2}, L_{0,3})\Big) = 0, \quad (25.2)$$

whenever the event $[(L_{0,4}, A_0, L_1, A_1, L_2, A_2, L_3) = (\ell_{0,4}, 1, \ell_1, 1, \ell_2, 1, \ell_3)]$ does not meet the encoding constraints. The objective of this chapter is to provide a point estimate and a 95% confidence interval for the statistical target parameter $\psi_0 = \Psi(P_0)$.

The parameter of interest $\psi_0 = \Psi(P_0)$ in (25.1) is a well-defined statistical parameter on the nonparametric statistical model $\mathcal{M}$. Its causal interpretation is enlightening, and can be derived in two different frameworks. Furthermore, it is not necessary to rely on the causal interpretation to justify the scientific interest of ψ_0 as a pure statistical estimand.

The first causal interpretation of (25.1) relies on the so-called counterfactual framework. Let us first introduce the set $\mathcal{A}$ of all possible realizations of $A_{0:2}$: $\mathcal{A} = \{(0,0,0), (1,0,0), (1,1,0), (1,1,1)\}$. By Theorem 2.1 in Yu and van der Laan (2002), there exists an *explicit* construction $L_a = f_a(O, P_0)$, $a \in \mathcal{A}$, involving augmenting the probability space with an independent draw of uniformly distributed random variables and quantile-quantile functions for discrete random variables, so that we have consistency, P_0–almost surely, $O = (A, L_A)$, and randomization, for all $0 \leq j \leq 2$, A_j, is independent of $X = (L_a : a \in xA)$ conditionally on the observed data history $(L_{0:j}, A_{0:j-1})$. Let $Y_{(1,1,1)}$ denote the last coordinate of $L_{(1,1,1)}$: $Y_{(1,1,1)} = 1$ if and only if the woman finally gives birth after four IVF cycles (the IVF program being interrupted if the woman gives birth mid-course).

Theorem 3.1 of Yu and van der Laan (2002), also guarantees that

$$\Pr(Y_{(1,1,1)} = 1) = E_{P_0}\Bigg(\sum_{\ell_{1:2}\in\{0,1\}^2} P_0\left(Y = 1 \mid A_{0:2} = 1_{0:2}, L_{1:2} = \ell_{1:2}, L_0\right) \\ \times P_0\left(L_2 = \ell_2 \mid A_{0:1} = 1_{0:1}, L_1 = \ell_1, L_0\right) \\ \times P_0\left(L_1 = \ell_1 \mid A_0 = 1, L_0\right)\Bigg). \quad (25.3)$$

This equality is an example of the g-computation formula. It relates the probability distribution of $Y_{(1,1,1)}$ to the probability distribution of the observed data structure O. In addition, it teaches us that $\psi_0 = \Psi(P_0)$ can be interpreted (at the cost of a weak assumption) as the probability of a successful outcome after four IVF cycles (the IVF program being interrupted if the woman gives birth mid-course). Note that when $L_{0,4} = 1$, the sum has only one nonzero term, whereas it has three nonzero terms when $L_{0,4} = 0$.

We need to emphasize that the counterfactuals whose existence is guaranteed by these theorems in Yu and van der Laan (2002), and Gill and Robins (2001) are not necessarily interesting nor have an interpretation that is causal *in the real world.* The structural equations framework that we present hereafter makes the definition of counterfactuals explicit and truly causal since they correspond with intervening on the system of equations (Chap. 2). Alternatively, as in the Neyman–Rubin counterfactual framework discussed in Chap. 21, one defines the counterfactuals in terms of an experiment, and one assumes the consistency and randomization assumption with respect to these user-supplied definitions of the counterfactuals.

It is possible, at the cost of untestable (and stronger) assumptions, to provide another interpretation of (25.1). This second interpretation is at the core of Pearl (2009). It is of course compatible with the previous one. Let us assume that the random phenomenon of interest has *no unmeasured confounders.* A causal graph is equivalent to the following system of structural equations: there exist ten independent random variables $(U^1_{L_0}, \ldots, U^4_{L_0}, U_{A_0}, U_{L_1}, \ldots, U_{A_2}, U_{L_3})$ and ten deterministic functions $(f^1_{L_0}, \ldots, f^4_{L_0}, f_{A_0}, f_{L_1}, \ldots, f_{A_2}, f_{L_3})$ such that

$$\begin{cases} L_{0,1} = f^1_{L_0}(U^1_{L_0}), \\ L_{0,2} = f^2_{L_0}(L_{0,1}, U^2_{L_0}), \\ L_{0,3} = f^3_{L_0}(L_{0,2}, L_{0,1}, U^3_{L_0}), \\ L_{0,4} = f^4_{L_0}(L_{0,3}, L_{0,2}, L_{0,1}, U^4_{L_0}), \\ \quad \text{and for every } 0 \le j \le 2, \\ A_j = f_{A_j}(L_{0:j-1}, A_{0:j-1}, U_{A_j}), \\ L_{j+1} = f_{L_{j+1}}(A_{0:j}, L_{0:j}, U_{L_{j+1}}). \end{cases} \quad (25.4)$$

One can intervene upon this system by setting the intervention nodes $A_{0:2}$ equal to some values $a_{0:2} \in \mathcal{A}$. Formally, this simply amounts to substituting the equality $A_j = a_j$ to $A_j = f_{A_j}(L_{0:j}, A_{0:j-1}, U_{A_j})$ for all $0 \le j \le 2$ in (25.4). This yields a new causal graph, the so-called graph under intervention $A_{0:2} = a_{0:2}$. The intervened, new, causal graph or system of structural equations describes how $Y = L_3$ is randomly generated under this intervention. Under the intervention $A_{0:2} = a_{0:2}$, this last (chronologically speaking) random variable is denoted by $Y_{a_{0:2}}$, naturally using the same notation. Moreover, it is known (see, for instance, Robins 1986, 1987a; Pearl 2009) that the g-computation formula (25.3) also holds in this nonparametric structural equation model framework, relating the probability distribution of $Y_{(1,1,1)}$ to the probability distribution of the observed data structure O.

Finally, even if one is not willing to rely on the causal assumptions in the SCM, and one is also not satisfied with the definition of an effect in terms of explicitly constructed counterfactuals, there is still a way forward. Assuming that the time ordering of observed variables $L_{0:4}$ and $A_{0:2}$ is correct (which it indeed is), the target parameter still represents an effect of interest aiming to get as close as possible to a causal effect as the data allow. In any case, $\psi_0 = \Psi(P_0)$ is a well-defined effect of an intervention on the distribution of the data, that can be interpreted as a variable importance measure (Chaps. 4, 22, and 23).

25.3 The TMLE

It can be shown that Ψ is a pathwise differentiable parameter (Appendix A). Therefore the theory of semiparametric models applies, providing a notion of asymptotically efficient estimation and, in particular, its key ingredient, the efficient influence curve. The TMLE procedure takes advantage of the pathwise differentiability and related properties in order to build an asymptotically efficient substitution estimator of $\psi_0 = \Psi(P_0)$.

Let $L_0^2(P)$ denote the set of measurable functions s mapping the set $\mathcal{O}$ (where the observed data structure takes its values) to $\mathbb{R}$, such that $Ps = 0$ and $Ps^2 < \infty$ [we recall that $P\varphi$ is shorthand notation for $E_P\varphi(O)$ for any $\varphi \in L^1(P)$]. A fluctuation model $\{P(\epsilon) : |\epsilon| < \eta\} \subset \mathcal{M}$ is a one-dimensional parametric model such that $P(0) = P$. Its score at $\epsilon = 0$ is $s \in L_0^2(P)$ if the derivative at $\epsilon = 0$ of the log-likelihood $\epsilon \mapsto \log P(\epsilon)(O)$ equals $s(O)$:

$$\frac{\partial}{\partial\epsilon} \log P(\epsilon)(O)\Big|_{\epsilon=0} = s(O).$$

As presented in Chap. 25 of van der Vaart (1998), the functional Ψ is pathwise differentiable at $\mathcal{M}$ with respect to $L_0^2(P)$ if there exists $D \in L_0^2(P)$ such that, for any fluctuation model $\{P(\epsilon) : |\epsilon| < \eta\}$ with score s, the function $\epsilon \mapsto \Psi(P(\epsilon))$ is differentiable at $\epsilon = 0$, with

$$\frac{\partial}{\partial\epsilon} \Psi(P(\epsilon))\Big|_{\epsilon=0} = PsD.$$

In the context of this chapter, if such a $D \in L_0^2(P)$ exists, then it is called the efficient influence curve. Remarkably, the asymptotic variance of a regular estimator of the pathwise differentiable parameter $\Psi(P)$ is lower-bounded by the variance of the efficient influence curve. For that reason in particular, it is important to determine if Ψ is pathwise differentiable and, if it is, to derive its efficient influence curve.

Let us introduce the shorthand notation $Q(L_0; P) = P(L_0)$, $Q(L_1 \mid A_0, L_0; P) = P(L_1 \mid A_0, L_0)$, $Q(L_2 \mid A_{0:1}, L_{0:1}; P) = P(L_2 \mid A_{0:1}, L_{0:1})$, $Q(Y \mid A_{0:2}, L_{0:2}; P) = P(Y \mid A_{0:2}, L_{0:2})$, $g(A_0 \mid X; P) = P(A_0 \mid L_0)$, $g(A_{0:1} \mid X; P) = g(A_0 \mid X; P) \times P(A_1 \mid L_{0:1}, A_0)$, and $g(A_{0:2} \mid X; P) = g(A_{0:1} \mid X; P) \times P(A_2 \mid L_{0:2}, A_{0:1})$. The likelihood $P(O)$ can be represented as

$$P(O) = \prod_{j=0}^{3} Q(L_j \mid A_{0:j-1}, L_{0:j-1}; P)$$
$$\times \prod_{j=0}^{2} g(A_j = 1 \mid A_{0:j-1}, L_{0:j}; P)^{A_j} (1 - g(A_j = 1 \mid A_{0:j-1}, L_{0:j}; P))^{1-A_j}$$

and thus factorizes as $P = Qg$. The parameter of interest at $P = Qg$ can be straightforwardly expressed as a function of Q:

$$\Psi(P) = E_P\Bigg(\sum_{\ell_{1:2} \in \{0,1\}^2} Q(Y = 1 \mid A_{0:2} = 1_{0:2}, L_{1:2} = \ell_{1:2}, L_0; P)$$
$$\times Q(L_2 = \ell_2 \mid A_{0:1} = 1_{0:1}, L_1 = \ell_1, L_0; P) \times Q(L_1 = \ell_1 \mid A_0 = 1, L_0; P)\Bigg).$$

Note that the outer expectation is with respect to the probability distribution $Q(L_0; P)$ of the baseline covariates L_0.

The following proposition states that Ψ is pathwise differentiable and it presents its efficient influence curve at $P \in \mathcal{M}$.

Proposition 25.1. *The functional Ψ is pathwise differentiable at every $P \in \mathcal{M}$. The efficient influence curve $D^*(\cdot \mid P)$ at $P \in \mathcal{M}$ is written*

$$D^*(\cdot \mid P) = \sum_{j=0}^{3} D_j^*(\cdot \mid P),$$

where

$$\begin{aligned} D_0^*(O \mid P) &= E_P(Y_{(1,1,1)} \mid L_0) - \Psi(P) \\ &= P(L_1 = 1 \mid A_0 = 1, L_0) \\ &\quad + P(L_1 = 0 \mid A_0 = 1, L_0) \times P(L_2 = 1 \mid A_{0:1} = 1_{0:1}, L_1 = 0, L_0) \\ &\quad + P(L_1 = 0 \mid A_0 = 1, L_0) \times P(L_2 = 0 \mid A_{0:1} = 1_{0:1}, L_1 = 0, L_0) \\ &\quad \times P(Y = 1 \mid A_{0:2} = 1_{0:2}, L_{1:2} = 0_{1:2}, L_0) - \Psi(P), \end{aligned}$$

$$\begin{aligned} D_1^*(O \mid P) &= \frac{I(A_0 = 1)}{g(A_0 = 1 \mid X; P)} \times (L_1 - P(L_1 = 1 \mid A_0, L_0)) \\ &\quad \times \{E_{Q_0}(Y_{(1,1,1)} \mid L_0, A_0 = 1, L_1 = 1) - E_{Q_0}(Y_{(1,1,1)} \mid L_0, A_0 = 1, L_1 = 0)\} \\ &= \frac{I(A_0 = 1)}{g(A_0 = 1 \mid X; P)} \times (1 - P(L_2 = 1 \mid A_{0:1} = 1_{0:1}, L_1 = 0, L_0) \end{aligned}$$

$$\times P(Y = 1 \mid A_{0:2} = 1_{0:2}, L_{1:2} = (0,1), L_0)$$
$$- P(L_2 = 0 \mid A_{0:1} = 1_{0:1}, L_1 = 0, L_0)$$
$$\times P(Y = 1 \mid A_{0:2} = 1_{0:2}, L_{1:2} = 0_{1:2}, L_0))$$
$$\times (L_1 - P(L_1 = 1 \mid A_0, L_0)),$$

$$D_2^*(O \mid P) = \frac{I(A_{0:1} = 1_{0:1})}{g(A_{0:1} = 1_{0:1} \mid X; P)} \times (L_2 - P(L_2 = 1 \mid A_{0:1}, L_{0:1}))$$
$$\times \{E_{Q_0}(Y_{(1,1,1)} \mid L_{0:1}, A_{0:1} = 1, L_2 = 1) - E_{Q_0}(Y_{(1,1,1)} \mid L_{0:1}, A_{0:1} = 1, L_2 = 0)\}$$
$$= \frac{I(A_{0:1} = 1_{0:1})}{g(A_{0:1} = 1_{0:1} \mid X; P)} \times (P(Y = 1 \mid A_{0:2} = 1_{0:2}, L_2 = 1, L_{0:1})$$
$$- P(Y = 1 \mid A_{0:2} = 1_{0:2}, L_2 = 0, L_{0:1}))$$
$$\times (L_2 - P(L_2 = 1 \mid A_{0:1}, L_{0:1})),$$

$$D_3^*(O \mid P) = \frac{I(A_{0:2} = 1_{0:2})}{g(A_{0:2} = 1_{0:2} \mid X; P)} \times (Y - P(Y = 1 \mid A_{0:2}, L_{0:2})),$$

and the latter equalities involve convention (25.2). Furthermore, the efficient influence curve $D^*(\cdot \mid P)$ is double robust: if $P_0 = Q_0 g_0$ and $P = Qg$, then

$$E_{P_0} D^*(O \mid P) = 0 \quad \textit{implies} \quad \Psi(P) = \Psi(P_0)$$

if either $Q = Q_0$ or $g = g_0$.

The theory of semiparametric models teaches us that the asymptotic variance of any regular estimator of ψ_0 is lower-bounded by the variance of the efficient influence curve, $E_{P_0} D^*(O \mid P_0)^2$. A regular estimator of ψ_0 having as limit distribution the mean-zero Gaussian distribution with variance $E_{P_0} D^*(O \mid P_0)^2$ is therefore said to be asymptotically efficient.

25.3.1 TMLE Procedure

We assume that we observe n independent copies $O^{(1)}, \ldots, O^{(n)}$ of the observed data structure O. The TMLE procedure takes advantage of the pathwise differentiability of the parameter of interest and bends an initial estimator, obtained as a substitution estimator $\Psi(P_n^0)$, into an updated substitution estimator $\Psi(P_n^*)$ (with P_n^* an update of P_n^0), which enjoys better properties.

Initial estimate. We start by constructing an initial estimate P_n^0 of the distribution P_0 of O, which could also be used to construct an initial estimate $\psi_n^0 = \Psi(P_n^0)$. The initial estimator of the probability distribution of the baseline covariates will be defined as the empirical probability distribution of $L_0^{(i)}$, $i = 1, \ldots, n$. The initial estimate of the other factors of P_n^0 is obtained by super learning, using the log-likelihood loss function for each of the binary conditional distributions in Q_0.

Updating the initial estimate. The optimal theoretical properties enjoyed by a super learner P_n^0 as an estimator of P_0 do not necessarily translate into optimal properties of $\Psi(P_n^0)$ as an estimator of the parameter of interest $\psi_0 = \Psi(P_0)$. In particular, writing $P_n^0 = Q_n^0 g_n^0$, due to the curse of dimensionality, $\Psi(Q_n^0)$ may still be overly biased due to an optimized tradeoff in bias and variance with respect to the infinite-dimensional parameter Q_0 instead of $\Psi(Q_0)$ itself.

The second step of the TMLE procedure stretches the initial estimate P_n^0 in the direction of the targeted parameter of interest, through a maximum likelihood step. If the initial estimate $\Psi(P_n^0)$ is biased, then this step removes all asymptotic bias for the target parameter whenever the g-factor of P_0, g_0, is estimated consistently: in fact, it maps an inconsistent $\Psi(P_n^0)$ into a consistent TMLE of ψ_0. Hence, the resulting updated estimator is said to be double robust: it is consistent if the initial first-stage estimator of the Q-factor of P_0, Q_0, is consistent or if the g-factor of P_0, g_0, is consistently estimated.

Let's now describe the specific TMLE. We first fluctuate P_n^0 with respect to the conditional distribution of Y given its past $(A_{0:2}, L_{0:2})$, i.e., construct a fluctuation model $\{P_n^0(\epsilon) : |\epsilon| < \eta\}$ through P_n^0 at $\epsilon = 0$ whose score at $\epsilon = 0$ is $D_3^*(\cdot \mid P_n^0)$. Fit ϵ with maximum likelihood. This yields an intermediate update $P_n^0(\epsilon_n^0)$ of P_n^0, which we denote by P_n^1. Then, iteratively from $j = 2$ to $j = 1$, we fluctuate P_n^{3-j} with respect to the conditional distribution of L_j given its past $(A_{0:j-1}, L_{0:j-1})$, using a fluctuation model $\{P_n^{3-j}(\epsilon) : |\epsilon| < \eta\}$ through P_n^{3-j} at $\epsilon = 0$ whose score at $\epsilon = 0$ is $D_j^*(\cdot \mid P_n^{3-j})$, and fitting ϵ with maximum likelihood. This produces a final estimate P_n^* of P_0 that is targeted toward the parameter of interest. The TMLE of ψ_0 is the corresponding substitution estimator $\psi_n^* = \Psi(P_n^*)$.

This TMLE corresponds with selecting the log-likelihood loss function $L(P) = -\log P$ and selecting a parametric model $\{P(\epsilon) : \epsilon\}$, ϵ multivariate, a separate ϵ-component for each factor of $Q(\cdot \mid P)$, no fluctuation of $g(\cdot \mid P)$, and using the recursive backwards MLE-updating algorithm that starts at the last factor and ends at first factor (as originally presented in van der Laan 2010a).

In this simple setting, the construction of the aforementioned fluctuations is easy. It is, for instance, possible to select as parametric fluctuation working models simple univariate logistic regression models. Indeed, let us introduce the so-called *clever covariate* for fluctuating the conditional distribution of Y under P_n^0, the last factor of $Q_n^0 = Q(\cdot \mid P_n^0)$, as $H_{n,3}^* = I(A_{0:2} = 1_{0:2})/g(A_{0:2} = 1_{0:2} \mid X; P_n^0)$. It is straightforward to check that the fluctuation model

$$P_n^0(\epsilon)(O) = \text{expit}\left(\text{logit}\, Q(Y \mid A_{0:2}, L_{0:2}; P_n^0) + \epsilon H_{n,3}^*\right)^Y \times\left[1 - \text{expit}\left(\text{logit}\, Q(Y \mid A_{0:2}, L_{0:2}; P_n^0) + \epsilon H_{n,3}^*\right)\right]^{(1-Y)} \times P_n^0(A_{0:2}, L_{0:2})$$

goes through P_n^0 at $\epsilon = 0$, with a score at $\epsilon = 0$ equal to $D_3^*(\cdot; P_n^0)$. Let $\epsilon_{n,3}$ denote the maximum likelihood estimate in the model, and let $P_n^1 = P_n^0(\epsilon_{n,3})$ be the update of P_n^0. Likewise, let us introduce the second clever covariate for fluctuating the conditional distribution of L_2 under P_n^1, the "next" factor of $Q_n^1 = Q(\cdot \mid P_n^1)$:

$$H^*_{n,2} = \frac{I(A_{0:1} = 1_{0:1})}{g(A_{0:1} = 1_{0:1} \mid X; P_n^1)} \times \left(P_n^1(Y = 1 \mid A_{0:2} = 1_{0:2}, L_2 = 1, L_{0:1}) - P_n^1(Y = 1 \mid A_{0:2} = 1_{0:2}, L_2 = 0, L_{0:1})\right)$$

and the related fluctuation model

$$P_n^1(\epsilon)(O) = Q(Y \mid A_{0:2}, L_{0:2}; P_n^1) \times g(A_2 = 1 \mid X; P_n^1)^{A_2}(1 - g(A_2 = 1 \mid X; P_n^1))^{1-A_2}$$
$$\times \text{expit}\left(\text{logit}\, Q(L_2 \mid A_{0:1}, L_{0:1}; P_n^1) + \epsilon H^*_{n,2}\right)^{L_2}$$
$$\times \left[1 - \text{expit}\left(\text{logit}\, Q(L_2 \mid A_{0:1}, L_{0:1}; P_n^1) + \epsilon H^*_{n,2}\right)\right]^{(1-L_2)} \times P_n^1(A_{0:1}, L_{0:1}).$$

Again, it is easy to verify that the latter fluctuation model goes through P_n^1 at $\epsilon = 0$, with a score at $\epsilon = 0$ equal to $D_2^*(\cdot \mid P_n^1)$. Let $\epsilon_{n,2}$ denote the maximum likelihood estimate in the model, and let $P_n^2 = P_n^1(\epsilon_{n,2})$ be the corresponding update. Finally, let us introduce the third clever covariate for fluctuating the conditional distribution of L_1 under P_n^2, the "next" factor of $Q_n^2 = Q(\cdot \mid P_n^2)$:

$$H^*_{n,1} = \frac{I(A_0 = 1)}{g(A_0 = 1 \mid X; P_n^2)} \times (1 - P_n^2(L_2 = 1 \mid A_{0:1} = 1_{0:1}, L_1 = 0, L_0)$$
$$\times P_n^2(Y = 1 \mid A_{0:2} = 1_{0:2}, L_{1:2} = (0,1), L_0) - P_n^2(L_2 = 0 \mid A_{0:1} = 1_{0:1}, L_1 = 0, L_0)$$
$$\times P_n^2(Y = 1 \mid A_{0:2} = 1_{0:2}, L_{1:2} = 0_{1:2}, L_0))$$

and the related fluctuation model

$$P_n^2(\epsilon)(O) = \prod_{j=2}^{3} Q(L_j \mid A_{0:j}, L_{0:j}; P_n^2)$$
$$\times \prod_{j=1}^{2} g(A_j = 1 \mid X; P_n^2)^{A_j}(1 - g(A_j = 1 \mid X; P_n^2))^{1-A_j}$$
$$\times \text{expit}\left(\text{logit}\, Q(L_1 \mid A_0, L_0; P_n^2) + \epsilon H^*_{n,1}\right)^{L_1}$$
$$\times \left[1 - \text{expit}\left(\text{logit}\, Q(L_1 \mid A_0, L_0; P_n^2) + \epsilon H^*_{n,1}\right)\right]^{(1-L_1)} P_n^2(A_0, L_0).$$

Once again, this fluctuation model goes through P_n^2 at $\epsilon = 0$, with its score at $\epsilon = 0$ equal to $D_1^*(\cdot \mid P_n^2)$. Let $\epsilon_{n,1}$ denote the maximum likelihood estimate in the model, and we define $P_n^* = P_n^2(\epsilon_{n,1})$. The first (and last) factor is the marginal distribution of L_0 under P_n^0, which is thus the empirical probability distribution of L_0. This is already a nonparametric maximum likelihood estimator, so that carrying out another updating step as above will result in an estimate of ϵ equal to zero. The TMLE of ψ_0 is the resulting substitution estimator $\Psi(P_n^*)$.

A closer look at the construction of P_n^* finally yields the following result:

Proposition 25.2. *It holds that*

(1) *For each* $1 \le j \le 3$, $D_j^*(\cdot \mid P_n^{3-j}) = D_j^*(\cdot \mid P_n^*)$.

(2) $Q(L_0; P_n^0) = \frac{1}{n} \sum_{i=1}^n I(L_0^{(i)} = L_0)$ *(expressed in words, the marginal distribution of* L_0 *is estimated with its empirical distribution), and* $P_n D^*(\cdot \mid P_n^*) = 0$.

(3) *The TMLE of* ψ_0, $\psi_n^* = \Psi(P_n^*)$, *satisfies*

$$\psi_n^* = \frac{1}{n} \sum_{i=1}^n \sum_{\ell_{1:2} \in \{0,1\}^2} Q(Y = 1 \mid A_{0:2} = 1_{0:2}, L_{1:2} = \ell_{1:2}, L_0^{(i)}; P_n^*)$$
$$\times Q(L_2 = \ell_2 \mid A_{0:1} = 1_{0:1}, L_1 = \ell_1, L_0^{(i)}; P_n^*) \times Q(L_1 = \ell_1 \mid A_0 = 1, L_0^{(i)}; P_n^*).$$

Item (1) in Proposition 25.2 is an example of the so-called *monotonicity* property of the clever covariates, which states that the clever covariate of the *j*th factor in Q_0 only depends on the future (later) factors of Q_0. This monotonicity property implies that the TMLE procedure presented above converges in one single step, referring to the iterative nature of the general TMLE procedure. A typical iterative TMLE procedure (Chap. 24 and Appendix A) would use the same logistic regression fluctuation models as presented above, but it would enforce a common ϵ across the different factors of Q_0, and thus updates all factors simultaneously at each maximum likelihood update step. This iterative TMLE converges very fast: in similar examples, experience shows that convergence is often achieved in two or three steps, and that most reduction occurs during the first step). Item (2) is of fundamental importance since it allows us to study the properties of $\Psi(P_n^*)$ from the point of view of the general theory of estimating equations. Item (3) just states that ψ_n^* is a plug-in estimator $\Psi(P_n^*)$ and provides a simple formula for evaluating ψ_n^*.

25.3.2 Merits of TMLE Procedure

Since the efficient influence curve $D^*(\cdot \mid P)$ is double robust and since P_n^* solves the efficient influence curve estimating equation, the general theory of estimating equations teaches us that the TMLE ψ_n^* enjoys remarkable asymptotic properties under certain assumptions. Stating the latter assumptions is outside the scope of this chapter. One often refers to such conditions as *regularity conditions*. Let $P_n^* = Q_n^* g_n^*$. The regularity conditions typically include the requirements that the sequence $(\psi_n^* : n = 1, \ldots)$ must belong to a compact set; that both Q_n^* and g_n^* must converge to some Q_1 and g_1 with at least one of these limits representing the truth; that the estimated efficient influence curve $D(\cdot \mid P_n^*)$ must belong to a P_0-Donsker class with P_0-probability tending to one; and that a second-order term that involves a product of $Q_n^* - Q_1$ and $g_n^* - g_1$ is $o_P(1/\sqrt{n})$. See Appendix A for more details.

The following classical result holds:

Proposition 25.3. *Under regularity conditions,*

(1) *The TMLE* ψ_n^* *consistently estimates* ψ_0 *as soon as either* Q_n^* *or* g_n^* *consistently estimates* Q_0 *or* g_0.

(2) If the TMLE consistently estimates ψ_0, then it is asymptotically linear: there exists D such that

$$\sqrt{n}(\psi_n^* - \psi_0) = \frac{1}{\sqrt{n}} \sum_{i=1}^{n} D(O^{(i)}) + o_P(1). \quad (25.5)$$

Equation (25.5) straightforwardly yields that $\sqrt{n}(\psi_n^* - \psi_0)$ is asymptotically Gaussian with mean zero and variance consistently estimated by

$$\frac{1}{n} \sum_{i=1}^{n} D_n(O^{(i)})^2,$$

where D_n is a consistent estimator of influence curve D.

If Q_n^* and g_n^* consistently estimate Q_0 and g_0 (hence P_n^* consistently estimates P_0), then $D = D^*(\cdot; P_0)$, so that the asymptotic variance is consistently estimated by

$$\frac{1}{n} \sum_{i=1}^{n} D^*(O^{(i)} \mid P_n^*)^2. \quad (25.6)$$

In this case, the TMLE is asymptotically efficient: its asymptotic variance is as small as possible (in the family of regular estimators).

Furthermore, if g_n^* is a maximum-likelihood-based consistent estimator of g_0, then (25.6) is a conservative estimator of the asymptotic variance of $\sqrt{n}(\psi_n^* - \psi_0)$ (it converges to an upper bound on the latter asymptotic variance).

Proposition 25.3 is the cornerstone of the TMLE methodology. It allows us to build confidence intervals. We assess how well such confidence intervals perform from a practical point of view through a simulation study in Sect. 25.4. For the estimation of the probability of success carried out in Sect. 25.5, we resort to the bootstrap to compute a confidence interval.

We emphasized how the TMLE benefits from advances in the theory of estimating equations. Yet, it enjoys some remarkable advantages over estimating equation methods. Let us briefly evoke the most striking in the context of this chapter:

(1) The TMLE is a substitution estimator. Thus, it automatically satisfies any constraint on the parameter of interest (here that the parameter of interest is a proportion and must therefore belong to the unit interval), and it respects the knowledge that the parameter of interest is a particular function of the data-generating distribution. On the contrary, solutions of an estimating equation may fail to satisfy such constraints.
(2) The TMLE methodology cares about the likelihood. The log-likelihood of the updated estimate of P_0, $\frac{1}{n}\sum_{i=1}^{n} \log P_n^*(O_i)$, is available, thereby allowing for the C-TMLE extension (Part VII).

25.3.3 Implementing TMLE

The TMLE procedure is implemented following the specification in Sect. 25.3.1. Only the details of the super learning procedure are missing. We chose to rely on a least squares loss functions, and on a collection of algorithms containing seven estimation procedures: generalized linear models, elastic net ($\alpha = 1$), elastic net ($\alpha = 0.5$), generalized additive models (degree = 2), generalized additive models (degree = 3), DSA, and random forest (ntree = 1000).

25.4 Simulations

The simulation scheme attempts to mimic the data-generating distribution of the DAIFI data set. We start with L_0 drawn from its empirical distribution based on the DAIFI data set and for $j = 0, \ldots, 2$, successively, $A_j \sim \text{Ber}(q_j(L_{0,1}, L_{0,2}, L_{0,3}))$ and $L_{j+1} \sim \text{Ber}(p_{j+1}(L_{0,1}, L_{0,2}, L_{0,3}))$, where for each $j = 0, 1, 2$, $p_{j+1}(L_{0,1}, L_{0,2}, L_{0,3}) = \text{expit}\,(\alpha_{1,L_{0,1}} + \alpha_{2,L_{0,1}} \log L_{0,2} + \alpha_{3,L_{0,1}} \log(5 + \min(L_{0,3}, 5)^5))$, and for each $j = 0, 1, 2$, $q_j(L_{0,1}, L_{0,2}, L_{0,3}) = \text{expit}\,(\beta_{1,L_{0,1}} + \beta_{2,L_{0,1}} L_{0,3})$. The values of the α- and β-parameters are reported in Table 25.1.

Regarding the empirical distribution of L_0, the IVF unit random variable $L_{0,1}$ follows a Bernoulli distribution with parameter approximately equal to 0.517. Both conditional distributions of age $L_{0,2}$ given the IVF unit are Gaussian-like, with means and standard deviations roughly equal to 33 and 4.4. The marginal distribution of the random number $L_{0,3}$ of embryos transferred or frozen has mean and variance approximately equal to 3.3 and 7.5, with values ranging between 0 and 23 (only 20% of the observed $L_{0,3}^{(i)}$ are larger than 5). We refer to Table 25.3 in Sect. 25.5 for a comparison of the empirical probabilities that $A_j = 1$ and $L_j = 1$ computed under the empirical distribution of a simulated data set with 10,000 observations and the empirical distribution of the DAIFI data set.

The super learning library is correctly specified for the estimation of the censoring mechanism, and misspecified for the estimation of the Q-factor. Indeed, $L_{0,2}$ plays a role in $p_{j+1}(L_{0,1}, L_{0,2}, L_{0,3})$ through its logarithm, and $L_{0,3}$ through $\log(5 + \min(L_{0,3}, 5)^5)$. We choose this expression because $x \mapsto \log(5 + \min(x, 5)^5)$ cannot be well approximated by a polynomial in x over $[0, 23]$. Furthermore, the true

Table 25.1 Values of the α- and β-parameters used in the simulation scheme

	IVF cycle j			
Parameters	0	1	2	3
$100 \times \alpha_{\cdot,0}$	–	(61, −55, 4.5)	(13, −45, 1.2)	(60, −40, 1.5)
$100 \times \alpha_{\cdot,1}$	–	(65, −70, 3.3)	(19, −49, 1.7)	(80, −50, 1)
$100 \times \beta_{\cdot,0}$	(40, 10)	(−45, 32)	(−30, 5)	–
$100 \times \beta_{\cdot,1}$	(40, 9)	(−50, 34)	(−40, 6)	–

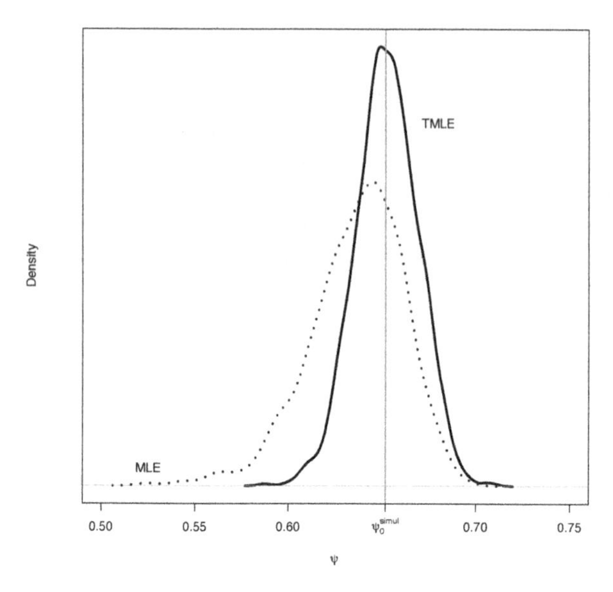

Fig. 25.1 MLE and TMLE empirical densities

Table 25.2 Simulation results

	Empirical		
Estimator	Bias	MSE	Cover (p-value)
MLE	−0.01571	0.00065	–
TMLE	0.00052	0.00027	0.958 (89%)

value of the parameter of interest for this simulation scheme can be estimated with great precision by Monte Carlo. Using a simulated data set of one million observations under the intervention (1,1,1) yields $\psi_0^{\text{simul}} = 0.652187$, with a 95% confidence interval equal to $(0.6512535, 0.6531205)$.

We repeat $B = 1000$ times the following steps: (1) simulate a data set with sample size $n = 3001$ according to the simulation scheme presented above and (2) estimate ψ_0^{simul} with $\Psi(P_{n,b}^*) = \psi_{n,b}^*$, the bth TMLE based on this bth data set. In order to shed some light one the properties of the TMLE procedure, we also keep track of the initial maximum-likelihood-based substitution estimator $\Psi(P_{n,b}^0)$, based on the bth data set.

We summarize the results of the simulation study in Table 25.2. They are illuminating: the MLE is biased, whereas the TMLE is unbiased. In the process of stretching the initial MLE into the updated TMLE in the direction of the parameter of interest, the update step not only corrects the bias but also diminishes the variance. Those key features are well illustrated in Fig. 25.1, where it is also seen that the TMLE is approximately normally distributed.

Let us now investigate the validity of the coverage guaranteed by the 95% confidence intervals based on the central limit theorem satisfied by ψ_n^*, using (25.6) as an estimate of the asymptotic variance. Since the super learner g_n^* is a consistent estimator of g_0, the latter estimate of the asymptotic variance of the TMLE is sensible, and may be slightly conservative due to the misspecification of Q_n^*. Among the $B = 1000$ 95% confidence intervals, 958 contain the true value ψ_0^{simul}. This is strongly in favor of the conclusion that the confidence intervals do meet their requirement. The probability for a binomial random variable with parameter $(B, 95\%)$ to be less than 958 equals 89%.

25.5 Data Application

We observe $n = 3001$ experimental units. We report in Table 25.3 the empirical probabilities of $A_j = 1$ (each $j = 0, 1, 2$) and $L_j = 1$ ($j = 0, 1, 2, 3$) for all IVF cycles. It is obvious from these numbers that the censoring mechanism plays a great role in the data-generating experiment. We applied the TMLE methodology and obtained a point estimate of ψ_0 equal to $\psi_n^* = 0.505$. The corresponding 95% confidence interval based on the central limit theorem, using (25.6) as an estimate of the asymptotic variance of $\sqrt{n}(\psi_n^* - \psi_0)$, is equal to $(0.480, 0.530)$.

However, we have no certainty of the convergence of g_n^* to g_0 (which would guarantee that the confidence interval is conservative). Therefore we also carried out a bootstrap study. Specifically, we iterated $B = 1000$ times the following procedure. First, draw a data set of $n = 3001$ observations from the empirical measure P_n; second, compute and store the TMLE $\psi_{n,b}^*$ obtained on this data set. This results in the following 95% confidence interval (using the original ψ_n^* as center of the interval): $(0.470, 0.540)$, which is wider than the previous one.

As a side remark, the MLE $\Psi(P_n^0)$ updated during the second step of the TMLE procedure (applied to the original data set) is equal to 0.490. We also note that the TMLE ψ_n^* falls between the estimates obtained in Soullier et al. (2008) by multiple imputation and the Kaplan–Meier method. The probability of success of a program of at most four IVF cycles may be slightly larger than previously thought. In conclusion, future participants in a program of at most four IVF cycles can be informed that approximately half of them may subsequently succeed in having a child.

Table 25.3 Empirical probabilities that $A_j = 1$ and $L_j = 1$ based on a simulated data set of 10,000 observations and the DAIFI data set

	Simulated data set		DAIFI data set	
	Empirical probability of		Empirical probability of	
IVF cycle j	$A_j = 1$	$L_j = 1$	$A_j = 1$	$L_j = 1$
0	73%	21%	75%	22%
1	57%	32%	59%	32%
2	46%	37%	49%	35%
3	–	40%	–	37%

25.6 Discussion

We studied the performance of IVF programs and provided the community with an accurate estimator of the probability of delivery during the course of a program of at most four IVF cycles in France (abbreviated to probability of success). We first expressed the parameter of interest as a functional $\Psi(P_0)$ of the data-generating distribution P_0 of the observed longitudinal data structure $O = (L_0, A_0, L_1, A_1, L_2, A_2, Y)$. Subsequently, we applied the TMLE. Under regularity conditions, the estimator is consistent as soon as at least one of two fundamental components of P_0 is consistently estimated; moreover, the central limit theorem allowed us to construct a confidence interval. These theoretical properties are illustrated by a simulation study. We obtained a point estimate that is approximately equal to 50%, with a 95% confidence interval given by (48%, 53%). Earlier results obtained by Soullier et al. (2008) based on the multiple-imputation methodology were slightly more pessimistic, with an estimated probability of success equal to 46% and (44%, 48%) as 95% confidence interval.

These authors also considered another approach that involves phrasing the problem of interest as the estimation of a survival function based on right-censored data. The key to this second approach is that the probability of success coincides with the probability $P(T \leq 3)$, where T is the number of IVF cycles attempted after the first one till the first successful delivery. Our observed longitudinal data structure O is equivalent to the right-censored data structure $O' = (W, \min(T, C), I(T \leq C))$, where $W = L_0$ and $C = \min(0 \leq j \leq 3 : A_j = 0)$ with the additional convention $A_3 = 0$. Neglecting the baseline covariates W and assuming that the dropout time C is independent of T, Soullier et al. (2008) estimated the probability of success by $1 - S_n(3)$, S_n being the Kaplan–Meier estimate of the survival function of T. Although the TMLE methodology to address the estimation of $P(T \leq 3)$ (incorporating the baseline covariates) is well understood (Chaps. 17 and 18), we choose to adopt the point of view of a longitudinal data structure rather than that of a right-censored data structure. From the survival analysis point of view, our contribution is to incorporate the baseline covariates in order to improve efficiency and to allow for informative censoring. We finally emphasize that an extension of the TMLE procedure presented in this chapter will allow, in future work, to take into account the successive number of embryos transferred or frozen at each IVF cycle (instead of the sole number at the first IVF cycle), thereby acknowledging the possibility that this time-dependent covariate may yield time-dependent confounding.

Acknowledgements

The author would like to thank E. de la Rochebrochard, J. Bouyer (Ined; Inserm, CESP; Univ Paris-Sud, UMRS 1018), and S. Enjalric-Ancelet (AgroParisTech, Unité Mét@risk) for introducing him to this problem, as well as the Cochin and Clermont-Ferrand IVF units for sharing the DAIFI data set.

Chapter 26
Individualized Antiretroviral Initiation Rules

Romain Neugebauer, Michael J. Silverberg, Mark J. van der Laan

In this chapter, TMLE is illustrated with a data analysis from a longitudinal observational study to investigate "when to start" antiretroviral therapy to reduce the incidence of AIDS-defining cancer (ADC), defined as Kaposi sarcoma, non-Hodgkin's lymphoma, or invasive cervical cancer, in a population of HIV-infected patients. A key clinical question regarding the management of HIV/AIDS is when to start combination antiretroviral therapy (ART), defined in the Department of Health and Human Services (2004) guidelines as a regimen containing three or more individual antiretroviral medications. CD4+ T-cell count levels have been the primary marker used to determine treatment eligibility, although other factors have also been considered, such as HIV RNA levels, history of an AIDS-defining illness (Centers for Disease Control and Prevention 1992), and ability of the patient to adhere to therapy. The primary outcomes considered in ART treatment guidelines described above have always been reductions in HIV-related morbidity and mortality. Until recently, however, guidelines have not considered the effect of CD4 thresholds on the risk of specific comorbidities, such as ADC. In this analysis, we therefore evaluate how different CD4-based ART initiation strategies influence the burden of ADC. We are analyzing ADC here since it is well established that these malignancies are closely linked to immunodeficiency.

We compare the effectiveness in delaying onset of ADC of two clinical guidelines regarding when to start ART. Specifically, the following research question is addressed: Should ART be initiated when a patient's CD4 count drops below 350 cells/μl (current guideline) or should ART initiation be instead delayed until his/her CD4 count drops below 200 cells/μl (official guideline for years 2001–2007)? The target population where this effect is of interest is composed of all patients who are HIV-infected, aged 18 years or older, ART-naive, never diagnosed with ADC and engaged in medical care as demonstrated by receipt of a CD4 test.

Addressing this research question involves the estimation of the effect of two personalized ART intervention rules (each based on the patients' CD4 count profile over time) on the distribution of the resulting failure times defined as the patients' times to cancer onset. A dynamic marginal structural model (dMSM) provides an adequate causal model for such an effect since dMSMs are models for the distribution of rule-specific counterfactual outcomes. More precisely, each of the two decision rules of interest for when to start ART are indexed by a CD4 count threshold denoted by θ (equal to 200 or 350) and can be described as follows: "Only initiate ART once the patient's CD4 count drops below θ and continue treatment with ART without interruption thereafter."

26.1 Longitudinal Data Structure

This analysis was conducted within Kaiser Permanente of Northern California (KPNC), a large integrated health care delivery system that provides comprehensive medical services to approx. 3.2 million members in a 14-county region in northern California, representing 30% of the surrounding population (N. Gordon, pers. comm.). KPNC maintains complete databases on hospitalizations, outpatient visits, laboratory tests, and prescriptions. Numerous disease registries are maintained at the KPNC Division of Research, including HIV and cancer. For additional details on KPNC's registries and members we refer readers to Selby et al. (2005) and our accompanying technical report: Neugebauer et al. (2010).

KPNC's databases were used to retrospectively identify a cohort of adult HIV-infected patients within KPNC followed between 1996 and 2007 who met the following eligibility criteria: HIV-infected, at least 18 years old, KPNC member during years 1996–2007, never previously treated with antiretrovirals, at least one CD4 count measurement available in the previous year, and never previously diagnosed with an ADC. Based on these eligibility criteria, a total of 6,250 HIV-infected patients were identified. The start of follow-up for patients was the first date at which they met all of the eligibility criteria defined above. Patients were then followed until they achieved the outcome of interest, i.e., incident ADC, or until right censored due to occurrence of a competing event: death, discontinuation of KPNC health insurance, or administrative censoring at the end of the study on December 31, 2007. Small gaps in KPNC health insurance of less than 3 months were ignored, which more likely represented administrative glitches as opposed to lack of health plan coverage. In addition, ART discontinuation lasting less than 6 months was also ignored.

The data for this analysis are viewed as realizations of 6250 i.i.d. copies of the following random longitudinal data structure:

$$O = (\tilde{T}, \Delta, L(0), A(0), L(1), A(1), \ldots, L(t), A(t), \ldots, L(\tilde{T}), A(\tilde{T}), L(\tilde{T}+1)),$$

where $\tilde{T}$ denotes the follow-up time, Δ denotes the indicator of $\tilde{T}$ being equal to the time till cancer onset, $L(0)$ denotes the baseline covariates, $L(t)$ denotes intermediate time-dependent covariates at time t, and $A(t) = (A_1(t), A_2(t) = I(\tilde{T} \leq t, \Delta = 0))$ denotes the indicator of receiving ART at time t ($A_1(t)$) and the indicator of being right-censored at time t ($A_2(t) = I(\tilde{T} \leq t, \Delta = 0)$). Let P_0 be the probability distribution of O.

In this data analysis the time scale is discretized in the sense that t denotes a discrete time stamp that indexes the consecutive intervals of $\tau = 180$ d following a patient's study entry. In particular, $t = 0$ represents the first τ days of a patient's follow-up, and $\tilde{T}$ is measured in units of τ days. The right-censoring time C is defined as the minimum time to a competing event (all expressed in units of τ days since study entry). Thus Δ is the indicator that cancer onset occurs prior to the right-censoring time C.

A patient was defined to initiate ART on the first day of a sequence of at least 2 consecutive months during which the patient was treated with three or more individual antiretroviral medications. The values for all treatment variables before ART initiation were set to 0, i.e., the value for each $A_1(t)$ such that t represents an interval of τ days all of which precede ART initiation was set to 0. Values for all other treatment variables, $A_1(t)$, were mapped to 1 except for all time points t that include or follow the first day of a sequence of 6 consecutive months when the patient had discontinued ART (discontinuation of ART is defined as being treated with less than three antiretroviral medications). For such time points, treatment with ART was deemed interrupted and the value for $A_1(t)$ was set to 0 for t representing the interval of τ days when the first discontinuation of ART was deemed to occur and was set to NA (i.e., considered missing) for all subsequent time points. Note that this missing treatment information could have been recovered but is irrelevant for the estimation of the causal estimand described below and was thus left indeterminate. We also note that $L(t)$ represents subject-matter attributes that occur before the action $A(t)$ at time t and otherwise are assumed not to be affected by the actions at time t or thereafter. In particular, the covariate $L(t)$ contains information on the failure time through the outcome variable $Y(t) = I(\tilde{T} \leq t - 1, \Delta = 1) \in L(t)$, which denotes the indicator of failure at or before time $t - 1$ for $t > 0$ and $Y(0) \equiv 0$ by convention since all patients are cancer free at study entry. The outcome variable, $Y(\tilde{T} + 1)$, is the only covariate relevant at time $\tilde{T} + 1$ for this analysis and information on other attributes at that time is thus ignored, i.e., $L(\tilde{T} + 1) \equiv Y(\tilde{T} + 1)$.

The number of time-independent (e.g., sex, race) and time-dependent (CD4 count, viral load, indicator of past clinical AIDS-defining events, indicator of past ADC diagnosis) covariate attributes are denoted respectively by $p = 15$ and $q = 4$. The covariates in $L(t)$ that represent time-independent attributes are denoted by $L_j(t)$ for $j = 1, \ldots, p$, where j represents an arbitrary order of the time-independent attributes. The covariates in $L(t)$ that represent time-dependent attributes are denoted by $L_j(t)$ for $j = p + 1, \ldots, p + q$ such that j represents an order of the time-dependent attributes, where $L_{p+1}(t)$ and $L_{p+2}(t)$ represent the indicator of past failure (i.e., $L_{p+1}(t) \equiv Y(t)$) and the CD4 count variable, respectively. We thus have $L_j(0)_{j=1,\ldots,p+q} \subset L(0)$, where $L_j(0)$ for $j = 1, \ldots, p$ represent the time-independent covariates collected at baseline and $L_j(0)$ for $j = p+1,\ldots,p+q$ represent the time-dependent covariates collected at baseline. Similarly, we have $L_j(t)_{j=p+1,\ldots,p+q} \subset L(t)$ for $t = 1,\ldots,\tilde{T}$, where $L_j(t)$ for $j = p+1,\ldots,p+q$ represent the time-dependent covariates collected at time t. Finally, we have $L(\tilde{T}+1) = L_{p+1}(\tilde{T}+1) = Y(\tilde{T}+1)$. Table 26.1 summarizes the link between the measurements of the subject-matter attributes and the notation adopted above to represent these data with the covariates in $L(t)$ for $t = 0,\ldots,\tilde{T}+1$. See the accompanying technical report for a full description of variables.

To respect the time-ordering assumption that imposes that covariates $L(t)$ are not affected by actions at time t and thereafter, the daily data on time-dependent attributes during follow-up were mapped to an observation of $L_j(t)$ for $j \in \{p+1,\ldots,p+q\}$. We will use the notation $[a,b[$ for $\{x : a \leq x < b\}$; thus all points between a and b, including a, but excluding b. For all time points t representing intervals $[t \times \tau, (t+1) \times \tau[$ that do not contain the day when ART is deemed to be initiated, $L_j(t)$ represents the last measurement for attribute j available: (1) at time

Table 26.1 Mapping of the subject-matter attribute measurements into the covariates, $L(t)$, and actions, $A(t)$, of the observed data process O

Attribute	Variable	Number of levels
sex	$L_1(0)$	2
race	$L_2(0)$	4
censusEdu	$L_3(0)$	4
censusPov	$L_4(0)$	4
censusInc	$L_5(0)$	4
riskHIV	$L_6(0)$	4
enrollYear	$L_7(0)$	12
yearsHIV	$L_8(0)$	4
ageAtEntry	$L_9(0)$	3
everSmoke	$L_{10}(0)$	2
everAlcohol	$L_{11}(0)$	2
everDrug	$L_{12}(0)$	2
everHepatitisB	$L_{13}(0)$	2
everHepatitisC	$L_{14}(0)$	2
everObese	$L_{15}(0)$	2
Y	$L_{16}(t)$ for $t = 0,\ldots,\tilde{T}+1$	$n(t,16) \equiv 2$
CD4	$L_{17}(t)$ for $t = 0,\ldots,\tilde{T}$	$n(t,17) \equiv 4$
VL	$L_{18}(t)$ for $t = 0,\ldots,\tilde{T}$	$n(t,18) \equiv 4$
clinicalAIDS	$L_{19}(t)$ for $t = 0,\ldots,\tilde{T}$	$n(t,19) \equiv 2$
I.CD4	$L_{20}(t)$ for $t = 0,\ldots,\tilde{T}$	$n(t,20) \equiv 2$
I.VL	$L_{21}(t)$ for $t = 0,\ldots,\tilde{T}$	$n(t,21) \equiv 2$
I.race	$L_{22}(0)$	2
I.censusEdu	$L_{23}(0)$	2
I.censusPov	$L_{24}(0)$	2
I.censusInc	$L_{25}(0)$	2
I.riskHIV	$L_{26}(0)$	2
ART	$A_1(t)$ for $t = 0,\ldots,\tilde{T}$	2

$t-1$ (i.e., the last measurement obtained during interval $[(t-1)\times\tau, t\times\tau[$) if $t > 0$ and (2) within the year preceding study entry if $t = 0$. For the time point t representing the interval $[t \times \tau, (t+1) \times \tau[$ that contains the day when ART is deemed to be initiated, $L_j(t)$ represents the last measurement for attribute j available (1) at time $t-1$ or time t but always prior to the actual day when ART was initiated if $t > 0$ and (2) within the year preceding study entry or at time point 0 but always prior to the actual day when ART was initiated if $t = 0$.

Once this mapping was implemented, some of the observations for $p' = 5$ time-independent attributes (race, censusEdu, censusPov, censusInc, and riskHIV) were missing. Similarly, some of the observations for $q' = 2$ time-dependent attributes (CD4 and VL) were missing. Such observations were imputed (e.g., with the mode or with the average of the nonmissing observations), and indicators of imputation (named I.censusEdu, I.censusPov, I.censusInc, I.race, I.riskHIV, I.CD4, and I.VL, respectively) were created. For the covariates race and riskHIV, the imputation was implemented conditional on the covariate sex. Each of these imputation indicators are denoted by $L_j(t)$ such that $L_j(t)$ for $j = p+q+1,\ldots,p+q+q'$ represent the indicators of imputation for the time-dependent attributes ordered arbitrarily (CD4 and VL), and $L_j(t)$ for $j = p+q+q'+1,\ldots,p+q+q'+p'$ represent the indicators of imputation for the time-independent attributes ordered arbitrarily (race, censusEdu, censusPov, censusInc, and riskHIV). These imputation indicators are included in the definition of $L(t)$.

The following forward imputation method was used for missing observations of time-dependent covariates at any time $t > 0$: the missing observation for $L_j(t)$ was imputed with the last nonmissing and nonimputed observation of the covariates $(L_j(0),\ldots,L_j(t-1))$ if available and otherwise with the imputed observation for $L_j(0)$. For additional detailed descriptions of the variables and a variety of summary statistics for the data, we refer to the accompanying technical report. Here, we suffice with mentioning that two thirds of the patients who experienced cancer onset before right censoring did so during the first two years of follow-up and that from the 118 patients who experienced a cancer-onset event in the first two years of follow-up, 13 occurred in patients who only followed the rule for starting ART indexed by a CD4 count threshold of 200, 12 occurred in patients who only followed the rule for starting ART indexed by the CD4 count threshold of 350, 51 occurred in patients who followed both rules for starting ART, and 42 occurred in patients who followed neither of these two when-to-start rules. This simple summary provides an indication that the data are sparse with respect to the scientific question of interest, and that the data lack a strong signal for favoring one dynamic treatment over the other. Nevertheless, it is of interest to determine if these data imply a narrow confidence interval around a zero treatment effect.

For conciseness, we adopt the following shorthand notation to represent the history of measurements on a given subject-matter attribute between time point 0 and t: for a time-dependent process $X()$, $\bar{X}(t) \equiv (X(0),\ldots,X(t))$ and by convention $X(t)$ is nil for $t < 0$. Using this notation, the observed data for one subject can be summarized as follows: $O = (\tilde{T}, \Delta, \bar{L}(\tilde{T}+1), \bar{A}(\tilde{T}))$.

26.2 Likelihood of the Observed Data Structure

Following the time ordering of actions and covariates encoded in the directed acyclic graph implied by Fig. 26.1, the likelihood of the observed data under a probability distribution P can be factorized as

$$P(O) = \prod_{t=0}^{\tilde{T}+\Delta} P(L(t) \mid \bar{L}(t-1), \bar{A}(t-1)) \prod_{t=0}^{\tilde{T}} P(A(t) \mid \bar{A}(t-1), \bar{L}(t)).$$

Note that the first product of conditional probabilities ends with the conditional probability of $L(\tilde{T})$ given all past actions, $\bar{A}(\tilde{T}-1)$, and past covariates, $\bar{L}(\tilde{T}-1)$, when the patient's data are right-censored, i.e., $\Delta = 0$, since $L(\tilde{T}+1) \equiv Y(\tilde{T}+1)$ is then 0 with probability one. If the patient's cancer onset is observed (i.e., $\Delta = 1$), the first product ends with the conditional probability of $L(\tilde{T}+1)$ given past actions, $\bar{A}(\tilde{T})$, and past covariates, $\bar{L}(\tilde{T})$.

The two products of the likelihood above are referred to as the Q-factor and g-factor of the likelihood. The Q-factor of the likelihood is composed of the product of the conditional probabilities of covariates given past covariates and actions, whereas the g-factor of the likelihood is composed of the product of the conditional probabilities of actions given past actions and covariates. The g-factor of the likelihood is also referred to as the action mechanism. Following this terminology, the notation for the likelihood of the observed data can be summarized as

$$P = \prod_{t=0}^{K} Q_{L(t)} \prod_{t=0}^{K} g_{A(t)}, \tag{26.1}$$

where the conditional probability distributions $P(L(t) \mid \bar{L}(t-1), \bar{A}(t-1))$ and $P(A(t) \mid \bar{A}(t-1), \bar{L}(t))$ are denoted by $Q_{L(t)}$ and $g_{A(t)}$, respectively, and K is the last possible time point so that $P(\tilde{T} < K) = 1$. After $t > \tilde{T} + \Delta$, all conditional distributions $Q_{L(t)}$

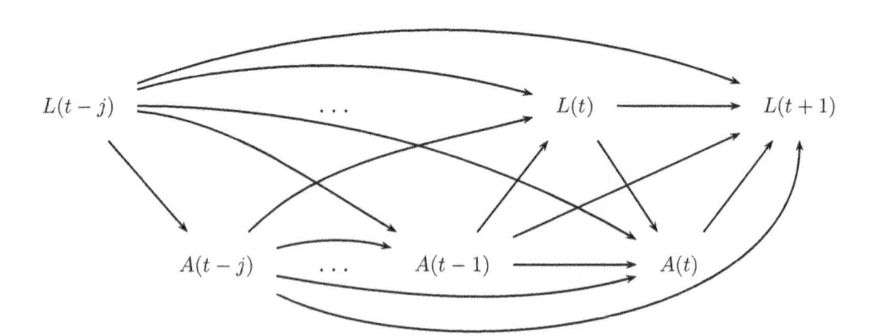

Fig. 26.1 Template of the directed acyclic graph that encodes the time ordering of all variables of the observed data process O. The complete graph can be derived by sequentially drawing the nodes and arcs implied by this template for $t = 0, \ldots, \tilde{T}$ and $j \leq t$

and $g_{A(t)}$ are degenerate at an arbitrarily defined value, such as the last measured value.

At each time point t, the covariate $L(t)$ is composed of a collection of discrete covariates denoted by $L_j(t)$. Specifically, $L(0) \equiv (L_j(0) : j = 1, \ldots, p+q+q'+p')$, $L(t) \equiv (L_j(t) : j = p+1, \ldots, p+q+q')$ for $t = 1, \ldots, \tilde{T}$, and $L(\tilde{T}+1) \equiv L_{p+1}(\tilde{T}+1)$, where, as described in Table 26.1, for $p = 15$, $q = 4$, $q' = 2$, and $p' = 5$: $j = 1, \ldots, p$ indexes the covariates that represent the time-independent attributes listed; $j = p+1, \ldots, p+q$ indexes the covariates that represent the time-dependent attributes listed such that $p+1$ represents Y and $p+2$ represents CD4; $j = p+q+1, \ldots, p+q+q'$ indexes the indicators of imputations for the q' time-dependent attributes that have missing observations; $j = p+q+q'+1, \ldots, p+q+q'+p'$ indexes the indicators of imputations for the p' time-independent attributes that have missing observations.

The factors $Q_{L(t)}$ of the likelihood for $t = 1, \ldots, \tilde{T} + \Delta$ can thus be factorized as $Q_{L(t)}(O) = \prod_{j=1}^{n_{\tilde{T}}(t)} Q_{L_{p+j}(t)}(O)$, where $n_{\tilde{T}}(t) \equiv q + q'$ for $t = 1, \ldots, \tilde{T}$, $n_{\tilde{T}}(\tilde{T}+1) \equiv 1$, and $Q_{L_{p+j}(t)}(O) \equiv P(L_{p+j}(t) \mid Pa(L_{p+j}(t)))$ with $Pa(L_{p+j}(t)) \equiv (\bar{L}(t-1), L_{p+1}(t), \ldots, L_{p+j-1}(t), \bar{A}(t-1))$. Note that the notation above makes implicit use of the convention that $(L_j(t), \ldots, L_{j'}(t))$ for $j' < j$ is nil.

Similarly, at each time point t, the action $A(t)$ is composed of a treatment, $A_1(t)$, and an indicator of right censoring, $A_2(t)$. The factors $g_{\bar{A}(t)}$ of the likelihood can thus be factorized as $g_{A(t)} = g_{A_1(t)} g_{A_2(t)}$, where $g_{A_1(t)}(O) \equiv P(A_1(t) \mid Pa(A_1(t)))$, $Pa(A_1(t)) = (\bar{A}(t-1), \bar{L}(t), A_2(t)))$, $g_{A_2(t)}(O) \equiv P(A_2(t) \mid Pa(A_2(t))$, and $Pa(A_2(t)) = (\bar{A}(t-1), \bar{L}(t))$. This yields the following factorization of likelihood (26.1):

$$P(O) = Q_{L(0)}(L(0) \prod_{t=1}^{\tilde{T}+\Delta} \prod_{j=1}^{n_{\tilde{T}}(t)} Q_{L_{p+j}(t)}(O) \prod_{t=0}^{\tilde{T}} g_{A_1(t)}(O) g_{A_2(t)}(O). \quad (26.2)$$

Since each covariate $L_{p+j}(t)$ for $t = 1, \ldots, \tilde{T} + \Delta$ and $j = 1, \ldots, n_{\tilde{T}}(t)$ is discrete with $n(t, p+j)$ categories, it can be recoded with $n(t, p+j) - 1$ binary variables: $L_{p+j,m}(t) \equiv I(L_{p+j}(t) = m)$ for $m = 1, \ldots, n(t, p+j) - 1$, i.e. $L_{p+j}(t) = (L_{p+j,m}(t))_{m=1,\ldots,n(t,p+j)-1}$. This recoding of the information in $L_{p+j}(t)$ leads to the following factorization $Q_{L_{p+j}(t)} = \prod_{m=1}^{n(t,p+j)-1} Q_{L_{p+j,m}(t)}$, where $Q_{L_{p+j,m}(t)}$ represents the conditional probability of $L_{p+j,m}(t)$ given $Pa(L_{p+j}(t))$ and $L_{p+j,l}(t)$ for $l = 1, \ldots, m-1$. Note that this conditional probability is degenerate, i.e., equal to 1 at $L_{p+j,m}(t) = 0$, if one of the indicators $L_{p+j,l}(t)$ in $Pa(L_{p+j,m}(t))$ is 1. Note also that if $L_{p+j}(t)$ is binary ($n(t, p+j) = 2$), then $L_{p+j,1}(t) = L_{p+j}(t)$ and $Q_{L_{p+j,1}(t)} = Q_{L_{p+j}(t)}$. This provides us with the following factorized likelihood in terms of conditional distributions of binary variables:

$$P(O) = Q_{L(0)}(L(0)) \prod_{t=1}^{\tilde{T}+\Delta} \prod_{j=1}^{n_{\tilde{T}}(t)} \prod_{m=1}^{n(t,p+j)-1} Q_{L_{p+j,m}(t)}(O) \prod_{t=0}^{\tilde{T}} g_{A_1(t)}(O) g_{A_2(t)}(O). \quad (26.3)$$

26.3 Target Parameter

In this section, the causal effect of interest in this analysis is defined as the effect of dynamic ART interventions on the cumulative risk of cancer in the first two years of follow-up. Under an identifiability assumption, this causal effect is expressed as a function of the likelihood of the observed data. This latter estimand is referred to as the target parameter. We can define an SCM for the full data (U, O) in terms of a nonparametric structural equation model: $L(0) = f_{L(0)}(U_{L(0)})$, $L(t) = f_{L(t)}(Pa(L(t)), U_{L(t)})$, $t = 1, \ldots, \tilde{T} + \Delta$, $A(t) = f_{A(t)}(Pa(A(t)), U_{A(t)})$, $t = 0, \ldots, \tilde{T}$. This SCM can also be defined for $t = 1, \ldots, K$, by defining the equations as degenerate for $t > \tilde{T} + \Delta$, and, it can also be extended to one equation for each univariate time-dependent covariate.

Clinical practice often involves treatment decisions that are continuously adjusted to the patient's evolving medical history (e.g., new diagnoses and laboratory values) and are not set a priori at baseline. Thus, it may often be less clinically relevant to compare the health effect of static treatment interventions than to compare the effectiveness of competing medical guidelines, i.e., adaptive treatment strategies that map the patient's unfolding medical history to subsequent treatment decisions. Following such treatment strategies leads to treatment interventions over time which are referred to as dynamic interventions since the treatment experienced by each patient at any point in time is not set a priori at baseline but is rather adjusted based on the patient's current circumstances.

Our aim was to evaluate the comparative effectiveness between ART initiation strategies guided by the patient's evolving CD4 count. These adaptive treatment strategies are referred to as individualized action rules. The individualized action rules of interest are each indexed by a CD4 count threshold, denoted by $\theta \in \Theta$, and are each defined as a vector function $d_\theta = (d_\theta(0), \ldots, d_\theta(K))$ where each function, $d_\theta(t)$ for $t = 0, \ldots, K$, is a decision rule for determining the action (treatment and right censoring) to be experienced by a patient during time interval t. A decision rule $d_\theta(t)$ maps the action and covariate history measured up to a given time interval t to an action regimen (i.e., an intervention) during time interval t: $d_\theta(t) : (\bar{L}(t), \bar{A}(t-1)) \mapsto (a_1(t), a_2(t))$. In this analysis, the decision rules of interest are defined such that $d_\theta(t)((\bar{L}(t), \bar{A}(t-1))$ is:

- $(a_1(t), a_2(t)) = (0, 0)$ (i.e., no ART use and no right censoring) if and only if the patient was not previously treated with ART [i.e. $\bar{A}(t-1) = 0$] and the previous CD4 count measurement was greater than or equal to the threshold θ (i.e., $L_{p+1}(t) \geq \theta$);
- $(a_1(t), a_2(t)) = (1, 0)$ (i.e., ART use and no right censoring) otherwise.

The individualized action rules, d_θ for $\theta \in \Theta$, implied by the time-specific decision rules above, $d_\theta(t)$ for $t = 0, \ldots, K$, are monotone in the sense that if a patient follows one of these rules, d_θ, then s/he is not treated with ART until his/her CD4 count falls below the threshold θ for the first time and from then on the patient remains treated with ART.

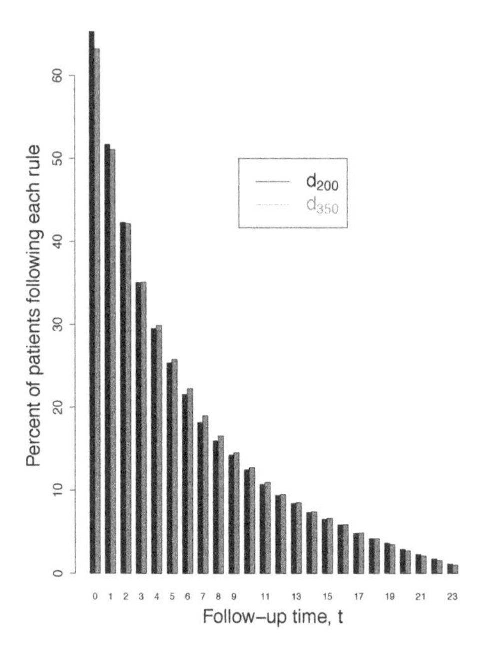

Fig. 26.2 Percentages of patients following each of the two individualized action rules of interest indexed by a CD4 count threshold of 200 and 350 cells per μl (reminder: $t = 0$ represents the first 180 d of follow-up)

The counterfactual covariate process that could be observed on a patient in an ideal experiment where interventions on the action process according to a decision rule d_θ are carried out through time K is denoted by $\bar{L}_{d_\theta}(K+1)$. Note that such dynamic treatment interventions through time K according to the adaptive treatment strategy d_θ are only functions of the observed covariate process $\bar{L}(K)$ and are thus denoted by $d_\theta(\bar{L}(K))$. Failure may occur during follow-up under any such dynamic treatment intervention. Such *counterfactual* failure times are denoted by $T_{d_\theta} \leq K$ and defined by $(\bar{Y}_{d_\theta}(T_{d_\theta}) = 0, Y_{d_\theta}(T_{d_\theta}+1) = 1, \ldots, Y_{d_\theta}(K+1) = 1)$. This random process $(T_{d_\theta}, L_{d_\theta} = \bar{L}_{d_\theta}(K+1))$ is defined in terms of the postintervention distribution of the above-stated SCM for the full-data (U, O). A causal effect can now be defined as a target parameter for the full-data SCM:

$$P(Y_{d_\theta}(t+1) = 1) - P(Y_{d_{\theta'}}(t+1) = 1) = P(T_{d_\theta} \leq t) - P(T_{d_{\theta'}} \leq t)$$

for $t = 0, \ldots, K$ and any two different individualized action rules d_θ with $\theta \in \Theta$ and $d_{\theta'}$ with $\theta' \in \Theta$.

For our research question, the comparative effectiveness between the two adaptive ART strategies indexed by the CD4 thresholds 200 and 350 is of interest. Figure 26.2 represents the percentages of patients following the corresponding two individualized action rules over time denoted by d_{200} and d_{350}. The empirical distribution of observed events indicates that two thirds of the observed cancers occurred in the first four time points of follow-up. To ease the computing time required for implementation of the TMLE procedure while illustrating the computing steps involved without loss of generality, we restrict the focus of this analysis to the evaluation of a single causal contrast between the cumulative risks of failure within 2 years of study entry under the individualized action rules d_{350} and d_{200}:

$$\begin{aligned}\psi^F &= P(T_{d_{350}} \leq 3) - P(T_{d_{200}} \leq 3)\\ &= P(Y_{d_{350}}(4) = 1) - P(Y_{d_{200}}(4) = 1).\end{aligned} \tag{26.4}$$

Note that this parameter is a function of the full-data distribution as is made explicit with the notation $\psi^F = \Psi^F(P_{X,U})$. This target parameter would be identifiable under this full-data SCM if we observed the full-data (U, O). However, we only observe the O-component of the full data.

Under the sequential randomization assumption (SRA)

$$A(t) \perp (Y_{d_\theta}, L_{d_\theta}) \mid \bar{L}(t), \bar{A}(t-1), \text{ for all } t = 0, \ldots, K,$$

the marginal distribution of the counterfactual process $(\bar{L}_{d_\theta}(t+1))$ with $t \leq K$ is identified by the g-computation formula:

$$P_{\bar{L}_{d_\theta}(t+1)} = Q_{L(0)} \prod_{t'=1}^{t+1} \prod_{j=1}^{n_t(t')} \prod_{m=1}^{n(t',p+j)-1} Q_{L_{p+j,m}(t'),d_\theta}, \tag{26.5}$$

where the conditional probabilities $Q_{L_{p+j,m}(t'),d_\theta}$ are the conditional probabilities $Q_{L_{p+j,m}(t')}$ defined in Sect. 26.2 where the action values are set according to the decision rule d_θ in the conditioning events. Recall that the covariate $L_{p+1,d_\theta}(t)$ of $L_{d_\theta}(t)$ corresponds with the outcome variable also denoted by $Y_{d_\theta}(t)$ and that $P(T_{d_\theta} = t) = P(\bar{Y}_{d_\theta}(t) = 0, Y_{d_\theta}(t+1) = 1)$. By integrating over all covariate values that are consistent with $T_{d_\theta} = t$ of the g-computation formula (26.5), the following probability $P(T_{d_\theta} = t)$ is obtained:

$$P(T_{d_\theta} = t) = \sum_{\{\bar{l}(t+1): y(t)=0, y(t+1)=1\}} Q_{L(0)}(l(0)) \prod_{t'=1}^{t+1} \prod_{j=1}^{n_t(t')} \prod_{m=1}^{n(t',p+j)-1} Q_{L_{p+j,m}(t'),d_\theta}(\bar{l}(t+1)). \tag{26.6}$$

We denote the right-hand side of equality (26.6) with $\Phi(Q, t, \theta)$ to make explicit that this parameter of P only depends on P through its $Q(P)$-factor. Using that $P(Y_{d_\theta}(t+1) = 1) = \sum_{t'=0}^{t} P(\bar{Y}_{d_\theta}(t') = 0, Y_{d_\theta}(t'+1) = 1)$ and equality (26.6), the causal estimand defined by (26.4) can be expressed as a function of the Q-factor of the observed data likelihood under the SRA:

$$\psi = \sum_{t=0}^{3} \Phi(Q, t, 350) - \sum_{t=0}^{3} \Phi(Q, t, 200). \tag{26.7}$$

The parameter $\psi = \Psi(Q)$, as defined by equality (26.7), is the target parameter in this analysis. It is a mapping from the Q-part of a probability distribution P of the observed data structure O into a one-dimensional euclidean parameter, as made explicit by the notation $\psi = \Psi(Q)$. We denote the true value of this target parameter by $\psi_0 = \Psi(Q_0)$ where Q_0 denotes the Q-part of the likelihood of the observed data under the true distribution P_0. Note that under the SRA, the target parameter value ψ_0 can be interpreted causally since it then corresponds to the causal parameter $\psi_0^F = \Psi^F(P_{X,U,0})$ from equality (26.4).

26.4 IPCW-R-TMLE

In this section, we develop an inverse probability of action-weighted reduced-data targeted maximum likelihood estimator (IPAW-R-TMLE) for estimation of the above-defined target parameter ψ_0. Implementation of this IPAW-R-TMLE is illustrated with data from the KPNC electronic medical record. The IPAW-R-TMLE is a weighted TMLE applied to so-called reduced data that corresponds to the original data where the time-dependent covariates are ignored, with the exception of the time-dependent CD4 count and the outcome process (van der Laan 2008b). The weights applied to the reduced-data TMLE (R-TMLE) permit adjustment for the other time-dependent confounders that could not be accounted for by the R-TMLE because of this data-reduction step.

The IPAW-R-TMLE is a targeted minimum-loss-based estimator as presented in Appendix A, where we provide detailed explanation and understanding of IPAW-R-TMLE (see also Chap. 24). The technical report provides additional detail regarding the specific implementation carried out here. It involves the following steps. Firstly, the observed data structure is reduced by replacing the time-dependent covariates L in O by a reduced-data time-dependent covariate L^r, resulting in a reduced observed data structure O^r. The causal quantity of interest is represented as a parameter of the probability distribution Q_0^r, a function of $O^r = (L^r, A)$, where $Q_0^r(l^r, a) = \prod_t Q_0^r(l^r(t) \mid \bar{l}^r(t-1), \bar{a}(t-1))$ represents the probability that the counterfactual L_a^r equals l^r. Thus Q_0^r is a function of the full data distribution of the counterfactuals $(L_a : a)$. A possible loss function for Q_0^r is given by $-g^r/g_0 log Q$, but more stable time-dependent weighting schemes will be employed, resulting in a specified loss function $L_{w_0}(Q)$ relying on a weight function $(w_0(t) : t)$, where $w_0(t) = \prod_{s \leq t-1} g_{0,A(s)}^r / \prod_{s \leq t-1} g_{0,A(s)}$ is indexed by g^r and g_0. Specifically, the minus log of the conditional distribution of $L_a^r(t)$, given $\bar{L}_a^r(t-1)$, in $Q^r(l^r, a) = \prod_t Q^r(l^r(t) \mid \bar{l}^r(t-1), \bar{a}(t-1))$ is weighted by the corresponding $w_0(t)$ for that time point. This loss function $L_{w_0}(Q)$ is valid for each choice of g^r, but it relies on correct specification of the true action mechanism g_0. Let w_n be an estimator of the weight function w_0, thereby using the actual observed data $O_1, \ldots, O_n$. We select a parametric model $(Q(\epsilon) : \epsilon)$ so that $\frac{d}{d\epsilon} \log Q(\epsilon)$ at $\epsilon = 0$ spans the efficient influence curve of the target parameter for the reduced data in the special case that there is no time-dependent confounding beyond L^r, or, equivalently, $w_0 = 1$. This now defines the quantity Q_0^r, the target parameter $\psi_0^r = \Psi(Q_0^r)$, the loss function $L_{w_0}(Q)$ for Q_0^r, and the parametric working model $\{Q(\epsilon) : \epsilon\}$, so that the targeted minimum-loss-based estimator is defined, and it will solve the so-called IPAW-R-efficient influence curve estimating equation:

$$0 = P_n \frac{d}{d\epsilon} L_{w_n}(Q_n^*(\epsilon))\Big|_{\epsilon=0}.$$

Section 26.4.1 describes the R-TMLE on which the IPAW-R-TMLE is based. The R-TMLE is identical to the actual targeted maximum likelihood estimator applied to the reduced data, relying on the log-likelihood loss function, using the parametric working logistic regression models defined by clever time-dependent covariates in order to fluctuate the conditional distributions of binary variables. This TMLE applied to reduced data would be consistent if $w_0 = 1$, but it is biased in general, due to ignoring the time-dependent covariates that were removed from the data structure. Section 26.4.2 describes the implementation of the corresponding IPAW-R-TMLE of ψ_0, which simply involves applying the estimated weights w_n to the R-TMLE. The results of the application of both the R-TMLE as well as the IPAW-R-TMLE are provided.

26.4.1 R-TMLE Implementation and Results

The R-TMLE described below corresponds with the TMLE applied to the simplified data where the only time-dependent covariates considered past baseline represent outcome and CD4 count measurements. Below, we describe the steps involved in the implementation of this R-TMLE starting with the presentation of the IPAW-estimating function, the corresponding derivation of the efficient influence curve, the parametric working model used to fluctuate the initial estimator defined in terms of logistic regression models for each binary conditional distribution, using a clever covariate, and, finally, the implementation of the iterative TMLE algorithm as defined by this parametric fluctuation model and the log-likelihood loss function.

For clarity, we abuse the notation previously introduced and associated with the original data structure to describe the R-TMLE based on the reduced-data structure. All reference to the covariates $L_{p+j}(t)$ for $j = 3, \ldots, q + q'$ and $t > 0$ in the notation below should thus be ignored since such variables are considered nil in this subsection.

IPAW estimating function. An IPAW estimating function for the target parameter ψ is defined as

$$D_{\mathrm{IPAW}}(g, \psi) \equiv \frac{I(\bar{A}(\check{T}) = d_{350}(\bar{L}(\check{T})))}{\prod_{t=0}^{\check{T}} g_{A_1(t)} g_{A_2(t)}} Y(\check{T} + 1)$$

$$-\frac{I(\bar{A}(\check{T}) = d_{200}(\bar{L}(\check{T})))}{\prod_{t=0}^{\check{T}} g_{A_1(t)} g_{A_2(t)}} Y(\check{T}+1) - \psi, \tag{26.8}$$

where $\check{T}$ is defined as the minimum between the follow-up time and 3, i.e., $\check{T} = \min(3, \tilde{T})$. Recall that the outcome variable $Y(t+1)$ is also denoted by $L_{p+1}(t+1)$ and $L_{p+1,1}(t+1)$ (Sect. 26.2). We use these three notations for the same variable interchangeably in the following sections.

Efficient influence curve and clever covariate. As described in Sect. 3.2 of van der Laan (2010a), the IPAW estimating function can be mapped into the efficient (relative to the reduced data) influence curve for ψ, denoted by $D^*(Q, g, \psi)$, by projecting it onto the tangent space of Q: $D^*(Q, g, \psi) = \Pi(D_{\mathrm{IPAW}} \mid T_Q)$, where D_{IPAW} is shorthand notation for $D_{\mathrm{IPAW}}(g, \psi)$ [definition (26.8)]. Theorem 2 in van der Laan (2010a) applied to factorization (26.3) of the likelihood of the reduced observed data leads to the following result:

$$\Pi(D_{\mathrm{IPAW}} \mid T_Q) = \Pi(D_{\mathrm{IPAW}} \mid T_{L(0)}) + \sum_{t=1}^{\tilde{T}} \sum_{j=1}^{2} \sum_{m=1}^{n(t,p+j)-1} \Pi(D_{\mathrm{IPAW}} \mid T_{L_{p+j,m}(t)}) + \Delta\Pi(D_{\mathrm{IPAW}} \mid T_{L_{p+1,1}(\tilde{T}+1)}),$$

where we have that $\Pi(D_{\mathrm{IPAW}} \mid T_{L(0)}) = E(D_{\mathrm{IPAW}} \mid L(0))$ and $\Pi(D_{\mathrm{IPAW}} \mid T_{L_{p+j,m}(t)}) = H^*_{L_{p+j,m}(t)}(L_{p+j,m}(t) - Q_{L_{p+j,m}(t)}(1))$ for $t = 1, \ldots, \tilde{T}$, $j = 1, 2$ and $m = 1, \ldots, n(t, p+j)-1$ or $(t, j, m) = (\tilde{T}+1, 1, 1)$, with $Q_{L_{p+j,m}(t)}(1)$ representing the conditional probability of $L_{p+j,m}(t)$ defined in Sect. 26.2 and evaluated at $L_{p+j,m}(t) = 1$. Here $H^*_{L_{p+j,m}(t)}$ is defined as the following function of $Pa(L_{p+j,m}(t))$:

$$E(D'_{\mathrm{IPAW}} \mid L_{p+j,m}(t) = 1, Pa(L_{p+j,m}(t))) - E(D'_{\mathrm{IPAW}} \mid L_{p+j,m}(t) = 0, Pa(L_{p+j,m}(t))), \tag{26.9}$$

where $D'_{\mathrm{IPAW}}(g)$ equals $D_{\mathrm{IPAW}}(g, \psi)$ with $\psi = 0$. Note that $D'_{\mathrm{IPAW}}(g)$ is only a function of the observed data collected up to $\check{T}+1$ which excludes $L_{p+j,m}(t)$ for $t > \check{T}+1$. As a result, equality (26.9) for $t > \check{T}+1$ becomes $H^*_{L_{p+j,m}(t)} = 0$. Note also that $D'_{\mathrm{IPAW}}(g)$ can be represented as

$$D'_{\mathrm{IPAW}}(O \mid g) = \frac{D_1(\bar{A}(\check{T}), \bar{L}(\check{T}+1))}{\prod_{t=0}^{\check{T}} g_{A_1(t)} g_{A_2(t)}},$$

with $D_1(\bar{A}(\check{T}), \bar{L}(\check{T}+1))$ defined as

$$\left(I(\bar{A}(\check{T}) = d_{350}(\bar{L}(\check{T}))) - I(\bar{A}(\check{T}) = d_{200}(\bar{L}(\check{T})))\right) Y(\check{T}+1).$$

From Theorem 2 in van der Laan (2010a), equality (26.9) can thus be rewritten as:

$$H^*_{L_{p+j,m}(t)} = \frac{1}{\prod_{t'=0}^{t-1} g_{A_1(t')} g_{A_2(t')}} \times \tag{26.10}$$

$$\Big(E(\sum_{\bar{a}(t,3)} D_1 \mid L_{p+j,m}(t) = 1, Pa(L_{p+j,m}(t))) - E(\sum_{\bar{a}(t,3)} D_1 \mid L_{p+j,m}(t) = 0, Pa(L_{p+j,m}(t)))\Big),$$

where D_1 is shorthand notation for $D_1(\bar{A}(t-1), \bar{a}(t, \check{T}), \bar{L}(\check{T}+1))$ and $\bar{a}(t,t') = (a(t), \ldots, a(t'))$ for $t' \geq t$ and nil otherwise. In addition, note that the second expectation in (26.10) is 0 when $j = 1$ and $t = 4$, and we have

$$H^*_{L_{p+1,1}(4)} = \frac{I(\bar{A}(\check{T}) = d_{350}(\bar{L}(\check{T}))) - I(\bar{A}(\check{T}) = d_{200}(\bar{L}(\check{T})))}{\prod_{t'=0}^{\check{T}} g_{A_1(t')} g_{A_2(t')}}.$$

Finally, note that both expectations in (26.10) are equal when $j = 2$ and $t = 4$. We thus have $H^*_{L_{p+2,m}(4)} = 0$.

From all the results above, the efficient (relative to the reduced data) influence curve for ψ, $D^*(Q, g, \psi)$ is defined as

$$\Pi(D_{\text{IPAW}} \mid T_{L(0)}) + \sum_{t=1}^{\check{T}} \sum_{j=1}^{2} \sum_{m=1}^{n(t,p+j)-1} \Pi(D_{\text{IPAW}} \mid T_{L_{p+j,m}(t)}) + \Delta^{I(\tilde{T} \leq 3)} \Pi(D_{\text{IPAW}} \mid T_{L_{p+1,1}(\check{T}+1)}), \qquad (26.11)$$

with $I(\tilde{T} \leq 3)$ representing the indicator that the follow-up time $\tilde{T}$ is lower than or equal to 3,

$$\Pi(D_{\text{IPAW}} \mid T_{L(0)}) = E(D_{\text{IPAW}} \mid L(0)),$$

$$\Pi(D_{\text{IPAW}} \mid T_{L_{p+j,m}(t)}) = H^*_{L_{p+j,m}(t)}(L_{p+j,m}(t) - Q_{L_{p+j,m}(t)}(1)), \text{ where}$$

for $t = 1, 2, 3$

$$H^*_{L_{p+j,m}(t)} = \frac{1}{\prod_{t'=0}^{t-1} g_{A_1(t')} g_{A_2(t')}} \times \qquad (26.12)$$

$$\Big(E_Q(\sum_{\bar{a}(t,3)} D_1 \mid L_{p+j,m}(t) = 1, Pa(L_{p+j,m}(t))) - E_Q(\sum_{\bar{a}(t,3)} D_1 \mid L_{p+j,m}(t) = 0, Pa(L_{p+j,m}(t)))\Big),$$

and

$$H^*_{L_{p+1,1}(4)} = \frac{I(\bar{A}(3) = d_{350}(\bar{L}(3))) - I(\bar{A}(3) = d_{200}(\bar{L}(3)))}{\prod_{t'=0}^{3} g_{A_1(t')} g_{A_2(t')}}. \qquad (26.13)$$

The variables $H^*_{L_{p+1,1}(t)}$ and $H^*_{L_{p+2,m}(t)}$ are the clever covariates that are used for updating the initial estimators of $Q_{L_{p+1,1}(t)}$ and $Q_{L_{p+2,m}(t)}$, respectively, during the implementation of the R-TMLE of the target parameter ψ_0.

Obtain an initial estimate Q_n^0 of Q_0. The efficient influence curve defined by equality (26.11) is a function of only a subset of the Q components of the reduced, observed data likelihood [see equality (26.3) tailored to the reduced-data structure]. Specifically, the following 14 components of Q are relevant for implementation of the R-TMLE of the target parameter and thus need to be estimated:

- $Q_{L(0)} \equiv P(L(0))$.
- $Q_{L_{p+1,1}(t)} \equiv P(Y(t) \mid \bar{L}(t-1), \bar{A}(t-1))$ for $t = 1, 2, 3, 4$ [only relevant at $\bar{Y}(t-1) = 0$, $\bar{A}_2(t-1) = 0$, and nonmissing $\bar{A}_1(t-1)$]. Recall that treatment is coded as missing after first ART discontinuation; see Sect. 26.1.
- $Q_{L_{p+2,m}(t)} \equiv P(I(L_{p+2}(t) = m) \mid \bar{L}(t-1), Y(t), \bar{A}(t-1), I(L_{p+2}(t) = 1), \ldots, I(L_{p+2}(t) = m-1))$ for $t = 1, 2, 3$ and $m = 1, 2, 3$ [only relevant at $\bar{Y}(t) = 0$, $\bar{A}_2(t-1) = 0$ and nonmissing $\bar{A}_1(t-1)$, and only unknown at $I(L_{p+2}(t) = 1) = 0, \ldots, I(L_{p+2}(t) = m-1) = 0$].

Thus, estimation of the target parameter $\psi_0 = \Psi(Q_0)$ with the R-TMLE relies on the initial estimation of the corresponding 14 Q_0-components of the true reduced-data-generating distribution, P_0. The initial estimate of $Q_{0,L(0)}$ is denoted by $Q^0_{L(0),n}$. It is defined based on nonparametric estimation of $Q_{0,L(0)}$ with the empirical distribution of $L(0)$. The initial estimates of $Q_{0,L_{p+1,1}(t)}$ and $Q_{0,L_{p+2,m}(t)}$ are denoted by $Q^0_{L_{p+1,1}(t),n}$ and $Q^0_{L_{p+2,m}(t),n}$, respectively. They are defined based on sieve estimation of $Q_{0,L_{p+1,1}(t)}$ and $Q_{0,L_{p+2,m}(t)}$ with the DSA algorithm as described below.

The initial estimate of $Q_{0,L_{p+1,1}(1)}$ (at $A_2(0) = 0$ and nonmissing $A_1(0)$) is obtained separately. The DSA algorithm was set so that it searched among main term logistic regression fits and reports the best fit of size s, $s = 1, \ldots, 10$, using deletion, substitution, and addition moves. Cross-validation was used to determine the best choice of size s.

This DSA algorithm was also used to obtain the remaining 12 estimates based on the following three data-pooling schemes:

- The initial estimates of $Q_{0,L_{p+1,1}(t)}$ for $t = 2, 3, 4$ (at $\bar{Y}(t-1) = 0$, $\bar{A}_2(t-1) = 0$, and nonmissing $\bar{A}_1(t-1)$) are obtained simultaneously through a DSA-selected, pooled estimator over the three time intervals, t.
- The initial estimates of $Q_{0,L_{p+2,m}(1)}$ for $m = 1, 2, 3$ (at $Y(1) = 0$, $A_2(0) = 0$, nonmissing $A_1(0)$, and $I(L_{p+2}(t) = 1) = 0, \ldots, I(L_{p+2}(t) = m-1) = 0$) are obtained simultaneously through a DSA-selected, pooled estimator over the three CD4 count levels, m.
- The initial estimates of $Q_{0,L_{p+2,m}(t)}$ for $t = 2, 3$ and $m = 1, 2, 3$ [at $\bar{Y}(t) = 0$, $\bar{A}_2(t-1) = 0$, nonmissing $\bar{A}_1(t-1)$, and $I(L_{p+2}(t) = 1) = 0, \ldots, I(L_{p+2}(t) = m-1) = 0$] are obtained simultaneously through a DSA-selected, pooled estimator over the three time intervals, t, and the three CD4 count levels, m.

We refer to the table in our technical report that lists the variables of the reduced data that were considered as candidate main terms in each of the four DSA estimators described above. With the exception of the variables enrollyear and m, no categorical variable with $l > 2$ levels was directly considered as a candidate main term. Instead, l binary variables, each of which represents the indicator that X is equal to m (denoted by $I(X = m)$) for $m = 1, \ldots, l$, were considered as potential main terms. The time-variable t was not only treated as a categorical variable but was also considered directly as a candidate main term. The initial estimates resulting from the application of the four DSA estimators described above are summarized in the accompanying technical report.

Calculate the optimal fluctuation. Estimation of the target parameter $\psi_0 = \Psi(Q_0)$ with the R-TMLE involves the fluctuation of the initial estimators of $Q_{0,L_{p+1,1}(t)}$ and $Q_{0,L_{p+2,m}(t)}$ obtained previously. The optimal fluctuation of each of these initial estimators is based on the clever covariates, H^*, defined by equalities (26.12) and (26.13). R-TMLE implementation thus requires calculation of these clever covariates. They are functions of $Q_{0,L_{p+1,1}(t)}$ for $t = 1, 2, 3, 4$ and $Q_{0,L_{p+2,m}(t)}$ for $t = 1, 2, 3$ and $m = 1, 2, 3$ but also the following components of the action mechanism defined in Sect. 26.2: $g_{0,A_1(t)}$ and $g_{0,A_2(t)}$ for $t = 0, 1, 2, 3$. Therefore, we first need to estimate $g_{0,A_1(t)}$ and $g_{0,A_2(t)}$ prior to computing the clever covariates. These estimates, combined with the initial estimates of $Q_{0,L_{p+1,1}(t)}$ and $Q_{0,L_{p+2,m}(t)}$, can then be mapped into an estimate of the clever covariates using Monte Carlo simulations.

Obtain an estimate g_n of g_0. The following eight components of the action mechanism, i.e., the g part of the reduced, observed data likelihood [see equality (26.3) tailored to the reduced-data structure], are relevant for implementation of the R-TMLE of the target parameter ψ_0 and need to be estimated:

- $g_{A_1(t)} \equiv P(A_1(t) \mid \bar{A}(t-1), \bar{L}(t), A_2(t))$ for $t = 0, 1, 2, 3$ [only relevant at $\bar{Y}(t) = 0$, $\bar{A}_2(t) = 0$, and nonmissing $\bar{A}_1(t)$];
- $g_{A_2(t)} \equiv P(A_2(t) \mid \bar{A}(t-1), \bar{L}(t))$ for $t = 0, 1, 2, 3$ [only relevant at $\bar{Y}(t) = 0$, $\bar{A}_2(t-1) = 0$, and nonmissing $\bar{A}_1(t-1)$].

Estimation of the target parameter $\psi_0 = \Psi(Q_0)$ with the R-TMLE relies on estimation of the corresponding 8 g_0-components of the true reduced-data-generating distribution, P_0. The 8 estimates of $g_{0,A_1(t)}$ and $g_{0,A_2(t)}$ are denoted by $g_{A_1(t),n}$ and $g_{A_2(t),n}$, respectively. They are obtained based on sieve estimation with the same estimator selection procedure adopted for initial estimation of the 14 Q_0 components described in the previous section. The following four data stratification/pooling schemes were applied to derive each of the 8 estimates:

- The estimate of $g_{0,A_1(0)}$ [at $A_2(0) = 0$ and nonmissing $A_1(0)$] is obtained separately.
- The estimates of $g_{0,A_1(t)}$ for $t = 1, 2, 3$ [at $\bar{Y}(t) = 0$, $\bar{A}_2(t) = 0$, and nonmissing $\bar{A}_1(t)$] are obtained simultaneously through a DSA-selected, pooled estimator over the three time intervals, t.
- The estimate of $g_{0,A_2(0)}$ is obtained separately.
- The estimates of $g_{0,A_2(t)}$ for $t = 1, 2, 3$ [at $\bar{Y}(t) = 0$, $\bar{A}_2(t-1) = 0$, and nonmissing $\bar{A}_1(t-1)$] are obtained simultaneously through a DSA-selected, pooled estimator over the three time intervals, t.

We refer to the table in the technical report that lists the variables of the reduced data that were considered as candidate main terms in each of the four DSA estimators described above. With the exception of the variables enrollyear and m, no categorical variable with $l > 2$ levels was directly considered as a candidate main term. Instead, l binary variables, each of which represents the indicator that X is equal to m (denoted by $I(X = m)$) for $m = 1, \ldots, l$, were considered as candidate main terms.

The variable t was not only treated as a categorical variable but was also considered directly as a candidate main term. The estimates resulting from the application of the DSA estimators are presented in our technical report.

Monte Carlo simulation based on g_n^0 and Q_n^0. The 13 clever covariates that need to be computed are defined by equalities (26.12) and (26.13): $H^*_{L_{p+1,1}(t)}$ for $t = 1, 2, 3, 4$ and $H^*_{L_{p+2,m}(t)}$ for $t = 1, 2, 3$ and $m = 1, 2, 3$. Each of these clever covariates are used to fluctuate the estimators of $Q_{0,L_{p+1,1}(t)}$ for $t = 1, 2, 3, 4$ and $Q_{0,L_{p+2,m}(t)}$ for $t = 1, 2, 3$ and $m = 1, 2, 3$ respectively.

By extending the definition of the observed outcome, $Y(t) = I(\tilde{T} \leq t-1, \Delta = 1)$, to time points t beyond the time of an event when it is observed, i.e., for $t > \tilde{T}$ when $\Delta = 1$, the clever covariate for updating the initial estimator of $Q_{0,L_{p+1,1}(t)}$ at $\bar{Y}(t-1) = 0, \bar{A}_2(t-1) = 0$, and nonmissing $\bar{A}_1(t-1)$ for $t = 1, 2, 3, 4$ can be rewritten

$$\begin{aligned} H^*_{L_{p+1,1}(t)} &= \frac{1}{\prod_{t'=0}^{t-1} g_{A_1(t')} g_{A_2(t')}} \\ &\times \Big[I(\bar{A}(t-1) = d_{350}(\bar{L}(t-1))) \Big(1 - E_Q(Y_{d_{350}}(4) \mid \bar{L}(t-1), \bar{A}(t-1), Y(t) = 0)\Big) \\ &- I(\bar{A}(t-1) = d_{200}(\bar{L}(t-1))) \Big(1 - E_Q(Y_{d_{200}}(4) \mid \bar{L}(t-1), \bar{A}(t-1), Y(t) = 0)\Big) \Big]. \end{aligned} \quad (26.14)$$

Note that at $t = 4$, equality (26.14) does indeed simplify to equality (26.13). Similarly, the clever covariate for updating the initial estimator of $Q_{0,L_{p+2,m}(t)}$ at $\bar{Y}(t) = 0$, $\bar{A}_2(t-1) = 0$, nonmissing $\bar{A}_1(t-1)$, and $L_{p+2,1}(t) = 0, \ldots, L_{p+2,m-1}(t) = 0$ for $t = 1, 2, 3$ and $m = 1, 2, 3$ can be rewritten as

$$\begin{aligned} H^*_{L_{p+2,m}(t)} &= \frac{1}{\prod_{t'=0}^{t-1} g_{A_1(t')} g_{A_2(t')}} \Big[I(\bar{A}(t-1) = d_{350}(\bar{L}(t-1))) \\ &\times \Big(E_Q(Y_{d_{350}}(4) \mid Pa(L_{p+2,m}(t)), L_{p+2,m}(t) = 1) - E_Q(Y_{d_{350}}(4) \mid Pa(L_{p+2,m}(t)), L_{p+2,m}(t) = 0) \Big) \\ &- I(\bar{A}(t-1) = d_{200}(\bar{L}(t-1))) \Big(E_Q(Y_{d_{200}}(4) \mid Pa(L_{p+2,m}(t)), L_{p+2,m}(t) = 1) \\ &\qquad - E_Q(Y_{d_{200}}(4) \mid Pa(L_{p+2,m}(t)), L_{p+2,m}(t) = 0) \Big) \Big], \end{aligned}$$

where $Pa(L_{p+2,m}(t)) \equiv (\bar{L}(t-1), \bar{A}(t-1), Y(t), L_{p+2,1}(t), \ldots, L_{p+2,m-1}(t))$.

The above formulation of the clever covariates makes explicit how they can be computed by first approximating each of the conditional expectations of $Y_{d_\theta}(4)$ by Monte Carlo simulations. Following the factorization of the reduced, observed data likelihood according to the time ordering of actions and covariates, 10,000 observations of the potential outcomes $Y_{d_\theta}(4)$ (for $\theta = 200, 350$) were simulated by sequentially generating future covariates starting at the fixed covariate and action history specified by the conditional event in each expectation and by setting future actions to the interventions implied by the individualized action rule d_θ. This simulation process ends when the outcome at time point 4 is simulated or earlier if the simulated event occurs before time point 4. The averages of these simulated potential outcomes approximate the desired conditional expectations of $Y_{d_\theta}(4)$. The value of the clever covariates needs to be calculated at each of the time points t, and for each of the n subjects in the sample. These values could also be computed analytically, using the above analytical expressions instead of the reliance on simulations.

The TMLE. The optimal fluctuations of the initial estimators of $Q_{0,L_{p+1,1}(t)}$ and $Q_{0,L_{p+2,m}(t)}$ based on the clever covariates computed previously, $H^*_{L_{p+1,1}(t)}$ and $H^*_{L_{p+2,m}(t)}$, result in the definition of updated, one-step estimates of $Q_{0,L_{p+1,1}(t)}$ and $Q_{0,L_{p+2,m}(t)}$ denoted by $Q^1_{L_{p+1,1}(t),n}$ and $Q^1_{L_{p+2,m}(t),n}$, respectively.

Specifically in this analysis, each updated estimate $Q^1_{L_{p+1,1}(t),n}$ for $t = 1, 2, 3, 4$ is defined by a separate, t-specific maximum likelihood regression of the outcome at time t, $L_{p+1,1}(t)$, on the clever covariate $H^*_{L_{p+1,1}(t)}$ based on a logistic model with offset equal to the logit transformation of the initial estimate $Q^0_{L_{p+1,1}(t),n}$ and based on the same observations at time t that contributed to the initial estimate of $Q_{0,L_{p+1,1}(t)}$, i.e., the updated estimate is defined by

$$Q^1_{L_{p+1,1}(t),n} = \frac{1}{1 + \exp\left(- (\text{logit}(Q^0_{L_{p+1,1}(t),n}) + \epsilon_n H^*_{L_{p+1,1}(t)})\right)},$$

where ϵ_n is the maximum likelihood estimate. Similarly, each updated estimate $Q^1_{L_{p+2,m}(t),n}$ for $t = 1, 2, 3$ and $m = 1, 2, 3$ is defined by a separate, (t, m)-specific maximum likelihood regression of the indicator of CD4 count at time t equal to level m, $L_{p+2,m}(t)$, on the clever covariate $H^*_{L_{p+2,m}(t)}$ based on a logistic model with offset equal to the logit transformation of the initial estimate $Q^0_{L_{p+2,m}(t),n}$ and based on the same observations at time t that contributed to the initial estimate of $Q_{0,L_{p+2,m}(t)}$. The value of the coefficient in front of the clever covariate in each of the logistic models defining the one-step estimates above is given in Table 26.2.

Implementation of the (iterative) R-TMLE relies on iteration of the updating process above until a convergence criterion is met. Starting with $k = 1$, the clever covariates are first recalculated by Monte Carlo simulations based on the latest updated estimates $Q^k_{L_{p+1,1}(t),n}$ and $Q^k_{L_{p+2,m}(t),n}$. Second, these latest updated estimates are fluctuated with the newly computed clever covariates to define newly updated estimates $Q^{k+1}_{L_{p+1,1}(t),n}$ and $Q^{k+1}_{L_{p+2,m}(t),n}$ using the updating process above where the initial estimates $Q^0_{L_{p+1,1}(t),n}$ and $Q^0_{L_{p+2,m}(t),n}$ are replaced with the latest updated estimates $Q^k_{L_{p+1,1}(t),n}$ and

Table 26.2 Estimates ϵ_n of the coefficients in front of the clever covariates in the logistic models defining the one-step, updated estimates of $Q_{0,L_{p+1,1}(t)}$ for $t = 1, 2, 3, 4$ and $Q_{0,L_{p+2,m}(t)}$ for $t = 1, 2, 3$ and $m = 1, 2, 3$

t	$L_{p+1,1}(t)$	$L_{p+2,1}(t)$	$L_{p+2,2}(t)$	$L_{p+2,3}(t)$
1	0.114	7.544	−24.694	34.977
2	−0.005	5.061	−20.949	29.879
3	0.031	1.886	−2.207	−1.892
4	0.013			

$Q^k_{L_{p+2,m}(t),n}$. Third, k is incremented by 1. The three-step process just described is repeated until a convergence criterion is met. The last updated estimates are referred to as the targeted estimates. A sensible convergence criterion is that the ϵ_n-values approximate zero, or that the empirical mean of the efficient influence curve at the current update approaches a value close enough to zero, taking into account the standard error of the estimator. In this analysis, only one step was carried out, so that the estimates $Q^1_{L_{p+1,1}(t),n}$ and $Q^1_{L_{p+2,m}(t),n}$ are deemed the targeted estimates of $Q_{0,L_{p+1,1}(t)}$ and $Q_{0,L_{p+2,m}(t)}$ denoted by $Q^*_{0,L_{p+1,1}(t),n}$ and $Q^*_{0,L_{p+2,m}(t),n}$, respectively. Practical evidence has suggested that most bias reduction occurs in the first step (Chap. 18). We also refer readers to the forthcoming Stitelman and van der Laan (2011a).

A substitution estimator of the parameter of interest. The R-TMLE estimate of the target parameter $\psi_0 = \Psi(Q_0)$ defined by equality (26.7) is derived by substitution of the relevant distributions Q_0 in the right hand-side of equality (26.7), i.e. $Q_{0,L(0)}$, $Q_{0,L_{p+1,1}(t)}$ for $t = 1, 2, 3, 4$, and $Q_{0,L_{p+2,m}(t)}$ for $t = 1, 2, 3$ and $m = 1, 2, 3$, with the empirical distribution $Q_{L(0),n}$, and the targeted estimates $Q^*_{L_{p+1,1}(t),n}$ and $Q^*_{L_{p+2,m}(t),n}$, respectively.

Concretely, this substitution estimate can be calculated using the following two-step procedure. First, the conditional expectations $E(Y_{d_\theta}(4) \mid L(0))$ (for $\theta = 200, 350$ and each unique observation of $L(0)$) are approximated by Monte Carlo simulation based on the targeted estimates $Q^*_{L_{p+1,1}(t),n}$ and $Q^*_{L_{p+2,m}(t),n}$ using the general simulation protocol described previously for the computation of the clever covariates. The resulting estimates of $E(Y_{d_\theta}(4) \mid L(0))$ are denoted by $E_{Q^*_n}(Y_{d_\theta}(4) \mid L(0))$. Second, these estimates are mapped into the R-TMLE estimate of ψ_0 denoted by $\Psi(Q^*_{0,n})$ using the formula

$$\Psi(Q^*_{0,n}) = \frac{1}{n}\sum_{i=1}^{n} E_{Q^*_{0,n}}(Y_{d_{350}}(4) \mid L(0) = l_i(0)) - \frac{1}{n}\sum_{i=1}^{n} E_{Q^*_{0,n}}(Y_{d_{200}}(4) \mid L(0) = l_i(0)).$$

This resulted in an R-TMLE estimate $\psi^*_n = 1.98\text{e}{-03}$ of ψ_0.

Influence curve based inference. Under regularity conditions, and under the assumption that g_n is a consistent estimator of action mechanism g_0, the R-TMLE estimator is asymptotically linear with influence curve that has a variance that is smaller than or equal to the variance (under P_0) of $D^*(Q^*, g_0, \psi_0)(O)$, where Q^* denotes the possibly misspecified limit of Q^*_n. A consistent estimator of the variance of the R-TMLE is thus obtained as follows:

$$Var_n(\Psi(Q^*_n)) = \frac{1}{n^2}\sum_{i=1}^{n}\{D^*_n(o_i) - \bar{D}^*_n\}^2, \tag{26.15}$$

where D^*_n is the estimated efficient influence curve, $\bar{D}^*_n$ is its empirical mean [which would equal zero if we plugged in the fully iterated TMLE (Q^*_n, g_n)]. The projection $\Pi(D_{IPAW} \mid L(0))$-term in the influence curve was estimated using the targeted estimates $Q^*_{L_{p+1,1}(t),n}$ and $Q^*_{L_{p+2,m}(t),n}$, while for the other (clever covariate) terms, we used the initial estimator Q_n^0. This simplification permits straightforward calculation of the influence curve evaluated at each observation i using the intermediate results from the previous computing steps, i.e., the clever covariate calculations based on the initial estimate of Q_0, and the Monte Carlo simulations based on the targeted estimate of Q_0 to derive the substitution estimator, without the need for additional computation. Based on this approach, the estimate of the standard error associated with the R-TMLE is $\sigma_{0,n} = 2.71e-03$ resulting in the following 95% confidence interval for ψ_0: [−3.32e−03, 7.28e−03].

Diagnosing sparse data bias. To mitigate the higher variability of the R-TMLE resulting from practical violation of the ETA assumption, truncation of the IPA weights can be used as part of the R-TMLE implementation to improve the mean squared error associated with R-TMLE estimation of the target parameter. Based on the distributions of the IPA weights in this analysis, as presented in the accompanying technical report, we used a truncation level of 20 for the implementation of the R-TMLE, i.e., the clever covariates on which implementation of the R-TMLE is based were computed based on IPA weights that were set to 20 if their values implied by the estimates $g_{0,A_1(t)}$ and $g_{0,A_2(t)}$ were greater than 20. The point estimate and estimate of the standard error associated with the R-TMLE based on truncated IPA weights is $\Psi(Q_n^*) = 1.44e-03$ and $\sigma_n = 2.68e-03$ respectively which results in the following 95% confidence interval for ψ_0: [−3.81e−03,6.69e−03].

26.4.2 IPAW-R-TMLE Implementation and Results

To account for potential time-dependent confounding that was ignored by the R-TMLE as a consequence of the data-reduction step, the IPAW-R-TMLE relies on an estimate of the true action mechanism, i.e., the components of the action mechanism, denoted by $g_{0,A_1(t)}$ and $g_{0,A_2(t)}$. These conditional distributions should not be confused with the components of the reduced-data action mechanism that were estimated in the previous section as part of the R-TMLE implementation and that we now denote by $g^r_{0,A_1(t)}$ and $g^r_{0,A_2(t)}$. The approach based on the DSA algorithm to derive the estimates of $g_{0,A_1(t)}$ and $g_{0,A_2(t)}$ is described in the accompanying technical report.

The initial estimates of $Q_{0,L_{p+1,1}(t)}$ and $Q_{0,L_{p+2,m}(t)}$ of the R-TMLE were recomputed, but now using weights equal to the plug-in estimator $w_n(t)$ of

$$w_0(t) \equiv \frac{\prod_{j=0}^{t-1} g^r_{0,A_1(t)} g^r_{0,A_2(t)}}{\prod_{j=0}^{t-1} g_{0,A_1(t)} g_{o,A_2(t)}}.$$

Similarly, the R-TMLE of the ϵ-coefficients was recomputed by now using these time-dependent weights $w_n(t)$. The resulting substitution estimate of the target parameter ψ_0 is equal to 1.41e-03 and corresponds to the one-step IPAW-R-TMLE point estimate. Note that the only difference in implementation of the R-TMLE point estimate vs. that of the IPAW-R-TMLE point estimate is in the use of the weights $w_n(t)$ to obtain the initial and updated estimates of $Q_{0,L_{p+1,1}(t)}$ and $Q_{0,L_{p+2,m}(t)}$. As explained in Appendix A, the weighted log-likelihood for the reduced data actually represents a valid loss function for the conditional counterfactual distributions of the reduced-data components $L^r_a(t)$ of the counterfactual $L_a(t)$, if g_0 is consistently estimated (i.e., w_n is consistent for w_0), or if the SRA holds with respect to the reduced data (i.e., there is no time-dependent confounding beyond the time-dependent covariates included in the reduced-data structure).

Inference with the IPAW-R-TMLE can be derived based on its influence curve (26.11) evaluated at the estimator of the action mechanism g_0 and the targeted estimator of Q_0 defined by the procedure above. Note that evaluation of formula (26.11) to derive inference with the IPAW-R-TMLE involves the estimates of $g_{0,A_1(t)}$ and $g_{0,A_2(t)}$ instead of the estimates of $g^r_{0,A_1(t)}$ and $g^r_{0,A_2(t)}$, i.e., the clever covariates used for fluctuation of the initial estimators of Q_0 in the implementation of the IPAW-R-TMLE should be multiplied by $w(t)$ to derive the clever covariates that appear in (26.11). Based on this approach and the same implementation shorcut employed earlier to simplify calculation of the R-TMLE influence curve evaluated at each observation i, the estimate of the standard error associated with the IPAW-R-TMLE is $\sigma_{0,n} = 2.48e{-}03$ resulting in the following 95% confidence interval for ψ_0: [−3.45e−03, 6.27e−03].

A few observations are characterized by relatively large IPA weights (>20) which suggests some practical violation of the ETA assumption. To mitigate the higher variability of the IPAW-R-TMLE resulting from practical violation of the ETA assumption, the IPAW-R-TMLE was implemented as described above with the difference that the clever covariates were computed based on reduced-data IPA weights, $\left(\prod_{t=0}^{\tilde{T}} g^r_{A_1(t)} g^r_{A_2(t)}\right)^{-1}$, that were truncated at 20. The point estimate and estimate of the standard error associated with this truncated IPAW-R-TMLE is $\Psi(Q^*_{0,n}) = 7.6e{-}04$ and $\sigma_{0,n} = 2.46e{-}03$ respectively which results in the following 95% confidence interval for ψ_0: [−4.07e−03, 5.59e−03].

Table 26.3 summarizes the results from the application of each estimator of the target parameter ψ_0 implemented in this analysis. Note that all inferences are consistent. The null hypothesis of a null effect ψ_0 may not be rejected based on the data

Table 26.3 Comparison of the results for each estimator of the target parameter ψ_0

Estimator	Estimate	SE	95% CI	p-value
R-IPAW (based on g^r)	1.42e−03	2.69e−03	[−3.86e−03, 6.69e−03]	0.60
R-TMLE	1.98e−03	2.71e−03	[−3.32e−03, 7.28e−03]	0.46
Truncated R-TMLE	1.44e−03	2.68e−03	[−3.81e−03, 6.69e−03]	0.59
IPAW (based on g)	6.9e−04	2.48e−03	[−4.16e−03, 5.54e−03]	0.78
IPAW-R-TMLE	1.41e−03	2.48e−03	[−3.45e−03, 6.27e−03]	0.57
Truncated IPAW-R-TMLE	7.6e−04	2.46e−03	[−4.07e−03, 5.59e−03]	0.76

from the KPNC electronic medical record and the three assumptions the IPAW-R-TMLE relies upon: SRA, positivity assumption, and consistent estimation of g_0.

The 95% confidence intervals suggest that the absolute value of the true causal risk difference is less than 1%. If the three assumptions on which these estimators rely for drawing a valid causal inference indeed hold, the null result may reflect a true null effect, a bias due to the erroneous inclusion of patients with a prevalent ADC at study entry, or a lack of power to detect a relatively small causal risk difference. In the accompanying technical report we comment on these three possible explanations before discussing possible reasons for potential bias due to violation of one or more of the three assumptions the IPAW-R-TMLE relies upon.

26.5 Discussion

In order to make progress in individualized medicine and comparative effectiveness research, one will need to understand outcome distributions under dynamic treatments. This chapter represents one very important application of dynamic treatments in comparative effectiveness research to inform the decision of when to start treatment in HIV patients.

The development of robust and efficient estimation methods that allow the data analyst to target clinically relevant causal quantities, and corresponding user friendly software implementations, will allow these methods to become prominent tools for analyzing longitudinal data. Furthermore, the roadmap for causal inference allows honest and careful interpretation of the results.

In response to the need to compare dynamic treatments, sequentially randomized controlled trials are also becoming more popular and provide a way to consistently estimate the causal effect of dynamic treatments such as dynamic treatments indexed by a choice of first line therapy, a cutoff for an intermediate biomarker, and a second line therapy to be assigned if the biomarker exceeds the cut-off (Thall et al. 2007; Bembom and van der Laan 2007b).

Possible important extensions of the analysis carried out in this chapter are to target dose-response curves defined as the survival curves under the when-to-start rule d_θ that starts HIV-treatment when the CD4-count drops below θ for a range of θ.By posing a working model for this dose-response curve in θ, one will be able to obtain more precise estimators of the projection of the true dose response curve on the working model, since all individuals will now contribute to the fit of this working model. Such an approach still allows for a valid test of a null hypothesis of interest about a certain contrast of this class of treatment rules as long as the working model is valid under the null hypothesis of interest. We refer to van der Laan (2010b) for details on formulation and the TMLE of the unknown parameters defined by this working model.

Part IX
Advanced Topics

Chapter 27
Cross-Validated Targeted Minimum-Loss-Based Estimation

Wenjing Zheng, Mark J. van der Laan

In previous chapters, we introduced targeted maximum likelihood estimation in semiparametric models, which incorporates adaptive estimation (e.g., loss-based super learning) of the relevant part of the data-generating distribution and subsequently carries out a targeted bias reduction by maximizing the log-likelihood, or minimizing another loss-specific empirical risk, over a "clever" parametric working model through the initial estimator, treating the initial estimator as offset. This updating process may need to be iterated to convergence. The target parameter of the resulting updated estimator is then evaluated, and is called the targeted minimum-loss-based estimator (also TMLE) of the target parameter of the data-generating distribution. This estimator is, by definition, a substitution estimator, and, under regularity conditions, is a double robust semiparametric efficient estimator.

However, we have seen in practice that the performance of the TMLE suffers when the initial estimator is too adaptive, leaving little signal in the data to fit the residual bias with respect to the initial estimator in the targeting step. Moreover, the use of adaptive estimators raises the question to what degree we can still rely on the central limit theorem for statistical inference. Our previous theorems (e.g., van der Laan and Robins 2003; van der Laan and Rubin 2006; van der Laan and Gruber 2010) show that under empirical process conditions and rate of convergence conditions, one can indeed still prove asymptotic linearity, and thereby obtain CLT-based inference. The empirical process conditions put some bounds on how adaptive the initial estimator can be.

We present a version of TMLE that uses V-fold sample splitting for the initial estimator in order to make the TMLE maximally robust in its bias reduction step. We refer to this estimator as the cross-validated targeted minimum-loss-based estimator (CV-TMLE). In a direct application, we formally establish its asymptotics under stated conditions that avoid such empirical process conditions.

We refer to our accompanying technical report (Zheng and van der Laan 2010) for the generalization of the theorem presented in this chapter to arbitrary semiparametric models and pathwise differentiable parameters.

27.1 The CV-TMLE

Let $O \sim P_0$. The probability distribution P_0 is known to be an element of a statistical model $\mathcal{M}$. We observe n i.i.d. copies $O_1, \ldots, O_n$ of O and wish to estimate a particular multivariate target parameter $\Psi(P_0) \in \mathbb{R}^d$, where $\Psi : \mathcal{M} \rightarrow \mathbb{R}^d$ and d denotes the dimension of the parameter. Let P_n denote the empirical probability distribution of $O_1, \ldots, O_n$ so that estimators can be represented as mappings from an empirical distribution to the parameter space of the parameter they are estimating. For example, $P_n \rightarrow \hat{\Psi}(P_n)$ denotes an estimator of $\psi_0 = \Psi(P_0)$.

We assume that Ψ is pathwise differentiable at each $P \in \mathcal{M}$ along a class of one-dimensional submodels $\{P_h(\epsilon) : \epsilon\}$ indexed by a choice h in an index set $\mathcal{H}$: i.e., there exists a fixed d-variate function $D(P) = (D_1(P), \ldots, D_d(P))$ so that for all $h \in \mathcal{H}$

$$\frac{d}{d\epsilon}\Psi(P_h(\epsilon))\Big|_{\epsilon=0} = PD(P)S(h),$$

where $S(h)$ is the score of $\{P_h(\epsilon) : \epsilon\}$ at $\epsilon = 0$. Here we used the notation $PS = \int S(o)dP(o)$ for the expectation of a function S of O.

We assume that a parameter $Q : \mathcal{M} \rightarrow \mathcal{Q}$ is chosen so that $\Psi(P_0) = \Psi^1(Q(P_0))$ for some mapping $\Psi^1 : \mathcal{Q} \rightarrow \mathbb{R}^d$. For convenience, we will refer to both mappings with Ψ, so we will abuse the notation by using interchangeably $\Psi(Q(P))$ and $\Psi(P)$. Let $g : \mathcal{M} \rightarrow \mathcal{G}$ be such that for all $P \in \mathcal{M}$

$$D^*(P) = D^*(Q(P), g(P)).$$

In other words, the canonical gradient only depends on P through a relevant part $Q(P)$ of P and a nuisance parameter $g(P)$ of P.

Let $\mathcal{L}^\infty(K)$ be the class of functions of O with bounded supremum norm over a set of K so that $P_0(O \in K) = 1$, endowed with the supremum norm. We assume there exists a uniformly bounded loss function $L : \mathcal{Q} \rightarrow \mathcal{L}^\infty(K)$ so that

$$Q(P_0) = \arg\min_{Q \in \mathcal{Q}} P_0 L(Q),$$

where, we remind the reader, $P_0 L(Q) = \int L(Q)(o)dP_0(o)$. In addition, we assume that for each $P \in \mathcal{M}$, for a specified d-dimensional (hardest) parametric model $\{P(\epsilon) : \epsilon\} \subset \mathcal{M}$ through P at $\epsilon = 0$ and with "score" at $\epsilon = 0$ for which the linear combinations of its components generates $D^*(P)$:

$$\langle D^*(P)\rangle \subset \langle \frac{d}{d\epsilon}L(Q(P(\epsilon)))\Big|_{\epsilon=0}\rangle.$$

Here we used the notation $\langle h \rangle$ for the linear span spanned by the components of $h = (h_1, \ldots, h_k)$.

We are now ready to define the CV-TMLE. Let $P_n \to \hat{Q}(P_n)$ be an initial estimator of $Q_0 = Q(P_0)$. Let $P_n \to \hat{g}(P_n)$ be an initial estimator of $g_0 = g(P_0)$. Given $\hat{Q}, \hat{g}$, let $P_n \to \hat{Q}_\epsilon(P_n)$ be a family of estimators indexed by ϵ chosen so that

$$\langle D^*(\hat{Q}(P_n), \hat{g}(P_n)) \rangle \subset \langle \frac{d}{d\epsilon} L(\hat{Q}_\epsilon(P_n)) \Big|_{\epsilon=0} \rangle. \tag{27.1}$$

One can think of $\{\hat{Q}_\epsilon(P_n) : \epsilon\} \subset \mathcal{M}$ as a submodel through $\hat{Q}(P_n)$ with parameter ϵ, chosen so that the derivative/score at $\epsilon = 0$ yields a function that equals or spans the efficient influence curve at the initial estimator $(\hat{Q}(P_n), \hat{g}(P_n))$. Note that this submodel for fluctuating $\hat{Q}(P_n)$ uses the estimator $\hat{g}(P_n)$ in its definition.

Let $B_n \in \{0, 1\}^n$ be a random vector indicating a split of $\{1, \ldots, n\}$ into a training and validation sample: $\mathcal{T} = \{i : B_n(i) = 0\}$ and $\mathcal{V} = \{i : B_n(i) = 1\}$. Let $P^0_{B_n,n}, P^1_{B_n,n}$ be the empirical probability distributions of the training and validation samples, respectively. For a given cross-validation scheme $B_n \in \{0, 1\}^n$, we now define

$$\epsilon_n^0 = \hat{\epsilon}(P_n) \equiv \arg\min_\epsilon E_{B_n} P^1_{B_n,n} L(\hat{Q}_\epsilon(P^0_{B_n,n})).$$

This now yields an update $\hat{Q}_{\epsilon_n^0}(P^0_{B_n,n})$ of $\hat{Q}(P^0_{B_n,n})$ for each split B_n.

It is important to point out that this cross-validated selector of ϵ equals the cross-validation selector among the library of candidate estimators $P_n \to \hat{Q}_\epsilon(P_n)$ of Q_0 indexed by ϵ. As a consequence, we can apply the results for the cross-validation selector that show that it is asymptotically equivalent with the so-called oracle selector. Formally, consider the oracle selector

$$\tilde{\epsilon}_n^0 \equiv \arg\min_\epsilon E_{B_n} P_0 L(\hat{Q}_\epsilon(P^0_{B_n,n})).$$

If, in addition to uniform boundedness, we assume that the loss function also satisfies

$$M_2 = \sup_{Q \in \mathcal{Q}} \frac{\mathrm{var}\{L(Q) - L(Q_0)\}}{E_0\{L(Q) - L(Q_0)\}} < \infty,$$

then the results in van der Laan and Dudoit (2003) and van der Vaart et al. (2006) imply that we have the following finite sample inequality:

$$\begin{aligned} 0 &\leq E E_{B_n} P_0 \{L(\hat{Q}_{\epsilon_n^0}(P^0_{n,B_n})) - L(\hat{Q}_{\tilde{\epsilon}_n^0})\} \\ &\leq 2\sqrt{c}\frac{1}{\sqrt{n}} \sqrt{E E_{B_n} P_0 \{L(\hat{Q}_{\tilde{\epsilon}_n^0}(P^0_{n,B_n})) - L(Q_0)\}}. \end{aligned}$$

Here c can be explicitly bounded by M_2 and an upper bound of L. This shows that under no conditions on the initial estimator does the selection of ϵ have good consistency properties.

One could iterate this updating process of the training-sample-specific estimators: define $\hat{Q}^1(P^0_{B_n,n}) = \hat{Q}_{\epsilon_n^0}(P^0_{B_n,n})$, define the family of fluctuations $P_n \to \hat{Q}^1_\epsilon(P_n)$

satisfying the derivative condition (27.1), and define

$$\epsilon_n^1 = \arg\min_{\epsilon} E_{B_n} P^1_{B_n,n} L(\hat{Q}^1_{\epsilon}(P^0_{n,B_n})),$$

resulting in another update $\hat{Q}^1_{\epsilon_n^1}(P^0_{B_n,n})$ for each B_n. This process is iterated till $\epsilon_n^k = 0$ (or close enough to zero). The final update will be denoted by $\hat{Q}^*(P^0_{B_n,n})$ for each split B_n. The TMLE of ψ_0 is now defined as

$$\psi_n^* = E_{B_n} \Psi(\hat{Q}^*(P^0_{B_n,n})).$$

In a variety of examples, the convergence occurs in one step (i.e., $\epsilon_n^1 = 0$ already). In this case, we write $\epsilon_n \equiv \epsilon_n^0$ and

$$\psi_n^* = E_{B_n} \Psi(\hat{Q}_{\epsilon_n}(P^0_{B_n,n})).$$

Linear components. This TMLE can also be generalized to the case where only one component of Q should be estimated using a parametric working fluctuation model, while the other component can be estimated using a substitution estimator plugging in the empirical probability distribution function (i.e., a nonparametric maximum likelihood estimator). In this case, it is not necessary to target the second component since it is already an unbiased estimator. Formally, consider a decomposition of Q into (Q_1, Q_2), such that $Q_2 \rightarrow \Psi(Q_1, Q_2)$ is linear and $Q_2(P)$ is linear in P itself so that it is sensible to estimate it with an empirical probability distribution. Suppose that the canonical gradient D^* can be decomposed as

$$D^*(P) = D_1^*(P) + D_2^*(P),$$

where $D_1^*(P_0)$ is the canonical gradient of the mapping

$$P \rightarrow \Psi(Q_1(P), Q_2(P_0)) \tag{27.2}$$

at $P = P_0$. Assume also that $D_1^*(P)$ does not depend on $Q_2(P)$. Then we may estimate (27.2) at P_0, viewed as a function of $Q_1(P_0)$, as if $Q_2(P_0)$ were known, with the above-defined CV-TMLE. In this case, the parametric fluctuation model needs to satisfy

$$\langle D_1^*(\hat{Q}_1(P_n), \hat{g}(P_n))\rangle \subset \langle \frac{d}{d\epsilon} L(\hat{Q}_{1,\epsilon}(P_n))\Big|_{\epsilon=0} \rangle.$$

The optimal ϵ at each step is selected using cross-validation as described above but now with respect to a loss function $L(Q_1)$. The procedure ends when ϵ_n^k converges to 0. This yields a CV-TMLE $\hat{Q}_1^*(P^0_{B_n,n})$ for each sample split B_n. The resulting CV-TMLE of ψ_0 is given by

$$\psi_n^* = E_{B_n} \Psi\left(\hat{Q}_1^*(P^0_{B_n,n}), \hat{Q}_2(P^1_{B_n,n})\right).$$

Note that we estimate Q_{20} on validation samples, which allows the asymptotics of the estimator to minimally depend on empirical process conditions, while the stated linearity in Q_2 makes this estimator behave well (just like it is fine to estimate a mean with the average of subsample specific empirical means over the subsamples that partition the whole sample). We illustrate this estimator with an application to the additive causal effect of a binary treatment on a continuous or binary outcome.

27.2 The CV-TMLE for the Additive Causal Effect

Let $O = (W, A, Y)$, W be a vector of baseline covariates, A a binary treatment variable, and Y an outcome of interest. Let $\mathcal{M}$ be the class of all probability distributions for O. We consider the parameter $\Psi : \mathcal{M} \to \mathbb{R}$:

$$\Psi(Q(P)) = E_P \left[E_P(Y \mid A = 1, W) - E_P(Y \mid A = 0, W) \right].$$

Here, $Q(P) = (\bar{Q}(P), Q_W(P))$, where $\bar{Q}(P)(A, W) \equiv E_P(Y \mid A, W)$ and $Q_W(P)$ is the density of the marginal probability distribution of W. For convenience, we will use $\bar{Q}(P)(W)$ to denote $E_P(Y \mid A = 1, W) - E_P(Y \mid A = 0, W)$. The distinctions will be clear from the arguments given to the function or from context. Let $g(P)(A \mid W) \equiv Pr_P(A \mid W)$. We also adopt the notations $\bar{Q}_0 = \bar{Q}(P_0)$ and $Q_{W,0} = Q_W(P_0)$.

Our parameter of interest is Ψ evaluated at the distribution $P_0 \in \mathcal{M}$ of the observed O:

$$\psi_0 = \Psi(Q_0) = E_{W,0} \left[E_0(Y \mid A = 1, W) - E_0(Y \mid A = 0, W) \right].$$

The canonical gradient of Ψ at $P \in \mathcal{M}$ is

$$\begin{aligned} D^*(Q(P), g(P))(O) &= \left\{ H^*_{g(P)}(A, W) \left(Y - \bar{Q}(P)(A, W) \right) \right\} \\ &\quad + \left\{ \bar{Q}(P)(W) - Q_W(P)\bar{Q}(P) \right\} \\ &\equiv D^*_Y(\bar{Q}(P), g(P)) + D^*_W(\bar{Q}(P), Q_W(P)), \end{aligned}$$

where

$$H^*_g(A, W) = \left(\frac{A}{g(1 \mid W)} - \frac{1 - A}{g(0 \mid W)} \right).$$

For convenience, we will also use the notation

$$H^*_g(W) = H^*_g(1, W) - H^*_g(0, W).$$

Firstly, note that the map $Q_W \mapsto \Psi(\bar{Q}, Q_W)$ is linear. Secondly, $D^*_Y(\bar{Q}_0, g_0)$ is the canonical gradient of the map $P \mapsto \Psi(\bar{Q}(P), Q_W(P_0))$ at $P = P_0$, and does not depend on $Q_W(P_0)$. In what follows we present a TMLE of Q_0 where only the initial estimator $\hat{\bar{Q}}(P_n)$ of $\bar{Q}_0$ is updated using a parametric working model $\hat{\bar{Q}}_\epsilon(P_n)$, while the marginal distribution of W is estimated with the empirical distribution, which is not updated. Given an appropriate loss function $L(\bar{Q})$ and initial estimators $\hat{\bar{Q}}$ and $\hat{g}$ of $\bar{Q}_0$ and g_0, respectively, the parametric working model $\{\hat{\bar{Q}}_\epsilon(P_n) : \epsilon\}$ will be selected such that

$$\frac{d}{d\epsilon} L(\hat{\bar{Q}}_\epsilon(P_n))\Big|_{\epsilon=0} = D^*_Y(\hat{\bar{Q}}(P_n), \hat{g}(P_n)).$$

We consider here two possible loss functions for binary outcome or continuous outcomes $Y \in [0,1]$.

Squared error loss function. The squared error loss function is given by

$$L(\bar{Q})(O) = (Y - \bar{Q}(A, W))^2,$$

with the parametric working model

$$\hat{\bar{Q}}_\epsilon(P_n) = \hat{\bar{Q}}(P_n) + \epsilon H^*_{\hat{g}(P_n)}.$$

Quasi-log-likelihood loss function. The quasi-log-likelihood loss function is given by:

$$L(\bar{Q})(O) \equiv -\left(Y \log(\bar{Q}(W,A)) + (1-Y)\log(1-\bar{Q}(W,A))\right),$$

with the parametric working model

$$\hat{\bar{Q}}_\epsilon(P_n) = \frac{1}{1 + e^{-\mathrm{logit}(\hat{\bar{Q}}(P_n)) - \epsilon H^*_{\hat{g}(P_n)}}}.$$

We note that we would use this loss function if Y were binary or Y were continuous with values in $[0,1]$. If Y is a bounded continuous random variable with values in $[a,b]$, then we can still use this loss function by using the transformed outcome $Y^* = (Y-a)/(b-a)$ and mapping the obtained TMLE of the additive treatment effect on Y^* (and confidence intervals) into a TMLE of the additive treatment effect on Y (and confidence intervals).

It is important to point out that the TMLE of $\bar{Q}_0$ corresponding with both fluctuation models will converge in one step, since the clever covariate $H^*_{\hat{g}(P_n)}$ in the update of $\hat{\bar{Q}}$ does not involve $\hat{\bar{Q}}$.

Let $B_n \in \{0,1\}^n$ be a random vector indicating a split of $\{1,\ldots,n\}$ into a training and a validation sample: $\mathcal{T} = \{i : B_n(i) = 0\}$ and $\mathcal{V} = \{i : B_n(i) = 1\}$. Let P^0_{n,B_n}, P^1_{n,B_n} be the empirical probability distributions of the training and validation samples, respectively. Given the parametric working model, the optimal ϵ_n is selected using cross-validation:

$$\epsilon_n = \arg\min_\epsilon E_{B_n} P^1_{n,B_n} L(\hat{\bar{Q}}_\epsilon(P^0_{B_n,n})).$$

In particular, the one-step convergence implies that ϵ_n satisfies

$$0 = E_{B_n} P^1_{B_n,n} D^*_Y(\hat{\bar{Q}}_{\epsilon_n}(P^0_{B_n,n}), \hat{g}(P^0_{B_n,n})). \tag{27.3}$$

The TMLE of ψ_0 is defined as

$$\psi_n^* = E_{B_n}\Psi\left(\hat{\bar{Q}}_{\epsilon_n}(P^0_{B_n,n}), \hat{Q}_W(P^1_{B_n,n})\right).$$

In the theorem and proof, at each sample split B_n, we define the TMLE of Q_0 at (P_n, B_n) as

$$\hat{Q}_{B_n}(P_n) \equiv \left(\hat{\bar{Q}}_{\epsilon_n}(P^0_{B_n,n}), \hat{Q}_W(P^1_{B_n,n})\right).$$

27.3 Asymptotics of the CV-TMLE

We will now use the squared error loss example to illustrate the theoretical advantages of CV-TMLE and the use of data-adaptive estimators for the initial estimators. We will show that under a natural rate condition on the initial estimators $\hat{\bar{Q}}$ and $\hat{g}$, the resulting TMLE ψ_n^* is asymptotically linear, and when $\hat{g}$ and $\hat{\bar{Q}}$ are consistent, its influence curve is indeed the efficient influence curve. For a similar theorem for the CV-TMLE using the quasi-log-likelihood loss function and its proof, we refer to the accompanying technical report (Zheng and van der Laan 2010).

Theorem 27.1. *Consider the setting above under the squared error loss function. Let $B_n \in \{0,1\}^n$ be a random vector indicating a split of $\{1,\ldots,n\}$ into a training and validation sample. Suppose B_n is uniformly distributed on a finite support. We will index the V possible outcomes of B_n with $v = 1,\ldots,V$. Let $\hat{\bar{Q}}$ and $\hat{g}$ be initial estimators of $\bar{Q}_0$ and g_0. In what follows, $\hat{\bar{Q}}(P_0)$ and $\hat{g}(P_0)$ denote limits of these estimators, not necessarily equal to $\bar{Q}_0$ and g_0, respectively. The CV-TMLE satisfies*

$$\begin{aligned}\psi_n^* - \psi_0 &= E_{B_n}\left(P^1_{B_n,n} - P_0\right)D^*\left(\hat{Q}_{B_n}(P_n), \hat{g}(P^0_{B_n,n})\right)\\ &+E_{B_n}P_0\left\{\frac{(-1)^{1+A}}{g_0\hat{g}(P^0_{B_n,n})}\left(\bar{Q}_0 - \hat{\bar{Q}}_{\epsilon_n}(P^0_{B_n,n})\right)\left(g_0 - \hat{g}(P^0_{B_n,n})\right)\right\}. \quad (27.4)\end{aligned}$$

Suppose now that there exists a constant $L > 0$ such that $P_0(|Y| < L) = 1$. Consider the following definition:

$$\epsilon_0 \equiv \arg\min_{\epsilon} P_0 L(\hat{\bar{Q}}_\epsilon(P_0)).$$

Suppose that these minima exist and satisfy the derivative equations

$$0 = P_0 D_Y(P_0, \epsilon_0),$$

where

$$\begin{aligned}D_Y(P,\epsilon)(O) &\equiv \frac{d}{d\epsilon}L(\hat{\bar{Q}}_\epsilon(P))(O)\\ &= \left(Y - \hat{\bar{Q}}(P)(A,W) - \epsilon H^*_{\hat{g}(P)}(A,W)\right)H^*_{\hat{g}(P)}(A,W)\\ &= D^*_Y\left(\hat{\bar{Q}}_\epsilon(P), \hat{g}(P)\right)(O).\end{aligned}$$

If there are multiple minima, then it is assumed that the argmin is uniquely defined and selects one of these minima. Suppose that $\hat{\bar{Q}}$ and $\hat{g}$ satisfy the following conditions:

1. *There exists a closed bounded set $K \subset \mathbb{R}^k$ containing ϵ_0 such that ϵ_n belongs to K with probability 1.*
2. *For some $\delta > 0$, $P(1 - \delta > \hat{g}(P_n)(1 \mid W) > \delta) = 1$.*
3. *For some $K > 0$, $P(|\hat{\bar{Q}}(P_n)(A, W)| < K) = 1$.*
4. $$\int_W (\hat{g}(P_n)(1|w) - \hat{g}(P_0)(1|w))^2 \, dQ_{W,0}(w) \to 0 \quad \text{in probability.}$$
5. *For $a = 0, 1$,*
$$\int_W \left(\hat{\bar{Q}}(P_n)(a, w) - \hat{\bar{Q}}(P_0)(a, w)\right)^2 dQ_{W,0}(w) \to 0 \quad \text{in probability.}$$

Then,

$$\begin{aligned}\psi_n^* - \psi_0 = &(P_n - P_0)\left\{D_Y^*\left(\hat{\bar{Q}}_{\epsilon_0}(P_0), \hat{g}(P_0)\right) + \hat{\bar{Q}}_{\epsilon_0}(P_0)\right\} \\ &+ E_{B_n} P_0 \left\{\frac{(-1)^{1+A}}{g_0 \hat{g}(P^0_{B_n,n})}\left(\bar{Q}_0 - \hat{\bar{Q}}_{\epsilon_n}(P^0_{B_n,n})\right)\left(g_0 - \hat{g}(P^0_{B_n,n})\right)\right\} \\ &+ o_P(1/\sqrt{n}). \end{aligned} \tag{27.5}$$

Furthermore, if $\hat{g}(P_n) = g_0$, the TMLE estimator ψ_n^* is an asymptotically linear estimator of ψ_0:

$$\psi_n^* - \psi_0 = (P_n - P_0)\, D^*(\hat{Q}_{\epsilon_0}(P_0), g_0) + o_P(1/\sqrt{n}), \tag{27.6}$$

where $\hat{Q}_{\epsilon_0}(P_0) = (\hat{\bar{Q}}_{\epsilon_0}(P_0), Q_{W,0})$.

If, in addition to $\hat{g}(P_n) = g_0$, $\hat{\bar{Q}}(P_0) = \bar{Q}_0$, which implies that $\hat{\bar{Q}}_{\epsilon_0}(P_0) = \bar{Q}_0$, then ψ_n^* is an asymptotically efficient estimator of ψ_0:

$$\psi_n^* - \psi_0 = (P_n - P_0)\, D^*(Q_0, g_0) + o_P(1/\sqrt{n}). \tag{27.7}$$

More generally, if the limits satisfy $\hat{g}(P_0) = g_0$ and $\hat{\bar{Q}}(P_0) = \bar{Q}_0$, and if the convergence satisfies

$$\sqrt{E_{B_n} P_0 \left(\frac{g_0 - \hat{g}(P^0_{B_n,n})}{g_0 \hat{g}(P^0_{B_n,n})}\right)^2} \sqrt{E_{B_n} P_0 \left(\hat{\bar{Q}}_{\epsilon_n}(P^0_{B_n,n}) - \bar{Q}_0\right)^2} = o_P(1/\sqrt{n}), \tag{27.8}$$

then ψ_n^* is an asymptotically efficient estimator of ψ_0:

$$\psi_n^* - \psi_0 = (P_n - P_0)\, D^*(Q_0, g_0) + o_P(1/\sqrt{n}).$$

Consider now the case where $\hat{g}(P_0) = g_0$, but $\hat{\bar{Q}}(P_0) \neq \bar{Q}_0$. If the convergence satisfies

$$\sqrt{E_{B_n} P_0 \left(\frac{g_0 - \hat{g}(P^0_{B_n,n})}{g_0 \hat{g}(P^0_{B_n,n})} \right)^2} \sqrt{E_{B_n} P_0 \left(\hat{\bar{Q}}_{\epsilon_n}(P^0_{B_n,n}) - \hat{\bar{Q}}_{\epsilon_0}(P_0) \right)^2} = o_P(1/\sqrt{n}), \quad (27.9)$$

and

$$P_0 \left\{ H^*_{\hat{g}(P_n)} \left(\hat{\bar{Q}}_{\epsilon_0}(P_0) - \bar{Q}_0 \right) \right\}$$

is an asymptotically linear estimator of

$$P_0 \left\{ H^*_{\hat{g}(P_0)} \left(\hat{\bar{Q}}_{\epsilon_0}(P_0) - \bar{Q}_0 \right) \right\},$$

with influence curve IC', then ψ^*_n is an asymptotically linear estimator of ψ_0:

$$\psi^*_n - \psi_0 = (P_n - P_0) \left\{ D^*(\hat{Q}_{\epsilon_0}(P_0), g_0) + IC' \right\} + o_P(1/\sqrt{n}).$$

For convenience of reference, we state several simple but useful results in the proof of the theorem.

Lemma 27.1. *If X_n converges to X in probability, and there exists $A > 0$ such that $P(|X_n| < A) = 1$, then $E|X_n - X|^r \to 0$ for $r \geq 1$.*

Definition 27.1. An envelope of a class of functions $\mathcal{F}$ is a function F such that $| f | \leq F$ for all $f \in \mathcal{F}$.

Definition 27.2. For a class of functions $\mathcal{F}$ whose elements are functions f that map O into a real number, we define the entropy integral

$$\text{Entro}(\mathcal{F}) \equiv \int_0^\infty \sqrt{\log \sup_Q N(\epsilon \parallel F \parallel_{Q,2}, \mathcal{F}, L_2(Q))} d\epsilon,$$

where $N(\epsilon, \mathcal{F}, L_2(Q))$ is the covering number, defined as the minimal number of balls of radius $\epsilon > 0$ needed to cover $\mathcal{F}$, using the $L_2(Q)$-norm when defining a ball of radius ϵ.

We refer to van der Vaart and Wellner (1996) for empirical process theory. Lemma 27.2 below is an application of Lemma 2.14.1 in van der Vaart and Wellner (1996).

Lemma 27.2. *Conditional on $P^0_{B_n,n}$, let $\mathcal{F}(P^0_{B_n,n})$ denote a class of measurable functions of O. Suppose that the entropy integral of this class is bounded and there is an envelope function $\mathbf{F}(P^0_{B_n,n})$ of $\mathcal{F}(P^0_{B_n,n})$ such that $EP_0\mathbf{F}(P^0_{B_n,n})^2 \to 0$. Then for any $\delta > 0$*

$$EP\left(\sup_{f \in \mathcal{F}(P^0_{B_n,n})} \left| \sqrt{n} \left(P^1_{B_n,n} - P_0 \right) f \right| > \delta \middle| P^0_{B_n,n} \right) \to 0.$$

Lemma 27.3. *Suppose $\hat{g}$ is such that for some $\delta > 0$, $P(1-\delta > \hat{g}(P_n)(1 \mid W) > \delta) = 1$. If $\hat{g}$ satisfies $P_{W,0}(\hat{g}(P_n) - \hat{g}(P_0))^2 \xrightarrow{P} 0$, then we have that $P_0\left(H^*_{\hat{g}(P_n)} - H^*_{\hat{g}(P_0)}\right)^2$, $P_0\left(H^*_{\hat{g}(P_n)} - H^*_{\hat{g}(P_0)}\right)$, and $P_0\left((H^*_{\hat{g}(P_n)})^2 - (H^*_{\hat{g}(P_0)})^2\right)$ also converge to zero in probability.*

Lemma 27.4. *Suppose $\hat{g}$ and $\hat{\bar{Q}}$ satisfy conditions 2–5 in Theorem 27.1. Then, for any $r \geq 1$:*

$$1.\ EP_0\left(\hat{\bar{Q}}(P^0_{B_n,n})H^*_{\hat{g}(P^0_{B_n,n})} - \hat{\bar{Q}}(P_0)H^*_{\hat{g}(P_0)}\right)^r \to 0;$$
$$2.\ EP_0\left((Y - \hat{\bar{Q}}(P^0_{B_n,n}))H^*_{\hat{g}(P^0_{B_n,n})} - (Y - \hat{\bar{Q}}(P_0))H^*_{\hat{g}(P_0)}\right)^r \to 0;$$
$$3.\ EP_0\left((H^*_{\hat{g}(P^0_{B_n,n})})^2 - (H^*_{\hat{g}(P_0)})^2\right)^r \to 0;$$
$$4.\ EP_0\left(H^*_{\hat{g}(P^0_{B_n,n})} - H^*_{\hat{g}(P_0)}\right)^r \to 0.$$

We are now ready to prove Theorem 27.1.

Proof. Firstly, we wish to establish that

$$\begin{aligned}\psi^*_n - \psi_0 = {} & E_{B_n}\left(P^1_{B_n,n} - P_0\right)D^*\left(\hat{Q}_{B_n}(P_n), \hat{g}(P^0_{B_n,n})\right) \\ & + E_{B_n}P_0\left\{\frac{(-1)^{1+A}}{g_0\hat{g}(P^0_{B_n,n})}\left(\bar{Q}_0 - \hat{\bar{Q}}_{\epsilon_n}(P^0_{B_n,n})\right)\left(g_0 - \hat{g}(P^0_{B_n,n})\right)\right\},\end{aligned}$$

where $\hat{Q}_{B_n}(P_n) = \left(\hat{\bar{Q}}_{\epsilon_n}(P^0_{B_n,n}), \hat{Q}_W(P^1_{B_n,n})\right)$.

Note that

$$\begin{aligned}-P_0D^*(Q(P), g_0) &\equiv -P_0\left\{\left(Y - \bar{Q}(P)\right)H^*_{g_0} + \bar{Q}(P) - Q_W(P)\bar{Q}(P)\right\} \\ &= -\left\{P_0YH^*_{g_0} - P_0\bar{Q}(P)H^*_{g_0} + P_{W,0}\bar{Q}(P) - Q_W(P)\bar{Q}(P)\right\} \\ &= Q_W(P)\bar{Q}(P) - P_0YH^*_{g_0} \\ &= \Psi(Q(P)) - \Psi(Q_0).\end{aligned}$$

Applying this result to each sample split B_n and averaging over its support, it follows that

$$\psi^*_n - \psi_0 \equiv E_{B_n}\Psi\left(\hat{Q}_{B_n}(P_n)\right) - \Psi(Q(P_0)) = -E_{B_n}P_0D^*\left(\hat{Q}_{B_n}(P_n), g_0\right). \tag{27.10}$$

On the other hand,

$$\begin{aligned}& E_{B_n}P^1_{B_n,n}D^*_W\left(\hat{Q}_W(P^1_{B_n,n}), \hat{\bar{Q}}_{\epsilon_n}(P^0_{B_n,n})\right) \\ &\equiv E_{B_n}P^1_{B_n,n}\left\{\hat{\bar{Q}}_{\epsilon_n}(P^0_{B_n,n}) - Q_W(P^1_{B_n,n})\hat{\bar{Q}}_{\epsilon_n}(P^0_{B_n,n})\right\} \\ &= E_{B_n}\left\{Q_W(P^1_{B_n,n})\hat{\bar{Q}}_{\epsilon_n}(P^0_{B_n,n}) - Q_W(P^1_{B_n,n})\hat{\bar{Q}}_{\epsilon_n}(P^0_{B_n,n})\right\} = 0.\end{aligned}$$

Moreover, it follows from the definition of ϵ_n and the one-step convergence of the chosen fluctuation model that $\left(\hat{\bar{Q}}_{\epsilon_n}(P^0_{B_n,n}), \hat{g}(P^0_{B_n,n})\right)$ satisfies (27.3). Therefore, we have

$$\begin{aligned}
&E_{B_n} P^1_{B_n,n} D^*\left(\hat{Q}_{B_n}(P_n), \hat{g}(P^0_{B_n,n})\right) \\
&\quad \equiv E_{B_n} P^1_{B_n,n} D^*_Y\left(\hat{\bar{Q}}_{\epsilon_n}(P^0_{B_n,n}), \hat{g}(P^0_{B_n,n})\right) + E_{B_n} P^1_{B_n,n} D^*_W\left(\hat{Q}_W(P^1_{B_n,n}), \hat{\bar{Q}}_{\epsilon_n}(P^0_{B_n,n})\right) \\
&\quad = 0. \qquad (27.11)
\end{aligned}$$

Combining (27.10), (27.11), and the robustness of D^*, $P_0 D^*(Q_0, g) = 0$ for all g, we may now rewrite $\psi^*_n - \psi_0$ as

$$\begin{aligned}
\psi^*_n - \psi_0 = &\, E_{B_n}\left(P^1_{B_n,n} - P_0\right) D^*\left(\hat{Q}_{B_n}(P_n), \hat{g}(P^0_{B_n,n})\right) \\
&+ E_{B_n} P_0 \left\{D^*\left(\hat{Q}_{B_n}(P_n), \hat{g}(P^0_{B_n,n})\right) - D^*\left(\hat{Q}_{B_n}(P_n), g_0\right)\right\} \\
&- E_{B_n} P_0 \left\{D^*\left(Q_0, \hat{g}(P^0_{B_n,n})\right) - D^*\left(Q_0, g_0\right)\right\}.
\end{aligned}$$

The last two summands in this equality can be combined as

$$\begin{aligned}
&E_{B_n} P_0 \left\{D^*\left(\hat{Q}_{B_n}(P_n), \hat{g}(P^0_{B_n,n})\right) - D^*\left(\hat{Q}_{B_n}(P_n), g_0\right)\right\} \\
&\quad - E_{B_n} P_0 \left\{D^*\left(Q_0, \hat{g}(P^0_{B_n,n})\right) - D^*\left(Q_0, g_0\right)\right\} \\
&\equiv E_{B_n} P_0 \left\{D^*_Y(\hat{\bar{Q}}_{\epsilon_n}(P^0_{B_n,n}), \hat{g}(P^0_{B_n,n})) + D^*_W(\hat{Q}_{B_n}(P_n))\right\} \\
&\quad - E_{B_n} P_0 \left\{D^*_Y(\hat{\bar{Q}}_{\epsilon_n}(P^0_{B_n,n}), g_0) + D^*_W(\hat{Q}_{B_n}(P_n))\right\} \\
&\quad - E_{B_n} P_0 \left\{D^*_Y(\bar{Q}_0, \hat{g}(P^0_{B_n,n})) + D^*_W(Q_0)\right\} \\
&\quad + E_{B_n} P_0 \left\{D^*_Y(\bar{Q}_0, g_0) + D^*_W(Q_0)\right\} \\
&= E_{B_n} P_0 \left(\bar{Q}_0 - \hat{\bar{Q}}_{\epsilon_n}(P^0_{B_n,n})\right)\left(H^*_{\hat{g}(P^0_{B_n,n})} - H^*_{g_0}\right) \\
&= E_{B_n} P_0 \left\{\left(\bar{Q}_0 - \hat{\bar{Q}}_{\epsilon_n}(P^0_{B_n,n})\right)(-1)^{1+A} \frac{\left(g_0 - \hat{g}(P^0_{B_n,n})\right)}{g_0 \hat{g}(P^0_{B_n,n})}\right\}.
\end{aligned}$$

Therefore, we indeed have the desired expression (27.4):

$$\begin{aligned}
\psi^*_n - \psi_0 = &\, E_{B_n}\left(P^1_{B_n,n} - P_0\right) D^*\left(\hat{Q}_{B_n}(P_n), \hat{g}(P^0_{B_n,n})\right) \qquad (27.12) \\
&+ E_{B_n} P_0 \left\{\frac{(-1)^{1+A}}{g_0 \hat{g}(P^0_{B_n,n})}\left(\bar{Q}_0 - \hat{\bar{Q}}_{\epsilon_n}(P^0_{B_n,n})\right)\left(g_0 - \hat{g}(P^0_{B_n,n})\right)\right\}. \qquad (27.13)
\end{aligned}$$

We now study each term separately. For convenience, we use the notation $D_Y(P, \epsilon) \equiv D^*_Y(\hat{\bar{Q}}_\epsilon(P), \hat{g}(P))$. Term (27.12) can be written as

$$\begin{aligned}
&E_{B_n}\left(P^1_{B_n,n} - P_0\right) D^*\left(\hat{Q}_{B_n}(P_n), \hat{g}(P^0_{B_n,n})\right) \\
&\quad = E_{B_n}\left(P^1_{B_n,n} - P_0\right) D^*_Y\left(\hat{\bar{Q}}_{\epsilon_n}(P^0_{B_n,n}), \hat{g}(P^0_{B_n,n})\right)
\end{aligned}$$

$$
\begin{aligned}
&+E_{B_n}\left(P^1_{B_n,n} - P_0\right)\left\{\hat{\bar{Q}}_{\epsilon_n}(P^0_{B_n,n}) - Q_W(P^1_{B_n,n})\hat{\bar{Q}}_{\epsilon_n}(P^0_{B_n,n})\right\} \\
&= E_{B_n}\left(P^1_{B_n,n} - P_0\right)\left\{D_Y\left(P^0_{B_n,n}, \epsilon_n\right) - D_Y(P_0, \epsilon_0)\right\} \qquad (27.14) \\
&+(P_n - P_0) D_Y(P_0, \epsilon_0) \\
&+E_{B_n}\left(P^1_{B_n,n} - P_0\right)\left\{\hat{\bar{Q}}_{\epsilon_n}(P^0_{B_n,n}) - \hat{\bar{Q}}_{\epsilon_0}(P_0)\right\} \qquad (27.15) \\
&+(P_n - P_0)\hat{\bar{Q}}_{\epsilon_0}(P_0).
\end{aligned}
$$

It follows from the following lemma that ϵ_n converges to ϵ_0 in probability.

Lemma 27.5. *Let ϵ_n and ϵ_0 be defined as in Theorem 27.1 and suppose they solve the derivative equations as stated in the theorem. If $\hat{g}$ and $\hat{\bar{Q}}$ satisfy conditions 1–5 in Theorem 27.1, then ϵ_n converges to ϵ_0 in probability.*

Now consider the following lemmas

Lemma 27.6. *If the initial estimators $\hat{\bar{Q}}$ and $\hat{g}$ satisfy conditions 1–5 in the theorem, then, conditional on a sample split B_n,*

$$\sqrt{n}(P^1_{n,B_n} - P_0)\left\{D_Y\left(P^0_{B_n,n}, \epsilon_n\right) - D_Y(P_0, \epsilon_0)\right\} = o_P(1).$$

Lemma 27.7. *If $\hat{\bar{Q}}$ and $\hat{g}$ satisfy conditions 1–5 of the theorem, then, conditional on a sample split B_n,*

$$\sqrt{n}(P^1_{B_n,n} - P_0)\left(\hat{\bar{Q}}_{\epsilon_n}(P^0_{B_n,n}) - \hat{\bar{Q}}_{\epsilon_0}(P_0)\right) = o_P(1).$$

Note that Lemmas 27.5–27.7 follow from Lemmas 27.2–27.4.

Lemmas 27.6 and 27.7 imply that (27.14) and (27.15) are $o_P(1/\sqrt{n})$. We thus have established that (27.12) is given by

$$
\begin{aligned}
&E_{B_n}\left(P^1_{B_n,n} - P_0\right) D^*\left(\hat{Q}_{B_n}(P_n), \hat{g}(P^0_{B_n,n})\right) \\
&= (P_n - P_0)\left\{D^*_Y\left(\hat{\bar{Q}}_{\epsilon_0}(P_0), \hat{g}(P_0)\right) + \hat{\bar{Q}}_{\epsilon_0}(P_0)\right\} + o_P(1/\sqrt{n}).
\end{aligned}
$$

Combining this result with (27.13), we have proved (27.5):

$$
\begin{aligned}
\psi^*_n - \psi_0 &= (P_n - P_0)\left\{D^*_Y\left(\hat{\bar{Q}}_{\epsilon_0}(P_0), \hat{g}(P_0)\right) + \hat{\bar{Q}}_{\epsilon_0}(P_0)\right\} \\
&+E_{B_n}P_0\left\{\frac{(-1)^{1+A}}{g_0\hat{g}(P^0_{B_n,n})}\left(\bar{Q}_0 - \hat{\bar{Q}}_{\epsilon_n}(P^0_{B_n,n})\right)\left(g_0 - \hat{g}(P^0_{B_n,n})\right)\right\} \\
&+o_P(1/\sqrt{n}).
\end{aligned}
$$

Note that up to this point we have only used the convergence of $\hat{\bar{Q}}(P_n)$ and $\hat{g}(P_n)$ to some limits, but we assumed neither consistency to the true Q_0, g_0, nor a rate of convergence for these initial estimators to such limits.

Finally, we study the remainder term (27.13):

$$E_{B_n} P_0 \left\{ \frac{(-1)^{1+A}}{g_0 \hat{g}(P^0_{B_n,n})} \left(\bar{Q}_0 - \hat{\bar{Q}}_{\epsilon_n}(P^0_{B_n,n})\right)\left(g_0 - \hat{g}(P^0_{B_n,n})\right) \right\}.$$

We consider several cases. Firstly, consider the case $\hat{g}(P_n) = g_0$. In this case, term (27.13) is exactly 0. Therefore, (27.5) now implies that ψ^*_n is asymptotically linear with influence curve $D^*(\hat{Q}_{\epsilon_0}(P_0), g_0)$. If, in addition, the initial estimator $\hat{\bar{Q}}$ is consistent for $\bar{Q}_0$, i.e., $\hat{\bar{Q}}(P_0) = \bar{Q}_0$, then

$$\begin{aligned} \epsilon_0 &\equiv \arg\min_{\epsilon} P_0(Y - \hat{\bar{Q}}(P_0) - \epsilon H^*_{\hat{g}(P_0)})^2 \\ &= \arg\min_{\epsilon} P_0(Y - Q_0 - \epsilon H^*_{\hat{g}(P_0)})^2 = 0. \end{aligned}$$

This implies that $\hat{\bar{Q}}_{\epsilon_0}(P_0)$ is simply Q_0. Consequently, ψ^*_n is asymptotically linear with influence curve $D^*(Q_0, g_0)$ and is thereby asymptotically efficient.

Let's now consider the case where $\hat{g}(P_0) = g_0$ and $\hat{\bar{Q}}(P_0) = \bar{Q}_0$. In this case, $\hat{\bar{Q}}_{\epsilon_n}(P^0_{B_n,n})$ converges to $\bar{Q}_0$ and $\hat{g}(P^0_{B_n,n})$ converges to g_0. In particular, these imply that (27.13) converges to 0. However, for ψ^*_n to be asymptotically linear, it is necessary that the convergence of this second order term occurs at a $\sqrt{n}$ rate, i.e.,

$$E_{B_n} P_0 \left\{ \frac{(-1)^{1+A}}{g_0 \hat{g}(P^0_{B_n,n})} \left(g_0 - \hat{g}(P^0_{B_n,n})\right)\left(\hat{\bar{Q}}_{\epsilon_n}(P^0_{B_n,n}) - \bar{Q}_0\right) \right\} = o_P(1/\sqrt{n}).$$

Applying the Cauchy–Schwartz inequality, it follows that if

$$\sqrt{E_{B_n} P_0 \left(\frac{g_0 - \hat{g}(P^0_{B_n,n})}{g_0 \hat{g}(P^0_{B_n,n})} \right)^2} \sqrt{E_{B_n} P_0 \left(\hat{\bar{Q}}_{\epsilon_n}(P^0_{B_n,n}) - \bar{Q}_0\right)^2} = o_P(1/\sqrt{n}),$$

then ψ^*_n will be asymptotically efficient.

Finally, consider the case where $\hat{g}(P_0) = g_0$, but $\hat{\bar{Q}}(P_0) \neq \bar{Q}_0$. We reconsider expression (27.13) to account for the limit $\hat{\bar{Q}}_{\epsilon_0}(P_0)$ of $\hat{\bar{Q}}_{\epsilon_n}(P^0_{B_n,n})$, which does not equal $\bar{Q}_0$:

$$\begin{aligned} &E_{B_n} P_0 \left\{ \frac{(-1)^{1+A}}{g_0 \hat{g}(P^0_{B_n,n})} \left(g_0 - \hat{g}(P^0_{B_n,n})\right)\left(\hat{\bar{Q}}_{\epsilon_n}(P^0_{B_n,n}) - \bar{Q}_0\right) \right\} \\ &\quad = E_{B_n} P_0 \left\{ \frac{(-1)^{1+A}}{g_0 \hat{g}(P^0_{B_n,n})} \left(g_0 - \hat{g}(P^0_{B_n,n})\right)\left(\hat{\bar{Q}}_{\epsilon_n}(P^0_{B_n,n}) - \hat{\bar{Q}}_{\epsilon_0}(P_0)\right) \right\} \quad (27.16) \\ &\quad + E_{B_n} P_0 \left\{ \frac{(-1)^{1+A}}{g_0 \hat{g}(P^0_{B_n,n})} \left(g_0 - \hat{g}(P^0_{B_n,n})\right)\left(\hat{\bar{Q}}_{\epsilon_0}(P_0) - \bar{Q}_0\right) \right\}. \quad (27.17) \end{aligned}$$

Firstly, we require again that the rate of convergence for the second order term in (27.16) be $\sqrt{n}$, that is,

$$E_{B_n} P_0 \left\{ \frac{(-1)^{1+A}}{g_0 \hat{g}(P^0_{B_n,n})} \left(g_0 - \hat{g}(P^0_{B_n,n})\right) \left(\hat{\bar{Q}}_{\epsilon_n}(P^0_{B_n,n}) - \hat{\bar{Q}}_{\epsilon_0}(P_0)\right) \right\} = o_P(1/\sqrt{n}).$$

Applying the Cauchy–Schwartz inequality, it suffices that

$$\sqrt{E_{B_n} P_0 \left(\frac{g_0 - \hat{g}(P^0_{B_n,n})}{g_0 \hat{g}(P^0_{B_n,n})} \right)^2} \sqrt{E_{B_n} P_0 \left(\hat{\bar{Q}}_{\epsilon_n}(P^0_{B_n,n}) - \hat{\bar{Q}}_{\epsilon_0}(P_0)\right)^2} = o_P(1/\sqrt{n}).$$

For (27.17) to be asymptotically linear, stronger requirements on the performance of $\hat{g}$ are needed in order to address the inconsistency of $\hat{\bar{Q}}$. For convenience of notation, we recall that

$$\begin{aligned} & E_{B_n} P_0 \left\{ \frac{(-1)^{1+A}}{g_0 \hat{g}(P^0_{B_n,n})} \left(\bar{Q}_0 - \hat{\bar{Q}}_{\epsilon_n}(P^0_{B_n,n})\right) \left(g_0 - \hat{g}(P^0_{B_n,n})\right) \right\} \\ & = E_{B_n} P_0 \left\{ \left(H^*_{\hat{g}(P^0_{B_n,n})} - H^*_{g_0}\right) \left(\bar{Q}_0 - \hat{\bar{Q}}_{\epsilon_n}(P^0_{B_n,n})\right) \right\}. \end{aligned}$$

Now, for the given initial estimator $\hat{\bar{Q}}$ and $\hat{g}$, let

$$\Phi(P) \equiv P_0 \left\{ H^*_{\hat{g}(P)} \left(\hat{\bar{Q}}_{\epsilon_0}(P_0) - \bar{Q}_0\right) \right\}.$$

If $\hat{g}$ is such that $\Phi(P_n) - \Phi(P_0)$ is asymptotically linear (with some influnce curve IC'), then (27.17) becomes

$$\begin{aligned} & E_{B_n} P_0 \left\{ \left(H^*_{\hat{g}(P^0_{B_n,n})} - H^*_{g_0}\right) \left(\hat{\bar{Q}}_{\epsilon_0}(P_0) - \bar{Q}_0\right) \right\} \\ & \equiv E_{B_n} \left(\Phi(P^0_{B_n,n}) - \Phi(P_0)\right) \\ & = E_{B_n} \left(P^0_{B_n,n} - P_0\right) IC' + o_P(1/\sqrt{n}) \\ & = (P_n - P_0) IC' + o_P(1/\sqrt{n}). \end{aligned}$$

Therefore, if $\hat{g}$ and $\hat{\bar{Q}}$ satisfy the convergence speed condition and $\Phi(P_n) - \Phi(P_0)$ is asymptotically linear, then it follows from (27.16) and (27.17) that the remainder (27.13) becomes

$$E_{B_n} P_0 \left\{ \frac{(-1)^{1+A}}{g_0 \hat{g}(P^0_{B_n,n})} \left(g_0 - \hat{g}(P^0_{B_n,n})\right) \left(\hat{\bar{Q}}_{\epsilon_n}(P^0_{B_n,n}) - \bar{Q}_0\right) \right\} = (P_n - P_0) IC' + o_P(1/\sqrt{n}).$$

This completes the proof.

27.4 Discussion of Conditions of the Theorem

Under no conditions we determined an exact identity (27.4) for the CV-TMLE minus its target ψ_0, which already provides the main insights about the performance of this estimator. It shows that the analysis of the CV-TMLE involves a cross-validated empirical process term applied to the efficient influence curve and a second-order remainder term. The cross-validated empirical process term is convenient because it involves, for each sample split, an empirical mean over a validation sample of an estimated efficient influence curve that is largely (up till a finite dimensional ϵ) estimated based on the training sample. Based on this, one would predict that one could establish a CLT for this cross-validated empirical process term without having to enforce restrictive entropy conditions on the support of (i.e., class of functions that contains) the estimated efficient influence curve (and thereby limit the adaptiveness of the initial estimators). This is formalized by our second result (27.5), which replaces the cross-validated empirical process term by an empirical mean of mean zero random variables $D^*(\hat{\bar{Q}}_{\epsilon_0}(P_0), \hat{g}(P_0))$ plus a negligible $o_P(1/\sqrt{n})$-term. This result only requires the positivity assumption and *that the estimators converge to a limit*. That is, under essentially no conditions beyond the positivity assumption does the CV-TMLE minus the true ψ_0 behave as an empirical mean of mean zero i.i.d. random variables (which thus converges to a normal distribution by CLT), plus a specified second-order remainder term.

The second-order remainder term predicts immediately that to make it negligible we will need for the product of the rates of convergence for $\hat{\bar{Q}}(P_n)$ and $\hat{g}(P_n)$ to their targets $\bar{Q}_0$ and g_0 to be $o(1/\sqrt{n})$. In an RCT, g_0 is known, and one might set $\hat{g}(P_n) = g_0$, so that the second-order remainder term is exactly equal to zero, giving us the asymptotic linearity (27.6) of the CV-TMLE under no other conditions than the positivity assumption and convergence of $\hat{\bar{Q}}(P_n)$ to some fixed function. This teaches us the remarkable lesson that in an RCT, one can use very aggressive super learning without causing any violations of the conditions, but one will achieve asymptotic efficiency for smaller sample sizes. In particular, in an RCT in which we use a consistent estimator $\hat{\bar{Q}}$ the CV-TMLE is asymptotically efficient, as stated in (27.7). That is, in an RCT, this theorem teaches us that CV-TMLE with adaptive estimation of $\bar{Q}_0$ is the way to go.

Let's now consider a study in which g_0 is not known, but one has available a correctly specified parametric model. For example, one knows that A is only a function of a discrete variable, and one uses a saturated model. If the initial estimator $\hat{\bar{Q}}$ is consistent for $\bar{Q}_0$, then the rate condition (27.8) holds, so that it follows that the CV-TMLE is asymptotically efficient. That is, in this scenario there is only benefit in using an adaptive estimator of $\bar{Q}_0$. If, by chance, the estimator $\hat{\bar{Q}}$ is actually inconsistent for $\bar{Q}_0$, then the rate condition (27.9) still holds, and the asymptotic linearity condition on $\hat{g}$ will also hold under minimal conditions, so that we still have that the CV-TMLE is asymptotically linear.

Finally, let's consider a case in which the assumed model for g_0 is a large semiparametric model. To have a chance at being consistent for g_0, one will need to utilize adaptive estimation to estimate g_0 such as a maximum-likelihood-based super learner respecting the semiparametric model. There are now two scenarios possible. Firstly, suppose that $\hat{\bar{Q}}$ converges to $\bar{Q}_0$ fast enough so that (27.8) holds. Then the CV-TMLE is asymptotically efficient. If, on the other hand, $\hat{\bar{Q}}$ converges fast enough to a misspecified $\bar{Q}$ so that (27.9) holds, then another condition is required. Namely, we now need for $\hat{g}$ to be such that the smooth functional $\Phi_{P_0}(\hat{g})$, indexed by P_0, is an asymptotically linear estimator of its limit $\Phi_{P_0}(g_0)$. This smooth functional can be represented as $\Phi_{P_0}(g) = P_0 H_g^*(\bar{Q}^* - Y)$, where $\bar{Q}^* = \hat{\bar{Q}}_{\epsilon_0}(P_0)$. A data-adaptive estimator $\hat{g}$ of g_0, only tailored to fit g_0 as a whole, may be too biased for this smooth functional (the whole motivation of TMLE!). Therefore, we suggest that the estimator $\hat{g}$ should be targeted toward this smooth functional. That is, one might want to work out a TMLE $\hat{g}^*$ that aims to target this parameter $\Phi_{P_0}(g_0)$. We leave this for future research.

The goal of this chapter was to present a TMLE that allows one to learn the truth ψ_0, while also providing statistical inference based on a CLT, *under as large a statistical model as possible*. For that purpose, adaptive estimation (super learning), targeted minimum-loss-based estimation, and cross-validated selection of the fluctuation parameter in the TMLE are *all* essential tools to achieve this goal. The CV-TMLE combines these tools in one machine that is able to utilize all the state-of-the-art algorithms in machine learning and still provide proper inference in terms of confidence intervals and type I error control for testing null hypotheses, under minimal conditions.

Chapter 28
Targeted Bayesian Learning

Iván Díaz Muñoz, Alan E. Hubbard, Mark J. van der Laan

TMLE is a loss-based semiparametric estimation method that yields a substitution estimator of a target parameter of the probability distribution of the data that solves the efficient influence curve estimating equation and thereby yields a double robust locally efficient estimator of the parameter of interest under regularity conditions. The Bayesian paradigm is concerned with including the researcher's prior uncertainty about the probability distribution through a prior distribution on a statistical model for the probability distribution, which combined with the likelihood yields a posterior distribution of the probability distribution that reflects the researcher's posterior uncertainty. Just like model-based maximum likelihood learning, Bayesian learning is intrinsically nontargeted by working with the prior and posterior distributions of the whole probability distribution of the observed data structure and is thereby very susceptible to bias due to model misspecification or nontargeted model selection.

In this chapter, we present a targeted Bayesian learning methodology mapping a prior distribution on the target parameter of interest into a valid posterior distribution of this target parameter. It relies on a marriage with TMLE, and we show that the posterior distribution of the target parameter inherits the double robust properties of the TMLE. In particular, we will apply this targeted Bayesian learning methodology to the additive causal effect, but our results can be generalized to any d-dimensional target parameter. For a general review of the proposed methodology, we refer the interested reader to van der Laan (2008b), p. 178.

Statistical theory is concerned with deriving inferences from observations (data) on a random variable about certain features of the probability mechanism that generates this random variable. Those features of interest are called parameters and can be described as mappings from a set of possible distributions of the data, called a *model*, to a d-dimensional real space. Models are at the core of statistical theory because they allow a description of the main features of the underlying probability mechanism based on prior knowledge about the experiment that generated the random variable. A model can be classified in three main categories: *parametric*, *semiparametric*, and *nonparametric* models. A parametric model is one in which the i.i.d. random variables $O_1, O_2, \ldots, O_n$ are assumed to be generated by a probability distribution P_0 that belongs to a set of the form $\{P_\theta : \theta \in \Theta\}$, where $\Theta \subset \mathbb{R}^k$. In a semiparametric model the parameter space Θ satisfies $\Theta \subset \mathbb{R}^k \times \mathbb{F}$, where $\mathbb{F}$ is an infinite-dimensional space. A nonparametric model poses no restrictions on P_0 and assumes that P_0 belongs to the set of all possible distributions. Note that a nonparametric model is a special case of a semiparametric model.

Statistical theory has been developed under two main paradigms: frequentist and Bayesian. In the context of inference, the main difference between these paradigms entails a conceptual distinction of the random nature of θ: in frequentist statistics θ is considered unknown but fixed, whereas Bayesian techniques treat it as a random variable. Besides the model, whose elements are P_θ, Bayesian techniques incorporate a *prior* distribution on θ in the statistical inference, whose density is denoted here by π. More important than the randomness of θ is the fact that Bayesian analysis incorporates an interpretation of the densities on θ as a way to summarize the current state of knowledge about it (Robert 2007, p. 34). Thus, $\pi(\theta)$ represents the certainty about the value of θ available prior to the collection of $\mathbf{O}' = (O_1, O_2, \ldots, O_n)$, and $p(\theta \mid \mathbf{O})$ represents the certainty about it once the evidence contained in $\mathbf{O}$ is extracted and the prior information is updated. The latter is called the *posterior* density. Bayes's theorem allows the calculation of the posterior density as

$$p(\theta \mid \mathbf{O}) = \frac{p(\mathbf{O} \mid \theta)\pi(\theta)}{\int p(\mathbf{O} \mid \theta)\pi(\theta)d\theta}.$$

Despite the revolutionary recourse of the prior and posterior distributions, parametric Bayesian analysis suffers from the same critical drawbacks as parametric frequentist analysis. First of all, the models used are typically very small (e.g., exponential families), and usually there is no justifiable reason to believe that the true probability distribution belongs to such small models. Choices of parametric models are often made based on the convenience of their analytical properties. Inferences about θ made according to such misspecified models are widely known to be biased.

Furthermore, the research interest usually rests in a parameter different from θ, that can be represented as a mapping from the model to a possibly multidimensional real space. In this article we analyze the particular case of the additive causal effect whose definition we now recall. Given a data set consisting of n identically distributed copies of $O = (W, A, Y)$, where A is a binary treatment, Y is a binary or continuous outcome, and W is a vector of covariates, the additive causal effect is defined as

$$\psi_0 = \Psi(P_0) = E_0[E_0(Y \mid A = 1, W) - E_0(Y \mid A = 0, W)], \tag{28.1}$$

where P_0 is the distribution of O. Any possible likelihood of O can be factorized as

$$P(O) = P(Y \mid A, W)P(A \mid W)P(W). \tag{28.2}$$

We define: $Q_W(W) \equiv P(W)$, $g(A \mid W) \equiv P(A \mid W)$, $Q_Y(Y \mid A, W) \equiv P(Y \mid A, W)$, and $\bar{Q}(P)(A, W) \equiv E_P(Y \mid A, W)$. We will occasionally use the notation $g(P)(A \mid W)$, to stress the dependence on P.

Standard Bayesian and frequentist techniques do well regarding inference for θ if the assumed model is small enough and contains the true distribution (consistency, efficiency, and central limit theorem), but, for general semiparametric models, substitution estimators and posterior distributions of the parameter of interest (i.e., additive causal effect) based on those techniques are not guaranteed to have optimal properties with respect to the target parameter.

Classical estimation techniques, such as maximum likelihood estimation or least squares estimation, fit densities to the data by minimizing the empirical risk $\sum_i L(Q)(O_i)$ implied by some loss function $L(Q)$. Here Q is the relevant part of P that is required to evaluate $\Psi(P) = \Psi(Q)$ [e.g., in the additive causal effect example, $Q = (\bar{Q}(P), Q_W)$]. For our parameter of interest, if Y is continuous, a common choice of loss function for the conditional mean $\bar{Q}_0$ is the square loss $L(\bar{Q})(O) = (Y - \bar{Q}(W, A))^2$. If one estimates $\bar{Q}(P_0)$ with $\bar{Q}_n$, and the marginal distribution of W by its empirical counterpart, then the substitution estimator of ψ_0 is given by

$$\frac{1}{n}\sum_{i=1}^{n}[\bar{Q}_n(1, W_i) - \bar{Q}_n(0, W_i)].$$

In the parametric Bayesian paradigm, models for the marginal distribution of W and conditional distribution of Y given (A, W) must be assumed in order to get a posterior distribution of the parameter ψ_0. Let $\{Q_W(W; \theta_W) : \theta_W\}$ and $\{Q_Y(Y \mid A, W; \theta_Y) : \theta_Y\}$ be such models, and let the prior densities for θ_W and θ_Y be given by π_{θ_W} and π_{θ_Y}, respectively. Bayesian standard procedures can be used to compute posterior densities $\pi_{\theta_W|\mathbf{O}}$ and $\pi_{\theta_Y|\mathbf{O}}$, which can be mapped into a posterior density on ψ_0 by (28.1).

Indeed, it is very likely that (1) prior information on the treatment effect ψ_0 itself is readily available and that (2) previous studies of the same treatment were analyzed based on different sets of covariates W, and different models for $Q_Y(Y \mid A, W)$ and $Q_W(W)$, thus providing information on different parameters θ'_W and θ'_Y. The Bayesian technique introduced here only requires a prior distribution on ψ_0, allows for realistic semiparametric models, and it maps it into a posterior distribution on ψ_0 with frequentist properties analogous to the TMLE.

28.1 Prior, Likelihood, and Posterior Distributions

In this section we determine the posterior distribution of ψ_0 when the likelihood of the parametric submodel employed in the TMLE is adopted as the likelihood of the data. For notational convenience, let $\bar{Q}_A(P)(W) \equiv \bar{Q}(P)(A, W)$. The parameter in (28.1) can be written as a mapping from $\mathcal{M}$ to $\mathbb{R}$, defined by

$$\Psi(P) = P\{\bar{Q}_1(P) - \bar{Q}_0(P)\}. \tag{28.3}$$

Treating P_n^0 as fixed, the fluctuation $\{P_n^0(\epsilon) : \epsilon\} \subset \mathcal{M}$ used in the TMLE is just a parametric model, and the likelihood under this parametric model can be used together with a prior distribution on ϵ to define the posterior distribution of ϵ. The corresponding posterior distribution of $\Psi(P_n^0(\epsilon))$ reflects the posterior uncertainty about the target parameter. It can be used to proceed to point and interval estimation of the target parameter of interest.

Firstly, we find a submodel $\mathcal{M}_\epsilon = \{P_n^0(\epsilon) : \epsilon\} \subset \mathcal{M}$ such that $P_n^0(0) = P_n^0$ and $\langle D^*(P_n^0)\rangle \subset \langle \frac{d}{d\epsilon} \log P_n^0(\epsilon)|_{\epsilon=0}\rangle$, where P_n^0 is the initial estimator of P_0 and is considered fixed. Here $D^*(P)$ is the efficient influence curve of Ψ at P, and we used the notation $\langle S \rangle$ for the linear span generated by the components of the function S of O. Secondly, we determine the prior distribution on ϵ yielded by the prior on the parameter ψ_0. For this purpose we define a mapping $f_n : \epsilon \to \Psi(P_n^0(\epsilon))$. Once the prior on ϵ is determined, its posterior can be computed and the mapping f_n can be used to map the posterior on ϵ into a posterior on ψ_0.

Fluctuation model. We consider a normal working model for $Q_{Y,n}(\epsilon)$ when Y is continuous and a logit regression model when Y is binary. If Y is continuous, the loss function $-\log Q_{Y,n}(\epsilon)$ corresponds with the squared error loss for the conditional mean $\bar{Q}_n(\epsilon)$. As a consequence, the TMLE and the proposed targeted posterior distribution of ψ_0 are not affected by the validity of this normal working model.

Consider an initial estimator P_n^0 of P_0: estimators $\bar{Q}_n^0$ and g_n can be obtained through standard procedures (e.g., logit or probit regression) or through more elaborated techniques, such as machine learning techniques. It is worth emphasizing that the efficiency and consistency of the TMLE depend on the choice of those initial estimators, which must be as close as possible to the real $\bar{Q}(P_0)$ and g_0. To achieve this goal, we encourage the use of the super learner. Let $Q_{W,n}$ be an initial estimator of Q_W (e.g., the empirical probability distribution of W). We fluctuate the initial estimator P_n^0 by finding a fluctuation of $\bar{Q}_n^0$ and $Q_{W,n}$ through ϵ, such that the score of $P_n^0(\epsilon)$ at $\epsilon = 0$ equals the efficient influence curve of Ψ at P_n^0, given by

$$D^*(P)(O) = (Y - \bar{Q}(P)(A, W))\frac{2A - 1}{g(A \mid W)} + \bar{Q}(P)(1, W) - \bar{Q}(P)(0, W) - \Psi(P). \quad (28.4)$$

We use either a binomial working model (case Y binary) or a constant variance normal working model (case Y continuous) for $Q_{Y,n}^0(\epsilon)$. The fluctuations adopted here are given by

$$\begin{aligned} m(\bar{Q}_n^0(\epsilon)) &= m(\bar{Q}_n^0) + \epsilon H_1^*, \\ Q_{W,n}(\epsilon) &= \frac{\exp(\epsilon H_2^*)}{Q_{W,n}\ \exp(\epsilon H_2^*)} Q_{W,n}, \end{aligned} \quad (28.5)$$

where

$$H_1^*(A, W) = \frac{2A - 1}{g_n(A, W)}, \quad (28.6)$$

$$H_2^*(W) = \bar{Q}(P_n^0)(1, W) - \bar{Q}(P_n^0)(0, W) - \Psi(P_n^0), \quad (28.7)$$

and m is the logit or identity link, depending on the type of outcome. It can be shown that the model $P_n^0(\epsilon)$ obtained by using these fluctuations has score $D^*(P_n^0)$ at $\epsilon = 0$. In contrast to the classic TMLE for this parameter, in which the fluctuations of $\bar{Q}_n^0$ and $Q_{W,n}$ are done independently through ϵ_1 and ϵ_2, and the maximum likelihood estimator of ϵ_2 happens to be zero, here we fluctuate both $\bar{Q}_n^0$ and $Q_{W,n}$ through a single ϵ. This is done in order to avoid dealing with a multivariate posterior distribution for $\epsilon^* = (\epsilon_1, \epsilon_2)'$. Ensuring that all the relevant parts of P_n^0 are fluctuated so that $d/d\epsilon \log P_n^0(\epsilon)\big|_{\epsilon=0} = D^*(P_n^0)$ results in a likelihood function with the right spread, which will ultimately result in the right coverage of the credible intervals if the initial estimator P_n^0 is consistent for P_0.

Prior Distribution on ϵ. For notational convenience, let $\bar{Q}_{n,A}(\epsilon)(W) \equiv \bar{Q}_n^0(\epsilon)(A, W)$. The substitution estimator based on $P_n^0(\epsilon)$ is given by

$$\begin{aligned}\Psi(P_n^0(\epsilon)) &= Q_{W,n}(\epsilon)[\bar{Q}_{n,1}(\epsilon) - \bar{Q}_{n,0}(\epsilon)] \qquad (28.8)\\ &= \sum_{i=1}^{n} \frac{\exp(\epsilon H_2^*(W_i))Q_{W,n}(W_i)}{\sum_{j=1}^{n} \exp(\epsilon H_2^*(W_j))Q_{W,n}(W_j)}[\bar{Q}_{n,1}(\epsilon)(W_i) - \bar{Q}_{n,0}(\epsilon)(W_i)].\end{aligned}$$

From the Bayesian perspective, the prior knowledge of ψ_0 can be incorporated into the inference procedure through a prior distribution on the latter parameter $\psi_0 = \Psi(P_0) \sim \Pi$.

Let π be the density of Π. Note that the prior distribution of ψ_0 defines a prior distribution on ϵ through the mapping $f_n : \epsilon \to \Psi(P_n^0(\epsilon))$. The fluctuation $p_n^0(\epsilon)$ must be chosen in a such way that this mapping is invertible. The prior on ϵ is given by

$$\pi^*(\epsilon) = \pi[\Psi(P_n^0(\epsilon))]J(\epsilon),$$

where $J(\epsilon)$ is the Jacobian of the transformation, defined as

$$J(\epsilon) = \left|\frac{d}{d\epsilon}\Psi(P_n^0(\epsilon))\right|.$$

Based on (28.8), we obtain

$$\begin{aligned}\frac{d}{d\epsilon}\Psi(P_n^0(\epsilon)) = \sum_{i=1}^{n}\Bigg\{&\frac{d\, Q_{W,n}(\epsilon)(W_i)}{d\epsilon}(\bar{Q}_{n,1}(\epsilon)(W_i) - \bar{Q}_{n,0}(\epsilon)(W_i))\\ &+ Q_{W,n}(\epsilon)(W_i)\frac{d}{d\epsilon}(\bar{Q}_{n,1}(\epsilon)(W_i) - \bar{Q}_{n,0}(\epsilon)(W_i))\Bigg\}, \qquad (28.9)\end{aligned}$$

where

$$\frac{d\, Q_{W,n}(\epsilon)(W)}{d\epsilon} = Q_{W,n}(\epsilon)(W)\left[H_2^*(W) - \frac{Q_{W,n}(H_2^* \exp(\epsilon H_2^*))}{Q_{W,n}\exp(\epsilon H_2^*)}\right],$$

and $Q_{W,n}(\epsilon)$ is defined in (28.5). It can also be shown that

$$\frac{d\, \bar{Q}_{n,A}(\epsilon)(W)}{d\epsilon} = H_1^*(A, W)$$

and

$$\frac{d\,\bar{Q}_{n,A}(\epsilon)(W)}{d\epsilon} = H_1^*(A,W)\,\bar{Q}_{n,A}(\epsilon)(W)[1-\bar{Q}_{n,A}(\epsilon)(W)],$$

for continuous and binary outcomes, respectively.

Targeted posterior distribution. Operating from a Bayesian perspective under the working fluctuation model, the conditional density of $O_1, O_2, \ldots, O_n$ given ϵ equals $\prod_{i=1}^n P_n^0(\epsilon)(O_i)$. Therefore, in our parametric working model $\{P_n^0(\epsilon) : \epsilon\}$, the posterior density of ϵ is proportional to

$$\pi^*(\epsilon)\prod_{i=1}^n P_n^0(\epsilon)(O_i). \tag{28.10}$$

Taking into account the factorization of the likelihood given in (28.2), and noting that the part of (28.10) corresponding to $g_n(A \mid W)$ does not involve ϵ, simulating from (28.10) is equivalent to simulating from the density proportional to

$$\pi^*(\epsilon)\prod_{i=1}^n Q_{Y,n}(\epsilon)(Y_i \mid A_i, W_i)Q_{W,n}(\epsilon)(W_i). \tag{28.11}$$

Standard Bayesian techniques such as the Metropolis–Hastings algorithm can be used to sample a large number of draws from this posterior distribution. Once a posterior sample ϵ_i $(i = 1, 2, \ldots, m)$ is drawn from (28.11), a sample from the targeted posterior distribution of ψ_0 can be computed as $\psi_i = \Psi(P_n^0(\epsilon_i))$. The estimated posterior mean of ψ_0 can be used as point estimator, and a 95% credible interval is $(\psi_{2.5}, \psi_{97.5})$, where ψ_k is the kth percentile of this posterior distribution.

Note that simulating observations from this posterior distribution is just one possible way of computing the quantities of interest. Alternatively, one can use the analytic formula of the posterior density of ϵ and the mapping f_n to find the analytical form of the posterior distribution of ψ. Recall that f_n is assumed to be invertible. Note that $\epsilon = f_n^{-1}(\psi)$. We have

$$P(\psi \mid O_1, \ldots, O_n) \propto \left|\frac{d\, f_n^{-1}(\psi)}{d\psi}\right| \pi^*(f_n^{-1}(\psi))\times \prod_{i=1}^n Q_{Y,n}(f_n^{-1}(\psi))(Y_i \mid A_i, W_i)Q_{W,n}(f_n^{-1}(\psi))(W_i), \tag{28.12}$$

where the constant of proportionality can be computed by using numerical integration. We can now calculate the value of the posterior distribution for any value ψ, plot the posterior distribution, or use numerical integration to find the analytical posterior mean or the posterior percentiles.

As a particular interesting case, the targeted posterior distribution when the TMLE procedure is implemented, as in van der Laan and Rubin (2006, p. 21), is presented in Appendix 2 of this chapter. In this posterior distribution, if the TMLE of P_0 is used as initial estimator P_n^0, the posterior mean is equal to

$$\mu_{\psi_0|O} = \frac{w_1\psi_n + w_2\mu_{\psi_0}}{w_1 + w_2},$$

where ψ_n is the TMLE, μ_{ψ_0} is the prior mean, and w_1 and w_2 are weights given in Appendix 2 of this chapter. It is important to note that $w_2/w_1 \rightarrow 0$ when either the sample size increases or the variance of the prior distribution is very large. This means that in those situations the posterior mean reduces to the TMLE, acquiring its double robustness and efficiency.

28.2 Convergence of Targeted Posterior Distribution

In standard Bayesian analysis, if X is a random variable distributed as the posterior, and θ_n is the maximum likelihood estimator of the parameter of the distribution of X, the variable $\sqrt{n}(X-\theta_n)$ can be shown to converge to a normal distribution with mean zero, and variance given by the inverse of the Fisher information, whenever the model is correct (Lindley 1980). This result is analogous to the central limit theorem and is very useful in establishing the asymptotic properties of the Bayesian point and interval estimators, such as their asymptotic bias and coverage probability. It also implies that as the sample size increases, the information given by the prior is neglected, and only the data are used to make inferences. An analogous result, presented in the next theorem, is valid in the case of the targeted posterior distribution when the TMLE P_n^* itself is used as initial estimator of P_0.

Theorem 28.1. *Let P_n^* be the TMLE of P_0, and let $\{P_n^*(\epsilon) : \epsilon\} \subset \mathcal{M}$ be a parametric fluctuation satisfying $P_n^*(0) = P_n^*$ and $d/d\epsilon \log P_n^*(\epsilon)|_{\epsilon=0} = D^*(P_n^*)$, where $D^*(P)$ is the efficient influence curve of $\Psi(P)$, defined in (28.4). Define the mapping $f_n^* : \epsilon \rightarrow \Psi(P_n^*(\epsilon))$ to be invertible. Assume that there exists a distribution P^* such that $P_0[h(\psi_n, P_n^*) - h(\psi_0, P^*)]^2$ converges to zero, where*

$$h(\psi_n, P_n^*)(O) \equiv \frac{d^2}{d\psi^2} \log p(f_n^{*-1}(\psi))(O)\Big|_{\psi=\psi_n}$$

and $h(\psi_0, P^*)$ is defined analogously. Assume that $h(\psi_n, P_n^*) - h(\psi_0, P^*)$ falls in a Glivenko–Cantelli class $\mathcal{F}$. Define $\psi_n = \Psi(P_n^*)$ (i.e., ψ_n is the TMLE of ψ_0). Note that $S(\psi_n) = 0$, where

$$S(\psi) = \sum_{i=1}^{n} \frac{d}{d\psi} \log P_n^*(f_n^{-1}(\psi))(O_i).$$

Assume that $\pi(\psi)$ is a prior density on ψ_0 such that $\pi(\psi) > 0$ for every possible value of ψ. Let $\tilde{\psi}_n$ be a random variable with posterior density proportional to (28.12). The sequence $\sqrt{n}(\tilde{\psi}_n - \psi_n)$ converges in distribution to T, where $T \sim N(0, \sigma^2)$ and

$$\sigma^2 = -\left(P_0 \frac{d^2}{d\psi_0^2} \log P^*(f^{*-1}(\psi_0))\right)^{-1}$$

$$= \frac{\left[P^*\left(\frac{\sigma^2(P^*)}{g^2(P^*)} + (\bar{Q}_1^* - \bar{Q}_0^* - \Psi(P^*))^2\right)\right]^2}{P_0\left(\frac{\sigma^2(P^*)}{g^2(P^*)} + (\bar{Q}_1^* - \bar{Q}_0^* - \Psi(P^*))^2\right)},$$

with $\sigma^2(P^*)(A, W) = Var_{P^*}(Y \mid A, W)$ *and* $\bar{Q}_A^*(W) = \bar{Q}(P^*)(A, W)$.

A proof is provided in Appendix 1 of this chapter. Since ψ_n is double robust, this theorem teaches us that the targeted posterior distribution is also double robust in the sense that it will be centered at ψ_0 if either g_n or $\bar{Q}_n^*$ (as used by the TMLE P_n^*) is consistent. Another important consequence is that if the limit P^* equals the true P_0, then the asymptotic variance of the posterior distribution is equal to

$$\sigma^2 = P_0\left(\frac{\sigma^2(P_0)}{g^2(P_0)} + (\bar{Q}_1(P_0) - \bar{Q}_0(P_0) - \Psi(P_0))^2\right),$$

where $\bar{Q}_A(P_0) = \bar{Q}(P_0)(A, W)$. This asymptotic variance equals the variance of the efficient influence curve $D^*(P_0)$ at P_0, providing the analogue of the standard result cited above (Lindley 1980). This means that asymptotic credible intervals are also confidence intervals [i.e., they have coverage probability $(1-\alpha)$]. A correction for the cases in which $P^* \neq P_0$ will be provided in the next section.

28.3 Frequentist Properties of Targeted Posterior Distribution

Once the posterior sample ψ_i $(i = 1, 2, \ldots, m)$ is obtained, point estimates and $(1 - \alpha)100\%$ credible intervals for ψ_0 can be computed as $\bar{\psi} = \frac{1}{m}\sum_{i=1}^m \psi_i$ and $(\psi_{[m\frac{\alpha}{2}]}, \psi_{[m(1-\frac{\alpha}{2})]})$, where the limits of the interval are given by order statistics and [ ] indicates rounding to the nearest integer. Recall that the TMLE is double robust under certain conditions. Assume that those conditions and the conditions of Theorem 28.1 hold. Then, we have that $E(\tilde{\psi}_n - \psi_0) = E(\tilde{\psi}_n - \psi_n) + E(\psi_n - \psi_0)$ converges to zero. This means that the estimated posterior mean is also double robust.

As mentioned in the previous section, $(1 - \alpha)100\%$ credible intervals only are guaranteed to have $(1 - \alpha)100\%$ asymptotic coverage if the initial estimator P_n^0 converges to the true P_0. We only wish to rely on the consistency of either g_n or $\bar{Q}_n$, so that the posterior mean is consistent (and asymptotically linear). We now provide a correction factor that can be applied to the credible intervals so that they preserve the desired $(1 - \alpha)$ asymptotic coverage when the TMLE is consistent and asymptotically linear.

Under the assumptions for asymptotic linearity, the TMLE satisfies

$$\psi_n - \psi_0 = \frac{1}{n}\sum_{i=1}^n IC(O_i) + o\left(\frac{1}{\sqrt{n}}\right),$$

where IC denotes the influence curve of ψ_n. Assume that the conditions of Theorem 28.1 hold, so that

$$\sqrt{n}(\tilde{\psi}_n - \psi_n) \to N(0, \sigma^2),$$
$$\sqrt{n}(\psi_n - \psi_0) \to N(0, \sigma^{2*}),$$

where σ^2 is given in Theorem 28.1 and $\sigma^{2*} = var_{P^*}(IC(O))$. Denote the β-percentile of the distribution of $\tilde{\psi}_n$ with q_β. Then

$$q_\beta \simeq \psi_n + z_\beta \frac{\sigma}{\sqrt{n}},$$

where z_β is the β-percentile of a standard normal distribution. This means that

$$\begin{aligned} P\left[(q_\beta, q_{1-\beta}) \ni \psi_0\right] &\simeq P\left(\psi_n - z_{1-\beta}\frac{\sigma}{\sqrt{n}} < \psi_0 < \psi_n + z_{1-\beta}\frac{\sigma}{\sqrt{n}}\right) \\ &= P\left(-z_{1-\beta}\frac{\sigma}{\sigma^*} < \frac{\sqrt{n}(\psi_n - \psi_0)}{\sigma^*} < z_{1-\beta}\frac{\sigma}{\sigma^*}\right). \end{aligned}$$

Therefore, for the credible interval $(q_\beta,\ q_{1-\beta})$ to have coverage probability $(1-\alpha)$, the value of β must be chosen such that

$$z_{1-\beta}\frac{\sigma}{\sigma^*} = z_{1-\alpha/2}, \tag{28.13}$$

hence

$$\beta = 1 - \Phi^{-1}\left(z_{1-\alpha/2}\frac{\sigma^*}{\sigma}\right),$$

where Φ is the $N(0,1)$ cumulative distribution function. Since P_0 and P^* are unknown, the values of σ^2 and σ^{2*} cannot be computed explicitly. However, estimates can be obtained by replacing P_0 with P_n and P^* with P_n^0. The variance σ^{2*} can also be estimated by the empirical variance of the estimated influence curve values $IC_n(O_i)$, $i = 1, \ldots, n$.

28.4 Simulations

In order to explore additional frequentist properties of the targeted posterior distribution, and, in particular, to compare the posterior mean of the targeted posterior distribution with the TMLE itself, a simulation study was performed. We only considered the case where Y is binary. The data were generated based on the following scheme:

1. Simulate W from $N_2\left(\begin{pmatrix} .5 \\ 2 \end{pmatrix}, \begin{pmatrix} 2 & .3 \\ .3 & .8 \end{pmatrix}\right)$.

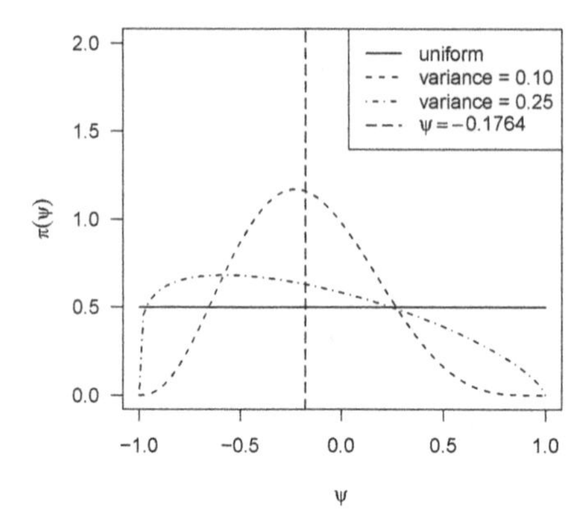

Fig. 28.1 Prior densities of ψ_0

2. Given $W = w$, simulate A from a Bernoulli distribution with probability $\text{expit}\,(-0.2 + 0.1w_1 - 0.2w_2 + .05w_1 \times w_2)$, where expit is the inverse of the logit function.
3. Given $W = w$ and $A = a$, draw Y from a Bernoulli distribution with probability $\text{expit}\,(-0.2 + 0.07a - 0.2w_1 + 0.02w_2 + 0.2a \times w_1 - 0.5a \times w_2 - 0.01w_1 \times w_2 - 0.003a \times w_1 \times w_2)$.

This probability distribution yields a parameter value of $\psi_0 = -.1764$. For each of the sample sizes 30, 50, 100, 150, 200, and 250, 1000 data sets were generated. We consider three different prior distributions on ψ_0, all from the beta family in the interval $(-1, 1)$. The first one boils down to a uniform prior, while the second and third ones have mean ψ_0 and variances 0.1 and 0.25, respectively. The uniform prior corresponds to the situation in which no prior information is available, and the other two correspond to situations in which there are different levels of certainty about the prior information. These three priors are plotted in Fig. 28.1.

Consider the following model:

$$W \sim N_2(\mu, \Sigma);\ A \mid W \sim Ber(\text{expit}\,(X'\beta_1));\ Y \mid A, W \sim Ber(\text{expit}\,(M'\beta_2)),$$

where $X' = (1, W_1, W_2, W_1 \times W_2)$ and $M' = (X', A, A \times X')$. Note that this model contains the real data-generating distribution. A misspecified model (i.e., a model that does not include true Q_0) was also considered by not including interaction terms in M'. The TMLE estimator based on these two models was used as initial estimator P_n^0, and the Metropolis–Hastings algorithm was used to draw 1000 observations from the posterior distribution given by (28.11). A brief description of this algorithm is presented in Appendix 3 of this chapter. The mean and variance of the posterior distribution were computed numerically, and a normal distribution was used as proposal density for the Metropolis–Hastings algorithm. The average acceptance rate of this procedure was 70%.

The estimated posterior mean was used as estimator of ψ_0. Its variance and bias were estimated for each sample size. The 2.5th and 97.5th percentiles of the posterior sample were used as estimators of the limits of the 95% credible intervals; corrected credible intervals based on (28.13) were also computed. The performance of these intervals was assessed through their average length and coverage probability, estimated by the percentage of times that the interval contained the true parameter value ψ_0. Bias, variance, coverage probability, and average length were also computed for the TMLE and its confidence interval. The results are shown in Figs. 28.2 and 28.3.

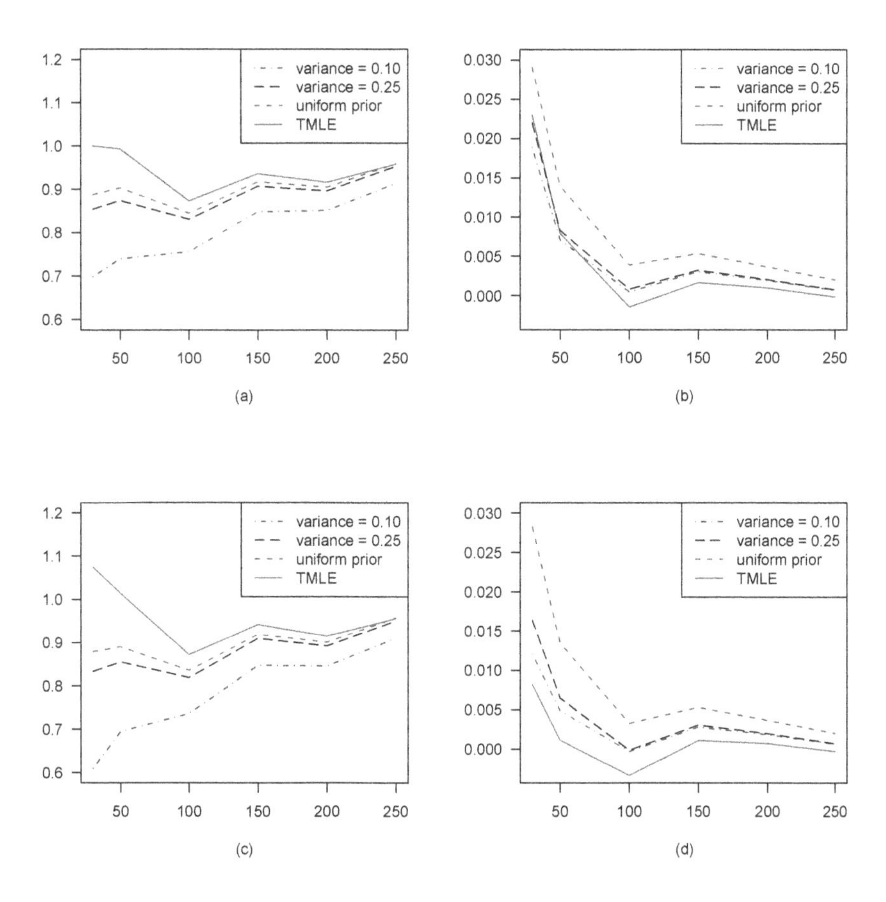

Fig. 28.2 Variance and bias of the posterior mean. (a) Variance (multiplied by n) for correctly specified $\bar{Q}$. (b) Bias for correctly specified $\bar{Q}$. (c) Variance (multiplied by n) for misspecified $\bar{Q}$. (d) Bias for misspecified $\bar{Q}$

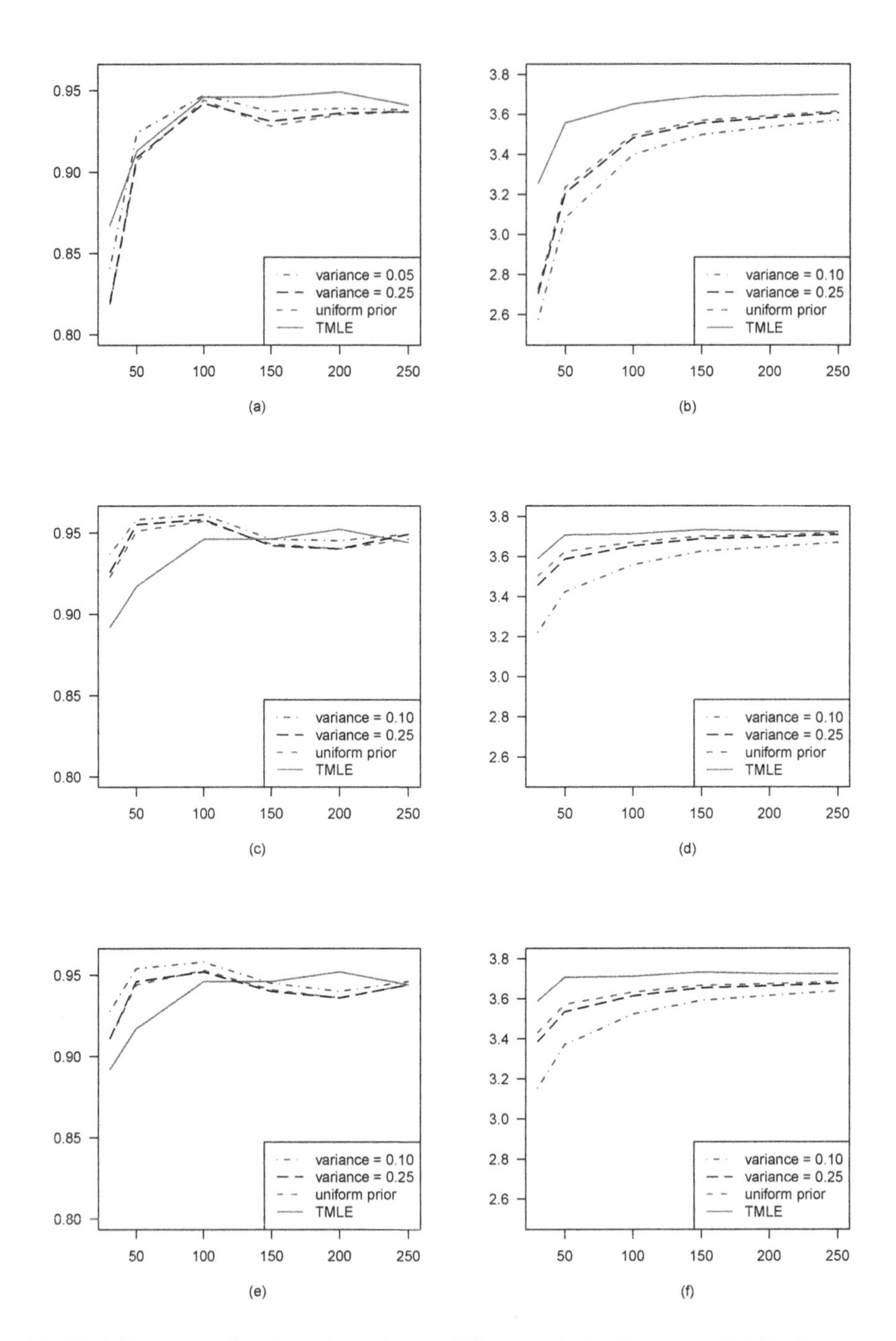

Fig. 28.3 Coverage probability and length of credible intervals. (a) Coverage probability for correctly specified $\bar{Q}_0$. (b) Length (multiplied by n) for correctly specified $\bar{Q}_0$. (c) Coverage probability for misspecified $\bar{Q}_0$. (d) Length (multiplied by n) for misspecified $\bar{Q}_0$. (e) Coverage probability of the corrected intervals. (f) Length (multiplied by n) of the corrected intervals

As expected, the inclusion of additional unbiased information reduces the variance of the estimators for small sample sizes, causing a bigger impact when the certainty about that additional knowledge is high. It is important to note that the variance of the posterior mean seems to be unaffected by the misspecification of the parametric model for $\bar{Q}_0$, though this simulation is not enough to believe that this type of robustness applies in general. The mean of the targeted posterior distribution appears to be more biased than the TMLE, especially if $\bar{Q}_0$ is misspecified and a uniform distribution is used as prior for ψ_0. However, all the estimators appear to be asymptotically unbiased.

Figure 28.3 shows the coverage probability and length of corrected and uncorrected credible intervals for cases in which the true and misspecified $\bar{Q}_0$ are used. Although all the intervals have asymptotic correct coverage, credible intervals with misspecified $\bar{Q}_0$ are somewhat conservative for some small sample sizes, having wider lengths and a coverage probability that is barely greater than the prespecified level 95%. This means that the variance of the posterior distribution is larger if $\bar{Q}_0$ is misspecified, thereby reflecting some kind of "inefficiency" of the posterior distribution due to misspecification of $\bar{Q}_0$. The correction to the credible intervals proposed in (28.13) operates, causing a slight and almost imperceptible decrease in the coverage probability and length of the intervals for all sample sizes, thereby providing an adjustment for the conservativeness of the intervals. The inclusion of an unbiased prior with small variance results in a significant reduction in the length of the credible intervals, especially for small sample sizes.

28.5 Discussion

A methodology to carry out targeted inference for an additive causal effect under the Bayesian paradigm is now available. Prior information on the effect of a binary treatment on an outcome can be directly used jointly with new data to update the knowledge about such an effect. This update involves the computation of a targeted posterior distribution of the parameter of interest whose mean has been found to be asymptotically double robust in the same sense as the TMLE. It is a consistent estimator of the parameter of interest if either the model for the conditional expectation of the outcome or the treatment mechanism is correctly specified. The frequentist can use the posterior mean as an estimator of the target parameter, thereby allowing the incorporation of a prior distribution, while proceeding with frequentist statistical inference.

The asymptotic variance of the targeted posterior distribution has been proven to be equal to the variance under the true distribution P_0 of the efficient influence curve at P_0 when the initial estimator of P_0 is consistent. This implies, amongst other characteristics, that credible intervals will also be frequentist confidence intervals for the target parameter in the sense that their credibility level will also be equal to their coverage probability. If consistency of the initial estimator is not a sensible assumption, but credible intervals are desired to have a specified coverage probability, a simple adjustment has been provided that provides the desired coverage under the assumption that the TMLE is asymptotically linear.

A simulation study showed that misspecification of the model for the expectation of the outcome leads to wider credible intervals. Moreover, it showed that in the particular case studied (notably for binary outcome Y), the uncorrected credible intervals based on misspecified $\bar{Q}_0$ also had the right asymptotic coverage probability, suggesting the possibility that for some cases, even if P_n^0 is not consistent, $(1-\alpha)$ credible intervals still have $(1-\alpha)$ coverage probability. Identification of those cases is an interesting issue for future work. The simulation also showed that the credible intervals for a misspecified $\bar{Q}_0$ were conservative for small sample sizes. The correction provided generated a slight correction of that conservativeness.

The methodology presented here is completely general, and is directly applicable to allow the computation of targeted posterior distribution for any pathwise differentiable parameter defined on any semiparametric model. Our formal asymptotic results for the targeted posterior distribution can be straightforwardly generalized. The targeted posterior distribution is defined by the TMLE, specifically, the loss function and parametric submodel that defined the TMLE, and a prior distribution on the target parameter. Future work in this area includes the determination of the analytical form of targeted posterior distributions for other interesting parameters, as well as simulations and formal theoretical studies that will provide a comprehensive understanding of the frequentist properties of the targeted posterior distribution.

Appendix 1

Proof (Theorem 28.1). Let $u_n^*(\psi)(O_i) \equiv P_n^*(f_n^{*-1}(\psi))(O_i)$, where $f_n^* : \epsilon \to \Psi(P_n^*(\epsilon))$. Let $u^*(\psi)(O_i) \equiv P^*(f_n^{*-1}(\psi))(O_i)$, for $f^* : \epsilon \to \Psi(P^*(\epsilon))$. Let $\tilde{\psi}_n$ be a random variable with distribution given by the targeted posterior distribution of ψ_0:

$$\pi(\psi) \prod_{i=1}^{n} u_n^*(\psi)(O_i),$$

and define $T_n = \sqrt{n}(\tilde{\psi}_n - \psi_n)$. The density of T_n is given by

$$p_{T_n}(t) \propto \pi\left(\psi_n + \frac{t}{\sqrt{n}}\right) \prod_{i=1}^{n} u_n^*\left(\psi_n + \frac{t}{\sqrt{n}}\right)(O_i).$$

We have that, for some positive constant c_n independent of ψ_n and t,

$$\log p_{T_n}(t) = \log c_n + \log \pi\left(\psi_n + \frac{t}{\sqrt{n}}\right) + \sum_{i=1}^{n} \log u_n^*\left(\psi_n + \frac{t}{\sqrt{n}}\right)(O_i).$$

The first two terms behave for n large as a constant function in t. We will now study the last term as a function in t for n large. A Taylor series expansion in t around zero yields the following asymptotic approximation for the last term:

$$\sum_{i=1}^{n} \log u_n^*\left(\psi_n + \frac{t}{\sqrt{n}}\right)(O_i) =$$

$$R_n^1 + R_n^2 + \frac{t^2}{2n}\sum_{i=1}^{n}\frac{d^2}{d\psi^2}\log u_n^*(\psi)(O_i)\bigg|_{\psi=\psi_n} + R_n^3, \quad (28.14)$$

where

- $R_n^1 = \sum_{i=1}^n \log u_n^*(\psi_n)(O_i) = \sum_{i=1}^n \log P_n^*(O_i)$ does not depend on t nor on ψ_n and satisfies $\log c_n + R_n^1 = \log c_n'$ for some constant c_n' independent of t and ψ_n;
- $R_n^2 = S(\psi_n) = 0$ because

$$\begin{aligned} S(\psi_n) &= \sum_{i=1}^{n}\frac{d}{d\psi}\log P_n^*(f_n^{*-1}(\psi))(O_i)\bigg|_{\psi=\psi_n} \\ &= \frac{d}{d\psi}f_n^{*-1}(\psi)\bigg|_{\psi=\psi_n}\sum_{i=1}^{n}\frac{d}{d\epsilon}\log P_n^*(\epsilon)(O_i)\bigg|_{\epsilon=0} = 0, \end{aligned}$$

  and $\epsilon_n = 0$ is the maximum likelihood estimator of ϵ in the model $\{P_n^*(\epsilon) : \epsilon\}$;
- The remainder R_n^3 can be written as

$$\frac{t^3}{6}\frac{1}{n^{3/2}}\sum_{i=1}^{n}\frac{d^3}{d\psi^3}\log u_n^*(\psi)(O_i)\bigg|_{\psi=\psi_1},$$

  for some ψ_1 between zero and ψ_n, and is thus of order $n^{-\frac{1}{2}}$. This shows that R_n^3 is negligible compared with the other term in (28.14) which is of order 1.

Recall the definition of $h(\psi, P)$ in the theorem, and note that

$$\frac{t^2}{2n}\sum_{i=1}^{n}\frac{d^2}{d\psi^2}\log u_n^*(\psi)(O_i)\bigg|_{\psi=\psi_n} = \frac{t^2}{2}P_n h(\psi_n, P_n^*).$$

Define $h_n = h(\psi_n, P_n^*)$ and $h_0 = h(\psi_0, P^*)$, and note that

$$P_n h_n - P_0 h_0 = (P_n - P_0)h_0 + (P_n - P_0)(h_n - h_0) + P_0(h_n - h_0).$$

The first term in this sum converges to zero by the law of large numbers, the second term converges to zero because $h_n - h_0$ falls in a Glivenko–Cantelli class, and the last term converges to zero because it is bounded by $P_0(h_n - h_0)^2$, which converges to zero. This proves that

$$P_n\frac{d^2}{d\psi^2}\log u_n^*(\psi)\bigg|_{\psi=\psi_n} \longrightarrow P_0\frac{d^2}{d\psi^2}\log u^*(\psi)\bigg|_{\psi=\psi_0},$$

which in turn proves that $p_{T_n}(t)$ converges, up to a constant, to

$$\exp\left(-\frac{t^2}{2\sigma^2}\right),$$

where

$$-\sigma^2 = \left(P_0 \frac{d^2}{d\psi^2} \log P^*(f^{*-1}(\psi))\Big|_{\psi=\psi_0}\right)^{-1}.$$

This asymptotic variance satisfies:

$$\begin{aligned}
-\sigma^{-2} &= P_0 \frac{d^2}{d\psi^2} \log P^*(f^{*-1}(\psi))\Big|_{\psi=\psi_0} \\
&= P_0 \left[\frac{d^2}{d\epsilon^2} \log P^*(\epsilon)\Big|_{\epsilon=0} \left(\frac{d}{d\psi} f^{*-1}(\psi)\Big|_{\psi=\psi_0}\right)^2 + \frac{d}{d\epsilon} \log P^*(\epsilon)\Big|_{\epsilon=0} \frac{d^2}{d\psi^2} f^{*-1}(\psi)\Big|_{\psi=\psi_0}\right] \\
&= P_0 \left[\frac{d^2}{d\epsilon^2} \log P^*(\epsilon)\Big|_{\epsilon=0} \left(\frac{d}{d\psi} f^{*-1}(\psi)\Big|_{\psi=\psi_0}\right)^2\right],
\end{aligned}$$

where $\frac{d}{d\epsilon} \log P^*(\epsilon)\big|_{\epsilon=0} = 0$ because $P_n D^*(P_n^*) = 0$ (a property of the frequentist TMLE), and because of the convergence of P_n and P_n^* to P_0 and P^*, respectively. Note that

$$-\frac{d^2}{d\epsilon^2} \log P^*(\epsilon)\Big|_{\epsilon=0} = \frac{\sigma^2(P^*)}{g^2(P^*)} + (\bar{Q}_1^* - \bar{Q}_0^* - \Psi(P^*))^2,$$

where $\sigma^2(P^*)(A, W) = Var_{P^*}(Y \mid A, W)$ and $\bar{Q}_A^* = \bar{Q}(P^*)(A, W)$. On the other hand, since Ψ is pathwise differentiable we know that

$$\frac{d}{d\epsilon} \Psi(P^*(\epsilon))\Big|_{\epsilon=0} = P^*[D^*(P^*) s(P^*)],$$

where $D^*(P^*)$ is the canonical gradient at P^* and $s(P^*)$ is the score of $P^*(\epsilon)$ at $\epsilon = 0$, which is precisely $D^*(P^*)$. Therefore:

$$\begin{aligned}
\left(\frac{d}{d\psi} f^{*-1}(\psi)\Big|_{\psi=\psi_0}\right)^2 &= (P^* D^2(P^*))^{-2} \\
&= \left[P^* \left(\frac{\sigma^2(P^*)}{g^2(P^*)} + (\bar{Q}_1^* - \bar{Q}_0^* - \Psi(P^*))^2\right)\right]^{-2},
\end{aligned}$$

and we conclude that

$$\sigma^2 = \frac{\left[P^* \left(\frac{\sigma^2(P^*)}{g^2(P^*)} + (\bar{Q}_1^* - \bar{Q}_0^* - \Psi(P^*))^2\right)\right]^2}{P_0 \left(\frac{\sigma^2(P^*)}{g^2(P^*)} + (\bar{Q}_1^* - \bar{Q}_0^* - \Psi(P^*))^2\right)}.$$

Appendix 2

Posterior distribution if only $\bar{Q}$ is fluctuated. If the outcome is continuous, we can consider a linear fluctuation model:

$$\bar{Q}_n^0(\epsilon) = \bar{Q}_n^0 + \epsilon H_1^*, \tag{28.15}$$

where H_1^* is defined in (28.6). In this case, the mapping $\Psi(P_n^0(\epsilon))$ can be written as

$$\begin{aligned}\Psi(P_n^0(\epsilon)) =& P_n\left(\bar{Q}_{n,1} - \bar{Q}_{n,0}\right) + \epsilon P_n\left(H_{1,1}^* - H_{1,0}^*\right) \\ =& \Psi\left(P_n^0\right) + \epsilon P_n\left(H_{1,1}^* - H_{1,0}^*\right),\end{aligned} \tag{28.16}$$

where $Q_{n,A}(W) \equiv \bar{Q}_n^0(A, W)$ and $H_{1,A}^*(W) \equiv H_1^*(A, W)$. The Jacobian of this transformation is

$$J(\epsilon) = |P_n(H_{1,1}^* - H_{1,0}^*)|.$$

If a normal distribution with mean μ_{ψ_0} and variance $\sigma_{\psi_0}^2$ is considered as prior on ψ_0, the prior distribution on ϵ is characterized by

$$\pi^*(\epsilon) = \frac{1}{\sigma_{\psi_0}}\phi\left(\frac{\Psi(P_n^0(\epsilon)) - \mu_{\psi_0}}{\sigma_{\psi_0}}\right)|P_n(H_{1,1}^* - H_{1,0}^*)|.$$

This implies that the prior on ϵ is a normal distribution with mean μ_ϵ and variance σ_ϵ^2, where

$$\mu_\epsilon = \frac{\mu_{\psi_0} - \Psi(P_n^0)}{P_n(H_{1,1}^* - H_{1,0}^*)} \text{ and } \sigma_\epsilon = \frac{\sigma_{\psi_0}}{|P_n(H_{1,1}^* - H_{1,0}^*)|}.$$

Let us consider $Q_{Y,n}(\epsilon)(Y \mid A, W)$ to be a normal distribution with mean $\bar{Q}_n^0(A, W) + \epsilon H_1^*(A, W)$ and variance $\sigma^2(\bar{Q}_n^0)(A, W)$, and let $\sigma_{\bar{Q}_n^0}^2 \equiv \sigma^2(\bar{Q}_n^0)$. The part of the likelihood corresponding to $Q_{Y,n}(\epsilon)(Y \mid A, W)$ can be written as follows:

$$\prod_{i=1}^n Q_{Y,n}(\epsilon)(Y_i \mid A_i, W_i) \propto \exp\left(-nP_n\frac{\left(Y - \bar{Q}_n^0 - \epsilon H_1^*\right)^2}{\sigma_{\bar{Q}_n^0}^2}\right).$$

Thus, the posterior density of ϵ is

$$\begin{aligned}p(\epsilon \mid O_1, \ldots O_n) &\propto \exp\left(-nP_n\frac{\left(Y - \bar{Q}_n^0 - \epsilon H_1^*\right)^2}{2\sigma_{\bar{Q}_n^0}^2} - \frac{(\epsilon - \mu_\epsilon)^2}{2\sigma_\epsilon^2}\right) \\ &\propto \exp\left(-\epsilon^2\left(nP_n\frac{H_1^{*2}}{2\sigma_{\bar{Q}_n^0}^2} + \frac{1}{2\sigma_\epsilon^2}\right) + \epsilon\left(nP_n\frac{H_1^*(Y - \bar{Q}_n^0)}{\sigma_{\bar{Q}_n^0}^2} + \frac{\mu_\epsilon}{\sigma_\epsilon^2}\right)\right).\end{aligned}$$

Now let

$$\sigma^2_{\epsilon|O} = \left(nP_n \frac{H_1^{*2}}{\sigma^2_{\bar{Q}_n^0}} + \frac{1}{\sigma^2_\epsilon} \right)^{-1} \quad \text{and} \quad \mu_{\epsilon|O} = \left(nP_n \frac{H_1^*(Y - \bar{Q}_n^0)}{\sigma^2_{\bar{Q}_n^0}} + \frac{\mu_\epsilon}{\sigma^2_\epsilon} \right) \sigma^2_{\epsilon|O}.$$

Then,

$$p(\epsilon \mid O_1, \ldots O_n) \propto \exp\left(-\frac{(\epsilon - \mu_{\epsilon|O})^2}{2\sigma^2_{\epsilon|O}} \right),$$

which is the normal distribution with mean $\mu_{\epsilon|O}$ and variance $\sigma^2_{\epsilon|O}$.

Note that the maximum likelihood estimator of ϵ in the model (28.15), under a normal distribution, is given by

$$\epsilon_n = \frac{P_n \frac{H_1^*(Y - \bar{Q}_n^0)}{\sigma^2_{\bar{Q}_n^0}}}{P_n \frac{H_1^{*2}}{\sigma^2_{\bar{Q}_n^0}}},$$

so that the posterior mean $\mu_{\epsilon|O}$ is, as expected, a weighted average of the maximum likelihood estimator ϵ_n and the prior mean μ_ϵ of ϵ.

The posterior distribution of ψ_0 is also normal with mean

$$\mu_{\psi_0|O} = \Psi(P_n^0) + \mu_{\epsilon|O} P_n \left(H_{1,1}^* - H_{1,0}^* \right)$$

and variance

$$\sigma^2_{\psi_0|O} = \sigma^2_{\epsilon|O} \left[P_n \left(H_{1,1}^* - H_{1,0}^* \right) \right]^2.$$

By plugging in $\mu_{\epsilon|O}$ and $\sigma^2_{\epsilon|O}$, and working out the algebraic details, we obtain:

$$\mu_{\psi_0|O} = \frac{w_1 \left[\Psi(p_n^0) + \epsilon_n P_n (H_{1,1}^* - H_{1,0}^*) \right] + w_2 \mu_{\psi_0}}{w_1 + w_2} = \frac{w_1 \hat{\psi}_n + w_2 \mu_{\psi_0}}{w_1 + w_2},$$

$$\sigma^2_{\psi_0|O} = \frac{w_2}{w_1 + w_2} \sigma^2_{\psi_0},$$

where

$$w_1 = nP_n \frac{H_1^{*2}}{\sigma^2_{Q_0}} \text{ and } w_2 = \frac{\left[P_n (H_{1,1}^* - H_{1,0}^*) \right]^2}{\sigma^2_{\psi_0}}.$$

Note the posterior mean of ψ_0 is just a weighted average of the TMLE of ψ_0 and its prior mean. Also, if the variance of the prior is very large compared to $[P_n(H_{1,1}^* - H_{1,0}^*)]^2$, the weight of the prior mean is very small, and the posterior mean of ψ_0 is just its TMLE.

Appendix 3

The Metropolis–Hastings algorithm is a Markov chain Monte Carlo method for sampling observations from a probability distribution whose analytic form is not easy to handle. Assume that $p(x)$ is the density from which observations are going to be drawn. The Metropolis–Hastings algorithm requires only that a function proportional to this density can be calculated. This is one of the most important aspects of the algorithm, since the constants of proportionality that arise in Bayesian applications are usually very difficult to compute. The algorithm generates a chain $x_1, x_2, \ldots, x_n$ by using a proposal density $q(x', x^i)$ at each step to generate a new proposed observation, x', that depends only on the previous state of the chain, x^i. This proposal is accepted as x^{i+1} if

$$\alpha < \min\left\{\frac{p(x')q(x^i, x')}{p(x^i)q(x', x^i)}, 1\right\},$$

where α is drawn from a uniform distribution in the interval (0, 1). If the proposal is not accepted, the previous value is preserved in the chain, $x^{i+1} = x^i$. For additional references on the Metropolis–Hastings algorithm, we refer readers to Robert (2007), p. 303.

For the sake of simulating observations from the targeted posterior distribution of ϵ, a normal distribution was used as proposal density. The mean and variance of the posterior were computed numerically and used as parameters of this normal distribution. The starting value of the chain was set to zero. The acceptance rate was computed as the proportion of times that the proposal was accepted.

The R function used to draw samples of size n from the posterior distribution of ϵ is described below.

```
mh.epsilon <- function (n, posterior, e0, sd0){
  n <- n + 1
  e <- numeric(n)
  e[1] <- e0
  z <- rnorm(n-1)
  for(i in 2:n){
      cand <- z[i-1]*sd0 + e[i-1]
      p <- (posterior(cand) * dnorm(e[i-1], mean = cand,
                sd = sd0))/(posterior(e[i-1]) * dnorm(cand,
                mean = e[i-1], sd = sd0))
      pr <- min(p, 1)
      e[i] <- sample(c(cand, e[i-1]), 1, prob = c(pr, 1-pr))
  }
  return(e[-1])}
```

Chapter 29
TMLE in Adaptive Group Sequential Covariate-Adjusted RCTs

Antoine Chambaz, Mark J. van der Laan

This chapter is devoted to group sequential covariate-adjusted RCTs analyzed through the prism of TMLE. By *adaptive covariate-adjusted design* we mean an RCT group sequential design that allows the investigator to dynamically modify its course through data-driven adjustment of the randomization probability based on data accrued so far, without negatively impacting the statistical integrity of the trial. Moreover, the patient's baseline covariates may be taken into account for the random treatment assignment. This definition is slightly adapted from Golub (2006). In particular, we assume following the definition of prespecified sampling plans given in Emerson (2006) that, prior to collection of the data, the trial protocol specifies the parameter of scientific interest, the inferential method, and confidence level to be used when constructing a confidence interval for the latter parameter.

Furthermore, we assume that the investigator specifies beforehand in the trial protocol a criterion of special interest that yields a notion of *optimal randomization scheme* that we therefore wish to target. For instance, the criterion could translate the necessity to minimize the number of patients assigned to their corresponding inferior treatment arm, subject to level and power constraints. Or the criterion could translate the necessity that a result be available as quickly as possible, subject to level and power constraints. The sole restriction on the criterion is that it must yield an optimal randomization scheme that can be approximated from the data accrued so far. The two examples above comply with this restriction.

We choose to consider specifically the second criterion cited above. Consequently, the optimal randomization scheme is the so-called *Neyman allocation*, which minimizes the asymptotic variance of the TMLE of the parameter of interest. We emphasize that there is nothing special about targeting the Neyman allocation, the whole methodology applying equally well to a large class of optimal randomization schemes derived from a variety of valid criteria.

By *adaptive group sequential design* we refer to the possibility of adjusting the randomization scheme only by blocks of c patients, where $c \geq 1$ is a prespecified integer (the case where $c = 1$ corresponds to a fully sequential adaptive design). The expression also refers to the fact that group sequential testing methods can be equally well applied on top of adaptive designs, an extension that we do not consider here. Although all our results (and their proofs) still hold for any $c \geq 1$, we consider the case $c = 1$ in the theoretical part of the chapter for simplicity's sake but the case where $c > 1$ is considered in the simulation study.

The literature on adaptive designs is vast, and our review is not comprehensive. The expression "adaptive design" has also been used in the literature for sequential testing and, in general, for designs that allow data-adaptive stopping times for the whole study (or for certain treatment arms) which achieve the desired type I and type II error requirements when testing a null hypothesis against its alternative. Data-adaptive randomization schemes go back to the 1930s, and we refer the interested reader to Hu and Rosenberger (2006, Sect. 1.2), Jennison and Turnbull (2000, Sect. 17.4), and Rosenberger (1996) for a comprehensive historical perspective.

Many articles have been devoted to the study of "response adaptive designs," an expression implicitly suggesting that those designs only depend on past responses of previous patients and not on the corresponding covariates. We refer readers to Hu and Rosenberger (2006) and Chambaz and van der Laan (2010) for a bibliography on that topic. On the contrary, covariate-adjusted response-adaptive (CARA) randomizations tackle the so-called issue of heterogeneity (i.e., the use of covariates in adaptive designs) by dynamically calculating the allocation probabilities on the basis of previous responses and current and past values of certain covariates. In this view, this chapter studies a new type of CARA procedure. The interest in CARA procedures is more recent, and there is a steadily growing number of articles dedicated to their study, starting with Rosenberger et al. (2001) and Bandyopadhyay and Biswas (2001), then Atkinson and Biswas (2005), Zhang et al. (2007), Zhang and Hu (2009), and Shao et al. (2010), among others. The latter articles are typically concerned with the convergence (almost sure and in law) of the allocation probabilities vector and of the estimator of the parameter *in a correctly specified parametric model*. The article by Shao et al. (2010) is devoted to the testing issue.

By contrast, the consistency and asymptotic normality results that we obtain here are robust to model misspecification. Thus, they notably contribute significantly to solving the question raised by the Food and Drug Administration (2006): "*When is it valid to modify randomization based on results, for example, in a combined phase 2/3 cancer trial?*" Finally, this chapter mainly relies on Chambaz and van der Laan (2010) and van der Laan (2008b), the latter technical report paving the way to robust and more efficient estimation based on adaptive RCTs in a variety of other setting (including the case that the outcome Y is a possibly censored time-to-event).

29.1 Statistical Framework

This chapter is devoted to the asymptotic study of *adaptive group sequential designs* in the case of RCTs with covariate, binary treatment and a one-dimensional primary outcome of interest. Thus, the experimental unit is $O = (W, A, Y)$, where $W \in \mathcal{W}$ consists of some baseline covariates, $A \in \mathcal{A} = \{0, 1\}$ denotes the assigned binary treatment, and $Y \in \mathcal{Y}$ is the primary outcome of interest. For example, Y can indicate whether the treatment has been successful or not ($\mathcal{Y} = \{0, 1\}$), or Y can count the number of times an event of interest has occurred under the assigned treatment during a period of follow-up ($\mathcal{Y} = \mathbb{N}$), or Y can measure a quantity of interest after a given time has elapsed ($\mathcal{Y} = \mathbb{R}$). Although we will focus on the last case in this chapter, the methodology applies equally well to each example cited above.

Let us denote by P_0 the true distribution of the observed data structure O in the population of interest. We see P_0 as a specific element of the nonparametric set $\mathcal{M}$ of all possible observed data distributions. Note that, in order to avoid some technicalities, we assume (or rather impose) that all elements of $\mathcal{M}$ are dominated by a common measure. The parameter of scientific interest is the marginal effect of treatment $a = 1$ relative to treatment $a = 0$ on the additive scale, or risk difference: $\psi_0 = E_{P_0}[E_{P_0}(Y \mid A = 1, W) - E_{P_0}(Y \mid A = 0, W)]$. Of course, other choices such as the log-relative risk (the counterpart of the risk difference on the multiplicative scale) could be considered, and dealt with along the same lines. The risk difference can be interpreted causally under certain assumptions.

For all $P \in \mathcal{M}$, $Q_W(W; P) = P(W), g(A \mid W; P) = P(A \mid W)$, and $Q_{Y|A,W}(O; P) = P(Y \mid A, W)$. We use the alternative notation $P = P_{Q,g}$ with $Q = Q(\cdot; P) \equiv (Q_W(\cdot; P), Q_{Y|A,W}(\cdot; P))$, and $g = g(\cdot \mid \cdot; P)$. Equivalently, $P_{Q,g}$ is the data-generating distribution such that $Q(\cdot; P_{Q,g}) = Q$ and $g(\cdot \mid \cdot; P_{Q,g}) = g$. In particular, we denote $Q_0 = Q(\cdot; P_0) = (Q_W(\cdot; P_0), Q_{Y|A,W}(\cdot; P_0))$. We also introduce the notation $\mathcal{Q} = \{Q(\cdot; P) : P \in \mathcal{M}\}$ for the nonparametric set of all possible values of Q, and $\mathcal{G} = \{g(\cdot \mid \cdot; P) : P \in \mathcal{M}\}$ for the nonparametric set of all possible values of g. Setting $\bar{Q}(A, W; P) = E_P(Y \mid A, W)$ and $\bar{Q}_0 = \bar{Q}(\cdot; P_0)$ [with a slight abuse, we also write sometimes $\bar{Q}(\cdot; Q)$ instead of $\bar{Q}(\cdot; P_{Q,g})$], we define in greater generality

$$\Psi(P) = E_P\left(\bar{Q}(1, W; P) - \bar{Q}(0, W; P)\right)$$

over the whole set $\mathcal{M}$, so that ψ_0 equivalently can be written as $\psi_0 = \Psi(P_0)$. This notation also emphasizes the fact that $\Psi(P)$ only depends on P through $\bar{Q}(\cdot; P)$ and $Q_W(\cdot; P)$, justifying the alternative notation $\Psi(P_{Q,g}) = \Psi(Q)$. The following proposition summarizes the most fundamental properties enjoyed by Ψ.

Proposition 29.1. *The functional Ψ is pathwise differentiable at every $P \in \mathcal{M}$. The efficient influence curve of Ψ at $P_{Q,g} \in \mathcal{M}$ is characterized by*

$$\begin{aligned} D^*(O; P_{Q,g}) &= D_1^*(W; Q) + D_2^*(O; P_{Q,g}), \text{ where} \\ D_1^*(W; Q) &= \bar{Q}(1, W) - \bar{Q}(0, W) - \Psi(Q), \text{ and} \\ D_2^*(O; P_{Q,g}) &= \frac{2A - 1}{g(A \mid W)}(Y - \bar{Q}(A, W)). \end{aligned}$$

The variance $\mathrm{var}_P D^*(O; P)^2$ *is the lower bound of the asymptotic variance of any regular estimator of $\Psi(P)$ in the i.i.d. setting. Furthermore, even if $Q \neq Q_0$,*

$$E_{P_0} D^*(O; P_{Q,g}) = 0 \quad \text{implies} \quad \Psi(Q) = \Psi(Q_0) \tag{29.1}$$

when $g = g(\cdot \mid \cdot; P_0)$.

The implication (29.1) is the key to the robustness of the TMLE introduced and studied in this chapter. It is another justification of our interest in the pathwise differentiability of the functional Ψ and its efficient influence curve.

29.2 Data-Generating Mechanism

In order to formally describe the data-generating mechanism, we need to state a starting assumption. During the course of a clinical trial, it is possible to recruit independently the patients from a stationary population. In the counterfactual framework, this is equivalent to supposing that it is possible to sample as many independent copies of the full-data structure as required. Let us denote the ith observed data structure by $O_i = (W_i, A_i, Y_i)$. We also find it convenient to introduce $\mathbf{O}_n = (O_1, \ldots, O_n)$, and for every $i = 0, \ldots, n$, $\mathbf{O}_n(i) = (O_1, \ldots, O_i)$ [with the convention $\mathbf{O}(0) = \emptyset$].

By adjusting the randomization scheme as the data accrue, we mean that the nth treatment assignment A_n is drawn from $g_n(\cdot \mid W_n)$, where $g_n(\cdot \mid W)$ is a conditional distribution (or treatment mechanism) given the covariate W, which additionally depends on past observations $\mathbf{O}_{n-1}$. Since the sequence of treatment mechanisms cannot reasonably grow in complexity as the sample size increases, we will only consider data-adaptive treatment mechanisms such that $g_n(\cdot \mid W)$ depends on $\mathbf{O}_{n-1}$ only through a finite-dimensional summary measure $Z_n = \phi_n(\mathbf{O}_{n-1})$, where the measurable function ϕ_n maps $\mathcal{O}^{n-1}$ onto $\mathbb{R}^d$ (where $\mathcal{O}$ is the set from which O takes its values) for some fixed $d \geq 0$ [$d = 0$ corresponds to the case where $g_n(\cdot \mid W)$ actually does not adapt]. For instance, $Z_{n+1} = \phi_{n+1}(\mathbf{O}_n) \equiv (n^{-1} \sum_{i=1}^n Y_i I(A_i = 0), n^{-1} \sum_{i=1}^n Y_i I(A_i = 1))$ characterizes a proper summary measure of the past, which keeps track of the mean outcome in each treatment arm. Another sequence of mappings ϕ_n will be at the core of the adaptive methodology that we study in depth in this chapter, see (29.4).

Formally, the data-generating mechanism is specified by the following factorization of the likelihood of $\mathbf{O}_n$:

$$\prod_{i=1}^n (Q_W(W_i; P_0) \times Q_{Y|A,W}(O_i; P_0)) \times \prod_{i=1}^n g_i(A_i \mid W_i),$$

which suggests the introduction of $\mathbf{g}_n = (g_1, \ldots, g_n)$, referred to as the *design of the study*, and the expression "$\mathbf{O}_n$ is drawn from $(Q_0, \mathbf{g}_n)$." Likewise, the likelihood of $\mathbf{O}_n$ under $(Q, \mathbf{g}_n)$ [where $Q = (Q_W, Q_{Y|A,W}) \in \mathcal{Q}$ is a candidate value for Q_0] is

$$\prod_{i=1}^n (Q_W(W_i) \times Q_{Y|A,W}(O_i)) \times \prod_{i=1}^n g_i(A_i \mid W_i),$$

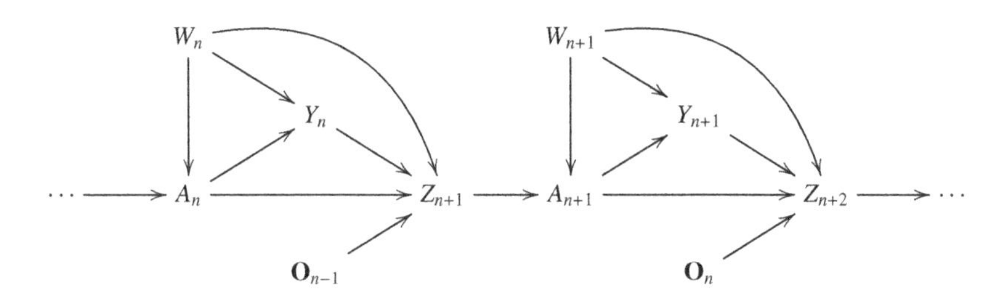

Fig. 29.1 A possible causal graph describing the data-generating mechanism

where we emphasize that the second factor is known. Thus we will refer with a slight abuse of terminology to $\sum_{i=1}^{n} \log Q_W(W_i) + \log Q_{Y|A,W}(O_i)$ as the log-likelihood of $\mathbf{O}_n$ under $(Q, \mathbf{g}_n)$. Furthermore, given $\mathbf{g}_n$, we introduce the notation $P_{Q_0,g_i} f \equiv E_{P_{Q_0,g_i}}(f(O_i) \mid \mathbf{O}_n(i-1))$ for any possibly vector-valued measurable f defined on O.

Another equivalent characterization of the data-generating mechanism involves the causal graph shown in Fig. 29.1. It is seen again that W_n is drawn independently from the past $\mathbf{O}_{n-1}$. Secondly, A_n is a deterministic function of W_n, the summary measure Z_n (which depends on $\mathbf{O}_{n-1}$), and a new independent source of randomness [in other words, it is drawn conditionally on (W_n, Z_n) and conditionally independently of the past $\mathbf{O}_{n-1}$]. Thirdly, Y_n is a deterministic function of (A_n, W_n) and a new independent source of randomness [it is drawn conditionally on (A_n, W_n) and conditionally independently of the past $\mathbf{O}_{n-1}$]. Then the next summary measure Z_{n+1} is obtained as a function of $\mathbf{O}_{n-1}$ and $O_n = (W_n, A_n, Y_n)$, and so on.

Finally, it is interesting in practice to adapt the design group sequentially. This can be simply formalized. For a given prespecified integer $c \geq 1$ ($c = 1$ corresponds to a fully sequential adaptive design), going forward c-group sequentially simply amounts to imposing $\phi_{(r-1)c+1}(\mathbf{O}_{(r-1)c}) = \ldots = \phi_{rc}(\mathbf{O}_{rc-1})$ for all $r \geq 1$. Then the c treatment assignments $A_{(r-1)c+1}, \ldots, A_{rc}$ in the rth c-group are all drawn from the same conditional distribution $g_{(r-1)c}(\cdot \mid W)$. Yet, although all our results (and their proofs) still hold for any $c \geq 1$, we prefer to consider in the rest of this section and in Sects. 29.4 and 29.5 the case where $c = 1$ for simplicity's sake. In contrast, the simulation study carried out in Sect. 29.6 involves some $c > 1$.

29.3 Optimal Design

One of the most important features of the adaptive group sequential design methodology is that it *targets* a *user-supplied* specific design of special interest. This specific design is generally an optimal design with respect to a criterion that translates what the investigator is most concerned about. Specifically, one could be most concerned with the well-being of the target population, wishing that a result be available as quickly as possible and aspiring therefore to the highest efficiency (i.e., the ability to reach a conclusion as quickly as possible subject to level and power constraints). Or one could be most concerned with the well-being of the subjects participating in the clinical trial, therefore trying to minimize the number of patients assigned to their corresponding inferior treatment arms, subject to level and power constraints. Obviously, these are only two important examples from a large class of potentially interesting criteria. The sole purpose of the criterion is to generate a random element in $\mathcal{G}$ of the form $g_n = g_{Z_n}$, where $Z_n = \phi_n(\mathbf{O}_{n-1})$ is a finite-dimensional summary measure of $\mathbf{O}_{n-1}$, and g_n converges to a desired or optimal fixed treatment mechanism. We decide to focus in this chapter on the first example, but it must be clear that the methodology applies to a variety of other criteria. See van der Laan (2008b) for other examples.

By Proposition 29.1, the asymptotic variance of any regular estimator of the risk difference $\Psi(Q_0)$ has lower bound $\mathrm{var}_{P_{Q_0,g}} D^*(O; P_{Q_0,g})$ if the estimator relies on data sampled independently from $P_{Q_0,g}$. We have that

$$\mathrm{var}_{P_{Q_0,g}} D^*(O; P_{Q_0,g}) = E_{Q_0}(\bar{Q}_0(1, W) - \bar{Q}_0(0, W) - \Psi(Q_0))^2 + E_{Q_0}\left(\frac{\sigma^2(Q_0)(1, W)}{g(1 \mid W)} + \frac{\sigma^2(Q_0)(0, W)}{g(0 \mid W)}\right),$$

where $\sigma^2(Q_0)(A, W)$ denotes the conditional variance of Y given (A, W) under Q_0. We use the notation E_{Q_0} above (for the expectation with respect to the marginal distribution of W under P_0) in order to emphasize the fact that the treatment mechanism g only appears in the second term of the right-hand side sum. Furthermore, it holds P_0–almost surely that

$$\frac{\sigma^2(Q_0)(1, W)}{g(1 \mid W)} + \frac{\sigma^2(Q_0)(0, W)}{g(0 \mid W)} \geq (\sigma(Q_0)(1, W) + \sigma(Q_0)(0, W))^2,$$

with equality if and only if

$$g(1 \mid W) = \frac{\sigma(Q_0)(1, W)}{\sigma(Q_0)(1, W) + \sigma(Q_0)(0, W)}, \tag{29.2}$$

P_0–almost surely. Therefore, the following lower bound holds for all $g \in \mathcal{G}$:

$$\mathrm{var}_{P_{Q_0,g}} D^*(O; P_{Q_0,g}) \geq E_{Q_0}(\bar{Q}_0(1, W) - \bar{Q}_0(0, W) - \Psi(Q_0))^2 + E_{Q_0}(\sigma(Q_0)(1, W) + \sigma(Q_0)(0, W))^2,$$

with equality if and only if $g \in \mathcal{G}$ is characterized by (29.2). This optimal design is known in the literature as the *Neyman allocation* (Hu and Rosenberger 2006, p. 13). This result makes clear that the most efficient treatment mechanism assigns with higher probability a patient with covariate vector W to the treatment arm with the largest variance of the outcome Y, regardless of the mean of the outcome (i.e., whether the arm is inferior or superior).

Due to logistical reasons, it might be preferable to consider only treatment mechanisms that assign treatment in response to a subvector V of the baseline covariate vector W. In addition, if W is complex, targeting the optimal Neyman allocation might be too ambitious. Therefore, we will consider the important case where V is a discrete covariate with finitely many values in the set $\mathcal{V} = \{1, \ldots, \nu\}$. The covariate V indicates subgroup membership for a collection of ν subgroups of interest. We decide to restrict the search for an optimal design to the set $\mathcal{G}_1 \subset \mathcal{G}$ of those treatment mechanisms that only depend on W through V. The same calculations as above yield straightforwardly that, for all $g \in \mathcal{G}_1$

$$\mathrm{var}_{P_{Q_0,g}} D^*(O; P_{Q_0,g}) \geq E_{Q_0}(\bar{Q}_0(1, W) - \bar{Q}_0(0, W) - \Psi(Q_0))^2 + E_{Q_0}(\bar{\sigma}(Q_0)(1, V) + \bar{\sigma}(Q_0)(0, V))^2,$$

where $\bar{\sigma}^2(Q_0)(a, V) = E_{Q_0}(\sigma^2(Q_0)(a, W) \mid V)$ for $a \in \mathcal{A}$, with equality if and only if g coincides with $g^*(Q_0)$, characterized by

$$g^*(Q_0)(1|V) = \frac{\bar{\sigma}(Q_0)(1, V)}{\bar{\sigma}(Q_0)(1, V) + \bar{\sigma}(Q_0)(0, V)},$$

P_0–almost surely. Hereafter, we refer to $g^*(Q_0)$ as *the optimal design.*

Because $g^*(Q_0)$ is characterized as the minimizer over $g \in \mathcal{G}_1$ of the variance under $P_{Q_0,g}$ of the efficient influence curve at $P_{Q_0,g}$, we propose to construct $g_{n+1} \in \mathcal{G}_1$ as the minimizer over $g \in \mathcal{G}_1$ of an estimator of the latter variance based on past observations $\mathbf{O}_n$. We proceed by recursion. We first set $g_1 = g^b$, the so-called balanced treatment mechanism such that $g^b(1 \mid W) = 1/2$ for all $W \in \mathcal{W}$, and assume that $\mathbf{O}_n$ has already been sampled from $(Q_0, \mathbf{g}_n)$, the sample size being large enough to guarantee $\sum_{i=1}^{n} I(V_i = \nu) > 0$ for all $\nu \in \mathcal{V}$ (if n_0 is the smallest sample size such that the previous condition is met, then we set $g_1 = \ldots = g_{n_0} = g^b$).

The issue is now to construct g_{n+1}. Let us assume for the time being that we already know how to construct an estimator Q_n of Q_0 based on $\mathbf{O}_n$ [hence the estimators $\bar{Q}_n = \bar{Q}(\cdot; Q_n)$ of $\bar{Q}_0$ and $\Psi(Q_n)$ of $\Psi(Q_0) = \psi_0$]. The reasoning is not circular by virtue of the chronological ordering as it is summarized in Fig. 29.1, for instance. Then, for all $g \in \mathcal{G}_1$,

$$\begin{aligned} S_n(g) &= \frac{1}{n}\sum_{i=1}^{n}\Bigg(D_1^*(W_i; Q_n)^2 + 2D_1^*(W_i; Q_n)D_2^*(O_i; P_{Q_n,g})\frac{g(A_i \mid V_i)}{g_i(A_i \mid V_i)} \\ &\quad + D_2^*(O_i; P_{Q_n,g})^2\frac{g(A_i \mid V_i)}{g_i(A_i \mid V_i)}\Bigg) \\ &\quad - \left(\frac{1}{n}\sum_{i=1}^{n} D_1^*(W_i; Q_n) + D_2^*(O_i; P_{Q_n,g})\frac{g(A_i \mid V_i)}{g_i(A_i \mid V_i)}\right)^2 \\ &= \frac{1}{n}\sum_{i=1}^{n}\frac{(Y_i - \bar{Q}_n(A_i, W_i))^2}{g(A_i|V_i)g_i(A_i|V_i)} \end{aligned}$$

$$+\left\{\frac{1}{n}\sum_{i=1}^{n} D_1^*(W_i;Q_n)^2 + 2D_1^*(W_i;Q_n)D_2^*(O_i;P_{Q_n,g_i}) - \left(\frac{1}{n}\sum_{i=1}^{n} D_1^*(W_i;Q_n) + D_2^*(O_i;P_{Q_n,g_i})\right)^2\right\}$$

estimates $\mathrm{var}_{P_{Q_0,g}} D^*(O;P_{Q_0,g})$ (the weighting provides the adequate tilt of the empirical distribution; it is not necessary to weight the terms corresponding to D_1^* because they do not depend on the treatment mechanism). Now, only the first term in the rightmost expression still depends on g. The same calculation as above straightforwardly yields that $S_n(g)$ is minimized at $g_{n+1} \in \mathcal{G}_1$ characterized by

$$g_{n+1}(1 \mid v) = \frac{s_{v,n}(1)}{s_{v,n}(1) + s_{v,n}(0)}$$

for all $v \in \mathcal{V}$, where for each $(v,a) \in \mathcal{V} \times \mathcal{A}$

$$s_{v,n}^2(a) = \frac{\frac{1}{n}\sum_{i=1}^{n} \frac{(Y_i - \bar{Q}_n(A_i,W_i))^2}{g_i(A_i|V_i)} I((V_i,A_i) = (v,a))}{\frac{1}{n}\sum_{i=1}^{n} I(V_i = v)}.$$

Yet, instead of considering the above characterization, we find it more convenient to define

$$g_{n+1}^*(1 \mid v) = \frac{\sigma_{v,n}(1)}{\sigma_{v,n}(1) + \sigma_{v,n}(0)}, \tag{29.3}$$

for all $v \in \mathcal{V}$, where for each $(v,a) \in \mathcal{V} \times \mathcal{A}$

$$\sigma_{v,n}^2(a) = \frac{\frac{1}{n}\sum_{i=1}^{n} \frac{(Y_i - \bar{Q}_n(A_i,W_i))^2}{g_i(A_i|V_i)} I((V_i,A_i) = (v,a))}{\frac{1}{n}\sum_{i=1}^{n} \frac{I((V_i,A_i)=(v,a))}{g_i(a|v)}}.$$

Note that $s_{v,n}^2(a)$ and $\sigma_{v,n}^2(a)$ share the same numerator, and that the different denominators converge to the same limit. Substituting $\sigma_{v,n}^2(a)$ for $s_{v,n}^2(a)$ is convenient because one naturally interprets the former as an estimator of the conditional variance of Y given $(A,V) = (a,v)$ based on $\mathbf{O}_n$, a fact that we use in Sect. 29.4.2. Finally, we emphasize that $g_{n+1}^* = g_{Z_{n+1}}$ for the summary measure of the past $\mathbf{O}_n$

$$Z_{n+1} = \phi_{n+1}(\mathbf{O}_n) \equiv ((\sigma_{v,n}^2(0), \sigma_{v,n}^2(1)) : v \in \mathcal{V}). \tag{29.4}$$

The rigorous definition of the design $\mathbf{g}_n^* = (g_1^*, \ldots, g_n^*)$ follows by recursion, but it is still subject to knowledge about how to construct an estimator Q_n of Q_0 based on $\mathbf{O}_n$. Because this last missing piece of the formal definition of the adaptive group sequential design data-generating mechanism is also the core of the TMLE procedure, we address it in Sect. 29.4.

29.4 TMLE Procedure

We assume hereafter that $\mathbf{O}_n$ has already been sampled from the $(Q_0, \mathbf{g}_n^*)$-adaptive sampling scheme. In this section, we construct an estimator Q_n (actually denoted by Q_n^*) of Q_0, thereby yielding the characterization of g_{n+1}^* and completing the formal definition of the adaptive design $\mathbf{g}_n^*$. In particular, the next data structure O_{n+1} can be drawn from (Q_0, g_{n+1}^*), and it makes sense to undertake the asymptotic study of the properties of the TMLE methodology based on adaptive group sequential sampling. As in the i.i.d. framework, the TMLE procedure maps an initial substitution estimator $\Psi(Q_n^0)$ of ψ_0 into an update $\psi_n^* = \Psi(Q_n^*)$ by fluctuating the initial estimate Q_n^0 of Q_0.

29.4.1 *Initial ML-Based Substitution Estimator*

The working model. In order to construct the initial estimate Q_n^0 of Q_0, we consider a *working model* Q_n^w. With a slight abuse of notation, the elements of Q_n^w are denoted by $(Q_W(\cdot; P_n), Q_{Y|A,W}(\cdot; \theta))$ for some parameter $\theta \in \Theta$, where $Q_W(\cdot; P_n)$ is the empirical marginal distribution of W. Specifically, the working model Q_n^w is chosen in such a way that

$$Q_{Y|A,W}(O; \theta) = \frac{1}{\sqrt{2\pi\sigma_V^2(A)}} \exp\left\{-\frac{(Y - m(A, W; \beta_V))^2}{2\sigma_V^2(A)}\right\}.$$

This implies that for any $P_\theta \in \mathcal{M}$ such that $Q_{Y|A,W}(\cdot; P_\theta) = Q_{Y|A,W}(\cdot; \theta)$, the conditional mean $\bar{Q}(A, W; P_\theta)$, which we also denote by $\bar{Q}(A, W; \theta)$, satisfies $\bar{Q}(A, W; \theta) = m(A, W; \beta_V)$, the right-hand side expression being a linear combination of variables extracted from (A, W) and indexed by the regression vector β_V (of dimension b). Defining

$$\theta(v) = (\beta_v, \sigma_v^2(0), \sigma_v^2(1))^\top \in \Theta_v \subset \mathbb{R}^b \times \mathbb{R}_+^* \times \mathbb{R}_+^* \tag{29.5}$$

for each $v \in \mathcal{V}$, the complete parameter is given by $\theta = (\theta(1)^\top, \ldots, \theta(\nu)^\top)^\top \in \Theta$, where $\Theta = \prod_{v=1}^{\nu} \Theta_v$. We impose the following conditions on the parameterization: The parameter set Θ is compact. Furthermore, the linear parameterization is identifiable; for all $v \in \mathcal{V}$, if $m(a, w; \beta_v) = m(a, w; \beta_v')$ for all $a \in \mathcal{A}$ and $w \in \mathcal{W}$ (compatible with v), then necessarily $\beta_v = \beta_v'$.

Characterizing Q_n^0. Let us set a reference fixed design $g^r \in \mathcal{G}_1$. We now characterize Q_n^0 by letting $Q_n^0 = (Q_W(\cdot; P_n), Q_{Y|A,W}(\cdot; \theta_n))$, where

$$\theta_n = \arg\max_{\theta \in \Theta} \sum_{i=1}^{n} \log Q_{Y|A,W}(O_i; \theta) \frac{g^r(A_i \mid V_i)}{g_i^*(A_i \mid V_i)} \tag{29.6}$$

is a *weighted* maximum likelihood estimator with respect to the working model. Thus, the νth component $\theta_n(\nu)$ of θ_n satisfies

$$\theta_n(\nu) = \arg\min_{\theta(\nu)\in\Theta_\nu} \sum_{i=1}^{n} \left(\log \sigma_\nu^2(A_i) + \frac{(Y_i - m(A_i, W_i; \beta_\nu))^2}{\sigma_\nu^2(A_i)} \right) \frac{g^r(A_i \mid V_i)}{g_i^*(A_i \mid V_i)} I(V_i = \nu)$$

for every $\nu \in \mathcal{V}$. Note that this initial estimate Q_n^0 of Q_0 yields the initial maximum-likelihood-based substitution estimator $\Psi(Q_n^0)$ of ψ_0:

$$\Psi(Q_n^0) = \frac{1}{n} \sum_{i=1}^{n} \bar{Q}(1, W_i; \theta_n) - \bar{Q}(0, W_i; \theta_n).$$

Studying Q_n^0 through θ_n. For simplicity, let us introduce, for all $\theta \in \Theta$, the additional notation: $\ell_{\theta,0} = \log Q_{Y|A,W}(\cdot; \theta)$, $\dot{\ell}_{\theta,0} = \frac{\partial}{\partial\theta}\ell_{\theta,0}$, and $\ddot{\ell}_{\theta,0} = \frac{\partial^2}{\partial\theta^2}\ell_{\theta,0}$. The first asymptotic property of θ_n that we derive concerns its consistency (see Theorem 5 in van der Laan 2008b).

Proposition 29.2. *Assume that*

A1. *There exists a unique interior point $\theta_0 \in \Theta$ such that*

$$\theta_0 = \arg\max_{\theta\in\Theta} P_{Q_0,g^r}\ell_{\theta,0};$$

A2. *The matrix $-P_{Q_0,g^r}\ddot{\ell}_{\theta_0,0}$ is positive definite.*

Provided that $\mathcal{O}$ is a bounded set, θ_n consistently estimates θ_0.

The limit in probability of θ_n has a nice interpretation in terms of projection of $Q_{Y|A,W}(\cdot; P_0)$ onto $\{Q_{Y|A,W}(\cdot; \theta) : \theta \in \Theta\}$. Preferring to discuss this issue in terms of the data-generating distribution rather than conditional distribution, let us set $Q_{\theta_0} = (Q_W(\cdot; P_0), Q_{Y|A,W}(\cdot; \theta_0))$ and assume that $P_{Q_0,g^r} \log Q_{Y|A,W}(\cdot; P_0)$ is well defined (this weak assumption concerns Q_0, not g^r, and holds for instance when $|\log Q_{Y|A,W}(\cdot; P_0)|$ is bounded). Then A1 is equivalent to $P_{Q_{\theta_0},g^r}$ being the unique Kullback–Leibler projection of P_{Q_0,g^r} onto the set

$$\{P \in \mathcal{M} : \exists\theta \in \Theta \text{ s.t. } Q_{Y|A,W}(\cdot; P) = Q_{Y|A,W}(\cdot; \theta), \\ \text{and } Q_W(\cdot; P) = Q_W(\cdot; P_0), g(\cdot \mid \cdot; P) = g^r\}.$$

In addition to being consistent, θ_n actually satisfies a central limit theorem if supplementary mild conditions are met. The latter central limit theorem is embedded in a more general result that we state in Sect. 29.4.3; see Proposition 29.5.

The cornerstone of the proof of Proposition 29.2 is to interpret θ_n as the solution in θ of the martingale estimating equation $\sum_{i=1}^{n} D_1(\theta)(O_i, Z_i) = 0$, where Z_i is the finite-dimensional summary measure of past observation $\mathbf{O}_n(i-1)$ such that g_i^* depends on $\mathbf{O}_n(i-1)$ only through Z_i (hence the notation $g_i^* = g_{Z_i}$) and $D_1(\theta)(O, Z) = \dot{\ell}_{\theta,0}(O) g^r(A \mid V)/g_Z(A \mid V)$ satisfies $P_{Q_0,g_i^*} D_1(\theta_0) = 0$ for all $i \leq n$.

By relying on a Kolmogorov strong law of large numbers for martingales (see Theorem 8 in Chambaz and van der Laan 2010), one obtains that $n^{-1}\sum_{i=1}^{n} P_{Q_0,g_i^*} D_1(\theta_n)$ converges to zero almost surely. This results in the convergence in probability of θ_n to θ_0 by a Taylor expansion of $\theta \mapsto P_{Q_0,g'}\dot{\ell}_{\theta,0}$ at θ_0 (hence assumption A2). The strong law of large numbers applies because the geometry of $\mathcal{F} = \{D_1(\theta) : \theta \in \Theta\}$ is moderately complex [heuristically, $\mathcal{F}$ can be covered by finitely many $\|\cdot\|_\infty$-balls because Θ is a compact set, (O, Z) is bounded, and the mapping $(o, z, \theta) \mapsto D_1(\theta)(o, z)$ is continuous; and the number of such balls of radius η needed to cover $\mathcal{F}$ does not grow too fast as η goes to zero].

Furthermore, maximizing a weighted version of the log-likelihood is a technical twist that makes the theoretical study of the properties of θ_n easier. Indeed, the unweighted maximum likelihood estimator $t_n = \arg\max_{\theta\in\Theta} \sum_{i=1}^{n} \log Q_{Y|A,W}(O_i; \theta)$ targets the parameter

$$T_{\bar{g}_n}(Q_0) = \arg\max_{\theta\in\Theta} \sum_{i=1}^{n} P_{Q_0,g_i^*} \log Q_{Y|A,W}(O_i; \theta) = \arg\max_{\theta\in\Theta} P_{Q_0,\bar{g}_n} \ell_{\theta,0},$$

where $\bar{g}_n = \frac{1}{n}\sum_{i=1}^{n} g_i^*$. Therefore, t_n asymptotically targets the limit, if it exists, of $T_{\bar{g}_n}(Q_0)$. Assuming that $\bar{g}_n$ converges itself to a fixed design $g_\infty \in \mathcal{G}$, then t_n asymptotically targets parameter $T_{g_\infty}(Q_0)$. The latter parameter is very difficult to interpret and to analyze as it depends directly and indirectly (through g_∞) on Q_0.

29.4.2 Convergence of the Adaptive Design

Consider the mapping G^* from Θ to $\mathcal{G}_1$ [respectively equipped with the Euclidean distance and, for instance, the distance $d(g, g') = \sum_{v\in\mathcal{V}} |g(1 \mid v) - g'(1 \mid v)|$] such that, for any $\theta \in \Theta$, for any $(a, v) \in \mathcal{A} \times \mathcal{V}$

$$G^*(\theta)(a \mid v) = \frac{\sigma_v(a)}{\sigma_v(1) + \sigma_v(0)}. \tag{29.7}$$

Equation (29.7) characterizes G^*, which is obviously continuous. Since $\mathbf{g}_n^*$ is adapted in such a way that $g_n^* = G^*(\theta_n)$, Proposition 29.2 and the continuous mapping theorem (see Theorem 1.3.6 in van der Vaart and Wellner 1996) straightforwardly imply the following result.

Proposition 29.3. *Under the assumptions of Proposition 29.2, the adaptive design* $\mathbf{g}_n^*$ *converges in probability to the limit design* $G^*(\theta_0)$.

The convergence of the adaptive design $\mathbf{g}_n^*$ is a crucial result. It is noteworthy that the limit design $G^*(\theta_0)$ equals the optimal design $g^*(Q_0)$ if the working model is correctly specified (which never happens in practical applications), but not necessarily otherwise. Furthermore, the relationship $g_n^* = G^*(\theta_n)$ also entails the possibility of deriving the convergence in distribution of $\sqrt{n}(g_n^* - G^*(\theta_0))$ to a centered Gaussian distribution with known variance by application of the delta method (G^* is differentiable) from a central limit theorem on θ_n (Proposition 29.5).

29.4.3 The TMLE

Fluctuating Q_n^0. The second step of the TMLE procedure stretches the initial estimate $\Psi(Q_n^0)$ in the direction of the parameter of interest, through a maximum likelihood step over a well-chosen fluctuation of Q_n^0. The latter fluctuation of Q_n^0 is just a one-dimensional parametric model $\{Q_n^0(\epsilon) : \epsilon \in \mathcal{E}\} \subset \mathcal{Q}$ indexed by the parameter $\epsilon \in \mathcal{E}$, $\mathcal{E} \subset \mathbb{R}$ being a bounded interval that contains a neighborhood of the origin. Specifically, we set, for all $\epsilon \in \mathcal{E}$, $Q_n^0(\epsilon) = (Q_W(\cdot; P_n), Q_{Y|A,W}(\cdot; \theta_n, \epsilon))$, where for any $\theta \in \Theta$:

$$Q_{Y|A,W}(O; \theta, \epsilon) = \frac{1}{\sqrt{2\pi\sigma_V^2(A)}} \exp\left\{-\frac{(Y - \bar{Q}(A, W; \theta) - \epsilon H^*(A, W; \theta))^2}{2\sigma_V^2(A)}\right\}, \quad (29.8)$$

with

$$H^*(A, W; \theta) = \frac{2A - 1}{G^*(\theta)(A \mid V)} \sigma_V^2(A).$$

In particular, the fluctuation goes through Q_n^0 at $\epsilon = 0$ (i.e., $Q_n^0(0) = Q_n^0$). Let $P_n^0(\epsilon) \in \mathcal{M}$ be a data-generating distribution such that $Q_{Y|A,W}(\cdot; P_n^0(\epsilon)) = Q_{Y|A,W}(\cdot; \theta_n, \epsilon)$. The conditional mean $\bar{Q}(A, W; P_n^0(\epsilon))$, which we also denote by $\bar{Q}(A, W; \theta_n, \epsilon)$, is $\bar{Q}(A, W; \theta_n, \epsilon) = \bar{Q}(A, W; \theta_n) + \epsilon H^*(A, W; \theta_n)$. Furthermore, the score at $\epsilon = 0$ of $P_n^0(\epsilon)$ equals

$$\frac{\partial}{\partial\epsilon} \log P_n^0(\epsilon)(O)\Big|_{\epsilon=0} = \frac{2A - 1}{G^*(\theta_n)(A \mid V)}(Y - \bar{Q}(A, W; \theta_n)) = D_2^*(O; P_{Q_n^0, G^*(\theta_n)}),$$

the second component of the efficient influence curve of Ψ at $P_{Q_n^0, G^*(\theta_n)} = P_{Q_n^0, g_n^*}$. Recall that $g_n^* = G^*(\theta_n)$.

Characterizing the TMLE Q_n^*. We characterize the update Q_n^* of Q_n^0 in the fluctuation $\{Q_n^0(\epsilon) : \epsilon \in \mathcal{E}\}$ by $Q_n^* = Q_n^0(\epsilon_n)$, where

$$\epsilon_n = \arg\max_{\epsilon \in \mathcal{E}} \sum_{i=1}^{n} \log Q_{Y|A,W}(O_i; \theta_n, \epsilon) \frac{g_n^*(A_i \mid V_i)}{g_i^*(A_i \mid V_i)} \quad (29.9)$$

is a *weighted* maximum likelihood estimator with respect to the fluctuation. It is worth noting that ϵ_n is known in closed form (we assume, without serious loss of generality, that $\mathcal{E}$ is large enough for the maximum to be achieved in its interior). Denoting the vth component $\theta_n(v)$ of θ_n by $(\beta_{v,n}, \sigma_{v,n}^2(0), \sigma_{v,n}^2(1))^\top$, it holds that

$$\epsilon_n = \frac{\sum_{i=1}^{n}(Y_i - \bar{Q}(A_i, W_i; \theta_n))\frac{2A_i-1}{g_i^*(A_i|V_i)}}{\sum_{i=1}^{n} \frac{\sigma^2_{V_i,n}(A_i)}{g_n^*(A_i|V_i)g_i(A_i|V_i)}}.$$

The notation Q_n^* for this first update of Q_n^0 is a reference to the fact that the TMLE procedure, which is in greater generality an iterative procedure, converges here in one single step. Indeed, suppose that one fluctuates Q_n^* as we fluctuate Q_n^0 i.e., by introducing $Q_n^1(\epsilon) = (Q_W(\cdot; P_n), Q_{Y|A,W}(\cdot; \theta_n, \epsilon_n, \epsilon))$ with $Q_{Y|A,W}(O; \theta, \epsilon', \epsilon)$ equal to the right-hand side of (29.8), where one substitutes $\bar{Q}(A, W; \theta, \epsilon')$ for $\bar{Q}(A, W; \theta)$. In addition, suppose that one then defines the weighted maximum likelihood ϵ_n' as the right-hand side of (29.9), where one substitutes $Q_{Y|A,W}(O_i; \theta_n, \epsilon_n, \epsilon)$ for $Q_{Y|A,W}(O_i; \theta_n, \epsilon)$. Then it follows that $\epsilon_n' = 0$ so that the "updated" $Q_n^*(\epsilon_n') = Q_n^*$. The updated estimator Q_n^* of Q_0 maps into the TMLE $\psi_n^* = \Psi(Q_n^*)$ of the risk difference $\psi_0 = \Psi(Q_0)$:

$$\psi_n^* = \frac{1}{n}\sum_{i=1}^{n} \bar{Q}(1, W_i; \theta_n, \epsilon_n) - \bar{Q}(0, W_i; \theta_n, \epsilon_n). \tag{29.10}$$

The asymptotics of ψ_n^* relies on a central limit theorem for (θ_n, ϵ_n), which we discuss in Sect. 29.5.

29.5 Asymptotics

We now state and comment on a consistency result for the stacked estimator (θ_n, ϵ_n), which complements Proposition 29.2 (see Theorem 8 in van der Laan 2008b). For simplicity, let us generalize the notation $\ell_{\theta,0}$ introduced in Sect. 29.4.1 by setting, for all $(\theta, \epsilon) \in \Theta \times \mathcal{E}, \ell_{\theta,\epsilon} = \log Q_{Y|A,W}(\cdot; \theta, \epsilon)$. Moreover, let us set, for all $(\theta, \epsilon) \in \Theta \times \mathcal{E}$: $Q_{\theta,\epsilon} = (Q_W(\cdot; P_0), Q_{Y|A,W}(\cdot; \theta, \epsilon))$.

Proposition 29.4. *Suppose that assumptions A1 and A2 from Proposition 29.2 hold. In addition, assume that:*

A3. *There exists a unique interior point $\epsilon_0 \in \mathcal{E}$ such that*

$$\epsilon_0 = \arg\max_{\epsilon \in \mathcal{E}} P_{Q_0,G^*(\theta_0)}\ell_{\theta_0,\epsilon}.$$

(1) It holds that $\Psi(Q_{\theta_0,\epsilon_0}) = \Psi(Q_0)$;
(2) Provided that O is a bounded set, (θ_n, ϵ_n) consistently estimates (θ_0, ϵ_0).

We already discussed the interpretation of the almost sure limit of θ_n in terms of the Kullback-Leibler projection. Likewise, the almost sure limit ϵ_0 of ϵ_n enjoys such an interpretation. Let us assume that $P_{Q_0,G^*(\theta_0)} \log Q_{Y|A,W}(\cdot; P_0)$ is well defined [this weak assumption concerns Q_0, not $G^*(\theta_0)$, and holds for instance when $|\log Q_{Y|A,W}(\cdot; P_0)|$ is bounded]. Then A3 is equivalent to $P_{Q_{\theta_0,\epsilon_0},G^*(\theta_0)}$ being the unique the Kullback–Leibler projection of $P_{Q_0,G^*(\theta_0)}$ onto the set $\{P \in \mathcal{M} : \exists \epsilon \in \mathcal{E}$ s.t. $Q(\cdot;P) = Q_{\theta_0,\epsilon}$ and $g(\cdot \mid \cdot; P) = G^*(\theta_0)\}$.

Of course, the most striking property that ϵ_0 enjoys is (1): Even if $\bar{Q}_0 \notin \{\bar{Q}(\cdot;\theta,\epsilon) : (\theta,\epsilon) \in \Theta \times \mathcal{E}\}$, it holds that $\Psi(Q_{\theta_0,\epsilon_0}) = \Psi(Q_0)$. This remarkable equality and the convergence of (θ_n, ϵ_n) to (θ_0, ϵ_0) are evidently the keys to the consistency of $\psi_n^* = \Psi(Q_n^*)$. We will also investigate how the consistency result stated in Proposition 29.4 translates into the consistency of the TMLE.

The proof of (1) in Proposition 29.4 is very simple and typical of robust statistical studies. Indeed, $0 = P_{Q_0,G^*(\theta_0)} \frac{\partial}{\partial \epsilon} \ell_{\theta_0,\epsilon}|_{\epsilon=\epsilon_0}$, while the latter expression simplifies as follows:

$$
\begin{aligned}
&E_{Q_0,G^*(\theta_0)}\left(\frac{2A-1}{G^*(\theta_0)(A \mid V)}(Y - \bar{Q}(A,W;\theta_0,\epsilon_0))\right)\\
&\quad = E_{Q_0,G^*(\theta_0)}\Big((\bar{Q}_0(1,W) - \bar{Q}(1,W;\theta_0,\epsilon_0)) - (\bar{Q}_0(0,W) - \bar{Q}(0,W;\theta_0,\epsilon_0))\Big)\\
&\quad = \Psi(Q_0) - \Psi(Q_{\theta_0.\epsilon_0}).
\end{aligned}
$$

This proves (1).

The proof of (2) in Proposition 29.4 fundamentally relies on the fact that (θ_n, ϵ_n) solves the martingale estimating equation $\sum_{i=1}^n D(\theta,\epsilon)(O_i, Z_i) = 0$, where

$$
D(\theta,\epsilon)(O,Z) = \frac{1}{g_Z(A \mid V)}\left(\dot{\ell}_{\theta,0}^{\top}(O) g^r(A \mid V), \frac{\partial}{\partial \epsilon}\ell_{\theta,\epsilon}(O) G^*(\theta)(A \mid V)\right)^{\top} \tag{29.11}
$$

satisfies $P_{Q_0,g_i^*} D(\theta_0, \epsilon_0) = 0$ for all $i \le n$. We have that

$$
D(\theta,\epsilon)(O,Z) = \left(D_1(\theta)^{\top}(O), \frac{\frac{\partial}{\partial \epsilon}\ell_{\theta,\epsilon}(O) G^*(\theta)(A \mid V)}{g_Z(A \mid V)}\right)^{\top}
$$

is an extension of $D_1(\theta)(O)$, which we introduced earlier when summarizing the proof of Proposition 29.2. Here, too, the proof involves the Kolmogorov strong law of large numbers for martingales (Chambaz and van der Laan 2010, Theorem 8), which yields that $n^{-1} \sum_{i=1}^n P_{Q_0,g_i^*} D(\theta_n, \epsilon_n)$ converges to zero almost surely. This results in the convergence in probability of (θ_n, ϵ_n) to (θ_0, ϵ_0) by a Taylor expansion of $(\theta, \epsilon) \mapsto (P_{Q_0,g^r} \dot{\ell}_{\theta,0}^{\top}, P_{Q_0,G^*(\theta)} \frac{\partial}{\partial \epsilon}\ell_{\theta,\epsilon})$ at (θ_0, ϵ_0). Note that assumption A3 is a clear counterpart of assumption A1 from Proposition 29.2 but that there is no counterpart of assumption A2 from Proposition 29.2 in Proposition 29.4. Indeed, it automatically holds in the framework of the proposition that $-P_{Q_0,G^*(\theta_0)} \frac{\partial^2}{\partial \epsilon^2}\ell_{\theta_0,\epsilon_0} > 0$, while the proof requires that the latter quantity be different from zero.

We now state and comment on a central limit theorem for the stacked estimator (θ_n, ϵ_n) (van der Laan 2008b, Theorem 9). Let us introduce, for all $(\theta, \epsilon) \in \Theta \times \mathcal{E}$,

$$
\widetilde{D}(\theta,\epsilon)(O) = (\dot{\ell}_{\theta,0}(O) g^r(A \mid V), \tfrac{\partial}{\partial \epsilon}\ell_{\theta,\epsilon}(O) G^*(\theta)(A \mid V)),
$$

so that $D(\theta,\epsilon)(O,Z)$, defined in (29.11), can be represented as $\widetilde{D}(\theta,\epsilon)(O)/g_Z(A \mid V)$.

Proposition 29.5. *Suppose that assumptions A1, A2 and A3 from Propositions 29.2 and 29.4 hold. In addition, assume that:*

A4. *Under Q_0, the outcome Y is not a deterministic function of (A, W).*

Then the following asymptotic linear expansion holds:

$$\sqrt{n}\,((\theta_n, \epsilon_n) - (\theta_0, \epsilon_0)) = S_0^{-1} \frac{1}{\sqrt{n}} \sum_{i=1}^{n} D(\theta_0, \epsilon_0)(O_i, Z_i) + o_P(1), \tag{29.12}$$

where

$$S_0 = E_{Q_0,G^*(\theta_0)} \begin{pmatrix} \ddot{\ell}_{\theta_0,0}(O) \frac{g^r(A|V)}{G^*(\theta_0)(A|V)} & 0 \\ \left[\frac{\partial^2}{\partial\theta\partial\epsilon} \ell_{\theta,\epsilon}(O) G^*(\theta)(A \mid V)\right]\Big|_{(\theta,\epsilon)=(\theta_0,\epsilon_0)}^{\top} \frac{1}{G^*(\theta_0)(A|V)} & \frac{\partial^2}{\partial\epsilon^2} \ell_{\theta_0,\epsilon}(O)|_{\epsilon=\epsilon_0} \end{pmatrix}$$

is an invertible matrix. Furthermore, (29.12) entails that $\sqrt{n}((\theta_n, \epsilon_n) - (\theta_0, \epsilon_0))$ converges in distribution to the centered Gaussian distribution with covariance matrix $S_0^{-1}\Sigma_0(S_0^{-1})^{\top}$, where

$$\Sigma_0 = E_{Q_0,G^*(\theta_0)} \left(\frac{\widetilde{D}(\theta_0, \epsilon_0)\widetilde{D}(\theta_0, \epsilon_0)^{\top}(O)}{G^*(\theta_0)(A \mid V)^2} \right)$$

is a positive definite symmetric matrix. Moreover, S_0 is consistently estimated by

$$S_n = \frac{1}{n} \sum_{i=1}^{n} \begin{pmatrix} \ddot{\ell}_{\theta_n,0}(O_i) \frac{g^r(A_i|V_i)}{g_{Z_i}(A_i|V_i)} & 0 \\ \left[\frac{\partial^2}{\partial\theta\partial\epsilon} \ell_{\theta,\epsilon}(O_i) G^*(\theta)(A_i \mid V_i)\right]\Big|_{(\theta,\epsilon)=(\theta_n,\epsilon_n)}^{\top} \frac{1}{g_{Z_i}(A_i|V_i)} & \frac{\partial^2}{\partial\epsilon^2} \ell_{\theta_n,\epsilon}(O_i)|_{\epsilon=\epsilon_n} g_{Z_i}(A_i \mid V_i) \end{pmatrix},$$

and Σ_0 is consistently estimated by

$$\Sigma_n = \frac{1}{n} \sum_{i=1}^{n} D(\theta_n, \epsilon_n) D(\theta_n, \epsilon_n)^{\top}(O_i, Z_i).$$

We will investigate how the above central limit theorem translates into a central limit theorem for the TMLE. The proof of Proposition 29.5 still relies on the fact that (θ_n, ϵ_n) solves the martingale estimating equation $\sum_{i=1}^{n} D(\theta, \epsilon)(O_i, Z_i) = 0$. It involves the Taylor expansion of $D(\theta, \epsilon)(O, Z)$ at (θ_0, ϵ_0), a multidimensional central limit theorem for martingales and again the Kolmogorov strong law of large numbers (Chambaz and van der Laan 2010, Theorems 8 and 10) . Assumption A4 guarantees that Σ_0 is positive definite.

TMLE is consistent and asymptotically Gaussian. In the first place, the TMLE ψ_n^* is robust: It is a consistent estimator even when the working model is misspecified.

Proposition 29.6. *Suppose that assumptions A1, A2, and A3 from Propositions 29.2 and 29.4 hold. Then the TMLE ψ_n^* consistently estimates the risk difference ψ_0.*

If the design of the RCT was fixed (and, consequently, the n first observations were i.i.d.), then the TMLE would be a robust estimator of ψ_0: Even if the working model is misspecified, then the TMLE still consistently estimates ψ_0 because the treatment mechanism is known (or can be consistently estimated, if one wants to gain in efficiency). Thus, the robustness of the TMLE stated in Proposition 29.6 is the *expected* counterpart of the TMLE's robustness in the latter i.i.d. setting: *Expected* because the TMLE solves a martingale estimating function that is unbiased for ψ_0 at misspecified Q and correctly specified g_i, $i = 1, \ldots, n$.

The proof of Proposition 29.6 is twofold and will now be described. Setting $Q_n^{\sim} = (Q_W(\cdot; P_0), Q_{Y|A,W}(\cdot; \theta_n, \epsilon_n))$, a continuity argument, and the convergence in probability of the stacked estimator (θ_n, ϵ_n) to (θ_0, ϵ_0) entail the convergence in probability of $\Psi(Q_n^{\sim})$ to $\Psi(Q_{\theta_0,\epsilon_0}) = \psi_0$ [see (1) in Proposition 29.4]. The conclusion follows because $\psi_n^* - \Psi(Q_n^{\sim})$ converges almost surely to zero by the Glivenko–Cantelli theorem [which, roughly speaking, guarantees that $P_n f$ converges almost surely to $P_0 f$ uniformly in $f \in \mathcal{F} = \{\bar{Q}(1, \cdot; \theta, \epsilon) - \bar{Q}(0, \cdot; \theta, \epsilon) : (\theta, \epsilon) \in \Theta \times \mathcal{E}\}$ because the set $\mathcal{F}$ is moderately complex].

The TMLE ψ_n^* is also asymptotically linear and therefore satisfies a central limit theorem. To see this, let us introduce the real-valued function ϕ on $\Theta \times \mathcal{E}$ such that $\phi(\theta, \epsilon) = \Psi(Q_{\theta,\epsilon})$. Because function ϕ is differentiable on the interior of $\Theta \times \mathcal{E}$, we denote its gradient at (θ, ϵ) with $\phi'_{\theta,\epsilon}$. The latter gradient satisfies

$$\phi'_{\theta,\epsilon} = E_{Q_{\theta,\epsilon},G^*(\theta)} \left\{ D^*(O; P_{Q_{\theta,\epsilon},G^*(\theta)}) \left(\tfrac{\partial}{\partial \theta} \ell^\top_{\theta,\epsilon}(O), \tfrac{\partial}{\partial \epsilon} \ell_{\theta,\epsilon}(O) \right)^\top \right\}.$$

Note that the right-hand-side expression cannot be computed explicitly because the marginal distribution $Q_W(\cdot; P_0)$ is unknown. By the law of large numbers (independent case), we can build an estimator ϕ'_n of $\phi'_{\theta_0,\epsilon_0}$ as follows. For B a large number (say $B = 10^4$), simulate B independent copies $\tilde{O}_b$ of O from the data-generating distribution $P_{Q_n^{\sim},G^*(\theta_n)}$, and compute

$$\phi'_n = \frac{1}{B} \sum_{b=1}^{B} D^*(O_b; P_{Q_n^{\sim},G^*(\theta_n)}) \left(\tfrac{\partial}{\partial \theta} \ell^\top_{\theta,\epsilon_n}(O_b)|_{\theta=\theta_n}, \tfrac{\partial}{\partial \epsilon} \ell_{\theta_n,\epsilon}(O_b)|_{\epsilon=\epsilon_n} \right)^\top.$$

Proposition 29.7. *Suppose that assumptions A1, A2, A3, and A4 from Propositions 29.2, 29.4, and 29.5 hold. Then the following asymptotic linear expansion holds:*

$$\sqrt{n}(\psi_n^* - \psi_0) = \frac{1}{\sqrt{n}} \sum_{i=1}^{n} \mathrm{IC}(O_i, Z_i) + o_P(1), \tag{29.13}$$

where

$$\mathrm{IC}(O, Z) = D_1^*(W; Q_{\theta_0,\epsilon_0}) + \phi'^\top_{\theta_0,\epsilon_0} S_0^{-1} D(\theta_0, \epsilon_0)(O, Z). \tag{29.14}$$

Furthermore, (29.13) entails that $\sqrt{n}(\psi_n^* - \psi_0)$ converges in distribution to the centered Gaussian distribution with a variance consistently estimated by

$$s_n^2 = \frac{1}{n}\sum_{i=1}^{n} D_1^*(W_i; Q_n^*)^2$$

$$+\frac{2}{n}\sum_{i=1}^{n} D_1^*(W_i; Q_n^*)\phi_n'^{\top} S_n^{-1} D(\theta_n, \epsilon_n)(O_i, Z_i) + (\phi_n'^{\top} S_n^{-1})\Sigma_n(\phi_n'^{\top} S_n^{-1})^{\top}.$$

Proposition 29.7 is the backbone of the statistical analysis of adaptive group sequential RCTs as constructed in Sect. 29.4. In particular, denoting the $(1-\alpha)$-quantile of the standard normal distribution by $\xi_{1-\alpha}$, the proposition guarantees that the asymptotic level of the confidence interval

$$\left[\psi_n^* \pm \frac{s_n}{\sqrt{n}}\xi_{1-\alpha/2}\right], \tag{29.15}$$

for the risk difference ψ_0 is $(1-\alpha)$.

The proof of (29.13) relies again on writing $\sqrt{n}(\psi_n^* - \psi_0) = \sqrt{n}(\psi_n^* - \Psi(Q_n^{\sim})) + \sqrt{n}(\Psi(Q_n^{\sim}) - \psi_0)$. It is easy to derive the asymptotic linear expansion of the first term [the influence function is $D_1^*(\cdot; Q_{\theta_0,\epsilon_0})$]. Moreover, the delta method and (29.12) provides the asymptotic linear expansion of the second term. Thus, the influence function IC is known in closed form. A central limit theorem for martingales (Chambaz and van der Laan 2010, Theorem 9) applied to (29.13) yields the stated convergence and validates the use of s_n^2 as an estimator of the asymptotic variance.

Extensions. We *conjecture* that the influence function IC computed at (O, Z), (29.14), is equal to

$$D_1^*(W; Q_{\theta_0,\epsilon_0}) + D_2^*(O; P_{Q_{\theta_0,\epsilon_0}, G^*(\theta_0)})\frac{G^*(\theta_0)(A \mid V)}{g_Z(A \mid V)}.$$

This conjecture is backed by the simulations that we carry out and present in Sect. 29.6. We will tackle the proof of the conjecture in future work. Let us assume for the moment that the conjecture is true. Then the asymptotic linear expansion (29.13) now implies that the asymptotic variance of $\sqrt{n}(\psi_n^* - \psi_0)$ can be consistently estimated by

$$s_n^{*2} = \frac{1}{n}\sum_{i=1}^{n}\left(D_1^*(W_i; Q_n^*) + D_2^*(O_i; P_{Q_n^*, G^*(\theta_n)})\frac{G^*(\theta_n)(A_i \mid V_i)}{g_{Z_i}(A_i \mid V_i)}\right)^2,$$

another independent argument showing that s_n^{*2} converges toward

$$\mathrm{var}_{Q_0, G^*(\theta_0)} D^*(O; P_{Q_{\theta_0,\epsilon_0}, G^*(\theta_0)}),$$

i.e., the variance under the fixed design $P_{Q_0, G^*(\theta_0)}$ of the efficient influence curve at $P_{Q_{\theta_0,\epsilon_0}, G^*(\theta_0)}$.

Furthermore, the most essential characteristic of the joint methodologies of design adaptation and TMLE is certainly the utmost importance of the role played by the *likelihood*. The targeted maximized log-likelihood of the data

$$\sum_{i=1}^{n} \left(\log Q_W(W_i; P_n) + \log Q_{Y|A,W}(O_i; \theta_n, \epsilon_n)\right),$$

provides us with a quantitative measure of the quality of the fit of the TLME of Q_0 (targeted toward the parameter of interest). It is therefore possible, for example, to use that quantity for the sake of selection among different working models for Q_0. As with TMLE for i.i.d. data, we can use likelihood-based cross-validation to select among more general initial estimators indexed by fine-tuning parameters. The validity of such TMLEs for the group sequential adaptive designs as studied in this chapter is outside the scope of this chapter.

29.6 Simulations

We characterize the component $Q_0 = Q(\cdot; P_0)$ of the true distribution P_0 of the data structure $O = (W, A, Y)$ as follows. The baseline covariate $W = (U, V)$ where U is uniformly distributed over the unit interval $[0, 1]$, and the subgroup membership covariate $V \in \mathcal{V} = \{1, 2, 3\}$ (hence $\nu = 3$) satisfies $P_0(V = 1) = 1/2, P_0(V = 2) = 1/3$, and $P_0(V = 3) = 1/6$. The conditional distribution of Y given (A, W) is the gamma distribution characterized by the conditional mean $\bar{Q}_0(Y \mid A, W) = 2U^2 + 2U + 1 + AV + (1 - A)/(1 + V)$ and the conditional standard deviation $\sqrt{\mathrm{var}_{P_0}(Y \mid A, W)} = U + A(1 + V) + (1 - A)/(1 + V)$. The risk difference $\psi_0 = \Psi(Q_0)$, our parameter of interest, is known in closed form $\psi_0 = 91/72 \simeq 1.264$, as is the variance: $v^b(Q_0) = \mathrm{var}_{Q_0,g^b} D^*(O; P_{Q_0,g^b})$ of the efficient influence curve under balanced sampling. The numerical value of $v^b(Q_0)$ is reported in Table 29.1.

We target the design that (a) depends on the baseline covariate $W = (U, V)$ only through V (i.e., belongs to $\mathcal{G}_1$) and (b) minimizes the variance of the efficient influence curve of the parameter of interest Ψ. The latter treatment mechanism $g^*(Q_0)$ and optimal efficient asymptotic variance $v^*(Q_0) = \mathrm{var}_{Q_0,g^*(Q_0)} D^*(O; P_{Q_0,g^*(Q_0)})$ are also known in closed form, and numerical values are reported in Table 29.1.

Table 29.1 Numerical values of the allocation probabilities and variance of the efficient influence curve. The ratio of the variances of the efficient influence curve under targeted optimal and balanced sampling schemes satisfies $R(Q_0) = v^*(Q_0)/v^b(Q_0) \simeq 0.762$

Sampling scheme (Q_0, g)	Allocation probabilities			Variance
	$g(1 \mid v = 1)$	$g(1 \mid v = 2)$	$g(1 \mid v = 3)$	$\mathrm{var}_{Q_0,g} D^*(O; P_{Q_0,g})$
(Q_0, g^b)-balanced	1/2	1/2	1/2	23.864
$(Q_0, g^*(Q_0))$-optimal	0.707	0.799	0.849	18.181

Let $n = (100, 250, 500, 750, 1000, 2500, 5000)$ be a sequence of sample sizes. We estimate $M = 1000$ times the risk difference $\psi_0 = \Psi(Q_0)$ based on $\mathbf{O}_{n_7}^m(n_i)$, $m = 1, \ldots, M$, $i = 1, \ldots, 7$, under i.i.d. (Q_0, g^b)-balanced sampling, i.i.d. $(Q_0, g^*(Q_0))$-optimal sampling, and $(Q_0, \mathbf{g}_{n_7}^*)$-adaptive sampling. Finally, we emphasize that the data structure $O = (W, A, Y)$ is not bounded, whereas O is assumed bounded in Propositions 29.2–29.7.

For each $v \in \mathcal{V}$, let us denote $\theta(v) = (\beta_v, \sigma_v^2(0), \sigma_v^2(1))^\top \in \Theta_v$, where $\Theta_v \subset \mathbb{R}^3 \times \mathbb{R}_+^* \times \mathbb{R}_+^*$ is compact, and $\beta_v = (\beta_{v,1}, \beta_{v,2}, \beta_{v,3})$ [$b = 3$ in (29.5)] is the vector of regression coefficients. Let $\theta = (\theta_1^\top, \theta_2^\top, \theta_3^\top)^\top \in \Theta = \Theta_1 \times \Theta_2 \times \Theta_3$. Following the description in Sect. 29.4.1, the working model Q_n^w that the TMLE methodology relieson is characterized by the conditional likelihood of Y given (A, W):

$$Q_{Y|A,W}(O; \theta) = \frac{1}{\sqrt{2\pi\sigma_V^2(A)}} \exp\left\{-\frac{(Y - m(A, W; \beta_V))^2}{2\sigma_V^2(A)}\right\},$$

where the conditional mean $\bar{Q}(Y; A, W; \theta)$ of Y given (A, W) is modeled as

$$\bar{Q}(Y; A = a, W = w; \theta) = m(a, w; \beta_v) = \beta_{v,1} + \beta_{v,2}u + \beta_{v,3}a,$$

for all $a \in \mathcal{A}$ and $w = (u, v) \in \mathcal{W} = \mathbb{R} \times \mathcal{V}$. As required, the parameterization condition is met. Obviously, the working model is heavily misspecified: a Gaussian conditional likelihood is used instead of a gamma conditional likelihood, and the parametric forms of the conditional expectation and variance are wrong, too.

Regarding the choice of a reference fixed design $g^r \in \mathcal{G}_1$ (Sect. 29.4.1), we select $g^r = g^b$, the balanced design. The parameter θ_0 only depends on Q_0 and the working model, but its estimator θ_n depends on g^r, which may negatively affect its performance. Therefore, we propose to dilute the impact of the choice of g^r as an initial reference design as follows. For a given sample size n, we first compute a first estimate θ_n^1 of θ_0 as in (29.6) but with $\lceil n/4 \rceil$ (the smallest integer not smaller than $n/4$) substituted for n in the sum. Then θ_n is computed as in (29.6), but this time with $G^*(\theta_n^1)(A_i|V_i)$ substituted for $g^r(A_i|V_i)$. The proofs can be adapted to incorporate this modification of the procedure. We refer the interested reader to van der Laan (2008b, Section 8.5).

We update the design each time $c = 25$ new observations are sampled. In addition, the first update only occurs when there are at least 5 completed observations in each treatment arm and for all V-strata. Thus, the minimal sample size at the first update is 30, and it can be shown that, under the balanced design, the expected sample size at the first sample size at which there are at least 5 observations in each arm equals 75. Finally, as a precautionary measure, we systematically apply a thresholding to the updated treatment mechanism: Using the notation of Sect. 29.4, we substitute $\max\{\delta, \min\{1 - \delta, g_i^*(A_i \mid V_i)\}\}$ to $g_i^*(A_i \mid V_i)$ in all computations. We arbitrarily choose $\delta = 0.01$.

We now invoke the central limit theorem stated in Proposition 29.7 to construct confidence intervals for the risk difference. Let us introduce, for all types of sampling and each sample size n_i, the confidence intervals

$$\mathcal{I}_{n_i,m} = \left[\psi^*_{n_i}(\mathbf{O}^m_{n_7}(n_i)) \pm \sqrt{\frac{v_{n_i}(\mathbf{O}^m_{n_7}(n_i))}{n_i}}\xi_{1-\alpha/2}\right], \quad m = 1,\ldots,M,$$

where the definition of the variance estimator $v_n(\mathbf{O}^m_{n_7}(n))$ based on the n first observations $\mathbf{O}^m_{n_7}(n)$ depends on the sampling scheme. Under i.i.d. (Q_0, g^b)-balanced sampling, $v_n(\mathbf{O}^m_{n_7}(n))$ is the estimator of the asymptotic variance of the TMLE $\Psi(Q^*_{n,\text{iid}})$:

$$v_n(\mathbf{O}^m_{n_7}(n)) = \frac{1}{n}\sum_{i=1}^{n} D^*(O^m_i; P_{Q^*_{n,\text{iid}},g^b})^2. \tag{29.16}$$

Under i.i.d. $(Q_0, g^*(Q_0))$-optimal sampling, $v_n(\mathbf{O}^m_{n_7}(n))$ is defined as in (29.16), replacing g^b with $g^*(Q_0)$. Lastly, under $(Q_0, \mathbf{g}^*_n)$-adaptive sampling, $v_n(\mathbf{O}^m_{n_7}(n)) = s^{*2}_n(\mathbf{O}^m_{n_7}(n))$, the estimator of the conjectured asymptotic variance of $\sqrt{n}(\psi^*_n(\mathbf{O}^m_{n_7}(n)) - \psi_0)$ computed on the n first observations $\mathbf{O}^m_{n_7}(n)$. We are interested in the empirical coverage (reported in Table 29.2, top rows) $c_{n_i} = 1/M\sum_{m=1}^{M} I(\psi_0 \in \mathcal{I}_{n_i,m})$ guaranteed for each sampling scheme and every $i = 1,\ldots,7$ by $\{\mathcal{I}_{n_i,m} : m = 1,\ldots,M\}$. The rescaled empirical coverage proportions Mc_{n_i} should have a binomial distribution with parameter $(M, 1-a)$ and $a = \alpha$ for every $i = 1,\ldots,7$. This property can be tested in terms of a standard binomial test, the alternative hypothesis stating that $a > \alpha$. This results in a collection of seven p-values for each sampling scheme, as reported in Table 29.2 (bottom rows).

Considering each sampling scheme (i.e., each row of Table 29.2) separately, we conclude that the $(1-\alpha)$-coverage cannot be declared defective under i.i.d. (Q_0, g^b)-balanced sampling for any sample size $n_i \geq n_3 = 500$, i.i.d. $(Q_0, g^*(Q_0))$-optimal sampling for any sample size $n_i \geq n_2 = 250$, and $(Q_0, \mathbf{g}^*_{n_7})$-adaptive sampling for any sample size $n_i \geq n_1 = 100$, adjusting for multiple testing in terms of the Benjamini–Yekutieli procedure for controlling the false discovery rate at level 5%.

This is a remarkable result that not only validates the theory but also provides us with insight into the finite sample properties of the TMLE procedure based on adaptive sampling. The fact that the TMLE procedure behaves better under an adaptive sampling scheme than under balanced i.i.d. sampling scheme at sample size $n_1 = 100$ may not be due to mere chance only. Although the TMLE procedure based

Table 29.2 Checking the validity of the coverage of our simulated confidence intervals, values c_{n_i} (top row), p-values (bottom row, between parentheses)

Sampling scheme	Sample size						
	n_1	n_2	n_3	n_4	n_5	n_6	n_7
i.i.d. (Q_0, g^b)-balanced	0.913	0.925	0.939	0.934	0.945	0.940	0.946
	$(p < 0.001)$	$(p < 0.001)$	(0.067)	(0.015)	(0.253)	(0.087)	(0.300)
i.i.d. $(Q_0, g^*(Q_0))$-optimal	0.894	0.941	0.940	0.953	0.954	0.947	0.947
	$(p < 0.001)$	(0.111)	(0.087)	(0.688)	(0.739)	(0.351)	(0.351)
adaptive $(Q_0, \mathbf{g}^*_{n_7})$	0.934	0.939	0.956	0.945	0.943	0.933	0.952
	(0.015)	(0.067)	(0.827)	(0.253)	(0.172)	(0.011)	(0.634)

on an adaptive sampling scheme is initiated under the balanced sampling scheme (so that each stratum consists at the beginning of comparable numbers of patients assigned to each treatment arm, allowing one to estimate, at least roughly, the required parameters), it starts deviating from it [as soon as every (A, V)-stratum counts 5 patients)] each time 25 new observations are accrued. The poor performance of the TMLE procedure based on an optimal i.i.d. sampling scheme at sample size n_1 is certainly due to the fact that, by starting directly from the optimal sampling scheme (a choice we would not recommend in practice), too few patients from stratum $V = 3$ are assigned to treatment arm $A = 0$ among the n_1 first subjects. At larger sample sizes, the TMLE procedure performs equally well under an adaptive sampling scheme and under both i.i.d. schemes in terms of coverage.

Now that we know that the TMLE-based confidence intervals based on $(Q_0, \mathbf{g}_n^*)$-adaptive sampling are valid confidence regions, it is of interest to compare the widths of the latter adaptive-sampling $(Q_0, \mathbf{g}_n^*)$-confidence intervals with their counterparts obtained under i.i.d. (Q_0, g^b)-balanced or $(Q_0, g^*(Q_0))$ optimal sampling schemes. For this purpose, we compare, for each sample size n_i, the empirical distribution of $\{\sqrt{v_n(\mathbf{O}_{n_7}^m(n_i))} : m = 1, \ldots, M\}$ as in (29.16) [i.e., the empirical distribution of width of the TMLE-based confidence intervals at sample size n_i obtained under i.i.d (Q_0, g^b)-balanced sampling, up to the factor $2\xi_{1-\alpha/2}/\sqrt{n_i}$] to the empirical distribution of $\{s_n^*(\mathbf{O}_{n_7}^m(n_i)) : m = 1, \ldots, M\}$ [i.e., the empirical distribution of the width of the TMLE-based confidence intervals at sample size n_i obtained under $(Q_0, \mathbf{g}_n^*)$-adaptive sampling, up to the factor $2\xi_{1-\alpha/2}/\sqrt{n_i}$] in terms of the two-sample Kolmogorov–Smirnov test, where the alternative states that the confidence intervals obtained under adaptive sampling are stochastically smaller than their counterparts under i.i.d. balanced sampling. This results in seven p-values, all equal to zero, which we nonetheless report in Table 29.3 (bottom row). In order to get a sense of how much narrower the confidence intervals obtained under adaptive sampling are, we also compute and report in Table 29.3 (top row) the ratios of empirical average widths:

$$\frac{\frac{1}{M}\sum_{m=1}^{M} s_n^*(\mathbf{O}_{n_7}^m(n_i))}{\frac{1}{M}\sum_{m=1}^{M} \sqrt{v_n(\mathbf{O}_{n_7}^m(n_i))}}, \tag{29.17}$$

for each sample size n_i. Informally, this shows a 12% gain in width.

On the other hand, we also compare, for each sample size n_i, the empirical distribution of $\{\sqrt{v_n(\mathbf{O}_{n_7}^m(n_i))} : m = 1, \ldots, M\}$, as in (29.16), but replacing g^b by $g^*(Q_0)$ [i.e., the empirical distribution of width of the TMLE-based confidence intervals at sample size n_i obtained under i.i.d. $(Q_0, g^*(Q_0))$-optimal sampling, up to the factor $2\xi_{1-\alpha/2}/\sqrt{n_i}$] to the empirical distribution of $\{s_n^*(\mathbf{O}_{n_7}^m(n_i)) : m = 1, \ldots, M\}$ [i.e., the empirical distribution of the width of the TMLE-based confidence intervals at sample size n_i obtained under $(Q_0, \mathbf{g}_n^*)$-adaptive sampling, up to the factor $2\xi_{1-\alpha/2}/\sqrt{n_i}$] in terms of the two-sample Kolmogorov–Smirnov test, the alternative stating that the confidence intervals obtained under adaptive sampling are stochastically larger than their counterparts under i.i.d. optimal sampling. This results in seven p-values that we report in Table 29.3 (bottom row). In order to get a sense of how similar the confidence intervals obtained under adaptive and i.i.d. optimal sampling schemes

Table 29.3 Comparing the width of our confidence intervals with the ratios of average widths as defined in (29.17) and p-values (bottom rows, between parentheses)

Comparison	Sample size						
	n_1	n_2	n_3	n_4	n_5	n_6	n_7
$(Q_0, \mathbf{g}^*_{n_7})$ vs. (Q_0, g^b)	0.856	0.871	0.879	0.880	0.878	0.877	0.876
	(0)	(0)	(0)	(0)	(0)	(0)	(0)
$(Q_0, \mathbf{g}^*_{n_7})$ vs. $(Q_0, g^*(Q_0))$	0.962	0.977	0.992	0.995	0.997	1.000	1.000
	(0.144)	(0.236)	(0.100)	(0.060)	(0.407)	(0.236)	(0.144)

are, we also compute and report for each sample size n_i in Table 29.3 (top row) the ratios of empirical average widths as in (29.17) replacing again g^b by $g^*(Q_0)$ in the definition (29.16) of $v_n(\mathbf{O}^m_{n_7}(n))$. Informally, this shows that the confidence intervals obtained under adaptive sampling are even slightly narrower in average than their counterparts obtained under i.i.d. optimal sampling.

Illustration. So far we have been concerned with distributional results, and we now investigate a particular arbitrarily selected simulated trajectory of the TMLE, the confidence intervals, and the adaptive design g^*_n as a function of sample size. Some interesting features of the selected simulated trajectory are apparent in Fig. 29.2 and Table 29.4. For instance, we can follow the convergence of the TMLE ψ^*_n toward the true risk difference ψ_0 in the top plot of Fig. 29.2 and in the fifth column of Table 29.4. Similarly, the middle plot of Fig. 29.2 and the second to fourth columns of Table 29.4 illustrate the convergence of $\mathbf{g}^*_n$ toward $G^*(\theta_0)$, as stated in Proposition 29.3. What these plots and columns also teach us is that, in spite of the misspecified working model, the learned design $G^*(\theta_0)$ seems very close to the optimal treatment mechanism $g^*(Q_0)$ for the chosen simulation scheme and working model used in our simulation study. Moreover, the last column of Table 29.4 illustrates how the confidence intervals $[\psi^*_n \pm s^*_n \xi_{1-0.05/2}/\sqrt{n}]$ shrink around the true risk difference ψ_0 as the sample size increases.

Yet, the bottom plot of Fig. 29.2 may be the most interesting of the three. It obviously illustrates the convergence of s^{*2}_n toward $\mathrm{var}_{Q_0,G^*(\theta_0)} D^*(O; P_{Q_{\theta_0,\epsilon_0},G^*(\theta_0)})$, i.e., toward the variance under the fixed-design $P_{Q_0,G^*(\theta_0)}$ of the efficient influence curve at $P_{Q_{\theta_0,\epsilon_0},G^*(\theta_0)}$. Hence, it also teaches us that the latter limit seems very close to the optimal asymptotic variance $v^*(Q_0)$ for the chosen simulation scheme and working model used in our simulation study. *More importantly, s^{*2}_n strikingly converges to $v^*(Q_0)$ from below.* This finite sample characteristic may reflect the fact that the true finite sample variance of $\sqrt{n}(\psi^*_n - \psi_0)$ might be lower than $v^*(Q_0)$. Studying this issue in depth is certainly very delicate and goes beyond the scope of this chapter.

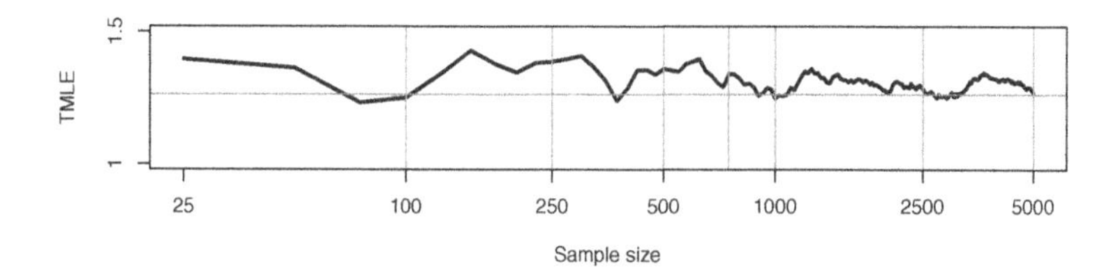

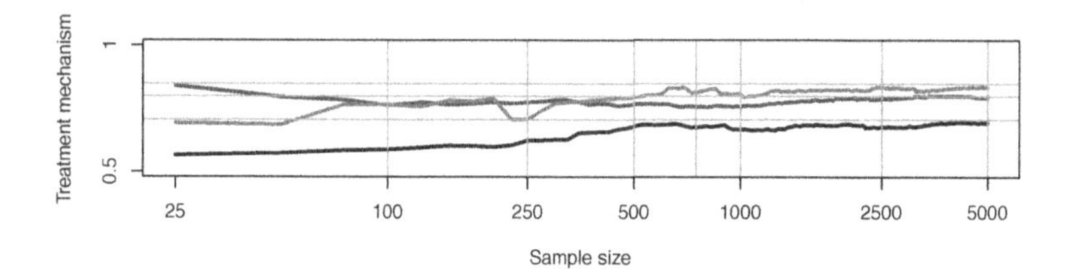

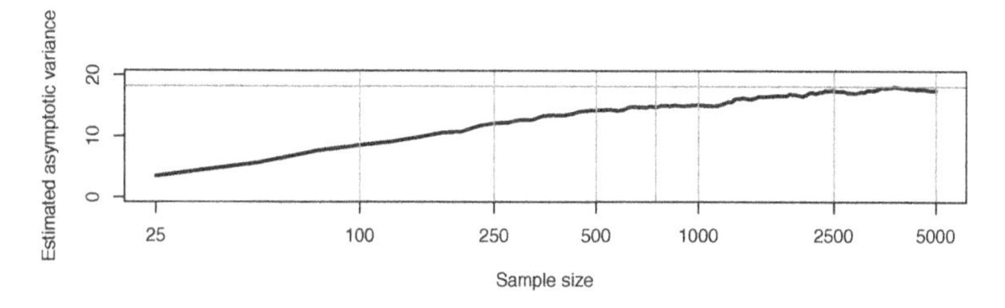

Fig. 29.2 Illustrating the TMLE procedure under $(Q_0, \mathbf{g}_n^*)$-adaptive sampling scheme. *Top plot*: The sequence $\psi_n^*(\mathbf{O}_{n_7}^1(n))$, *horizontal gray line* indicates true value of risk difference ψ_0. *Middle plot*: Three sequences $g_n^*(1 \mid 1) = G^*(\theta_n(\mathbf{O}_{n_7}^1(n)))(1 \mid 1)$ (*bottom curve*), $g_n^*(1 \mid 2) = G^*(\theta_n(\mathbf{O}_{n_7}^1(n)))(1 \mid 2)$ (*middle curve*), and $g_n^*(1 \mid 3) = G^*(\theta_n(\mathbf{O}_{n_7}^1(n)))(1 \mid 3)$ (*top curve*). The three *horizontal gray lines* indicate the optimal allocation probabilities $g^*(Q_0)(1 \mid 1)$ (*bottom line*), $g^*(Q_0)(1 \mid 2)$ (*middle line*), and $g^*(Q_0)(1 \mid 3)$ (*top line*). *Bottom plot*: The sequence s_n^{*2} of estimated asymptotic variance of $\sqrt{n}(\psi_n^* - \psi_0)$, *horizontal gray line* indicates the value of the optimal variance $v^*(Q_0)$. (The x-axis is on a logarithmic scale for all plots)

Table 29.4 Simulation results of the TMLE procedure under a $(Q_0, \mathbf{g}_n^*)$-adaptive sampling scheme

Sample size	Allocation probabilities			TMLE	confidence interval
n	$g_n^*(1 \mid 1)$	$g_n^*(1 \mid 2)$	$g_n^*(1 \mid 3)$	ψ_n^*	$(\psi_n^* \pm s_n^* \xi_{1-0.05/2}/\sqrt{n})$
n_1	0.589	0.764	0.766	1.252	(0.722,1.783)
n_2	0.624	0.775	0.707	1.388	(0.974,1.802)
n_3	0.679	0.767	0.795	1.361	(1.037,1.685)
n_4	0.677	0.757	0.813	1.341	(1.068,1.615)
n_5	0.670	0.760	0.806	1.250	(1.012,1.488)
n_6	0.677	0.788	0.835	1.288	(1.126,1.451)
n_7	0.694	0.793	0.834	1.273	(1.157,1.389)

Concluding Remarks

We developed the TMLE in group sequential adaptive designs for the data structure $O = (W, A, Y)$. This generalizes the TMLE for the i.i.d. design for this data structure O as covered in depth by the first part of this book. In addition, we showed that targeted learning goes beyond targeted estimation and starts with the choice of design. Our targeted adaptive designs combined with the TMLE provides a fully targeted methodology, including design, for statistical inference with respect to a causal effect of interest. In the previous two chapters, we demonstrated (1) how to fully integrate the state of the art in machine learning while fully preserving the CLT for statistical inference and (2) the application of TMLE for the purpose of obtaining a targeted posterior distribution of the target parameter of interest, thereby improving on the current standard in Bayesian learning.

This book demonstrated that targeted learning with TMLE represents a unified optimal approach for learning from data that can be represented as realizations of n i.i.d. random variables. However, these last three chapters provide insight into the enormous reach of targeted learning, covering Bayesian learning, integrating the most adaptive machine learning algorithms, targeted designs, and statistical inference for targeted adaptive designs that generate dependent data. Further exciting research in these areas is needed, but it appears that targeted learning based on super learning and TMLE provides a road map for developing optimal tools to attack upcoming statistical challenges.

Part X
Appendices

Appendix A
Foundations of TMLE

A.1 Asymptotic Linearity: The Functional Delta Method

Summary. An estimator of a parameter is a mapping from the data set to the parameter space. Estimators that are empirical means of a function of the unit data structure are asymptotically consistent and normally distributed due to the CLT. Such estimators are called linear in the empirical probability distribution. Most estimators are not linear, but many are approximately linear in the sense that they are linear up to a negligible (in probability) remainder term. One states that the estimator is asymptotically linear, and the relevant function of the unit data structure, centered to have mean zero, is called the influence curve of the estimator. How does one prove that an estimator is asymptotically linear? One key step is to realize that an estimator is a mapping from a possibly very large collection of empirical means of functions of the unit data structure into the parameter space. Such a collection of empirical means is called an empirical process whose behavior with respect to uniform consistency and the uniform CLT is established in empirical process theory. In this section we present succinctly that (1) a uniform central limit theorem for the vector of empirical means, combined with (2) differentiability of the estimator as a mapping from the vector of empirical means into the parameter space yields the desired asymptotic linearity. This method for establishing the asymptotic linearity and normality of the estimator is called the functional delta method (van der Vaart and Wellner 1996; Gill 1989).

Consider a sample of n i.i.d. observations $O_1, \ldots, O_n$ from a probability distribution P_0 that is known to be an element of a statistical model $\mathcal{M}$. Let $\Psi : \mathcal{M} \rightarrow \mathbb{R}^d$ be the parameter of interest, and let $\psi_0 = \Psi(P_0)$ be the true parameter value. We assume that the parameter Ψ is pathwise differentiable so that it is reasonable to assume asymptotically linear estimators of ψ_0 exist.

Let $\mathcal{M}_{NP}$ denote a nonparametric model that includes the empirical distribution P_n of $O_1, \ldots, O_n$. Let $\hat{\Psi} : \mathcal{M}_{NP} \rightarrow \mathbb{R}^d$ be an estimator of ψ_0 that maps the empirical distribution P_n of $O_1, \ldots, O_n$ into an estimate $\hat{\Psi}(P_n)$. First, we will assume that $\hat{\Psi}(P_0) = \psi_0$ so that the estimator targets the desired target parameter ψ_0. This estimator is asymptotically linear at P_0 if $\hat{\Psi}(P_n) - \hat{\Psi}(P_0) = (P_n - P_0)IC(P_0) + o_P(1/\sqrt{n})$ for some mean zero function $IC(P_0)$ of O: i.e., $P_0 IC(P_0) = 0$. This function $IC(P_0)$ of O is called the influence curve of the estimator $\hat{\Psi}$. Notice that $(P_n - P_0)IC(P_0) = \frac{1}{n}\sum_{i=1}^n IC(P_0)(O_i)$ is thus an empirical mean of mean zero i.i.d. random variables, so that the CLT immediately implies that this empirical mean is asymptotically normally distributed.

Instead of simply representing an estimator as a function of P_n, we need to be more specific by representing the estimator as a function of an empirical process $(P_n f : f \in \mathcal{F})$ for some class $\mathcal{F}$ of functions of O; that is, the estimator maps a "vector" of empirical means into the estimate. Some simple estimators, such as the sample variance, are only a function of a few empirical means, but most estimators are functions of an infinite collection of empirical means, such as whole cumulative empirical distribution functions. Similarly, $\psi_0 = \Psi(P_0 f : f \in \mathcal{F})$ is a function of the corresponding true means $P_0 = (P_0 f : f \in \mathcal{F})$. For example, in a nonparametric model $\mathcal{M}$ for a probability distribution P_0 of a multivariate Euclidean valued random variable O, ψ_0 might depend on $P_0 I(O \leq o)$ for each possible o. We will let P_0 denote the "vector" $(P_0 f : f \in \mathcal{F})$ and P_n will denote the "vector" $(P_n f : f \in \mathcal{F})$.

P_n and P_0 will be viewed as elements in a function space $\ell^\infty(\mathcal{F})$, where the latter space consists of all functions $G : \mathcal{F} \rightarrow \mathbb{R}$, endowed with the supremum norm $\|G\|_\infty = \sup_{f \in \mathcal{F}} \mid G(f) \mid$. This allows us to write $\hat{\Psi} : \ell^\infty(\mathcal{F}) \rightarrow \mathbb{R}^d$ and $\Psi : \ell^\infty(\mathcal{F}) \rightarrow \mathbb{R}^d$. With this framework in mind, we ask ourselves: Why would $\hat{\Psi}(P_n)$ be an asymptotically linear estimator of $\hat{\Psi}(P_0)$? To start with, why would $\hat{\Psi}(P_n)$ be a consistent estimator?

Formally, consistency is proven as follows. In the space $\ell^\infty(\mathcal{F})$, for a small enough class of functions $\mathcal{F}$, one has that $\|P_n - P_0\|_\infty = \sup_{f \in \mathcal{F}} \mid (P_n - P_0)f \mid$ converges to 0 in probability (as n converges to infinity). *Small enough* is measured by the entropy function of the class of functions, which is defined as the logarithm of the covering number $N(\epsilon, \mathcal{F}, \|\cdot\|)$ as a function of ϵ. The covering number $N(\epsilon, \mathcal{F}, \|\cdot\|)$ is defined as the number of balls/spheres of size ϵ, with respect to norm $\|\cdot\|$, one needs in order to cover this set $\mathcal{F}$. Specifically, if $\sup_Q N(\epsilon \|F\|_\infty, \mathcal{F}, L_1(Q)) < \infty$ for all $\epsilon > 0$ (supremum is taken over all probability measures Q), where the function $F = \sup_{f \in \mathcal{F}} f$ is called the envelope of this class $\mathcal{F}$ of functions, then $\|P_n - P_0\|_\infty$ converges to 0 in probability. Here $L_1(Q)$ is endowed with the norm $\|f\| = \int \mid f \mid dQ$. A class $\mathcal{F}$ that satisfies this entropy condition is called a Glivenko–Cantelli class of functions. Suppose now that $\hat{\Psi} : \ell^\infty(\mathcal{F}) \rightarrow \mathbb{R}^d$ is a continuous function at P_0: i.e., if a sequence P_n converges to P_0 in $\ell^\infty(\mathcal{F})$ (i.e., with respect to the supremum norm), then $\hat{\Psi}(P_n) \rightarrow \hat{\Psi}(P_0)$. This continuity property of the mapping $\hat{\Psi}$, and the stochastic convergence $\|P_n - P_0\|_\infty \rightarrow 0$ in probability, implies now that $\hat{\Psi}(P_n)$ converges to $\hat{\Psi}(P_0)$ in probability. This is implied by the continuous mapping theorem. That is, continuity of the estimator as a mapping and $\mathcal{F}$'s being a Glivenko–Cantelli class imply the consistency of the estimator. This typically represents the first important step proving that the estimator is also asymptotically linear, which is a stronger and much more useful statement than stating that the estimator is consistent.

For the purpose of proving asymptotic linearity, we view $G_n = \sqrt{n}(P_n - P_0)$ as a random variable in $\ell^\infty(\mathcal{F})$. In this space, for a small enough class of functions $\mathcal{F}$, one can prove that the probability distribution of G_n converges to the distribution of a Gaussian process G_0, where this Gaussian process is identified by the fact that for any finite set of functions $(f_j : j)$, $(G_0 f_j : j)$ has a multivariate normal distribution with covariances $\Sigma(f_k, f_l) = P_0(f_k - P_0 f_k)(f_l - P_0 f_l)$. Specifically, if $\int_0^\infty \sqrt{\sup_Q \log N(\epsilon, \mathcal{F}, L_2(Q))} d\epsilon < \infty$, then G_n converges in probability distribution to G_0 in $\ell^\infty(\mathcal{F})$, which is also called weak convergence and denoted by $G_n \Rightarrow_d G_0$. A class $\mathcal{F}$ for which $G_n \Rightarrow_d G_0$, such as a class satisfying this entropy condition, is called a P_0–Donsker class. Thus, whether or not $\mathcal{F}$ is a Donsker class is again determined by its entropy function. Establishing what classes of functions constitute a Donsker class is of utmost importance and is covered by empirical process theory. Beyond that the Donsker class property yields convergence of G_n to the Gaussian process G_0 in probability distribution; it also implies $\| P_n - P_0 \|_{\mathcal{F}} = O_P(1/\sqrt{n})$, and that, for any sequence $f_n \in \mathcal{F}$ so that $P_0 f_n^2 \to 0$ in probability, we have $(P_n - P_0) f_n = o_P(1/\sqrt{n})$. These types of properties are fundamental ingredients in any study of the asymptotic behavior of an estimator.

Suppose now that $\hat{\Psi} : \ell^\infty(\mathcal{F}) \to \mathbb{R}^d$ is a differentiable function at P_0. Specifically, for any sequence P_n (which can occur as a random realization of the actual empirical distribution P_n) satisfying that $\sqrt{n}(P_n - P_0) \to G_0$ in $\ell^\infty(\mathcal{F})$, we have $\sqrt{n}(\hat{\Psi}(P_n) - \hat{\Psi}(P_0)) \to \hat{\Psi}'(P_0)(G_0)$, where $\hat{\Psi}'(P_0)(G_0) = \sum_{f \in \mathcal{F}} \frac{d}{dP_0 f} \hat{\Psi}(P_0) G_0(f)$ is the directional derivative of $\hat{\Psi}$ at P_0 applied to direction G_0. Note that $\frac{d}{dP_0 f} \hat{\Psi}(P_0)$ is just the partial derivative of a function of a vector. This differentiability property of the mapping $\hat{\Psi}$ at P_0, and the stochastic convergence $G_n = \sqrt{n}(P_n - P_0) \Rightarrow_d G_0$ in distribution as random elements in $\ell^\infty(\mathcal{F})$, implies now that $\sqrt{n}(\hat{\Psi}(P_n) - \hat{\Psi}(P_0)) \Rightarrow_d \hat{\Psi}'(P_0)(G_0)$, i.e., it implies weak convergence of the standardized estimator to a d-variate normally distributed random variable $Z = \hat{\Psi}'(P_0)(G_0)$. This result is implied by the generalized continuous mapping theorem as presented in van der Vaart and Wellner (1996), applied to the functions $f_n(G_n) = \hat{\Psi}(P_0 + 1/\sqrt{n} G_n) - \hat{\Psi}(P_0)$ and its limit $f(G_0) = \hat{\Psi}'(P_0)(G_0)$. That is, an analytic differentiability property of the estimator as a mapping, and $\mathcal{F}$'s being a Donsker class imply the desired convergence in distribution of the (mean and variance-)standardized estimator to a Gaussian process. The differentiability condition and stochastic convergence of the standardized empirical process G_n, also implies

$$\sqrt{n}(\hat{\Psi}(P_n) - \hat{\Psi}(P_0)) = \hat{\Psi}'(P_0)(G_n) + o_P(1),$$

where, by linearity of the derivative $\hat{\Psi}'(P_0) : \ell^\infty(\mathcal{F}) \to \mathbb{R}^d$ and (linearity of)

$$G_n = \left(\frac{1}{\sqrt{n}} \sum_{i=1}^n f(O_i) - P_0 f : f \in \mathcal{F} \right),$$

we have

$$\hat{\Psi}'(P_0)(G_n) = \frac{1}{\sqrt{n}} \sum_{i=1}^{n} \hat{\Psi}'(P_0)(f(O_i) - P_0 f : f).$$

Thus, $\hat{\Psi}(P_n)$ is asymptotically linear with d-dimensional influence curve

$$IC(P_0)(O) = \hat{\Psi}'(P_0)(f(O) - P_0 f : f) = \sum_{f \in \mathcal{F}} \frac{d\hat{\Psi}(P_0)}{dP_0 f}(f(O) - P_0 f).$$

Clearly, serious mathematics/functional analysis is needed to formally prove that an estimator is asymptotically linear, but it is beautiful to see that some pure analytical properties of the estimator as a mapping, and stochastic properties of the empirical process as established in empirical process theory, translate into the desired consistency and convergence in probability distribution of the standardized estimator to a normal distribution, providing a firm basis for statistical inference. In addition, the mathematics also results in the influence curve of the estimator, which has great utility in robustness analysis and estimation of the asymptotic covariance matrix of the standardized estimator $\sqrt{n}(\psi_n - \psi_0)$.

A.2 Influence Curve of an Asymptotically Linear Estimator

Summary. The functional delta method also provides us with the influence curve of the estimator. The influence curve allows robustness analysis and provides an estimator of the variance of the estimator, and thereby construction of confidence intervals and tests of null hypotheses of interest. It is a function of the unit data structure, indexed by the true probability distribution. If the true probability distribution is such that the influence curve is a nicely bounded function, then the estimator will generally behave well. This insight allows one to inspect the influence curve for necessary practical assumptions in order to have a reliable and robust estimator, without the need to formally prove mathematical theorems. One can calculate the influence curve of an estimator without formally analyzing the estimator; the influence curve is expressed in terms of the derivative of the estimator viewed as a mapping from a vector of means into the parameter space. That is, the influence curve of the estimator is expressed as a linear combination of the influence curves of the empirical means that were inputted into the estimator.

Why are we interested in calculation of the influence curve of an estimator? Given the asymptotic linearity of the estimator, the influence curve allows one to identify observations O_i that have a disproportional effect on the estimator. It teaches us under what assumptions about P_0 the influence curve $IC(P_0)$ is a nicely bounded function of O (these will be required assumptions to claim asymptotic linearity), and its covariance matrix equals the asymptotic covariance matrix of the estimator, thereby providing confidence intervals and tests of null hypotheses of interest. This will be discussed in more detail below. In addition, if one has the influence curve

IC_j of an estimator ψ_{nj} of a parameter ψ_{0j}, for each $j = 1, \ldots, d$, then one also obtains the influence curve of a function $f(\psi_{nj} : j)$ as an estimator of $f(\psi_{0j} : j)$: It is given by $\sum_j d/d\psi_{0j} f(\psi_0) IC_j$. That is, an influence curve of an estimator is a building block for calculating the influence curve of an estimator that uses this estimator as an ingredient.

Recall that P_0 denotes the "vector" $(P_0 f : f \in \mathcal{F})$ and P_n will denote the "vector" $(P_n f : f \in \mathcal{F})$. Since $\hat{\Psi}$ is a function of a vector, one needs to define directional derivatives of this function in a direction defined by a "vector" $h = (h(f) : f \in \mathcal{F})$. This directional derivative is defined as

$$\hat{\Psi}'(P_0)(h) \equiv \frac{d}{d\epsilon} \hat{\Psi}(P_0 + \epsilon h)\Big|_{\epsilon=0} .$$

Since we can think of $\hat{\Psi}$ as a function of a vector with components indexed by $f \in \mathcal{F}$, we can define a partial derivative with respect to to its fth component at $(P_0 f : f)$:

$$\frac{d\hat{\Psi}(P_0)}{dP_0 f} = \frac{d}{d\epsilon} \hat{\Psi}(P_0 + \epsilon h_f)\Big|_{\epsilon=0} ,$$

with $h_f(f) = 1$ and $h_f(f_1) = 0$ for $f_1 \neq f$. This partial derivative is d-dimensional, one for each component of $\hat{\Psi}$. The directional derivative in the direction of h can then be presented as a gradient (one for each of the d components of $\hat{\Psi}$) applied to vector h:

$$\begin{aligned} \hat{\Psi}'(P_0)(h) &= \frac{d}{d\epsilon} \hat{\Psi}(P_0 + \epsilon h)\Big|_{\epsilon=0} \\ &= \sum_{f \in \mathcal{F}} \frac{d\hat{\Psi}(P_0)}{dP_0 f} h(f). \end{aligned}$$

The influence curve of $\hat{\Psi}(P_n)$ under i.i.d. sampling from P_0 can be represented as the directional derivative in direction h_O defined componentwise as $h_O(f) = f(O) - P_0 f$. Note that h_O is the centered empirical process $P_{n=1} - P_0$ of one observation O, and $(P_n - P_0)(f) = 1/n \sum_{i=1}^n h_{O_i}(f)$. Thus, the influence curve can be defined as

$$\begin{aligned} IC(P_0)(O) &= \frac{d}{d\epsilon} \hat{\Psi}(P_0 + \epsilon h_O)\Big|_{\epsilon=0} \\ &= \sum_{f \in \mathcal{F}} \frac{d\hat{\Psi}(P_0)}{dP_0 f} \{f(O) - P_0 f\}. \end{aligned}$$

To summarize what we have learned, let us restate the basic delta method argument. A first-order Taylor expansion of $\hat{\Psi}$ at $P_0 = (P_0 f : f \in \mathcal{F})$ yields

$$\hat{\Psi}(P_n) - \hat{\Psi}(P_0) \approx \hat{\Psi}'(P_0)(P_n - P_0),$$

where the additional second-order term often involves differences such as $\|P_n - P_0\|^2$ or $(P_n - P_0) f_n$ with a sequence of functions f_n (depending on P_n) converging to 0 in probability. Formally, as presented previously, the functional delta method and empirical process theory can be used to show that the remainder is $o_P(1/\sqrt{n})$, which is also the condition under which we can claim that the estimator $\hat{\Psi}(P_n)$ is asymptotically linear under i.i.d. sampling from P_0. Under this asymptotic linearity condition we have

$$\begin{aligned}\hat{\Psi}(P_n) - \hat{\Psi}(P_0) &= \hat{\Psi}'(P_0)(P_n - P_0) + o_P(1/\sqrt{n}) \\ &= \frac{1}{n}\sum_{i=1}^{n} \hat{\Psi}'(P_0)(f(O_i) - P_0 f : f \in \mathcal{F}) + o_P(1/\sqrt{n}) \\ &= \frac{1}{n}\sum_{i=1}^{n} IC(P_0)(O_i) + o_P(1/\sqrt{n}).\end{aligned}$$

The influence curve of an estimator is of great importance. Firstly, it provides us with an estimator of the asymptotic covariance matrix of the estimator, which can be used for testing null hypotheses, sequential testing, sample size calculations, and the construction of confidence intervals. Specifically, $\sqrt{n}(\hat{\Psi}(P_n) - \hat{\Psi}(P_0))$ converges in distribution to $N(0, \Sigma_0)$, where $\Sigma_0 = P_0 IC(P_0) IC(P_0)^\top$. This covariance matrix can be estimated with the empirical covariance matrix of $\widehat{IC}(O_i)$, $i = 1, \ldots, n$, where $\widehat{IC}$ is an estimate of $IC(P_0)$. The asymptotically valid working model $\hat{\Psi}(P_n) \sim N(\psi_0, \hat{\Sigma})$ provides a basis for statistical inference. In addition, the influence curve values $\widehat{IC}(O_i)$, $i = 1, \ldots, n$, provide a tool for investigating the influence of one observation O_i on the estimator, and is thus also helpful for detecting outliers (robustness analysis).

Beyond its utility for assessing uncertainty and evaluating robustness, the theoretical investigation of $IC(P_0)$ allows one to determine the conditions on P_0 under which it is uniformly bounded as a function of O. These conditions will be required assumptions under which the estimator $\hat{\Psi}(P_n)$ is a reliable robust and consistent estimator of ψ_0, and these assumptions will suggest truncations or other modifications of the data so that these assumptions are met. As a consequence of this theoretical utility, a nontheoretician is able to assess quickly the situations in which the estimator is unreliable and the required conditions under which it is a trustworthy estimator. In particular, it provides insight into the amount of information, or lack of information (i.e., sparsity), in the data with respect to the target parameter ψ_0.

A.3 Computation of the Influence Curve: An Example

Summary. We present two concrete examples where we demonstrate the computation of an influence curve of an estimator. A first important step is to represent the estimator as a function of a large collection of empirical means (i.e., linear estimators), or, more generally, as a function of a collection of asymptotically linear estimators with known influence curves. Given this formulation of the estimator, for the sake of determining the influence curve of the estimator, one should only be concerned with a first-order Taylor expansion of the estimator, viewed as a function of this collection of asymptotically linear estimators, so that one can ignore all second- and higher-order terms. In this way, the influence curve follows naturally as a linear combination of the influence curves of the inputted estimators. That is, the influence curve equals the (functional) derivative of the estimator applied to the vector of influence curves of the inputted estimators.

We demonstrate the computation of an influence curve of an estimator. Let $O = (W, A, Y) \sim P_0$, and let $\Psi(P) = E_P[E_P(Y \mid W, A = 1) - E_P(Y \mid W, A = 0)]$ be the parameter of interest, $O_1, \ldots, O_n$ be n i.i.d. observations of O, and P_n be the empirical probability distribution.

Influence curve of MLE based on parametric model. Suppose that we use a parametric model $\{\bar{Q}_\beta : \beta\}$ for $\bar{Q}_0$, where $\bar{Q}_0(A, W) = E_0(Y \mid W, A)$. For example, $\bar{Q}_\beta(A, W) = \beta^\top(A, W)$ is a main term linear regression model. Let β_n be an estimator of β according to this parametric model. Such an estimator β_n solves an estimating equation such as $P_n D_{\beta_n} = 0$. For example, if $L(\bar{Q})$ is a loss function for $\bar{Q}_0$, such as $L(\bar{Q})(O) = (Y - \bar{Q}(W, A))^2$, and $\beta_n = \arg\min_\beta P_n L(\bar{Q}_\beta)$, then $D(\beta) = \frac{d}{d\beta} L(\bar{Q}_\beta)$. Let β_0 be the limit of β_n satisfying $P_0 D_{\beta_0} = 0$. Then, under regularity conditions, it follows that $\beta_n - \beta_0 = (P_n - P_0) IC_{\beta_0} + o_P(1/\sqrt{n})$, where $IC_{\beta_0} = c_0^{-1} D_{\beta_0}$, with $c_0 = -\frac{d}{d\beta_0} P_0 D_{\beta_0}$.

We will also use the notation $\tilde{Q}_\beta(W) \equiv \bar{Q}_\beta(W, 1) - \bar{Q}_\beta(W, 0)$. Let $\psi_0 = P_{W,0} \tilde{Q}_{\beta_0}$ be the target parameter of interest. Thus, if the parametric model is correctly specified, we have $\psi_0 = E_0[E_0(Y \mid W, A = 1) - E_0(Y \mid W, A = 0)]$. Let $\psi_n = P_{W,n} \tilde{Q}_{\beta_n}$ be the estimator of ψ_0. We wish to determine the influence curve of ψ_n as an estimator of ψ_0. We have

$$
\begin{aligned}
\psi_n - \psi_0 &= P_{W,n} \tilde{Q}_{\beta_n} - P_{W,0} \tilde{Q}_{\beta_0} \\
&= (P_{W,n} - P_{W,0}) \tilde{Q}_{\beta_0} + P_{W,n} \{\tilde{Q}_{\beta_n} - \tilde{Q}_{\beta_0}\} \\
&= (P_{W,n} - P_{W,0}) \tilde{Q}_{\beta_0} + P_{W,0} \{\tilde{Q}_{\beta_n} - \tilde{Q}_{\beta_0}\} + (P_{W,n} - P_{W,0}) \{\tilde{Q}_{\beta_n} - \tilde{Q}_{\beta_0}\}.
\end{aligned}
$$

The last term is a second-order term and can therefore be ignored for the purpose of calculating of an influence curve. The second term can be approximated by applying first-order Taylor expansions in β and the asymptotic linearity of β_n:

$$
\begin{aligned}
P_{W,0} \{\tilde{Q}_{\beta_n} - \tilde{Q}_{\beta_0}\} &\approx \left\{ P_{W,0} \frac{d}{d\beta_0} \tilde{Q}_{\beta_0} \right\}^\top (\beta_n - \beta_0) \\
&\approx (P_n - P_0) \left\{ P_{W,0} \frac{d}{d\beta_0} \tilde{Q}_{\beta_0} \right\}^\top IC_{\beta_0}.
\end{aligned}
$$

We can conclude that $\psi_n - \psi_0 \approx (P_n - P_0) IC$ with influence curve

$$
IC = \tilde{Q}_{\beta_0} - \psi_0 + P_{W,0} \left\{ \tfrac{d}{d\beta_0} \tilde{Q}_{\beta_0} \right\}^\top IC_{\beta_0}.
$$

Influence curve of nonparametric MLE. Let us now consider a nonparametric estimator $\psi_n = P_{W,n}\tilde{Q}_n$ of $\psi_0 = P_{W,0}\tilde{Q}_0$, where $\tilde{Q}_n(W) = \bar{Q}_n(W,1) - \bar{Q}_n(W,0)$ and $\tilde{Q}_0(W) = E_0(Y \mid W, A = 1) - E_0(Y \mid W, A = 0)$. It is assumed that W is discrete. Note that

$$\bar{Q}_n(w,a) = \textstyle\sum_y y(P_n f_{y,w,a}/P_n f_{w,a}),$$

with $f_{w,a}(O) = I(W = w, A = a)$ and $f_{y,w,a}(O) = I(W = w, A = a, Y = Y)$. We will focus on deriving the influence curve IC_1 of $\psi_n(1) = P_{W,n}\bar{Q}_{1,n}$ as an estimator of $\psi_0(1) = P_W\bar{Q}_{1,0}$, where $\bar{Q}_{1,0}(W) = E_0(Y \mid W, A = 1)$. Since $\psi_n = \psi_n(1) - \psi_n(0)$, this will yield the influence curve $IC_1 - IC_0$ of ψ_n. Note that $\psi_n(1)$ can be represented as a function Φ of $(P_n f : f \in \mathcal{F})$ with $\mathcal{F} = \{f_{w,a}, f_{y,w,a} : w, a, y\}$. Thus $\psi_n(1) = \Phi(P_n) = \Phi(P_n f : f)$. The functional delta method teaches us that we can use the first order linear approximation $\Phi(P_n) - \Phi(P_0) = \Phi'(P_0)(P_n - P_0)$, where $\Phi'(P_0) = (\frac{d}{dP_0 f}\Phi(P_0 f : f) : f)$ and $(P_n - P_0) = ((P_n - P_0)f : f)$. In particular, it follows that the influence curve of $\psi_n(1) = \Phi(P_n)$ as an estimator of $\psi_0(1)$ is given by

$$IC_1 = \left(\frac{d\Phi(P_0)}{dP_0 f} : f\right)(P_{n=1} - P_0),$$

where $P_{n=1} = (f(O) - P_0 f : f \in \mathcal{F})$ is the empirical process based on a single observation $O = (W, A, Y)$. One can also carry out this process of determining the linear approximation in a stepwise fashion. Firstly, we linearize $\Phi(P_n)$ in terms of $P_{W,n} - P_{W,0}$ and $\bar{Q}_{1n} - \bar{Q}_{1,0}$:

$$P_{W,n}\bar{Q}_{1,n} - P_{W,0}\bar{Q}_{1,0} \approx (P_{W,n} - P_{W,0})\bar{Q}_{1,0} + P_{W,0}(\bar{Q}_{1,n} - \bar{Q}_{1,0}).$$

Note that the first term equals the empirical mean of $\bar{Q}_{1,0}(W) - \psi_0(1)$. Secondly, we linearize the latter term:

$$\bar{Q}_{1,n}(w) - \bar{Q}_{1,0}(w) \approx \textstyle\sum_y y \frac{1}{P_0 f_{w,1}}(P_n - P_0)f_{y,w,1} - \frac{P_0 f_{y,w,1}}{P_0^2 f_{w,1}}(P_n - P_0)f_{w,1}.$$

Thus,

$$\begin{aligned}\sum_w P_{W,0}(w)(\bar{Q}_{1,n} - \bar{Q}_{1,0})(w) &\approx (P_n - P_0)\left\{\sum_w P_{W,0}(w)\sum_y y\left\{\frac{1}{P_0 f_{w,1}}f_{y,w,1} - \frac{P_0 f_{y,w,1}}{P_0^2 f_{w,1}}f_{w,1}\right\}\right\} \\ &\equiv (P_n - P_0)IC_1'.\end{aligned}$$

Since $f_{y,w,1} = I(Y = y, W = w, A = a)$ and $f_{w,1} = I(W = w, A = 1)$, the integrals/sums over w, y simplify:

$$\begin{aligned}IC_1' &= \frac{P_0(W)}{P_0(W, A = 1)}YI(A = 1) - P_0(W)\sum_y y\frac{P_0(y, W, 1)}{P_0^2(W, 1)}I(A = 1) \\ &= \frac{I(A = 1)}{g_0(1 \mid W)}Y - \frac{I(A = 1)}{g_0(1 \mid W)}E_0(Y \mid W, A = 1) \\ &= \frac{I(A = 1)}{g_0(1 \mid W)}(Y - E_0(Y \mid W, A = 1)),\end{aligned}$$

where we used the notation $g_0(1 \mid W) = P_0(A = 1 \mid W)$. Thus, the influence curve IC_1 of $\psi_n(1)$ is given by $\bar{Q}_{1,0}(W) - \psi_0(1) + IC_1'(O)$. The above proof also yields the analog influence curve IC_0 of $\psi_n(0)$. As a consequence, we have shown that the influence curve IC of $\psi_n = \psi_n(1) - \psi_n(0)$ is given by $IC_1 - IC_0$, which can be represented as

$$IC(P_0)(O) = \left\{\frac{I(A=1)}{g_0(1|W)} - \frac{I(A=0)}{g_0(0|W)}\right\}(Y - \bar{Q}_0(W, A)) + \tilde{Q}_0(W) - \Psi(Q_0).$$

We note that this influence curve equals the efficient influence curve of ψ_0 in the nonparametric model for P_0. Because the nonparametric MLE is asymptotically linear with influence curve equal to the efficient influence curve, by definition, it is an efficient estimator. Computing the influence curve of the (nonparametric) MLE of a target parameter in a nonparametric or semiparametric model, ignoring second-order terms and assuming the data structure is discrete, is a general tool for deriving the efficient influence curve of the target parameter. The resulting expression will have a natural analog for the general (e.g., continuously valued) data structure since each continuous data structure can be approximated by discrete data structures, and this generalized expression will then be the efficient influence curve.

Estimation of the influence curve of the nonparametric MLE, or any other efficient estimator, requires an estimator of the treatment mechanism. If one used a data-adaptive machine learning algorithm to estimate $E_0(Y \mid A, W)$ instead of a nonparametric MLE, and claimed that the resulting MLE-based estimator of the target parameter are still unbiased *enough*, then one would claim that it was asymptotically linear with influence curve equal to the efficient influence curve. Thus, estimation of the influence curve requires estimation of the treatment mechanism, again. Overall, one can conclude that statistical inference based on an MLE in a nonparametric model still requires implicit or explicit estimation of the treatment mechanism. From this point of view, the TMLE is not asking for more than what a nontargeted MLE already requires; the TMLE just utilizes the estimator of the treatment mechanism to target the estimator so that the desired asymptotic linearity is a more reasonable assumption.

A.4 Cramer–Rao Lower Bound

Summary. We prove that the influence curve of an asymptotically linear estimator of a statistical parameter that also satisfies a regularity property has a variance that is larger than the variance of the canonical gradient of the pathwise derivative of the statistical parameter. As a consequence, we can state that an estimator is optimal/efficient among all such asymptotically linear estimators if and only if its influence curve equals the canonical gradient. This explains why the latter is also-called the efficient influence curve. This result is implied by the more general convolution theorem for regular estimators (Bickel et al. 1997), but it provides a self-contained understanding of efficiency theory for asymptotically linear estimators. Given the efficiency theory, one should always be highly motivated to determine the efficient influence curve of the target parameter. Indeed, it provides the ingredient for the construction of an efficient substitution estimator, such as the TMLE.

We provide a basic understanding of the result that an estimator is efficient among regular estimators if and only if it is asymptotically linear with influence curve equal to the efficient influence curve. We will prove a result stating that an asymptotically linear estimator at P_0 that maintains low negligible bias in local neighborhoods of P_0 has an influence curve that equals a gradient of the pathwise derivative. As a consequence, the best estimator among such asymptotically linear estimators is the one with an influence curve equal to the canonical gradient of the pathwise derivative.

Let $O \sim P_0 \in \mathcal{M}$, and let $\Psi : \mathcal{M} \to \mathbb{R}^d$ be the target parameter. For each $P \in \mathcal{M}$, consider a class of parametric models $\{P_h(\epsilon) : \epsilon\} \subset \mathcal{M}$ through a $P \in \mathcal{M}$ at $\epsilon = 0$, indexed by an h in an index set $\mathcal{H}$, and with score $S(h) = \frac{d}{d\epsilon} \log P_h(\epsilon)\big|_{\epsilon=0}$ at $\epsilon = 0$. It is assumed that these scores $\{S_h : h \in \mathcal{H}\}$ are an element of the Hilbert space $L_0^2(P)$ of mean 0 functions of O, endowed with the inner product $\langle f, g\rangle = Pfg$, the covariance operator. The set of scores generated by this class of parametric models spans a linear subspace of $L_0^2(P)$, and by taking the closure of this linear subspace we obtain the tangent space $T(P) \subset L_0^2(P)$ at P, which is itself a Hilbert space. We state that $\Psi : \mathcal{M} \to \mathbb{R}^d$ is pathwise differentiable at P if there exists a D^* in the tangent space $T(P) \subset L_0^2(P)$ at P so that for each of these submodels through P we have

$$\frac{d}{d\epsilon} \Psi(P(\epsilon))\Big|_{\epsilon=0} = PD^*(P)S.$$

This inner product representation of the derivative can be expected since 1) the left-hand side is linear in $\frac{d}{d\epsilon}P(\epsilon)\big|_{\epsilon=0}$, so that at this fixed P, it should also be linear in the score $S = \frac{d}{d\epsilon}P(\epsilon)\big|_{\epsilon=0}/P$, and 2) by the Riesz representation theorem, a bounded linear operator on a Hilbert space (i.e., $T(P)$) can be represented as an inner product as above. One refers to $D^*(P)$ as the canonical gradient of the pathwise derivative of $\Psi : \mathcal{M} \to \mathbb{R}^d$ at P. If the inner-product representation applies for a $D(P) \in L_0^2(P)$, then such a $D(P)$ is called a gradient. We note that for any $D^\perp$ in the orthogonal complement of the tangent space, $T(P)$, $D^*(P)+D^\perp$ is a gradient: $P(D^*(P)+D^\perp)S = PD^*(P)S$ for all $S \in T(P)$. Since a gradient has to yield the same pathwise derivative on the tangent space $T(P)$ as the canonical gradient, it follows that any gradient can be represented as $D^*(P)+D^\perp$. This shows that the set of all gradients is any function in $L_0^2(P)$ whose projection on $T(P)$ equals the canonical gradient.

Thus the canonical gradient is the unique gradient of the pathwise derivative that is an element of the tangent space, and it is also the gradient that has the smallest variance among all gradients:

$$P\{D^*(P)(O) + D^\perp\}^2 = P\{D^*(P)\}^2 + P\{D^\perp\}^2 \geq P\{D^*(P)\}^2.$$

Since an asymptotically linear estimator is efficient if and only if its influence curve equals the canonical gradient, the canonical gradient is also called the efficient influence curve.

Let us formalize the latter statement. Consider an estimator $\hat{\Psi} : \mathcal{M}_{NP} \rightarrow \mathbb{R}^d$ that maps the empirical distribution of the data set $O_1, \ldots, O_n$ into the parameter space of Ψ. Suppose the estimator is asymptotically linear under i.i.d. sampling from P with influence curve $IC(P)$:

$$\hat{\Psi}(P_n) - \Psi(P) = (P_n - P)IC(P) + R(P_n, P),$$

where $R(P_n, P) = o_P(1/\sqrt{n})$. We now argue that, for any parametric model $\{P(\epsilon) : \epsilon\}$ (one of the models used in the pathwise derivative) this linear approximation in the data P_n should still be valid under i.i.d. sampling from $P(\epsilon_n)$ with $\epsilon_n = 1/\sqrt{n}$. That is, if $P(\epsilon_n)_n$ is the empirical distribution of n i.i.d. observations from $P(\epsilon_n)$, then

$$\hat{\Psi}(P(\epsilon_n)_n) - \Psi(P) = (P(\epsilon_n)_n - P)IC(P) + R(P(\epsilon_n)_n, P),$$

where $R(P(\epsilon_n)_n, P) = o_P(1/\sqrt{n})$. This is indeed expected since $P(\epsilon_n)_n - P = (P(\epsilon_n)_n - P(\epsilon_n)) + (P(\epsilon_n) - P)$, and, if $\epsilon_n = 1/\sqrt{n}$, then $\sup_{f \in \mathcal{F}} \mid (P(\epsilon_n)_n - P(\epsilon_n))f \mid = O_P(1/\sqrt{n})$ for a Donsker class $\mathcal{F}$, while also $\| P(\epsilon_n) - P \|_{\mathcal{F}} = O(1/\sqrt{n})$. For example, to use simplistic notation, if $R(P_n, P) = \|P_n - P\|^2$, then $R(P(\epsilon_n)_n, P) = \|P(\epsilon_n)_n - P\|^2$ will converge to zero in probability at same rate as $R(P_n, P)$. As a consequence, it is reasonable to state that the linear approximation of $\hat{\Psi}(P_n)$ in the data P_n at P also holds up under sampling from $P(\epsilon_n)$, that is, under i.i.d. sampling from $P(\epsilon_n)$, we have

$$\hat{\Psi}(P(\epsilon_n)_n) - \Psi(P) = \tfrac{1}{n} \textstyle\sum_{i=1}^n IC(P)(O_i) + R_n,$$

where $R_n = o_P(1/\sqrt{n})$. Suppose we now also require that the estimator $\hat{\Psi}(P(\epsilon_n)_n)$ has a bias that is $o(1/\sqrt{n})$ under i.i.d. sampling from $P(\epsilon_n)$ for $\epsilon_n = 1/\sqrt{n}$ in the sense that

$$\frac{E_{P(\epsilon_n)}\hat{\Psi}(P(\epsilon_n)_n) - \Psi(P(\epsilon_n))}{\epsilon_n} \rightarrow 0 \text{ as } n \rightarrow \infty, \tag{A.1}$$

$$\frac{E_{P(\epsilon_n)}R_n}{\epsilon_n} \rightarrow 0, \tag{A.2}$$

and these two statements need to hold for each of the parametric submodels. We will now show that this requirement implies that $IC(P) = D^*(P) + D^{\perp}$ for some $D^{\perp} \perp T(P)$, i.e., it implies that $IC(P)$ is a gradient of the pathwise derivative at P. This then also proves that an estimator, among the class of asymptotically linear estimators that are locally uniformly unbiased in the above sense, is efficient if and only if $IC(P) = D^*(P)$. Note that if (A.1) does not hold for a particular parametric submodel, then for this submodel $\sqrt{n}(\hat{\Psi}(P(\epsilon_n)_n) - \Psi(P(\epsilon_n)))$ will converge to a normal distribution with a bias term, possibly even a bias term of infinite magnitude, so that statistical inference based on the CLT under sampling from $P(\epsilon_n)$ will not be valid.

The fact that this "negligible bias" requirement under $P(\epsilon_n)$ implies that $IC(P)$ is a gradient is shown as follows. Firstly, substitute $\hat{\Psi}(P(\epsilon_n)_n) = \Psi(P) + P(\epsilon_n)_n IC(P) + R_n$ in (A.1) to obtain

$$\begin{aligned}\frac{E_{P(\epsilon_n)}\hat{\Psi}(P(\epsilon_n)_n) - \Psi(P(\epsilon_n))}{\epsilon_n} &= \frac{P(\epsilon_n)IC(P)}{\epsilon_n} - \frac{\Psi(P(\epsilon_n)) - \Psi(P)}{\epsilon_n} + E_{P(\epsilon_n)}\frac{R_n}{\epsilon_n}\\ &= P\frac{P(\epsilon_n) - P}{\epsilon_n P}IC(P) - \{PD^*(P)S + o(1)\} + o(1),\end{aligned}$$

where we used (A.2) and the definition of the pathwise differentiability of Ψ. Note that

$$P\tfrac{P(\epsilon_n)-P}{\epsilon_n P}IC(P) = P\,IC(P)S + o(1).$$

Thus, we obtain that the limit for $\epsilon_n \to 0$ (i.e., A.1) equals:

$$P\{IC(P) - D^*(P)\}S \text{ for each } S \in T(P).$$

By assumption (A.1), this limit must equal zero for all S. This proves the statement that the projection of the influence curve onto the tangent space at P is unique, and equals the canonical gradient: $\Pi(IC(P) \mid T(P)) = D^*(P)$. We will state what we just proved as a theorem.

Theorem A.1. *Let $O \sim P \in \mathcal{M}$, and $\Psi : \mathcal{M} \to \mathbb{R}^d$. Consider a class of parametric submodels $\{P_h(\epsilon) : \epsilon\} \subset \mathcal{M}$ through $P \in \mathcal{M}$ at $\epsilon = 0$, with score $S(h) = \frac{d}{d\epsilon}\log P_h(\epsilon)\big|_{\epsilon=0}$ at $\epsilon = 0$, indexed by h in an index set $\mathcal{H}$. Let $T(P) \subset L_0^2(P)$ be the tangent space at P of this class of parametric submodels. Assume that Ψ is pathwise differentiable at P with respect to this class of parametric submodels; we have that there exists a D^* in the tangent space $T(P) \subset L_0^2(P)$ at P so that for each of these submodels through P, we have*

$$\tfrac{d}{d\epsilon}\Psi(P(\epsilon))\big|_{\epsilon=0} = PD^*(P)S.$$

Here we use the notation $Pf = \int f(o)dP(o)$.

Consider an estimator $\hat{\Psi} : \mathcal{M}_{NP} \to \mathbb{R}^d$ that maps an empirical distribution P_n of $O_1, \ldots, O_n \sim P$ (for any P) into $\mathbb{R}^d$. Assume that for each of the above submodels $\{P_h(\epsilon) : \epsilon\}$, $h \in \mathcal{H}$, under i.i.d. sampling from $P(\epsilon_n)$ (suppressing h) with $\epsilon_n = 1/\sqrt{n}$, we have

$$\hat{\Psi}(P(\epsilon_n)_n) - \Psi(P) = P(\epsilon_n)_n IC(P) + R_n,$$

with

$$\frac{E_{P(\epsilon_n)}\hat{\Psi}(P(\epsilon)_n) - \Psi(P(\epsilon_n))}{\epsilon_n} \to 0 \text{ as } n \to \infty, \tag{A.3}$$

$$E_{P(\epsilon_n)}R_n = o(\epsilon_n). \tag{A.4}$$

Here $P(\epsilon)_n$ is the empirical distribution of an i.i.d. sample of size n from $P(\epsilon)$. Then the projection of $IC(P)$ onto $T(P)$ in the Hilbert space $L_0^2(P)$ equals the canonical gradient $D^*(P)$:

$$\Pi(IC(P) \mid T(P)) = D^*(P).$$

In particular,

$$VAR_P\{IC(P)(O)\} \geq VAR_P\{D^*(P)(O)\}.$$

Why the variance of the efficient influence curve is a generalized Cramer–Rao lower bound: An informal explanation. If one assumes a parametric model $\{P(\epsilon) : \epsilon\}$ so that $O \sim P(\epsilon_0)$, and one wishes to estimate $f(\epsilon_0) = \Psi(P(\epsilon_0))$, where we let $\epsilon_0 = 0$ (unknown to the user), then the Cramer–Rao lower bound for the variance of an unbiased estimator of $f(\epsilon_0)$ is given by

$$\frac{\left(\frac{d}{d\epsilon_0} f(\epsilon_0)\right)^2}{PS^2} = \frac{P^2 D^*(P)S}{PS^2}.$$

Here S is the score of $P(\epsilon)$ at $\epsilon = 0$. Since each such parametric models is a submodel, it makes sense to define as the Cramer–Rao bound for the actual model $\mathcal{M}$, the worst-case bound obtained by selecting the hardest among a class of parametric submodels. For most models $\mathcal{M}$, if one has univariate submodels with scores S_1 and S_2, then one can also construct a submodel with two parameters whose score is any linear combination of S_1 and S_2. In that case, the worst-case bound is given by

$$\sup_{S \in T(P)} \frac{P^2 D^*(P)S}{PS^2}.$$

By the Cauchy–Schwarz inequality, it follows that this supremum is attained at $S = D^*(P)$ and it equals $PD^*(P)^2$, the variance of the efficient influence curve.

A.5 Invariance of Statistical Properties

Summary. Given the statistical model and target parameter, we emphasize that statistical properties, such as the pathwise derivative of the target parameter, the gradient and canonical gradient/efficient influence curve, and robustness of this efficient influence curve, are invariant to additional nontestable assumptions that do not change the statistical model. This insight is useful, since it allows one to borrow from previously obtained statistical results.

Consider a random variable (U, X), a model $\mathcal{M}^F$ for its distribution $P_{U,X}$, and a mapping from $P_{U,X} \in \mathcal{M}^F$ into a probability distribution $P_O(P_{U,X})$ for an observed data structure O (e.g., $O = \Phi(U, X)$ for some mapping Φ). We use the notation (U, X) for the underlying random variable because we have used this notation to describe the random variables modeled by an SCM. However, (U, X) can denote any underlying random variable; for example, U might be the censoring variable, X a full data structure, and $O = \Phi(U, X)$ the observed data structure. Let

$\mathcal{M} = \{P_O(P_{U,X}) : P_{U,X} \in \mathcal{M}^F\}$ be the corresponding observed data statistical model. Consider a random variable (U^*, X^*), a model $\mathcal{M}^{F*}$ for its distribution P_{U^*,X^*}, and a mapping from $P_{U^*,X^*} \in \mathcal{M}^{F*}$ into a probability distribution $P_O(P_{U^*,X^*})$ for the observed data structure O. Let $\mathcal{M}^* = \{P_O(P_{U^*,X^*}) : P_{U^*,X^*} \in \mathcal{M}^{F*}\}$ be the corresponding observed data statistical model. If we write $\mathcal{M}$ we also refer to the actual model assumptions coded by the parameterization $P_O(P_{U,X})$ and underlying model $\mathcal{M}^F$, and similarly for $\mathcal{M}^*$. Although models $\mathcal{M}$ and $\mathcal{M}^*$ can be very different in their underlying assumptions, we assume that their statistical models are identical: $\mathcal{M}^* = \mathcal{M}$.

In general, if one proves statistical properties that concern the probability distribution of the observed data structure O under one of these models, it will also apply to the other model. This might sound too trivial to even mention, but it is a useful fact. In order to be concrete, let us consider a number of scenarios in which we apply this invariance principle.

Suppose that one has proven the following double robustness results for an observed data estimating function $(Q, g) \to D(Q, g)$, with respect to nuisance parameters $Q(P)$ and $g(P)$, based on model $\mathcal{M}$ [i.e., the proof might have used the parameterization $P_O(P_{U,X})$ and assumptions $P_{U,X} \in \mathcal{M}^F$]. For each $P \in \mathcal{M}$ and $Q \in \mathcal{Q}$, there is a set $\mathcal{G}(Q, P)$ of distributions such that $E_P D(Q, g)(O) = 0$ for $g \in \mathcal{G}(Q, P)$. Then, we also have for each $P \in \mathcal{M}^*$ and $Q \in \mathcal{Q}$, $E_P D(Q, g)(O) = 0$ for $g \in \mathcal{G}(Q, P)$.

For example, consider the CAR missing-data model for $O = (W, A, Y = Y_A) \sim P_0$ with $X = (Y_0, Y_1, W)$ nonparametrically modeled, and the treatment assignment mechanism $g_0(a \mid X) = P_0(A = a \mid X) = P_0(A = a \mid W)$ only assumed to satisfy CAR. Let $D^*(P_0) = D^*(Q_0, g_0)$ be the efficient influence curve of the target parameter $\Psi(P_0) = E_0[E_0(Y \mid A = 1, W) - E(Y \mid A = 0, W)]$, with Q_0 representing $E_0(Y \mid A, W)$ and the marginal distribution of W, so that both Q_0, g_0 represent parameters of P_0. Suppose that one has proven a desired double robustness result in this CAR missing-data model such as $P_0 D^*(Q, g) = 0$ if either $Q = Q_0$ or $g = g_0$ (van der Laan and Robins 2003). Then this same double robustness result applies to other causal underlying models that result in the same nonparametric observed data model, including the pure statistical model for $O = (W, A, Y) \sim P_0$ that makes no assumptions at all.

One possible example is that model $\mathcal{M}$ makes stronger assumptions than $\mathcal{M}^*$ (e.g., $\mathcal{M}^F \subset \mathcal{M}^{F*}$ or $\mathcal{M}^*$ is a pure statistical model); apparently, proving a result under stronger assumptions implies the result under weaker assumptions if these stronger assumptions do not shrink the statistical model. For example, if one proves statistical properties under the causal model for a longitudinal data structure $(\bar{A}, \bar{L}_A)$ that assumes a strong SRA, $A(t) \perp L_{\bar{A}(t-1),\underline{a}(t)} \mid \bar{A}(t-1), \bar{L}(t)$, then these same statistical properties apply under the causal model that assumes the weaker randomization with respect to the Y outcome, where the Y outcome is included in the L process. We know the latter randomization assumption is sufficient for identification of marginal distributions of Y_a (but not for L_a), but it might prevent us from doing calculations and engaging in reasoning that feels natural to us.

Similarly, suppose that one has proven that, given a loss function $L(Q)$, for each $P \in \mathcal{M}$ and $Q(P) = \arg\min_{Q \in \mathcal{Q}} PL(Q)$, we have that $\Psi(Q(P))$ is a desired number $\Phi(P)$, and this proof used model $\mathcal{M}$. Then this also implies that for each $P \in \mathcal{M}^*$, and $Q(P) = \arg\min_{Q \in \mathcal{Q}} PL(Q)$, we have that $\Psi(Q(P)) = \Phi(P)$. For example, consider the CAR missing-data model for $O = (W, A, Y = Y_A)$ again. Consider the loss function $L(Q) = -\log Q(Y \mid A) g_0(A)/g_0(A \mid X)$. Using the CAR censored-data model, it follows that this is a valid IPTW loss function for $Q_0(y \mid a) = P_0(Y(a) = y)$, i.e., for the marginal distribution of the counterfactual Y_a for each a: $Q_0 = \arg\min_Q E_0 L(Q)$. As a consequence, we can identify the additive causal effect as follows: $E_0\{Y_1 - Y_0\} = \sum_y y\{Q_0(y \mid a = 1) - Q_0(y \mid a = 0)\}$. The right-hand side defines now a mapping Φ from P_0 into a desired value $\Phi(P_0) = \Psi(P_0) = E_0[E_0(Y \mid A = 1, W) - E_0(Y \mid A = 0, W)]$. Now, suppose we are not willing to make any causal assumptions. Then we still have $\Phi(P_0) = \Psi(P_0)$, allowing one to construct estimators based on the mapping Φ, even though Q_0 no longer represents a counterfactual distribution.

Another application of this invariance principle is the following. Suppose we have shown that $D(P)$ is a gradient of a parameter $\Psi : \mathcal{M} \to \mathbb{R}$ at $P \in \mathcal{M}$. That is, for each one-dimensional submodel $\{P(\epsilon) : \epsilon\}$ through P at $\epsilon = 0$, $\frac{d}{d\epsilon}\Psi(P(\epsilon))\big|_{\epsilon=0} = E_P D(P) S$, where S is the score of $P(\epsilon)$ at $\epsilon = 0$. Suppose this proof (seemingly) relied on the model $\mathcal{M}$, including its nontestable assumptions. Then, $D(P)$ is also a gradient of the parameter $\Psi : \mathcal{M}^* \to \mathbb{R}$. Thus, the strategy for deriving the set of all gradients or the canonical gradient might be to assume various nontestable assumptions, such as representing the observed data structure as a CAR censored data structure. If one determines a gradient or canonical gradient under these assumptions, then one has also determined a gradient or canonical gradient under another model that maps into the same statistical model for the distribution of O.

This strategy allows us to utilize results from the literature. In particular, van der Laan and Robins (2003) present a theory for determining the class of gradients of a target parameter for a statistical model for the observed data structure under the assumption that the observed data structure is a function of a full-data random variable and censoring variable and that the conditional distribution of the censoring variable, given the full-data random variable, satisfies coarsening at random. In particular, it shows how to map the gradients of an identifiable target parameter in the full-data model into the gradients for the corresponding target parameter in the observed data model. Because of the invariance principle, this provides us with the set of gradients and the canonical gradient of the target parameter of the observed data distribution for the statistical model for O, regardless of the nontestable underlying assumptions one makes. This insight allows us to borrow from the rich literature on CAR censored-data models. For example, the censored-data literature provides us with IPCW estimating functions that were shown to be gradients of the pathwise derivative in the observed data model in which the censoring mechanism is assumed known. By projecting a gradient on the tangent space of the model one obtains the canonical gradient, so that these IPTW estimating functions can be used to derive the canonical gradient. If one does not assume that the observed data are represented as a censored-data structure, it does not make sense to use such naming or talk about full data estimating functions, but nevertheless, we can still temporarily move ourselves into this world to make progress by building on theory developed in that world, and use IPCW estimating functions (that were developed and presented in this CAR censored data world) as functions of the observed data that are gradients of the statistical target parameter.

In the CAR censored-data model for $O = (W, A, Y = Y_A)$, with full data structure $X = (W, Y_0, Y_1)$ nonparametrically modelled, and g_0 known, $\{I(A = 1) - I(A = 0)\}/g_0(A \mid X)Y - \psi_0$ represents an IPTW estimating function for ψ_0 (which is verified by showing that its conditional expectation, given X, yields a gradient in the full data model), so that we can also use this gradient in the pure statistical model, but one now represents g_0 as the conditional distribution of A, given W.

Suppose that one assumes a time-ordering $A \rightarrow W \rightarrow Y$, where A might be gender, W intermediate variables, and Y a final outcome of interest. One assumes an SCM according to this time ordering, and one assumes that (A, W) is randomized. Suppose that one is interested in a direct effect of gender on salary, controlled by the intermediate variables W, of the type $E_0 \sum_w \{Y(1, w) - Y(0, w)\} P_0(w \mid A = 0)$. This parameter can be identified from the observed data as

$$E_0 \sum_w \{Y(1, w) - Y(0, w)\} P_0(w \mid A = 0) = \\ E_0[E_0(Y \mid A = 1, W) - E_0(Y \mid A = 0, W) \mid A = 0].$$

Suppose one has derived the canonical gradient of this target parameter of the observed data distribution, as presented in van der Laan (2010c).

Consider now a new causal model in which one wishes to estimate the effect of treatment among the nontreated. That is, one assumes the time ordering $A \rightarrow W \rightarrow Y$, where W are baseline covariates, A is a binary treatment, and Y is a final outcome of interest. One assumes an SCM according to this ordering, and one assumes that A is randomized, conditional on W. Suppose that one is interested in the causal effect of treatment among the nontreated $E_0(Y_1 - Y_0 \mid A = 0)$. This parameter is identified from the observed data $O = (W, A, Y)$ as

$$E_0(Y_1 - Y_0 \mid A = 0) = E_0[E_0(Y \mid A = 1, W) - E_0(Y \mid A = 0, W) \mid A = 0].$$

Even though the two causal models and the causal quantities are very different, the observed data structures are identical, the statistical models are identical, and the statistical target parameters are identical. As a consequence, we now also have the canonical gradient for the latter causal model and target parameter.

Finally, let us consider another kind of application of this invariance of statistical properties under varying nontestable assumptions. Suppose that, given a parameter $\Psi^{F*} : \mathcal{M}^{F*} \rightarrow \mathbb{R}$, one has shown that $\Psi^{F*}(P_{U^*,X^*}) = \Psi^*(P_O(P_{U^*,X^*}))$ for each $P_{U^*,X^*} \in \mathcal{M}^{F*}$ for some mapping $\Psi^* : \mathcal{M} \rightarrow \mathbb{R}$. In other words, one has established the identifiability of the causal parameter Ψ^{F*} in model $\mathcal{M}^*$ through the statistical parameter Ψ^*. Suppose that one has proposed a new mapping $\hat{\Psi} : \mathcal{M} \rightarrow \mathbb{R}$ and one is able to show: for each $P \in \mathcal{M}$, $\hat{\Psi}(P) = \Psi^*(P)$. Thus the two parameters $\hat{\Psi}$ and Ψ^* defined in the two models $\mathcal{M}$ and $\mathcal{M}^*$ are identical as statistical parameters. Then, $\Psi^{F*}(P_{U^*,X^*}) = \hat{\Psi}(P_O(P_{U^*,X^*}))$ for each $P_{U^*,X^*} \in \mathcal{M}^{F*}$: i.e., one also has the identifiability of the causal parameter Ψ^{F*} in model $\mathcal{M}^*$ through the statistical parameter $\hat{\Psi}$. This can be used to establish that a particular estimator is indeed valid for estimating a desired causal effect; one shows that it statistically agrees with the mapping Ψ^* that came out of an original identifiability result.

A.6 Targeted Minimum-Loss-Based Estimation

Summary. We present a natural generalization of targeted maximum likelihood estimation, demonstrating that TMLE requires specifying an appropriate loss function and fluctuation working model so that the derivative at zero fluctuation of the loss yields the desired estimating function, such as the efficient influence curve.

Let O be the observed data structure, and let P_0 be its probability distribution. In addition, let $\mathcal{M}$ be the statistical model for P_0, and let $\Psi : \mathcal{M} \to \mathbb{R}^d$ be a pathwise differentiable d-dimensional parameter. One observes n i.i.d. copies $O_1, \ldots, O_n$ of O and one wishes to construct an estimator of $\Psi(P_0)$. Suppose that $Q_0 = Q(P_0)$ represents a parameter $Q : \mathcal{M} \to \mathcal{Q}$ so that for some Ψ^1 we have $\Psi(P) = \Psi^1(Q(P))$ for all $P \in \mathcal{M}$. Let $\mathcal{Q} = \{Q(P) : P \in \mathcal{M}\}$ be the parameter space for Q. For notational convenience, we will use notation $\Psi(P)$ and $\Psi(Q)$ interchangeably. We wish to construct a substitution estimator $\Psi(Q_n^*)$ of ψ_0 obtained by substitution of an estimator Q_n^* of Q_0 into the parameter mapping Ψ. Let $L(Q)$ be a loss function for Q_0 so that $Q_0 = \arg\min_{Q \in \mathcal{Q}} P_0 L(Q)$. We will allow this loss function to be indexed by a nuisance parameter: $L(Q) = L_{\eta_0}(Q)$ for some unknown nuisance parameter $\eta_0 = \Gamma(P_0)$. Given an estimator of η_0, one can use loss-based (e.g., super) learning to construct an estimator Q_n^0 of Q_0 (e.g., van der Laan and Dudoit 2003).

We are not satisfied with a good estimator of Q_0. Instead, we wish to construct an updated estimator Q_n^* so that Q_n^* and η_n solve a particular estimating equation $P_n D(Q_n^*, \eta_n) = 0$ for a user-supplied target-parameter-specific estimating function $D(Q, \eta)$. The choice of this estimating function D is tailored so that solving this equation implies good properties for the substitution estimator $\Psi(Q_n^*)$ of ψ_0. For example, $D(Q_0, \eta_0)$ might be the canonical gradient (i.e., efficient influence curve) of the pathwise derivative of Ψ at P_0, and solving the efficient influence curve estimating equation is known to imply that $\Psi(Q_n^*)$ is asymptotically linear with influence curve equal to the efficient influence curve under appropriate conditions.

For any possible (Q, η), let $\{Q_\eta(\epsilon) : \epsilon\} \subset \mathcal{Q}$ be a submodel with a finite-dimensional parameter ϵ that contains Q at $\epsilon = 0$, typically indexed by η, that satisfies the following local condition at $\epsilon = 0$:

$$\frac{d}{d\epsilon} L_\eta(Q_\eta(\epsilon))\Big|_{\epsilon=0} = D(Q, \eta).$$

The targeted minimum loss based estimator (also TMLE) is now defined by the following iterative algorithm. Start with initial estimator Q_n^0, and for $k = 1, \ldots,$

define $Q_n^k = Q_{n,\eta_n}^{k-1}(\epsilon_n^k)$, where $\epsilon_n^k = \arg\min_\epsilon P_n L_{\eta_n}(Q_{n,\eta_n}^{k-1}(\epsilon))$, and stop at step k when $\epsilon_n^k \approx 0$. If $\epsilon_n^k = 0$ and it is a local minima at an interior point, then it follows that the final update $Q_n^* = Q_n^k$ solves $0 = P_n D(Q_n^*, \eta_n)$. The substitution estimator $\Psi(Q_n^*)$ is the targeted minimum-loss-based estimator of ψ_0.

Suppose $\frac{d}{d\epsilon_j} L_\eta(Q_\eta(\epsilon))\Big|_{\epsilon=0} = D_j(Q,\eta)$, while $D(Q,\eta) = \sum_j D_j(Q,\eta)$. One can also select an ordering for $(\epsilon_1, \ldots, \epsilon_J)$ (e.g., starting at ϵ_J and going backwards) and, according to this ordering, iteratively carry out the update step $Q_n^k = Q_{n,\eta_n}^{k-1}(\epsilon_n^k)$, but where ϵ_n^k is now obtained by minimizing $P_n L_{\eta_n}(Q_{n,\eta_n}^{k-1}(\epsilon))$ only over the next ϵ-component according to the ordering of the ϵ-components, using the previous value ϵ_n^{k-1} for all other components. The next ϵ-component of the last ϵ-component in this ordering is defined as the first ϵ-component in the ordering, so that one keeps circling through all ϵ-components. At convergence, we have that ϵ_n solves $P_n D_j(Q_n^*, \eta_n) = 0$ for all j, and thus $P_n D(Q_n^*, \eta_n) = 0$ as well.

The asymptotic linearity of $\Psi(Q_n^*)$ can now be based on the fact that Q_n^* solves this estimating equation, and on statistical properties of (Q_n^*, g_n) as an estimator of Q_0, g_0 (see the asymptotic linearity theorem in Appendix A.1). By selecting a loss function for Q_0 (e.g., log-likelihood loss function), and a fluctuation working model so that the linear span of the derivative of $L(Q(\epsilon))$ at $\epsilon = 0$ includes the components of the efficient influence curve of Ψ at P, one obtains a TMLE that is asymptotically efficient under appropriate conditions.

A.7 Efficient Influence Curve for Longitudinal Data Structures

Summary. We demonstrate how one calculates the efficient influence curve of a target parameter of interest for the longitudinal data structures covered in this book. The canonical gradient is a projection of an initial gradient onto the tangent space generated by scores of parametric submodels through the data-generating distribution, where this projection is carried out in the Hilbert space of mean zero functions of the unit data structure O, endowed with an inner product equal to the covariance operator. We show that a factorization of the likelihood of the unit data structure yields an orthogonal decomposition of this tangent space, and thereby of this projection as a sum of projections on orthogonal subtangent spaces. We show that these projections on the subtangent spaces can be represented in terms of conditional expectations.

Consider a set of variables $O = (O(j) : j)$ and corresponding parent variables $(Pa(O(j)) : j)$ and suppose that the probability distribution of O is given by

$$P_0(O) = \prod_j P_0(O(j) \mid Pa(O(j))).$$

For example, O could be represented by an ordered sequence of variables, and the jth variable $O(j)$ in the sequence has corresponding parents $Pa(O(j)) = \bar{O}(j-1) =$

$O(1), \ldots, O(j-1)$. Typically, $O(0)$ represents the baseline covariates. Consider the statistical model $\mathcal{M}$ implied by all such possible probability distributions, without putting any constraints on $P_0(O(j) \mid Pa(O(j)))$. In the special case where $Pa(O(j)) = \bar{O}(j-1)$, this statistical model is completely nonparametric. We use the short-hand notation $P_{O(j)}$ for the conditional distribution of $O(j)$, given $Pa(O(j))$, under P.

Let $\Psi : \mathcal{M} \rightarrow \mathbb{R}^d$ be the d-dimensional statistical parameter of interest, so that $\Psi(P_0)$ is the target parameter value we wish to learn from the data consisting of n i.i.d. draws $O_1, \ldots, O_n$ of the random variable O. We wish to determine the efficient influence curve/canonical gradient $D^*(P)$ of the pathwise derivative of Ψ at P. The canonical gradient $D^*(P)$ equals the projection $\Pi(D(P) \mid T(P))$ of an initial gradient $D(P)$ of the pathwise derivative of Ψ at P onto the tangent space $T(P)$.

Consider a rich class of submodels $P(\epsilon)$ that only vary $P_{O(j)|Pa(O(j))}$, and denote the tangent space generated by this class of submodels by $T_{O(j)}(P)$. We can do this for each of the factors indexed by $j = 1, \ldots, J$. The resulting union of parametric submodels generates a tangent space $T(P)$ at P, given by the sum space $T(P) = \sum_j T_{O(j)}(P)$. One can also observe that by adding parametric submodels that simultaneously fluctuate multiple factors in the factorization of P one generates scores that are sums of scores that are thus still contained in this sum space $\sum_j T_{O(j)}(P)$. These subtangent spaces $T_{O(j)}(P)$ are pairwise orthogonal due to the factorization of the probability density in terms of these conditional distributions $P_{O(j)}$. This shows that $T(P) = \sum_j T_{O(j)}(P)$ is an orthogonal decomposition in subspaces. The tangent space of $P_{O(j)}$ can be generated by the following parametric submodels through $P_{O(j)}$: $P_{O(j),\epsilon} = (1 + \epsilon S(O(j) \mid Pa(O(j)))P_{O(j)}$, where S is any function of $(O(j), Pa(O(j)))$ with conditional mean zero, given $Pa(O(j))$. The scores S of these parametric fluctuations at $\epsilon = 0$ generate the tangent space $T_{O(j)}(P)$, so that we have

$$T_{O(j)}(P) = \{S(O(j), Pa(O(j)) : E_P(S \mid Pa(O(j)) = 0\} \subset L_0^2(P).$$

The projection of a function D onto $T_{O(j)}(P)$ is obtained by first projecting onto all functions of $(O(j), Pa(O(j)))$, which is given by $E(D \mid O(j), Pa(O(j)))$, and subsequently projecting this projection onto all functions which also have conditional mean zero, given $Pa(O(j))$, resulting in

$$\Pi(D(P) \mid T_{O(j)}(P)) = E(D(P) \mid O(j), Pa(O(j))) - E(D(P) \mid Pa(O(j))).$$

The reader can directly verify the validity of this formula by proving that it is an element of the space $T_{O(j)}(P)$, and that $D(P)$ minus this projection is orthogonal to $T_{O(j)}(P)$. We conclude that, if $D(P)$ is a gradient of the pathwise derivative of Ψ at P, then the canonical gradient $D^*(P)$ can be determined as

$$D^*(P) = \textstyle\sum_j \{E(D(P) \mid O(j), Pa(O(j))) - E(D(P) \mid Pa(O(j)))\}.$$

The efficient influence curves presented in this book have all been determined with this recipe.

One might now wonder, how do I obtain this initial gradient? One approach is to come up with an ad hoc estimator of ψ_0 that is regular and asymptotically linear, and derive its influence curve. As shown in Theorem A.1, this influence curve is now a gradient and can thus be used as initial gradient $D(P)$. We can make this more specific by adding some additional structure by defining $\mathcal{I}$ as the index set that identifies the intervention nodes $(O(j) : j \in \mathcal{I})$, and by assuming that $\Psi(P_0)$ is only a function of $P_{O(j),0}$ for $j \in \mathcal{I}^c$. Let $Q_0 = \prod_{j\in\mathcal{I}^c} P_{O(j),0}$, and let $g_0 = \prod_{j\in\mathcal{I}} P_{O(j),0}$, and note that $P_0 = Q_0 g_0$. We will use the notation $\Psi(Q_0)$ for the target parameter to stress that it only depends on P_0 through Q_0. For example, if our target parameter represents a parameter of the g-computation formula for the counterfactual distribution of O under interventions on the intervention nodes, then, indeed, $\Psi(P_0)$ is only a function of these conditional distributions $P_{O(j),0}$ with $j \in \mathcal{I}^c$.

In this case, we can use the following trick to determine a gradient. We consider the submodel $\mathcal{M}(g_0)$ of $\mathcal{M}$, which assumes that Q_0 is unspecified as in the actual model $\mathcal{M}$ but that g_0 is known. Due to the factorization of $P_0 = Q_0 g_0$ and that Ψ is only a function of P_0 through Q_0, it follows that the canonical gradient of $\Psi : \mathcal{M} \to \mathbb{R}^d$ is identical to the canonical gradient of $\Psi : \mathcal{M}(g_0) \to \mathbb{R}^d$. As a consequence, we can now act as if $\mathcal{M}(g_0)$ is the statistical model and determine the canonical gradient in this smaller model, which will then also equal the desired canonical gradient for the actual model $\mathcal{M}$. Note that the tangent space, say, $T_{g_0}(P)$ of $\mathcal{M}(g_0)$, is now only generated by fluctuations of the conditional distributions of $O(j)$, $j \in \mathcal{I}^c$ since g_0 is known. Thus the tangent space $T_{g_0}(P)$ at $P \in \mathcal{M}(g_0)$ for this model $\mathcal{M}(g_0)$ is given by $T_{g_0}(P) = \sum_{j\in\mathcal{I}^c} T_{O(j)}(P)$. In this model, with g_0 known, it is often easy to determine an ad hoc regular asymptotically linear estimator of ψ_0 that utilizes the known g_0, so that its influence curve gives us the desired initial gradient $D(P)$, whose projection onto the tangent space $T_{g_0}(P)$ of model $\mathcal{M}(g_0)$ yields the canonical gradient. Specifically, relying on the invariance of statistical properties under varying nontestable assumptions and the theory presented in van der Laan and Robins (2003), one can construct the inverse probability of censoring (g_0)-weighted estimators of the type

$$\psi_{IPCW,n} = \frac{1}{n}\sum_{i=1}^{n} \frac{h(O_i)}{g_0(O_i)},$$

where h is chosen such that $E_0 h(O)/g_0(O) = \psi_0$. This estimator has influence curve $D(P) = h/g_0 - \psi_0$. Or, more generally, one might define $\psi_{IPCW,n}$ as a solution of an estimating equation $P_n h(\psi)/g_0 = 0$, so that the influence curve of $\psi_{IPCW,n}$ is given by

$$D(P_0) = -\left[\frac{d}{d\psi_0} P_0 h(\psi_0)/g_0\right]^{-1} \frac{h(\psi_0)}{g_0}.$$

One can also apply the inverse weighting to the different components of a sum representation $h = \sum_j h_j$, so that $\psi_{IPCW,n}$ is defined as the solution of

$$0 = \frac{1}{n}\sum_{i=1}^{n} \sum_j \frac{h_j(\bar{O}_i(j),\psi)}{\prod_{l\in\mathcal{I},l<j} g_{0(l),0}}(\bar{O}_i(l)),$$

and its influence curve is the standardized version of $\sum_j h_j(\psi_0)/\prod_{l\in\mathcal{I}:l<j} g_{O(l),0}$.

Thus, for example, if we take the initial gradient of the form $D(P) = h/g_0 - \psi_0$, then we obtain the following explicit representation of the canonical gradient:

$$D^*(P) = E\left(\frac{h}{g_0} \mid O(0)\right) - \psi + \sum_{j \in \mathcal{I}^c} E\left(\frac{h}{g_0} \mid O(j), Pa(O(j))\right) - E\left(\frac{h}{g_0} \mid Pa(O(j))\right).$$

Let us assume that $Pa(O(j))$ includes all the intervention nodes $(O(l) : l \in \mathcal{I}(j))$, where, for notational convenience, we defined $\mathcal{I}(j) = \{l \in \mathcal{I} : l < j\}$. In this case, these conditional expectations can always be factorized as $1/\prod_{l \in \mathcal{I}(j)} g_{O(l),0}$, times a conditional expectation that is determined by the Q_0-factor only. For example, if $Pa(O(j)) = \bar{O}(j-1)$, then

$$E_0(h/g_0 \mid O(j), Pa(O(j))) = \frac{1}{\prod_{l \in \mathcal{I}(j)} g_{O(l),0}} E_{Q_0}\left(\sum_{o(l):l \in \mathcal{I}(j)^c} h \mid O(j), Pa(O(j))\right),$$

where the sum sums up over all possible realizations of the intervention nodes $(O(l) : l \in \mathcal{I}(j)^c)$ after j. We used notation $\mathcal{I}(j)^c = \{l \in \mathcal{I} : l \notin \mathcal{I}(j)\}$ for the intervention nodes with index larger than j. The conditional expectation corresponds with taking the expectation of h with respect to to the counterfactual distribution of $(O(l) : l > j)$ under which the intervention nodes $l \in \mathcal{I}(j)^c$ are set to a fixed value $o(l)$, summed up over all possible realizations of the intervention nodes. Thus,

$$E_{Q_0}\left(\sum_{o(l):l \in \mathcal{I}(j)^c} h \mid O(j), Pa(O(j))\right) = \sum_{o(l):l>j} h(o) \prod_{l>j} Q_{0,O(l)}(\bar{o}(l)) \prod_{l \in \mathcal{I}(j)^c} g^*_{O(l)}(\bar{o}(l)),$$

where $g^*_{O(l)}(\bar{o}(l)) = 1$. The same applies to the conditional expectation of h/g_0, given $Pa(L(j))$. Thus, this yields the following explicit representation of the canonical gradient:

$$\begin{aligned} D^*(P_0)(O) &= E_{Q_0}\left(\sum_{o(l):l \in \mathcal{I}} h \mid O(0)\right) - \Psi(Q_0) \qquad (A.5) \\ &+ \sum_{j \in \mathcal{I}^c} \frac{1}{\prod_{l \in \mathcal{I}(j)} g_{O(l),0}} \left\{ E_{Q_0}\left(\sum_{o(l):l \in \mathcal{I}(j)^c} h \mid O(j), Pa(O(j)\right) \right. \\ &\left. - E_{Q_0}\left(\sum_{o(l):l \in \mathcal{I}(j)^c} h \mid Pa(O(j)\right) \right\}. \end{aligned}$$

Representation of the efficient influence curve based on factorization of the likelihood in terms of binary conditional distributions. One can always represent a longitudinal data structure in terms of an ordered sequence of binary random variables. Let $L(k)$ be a particular variable measured as part of the longitudinal data structure. One can decompose $L(k)$ in terms of binaries $(L(k,l) : l = 1, \ldots, l_k)$. For example, for a univariate continuous covariate $L(k)$, we could partition its range, and set $L(k,l) = I(L(k) = (a_l, a_{l+1}])$ for the lth interval $(a_l, a_{l+1}]$ in the partitioning of its range. If $L(k)$ consists of several univariate covariates, then one first orders these covariates, discretizes each of them, and creates corresponding indicator variables. It follows that, given a certain ordering for all the binary variables coding $L(k)$, one can parameterize the conditional distribution of $L(k)$, given $Pa(L(k))$, as

$$P_{L(k)}(L(k)) = \prod_l P_{L(k,l)}(L(k,l) \mid Pa(L(k,l))),$$

where $Pa(L(k,l)) = (Pa(L(k)), L(k,1), \ldots, L(k,l-1))$.

Therefore, we will assume that this kind of preprocessing of the data has been carried out, so that $O(l)$ for $l \geq 1$ are all binary random variables, while the baseline covariates $O(0)$ can be a vector of continuous and discrete covariates. Since $O(l)$ is a binary variable, we can represent any function S of $O(l)$ and $(O(l))$ with conditional mean zero, given $Pa(O(l))$, as

$$S = \{S(1 \mid Pa(O(l)) - S(0 \mid Pa(O(l))\}\{O(l) - P_{O(l)}(1 \mid Pa(O(l)))\}.$$

The projection of an initial gradient D (or any other function) onto $T_{O(l)}(P)$ is given by

$$D^*_{O(l)}(P) = H^*_{O(l}(Pa(O(l)))\{O(l) - P_{O(l)}(1 \mid Pa(O(l))\},$$

where the term $H^*_{O(l)}$ in front of the residual of $O(l)$ plays a crucial role as the clever covariate in the TMLE algorithm, and is given by

$$H^*_{O(l}(Pa(O(l))) \equiv E(D \mid O(l) = 1, Pa(O(l))) - E(D \mid O(l) = 0, Pa(O(l))).$$

The efficient influence curve can thus be represented as

$$D^*(P) = \sum_{k \in \mathcal{I}^c} D^*_{O(k)}(P) = \sum_{k \in \mathcal{I}^c} H^*_{O(k)}(O(k) - P_{O(k)}(1)),$$

where we used short-hand notation. Above we showed that

$$H^*_{O(k)}(Q, g) = H^*_{O(k),g} H^*_{O(k),Q}$$

factorizes in a g-factor $H^*_{O(k),g}$ and a Q-factor $H^*_{O(k)}(Q)$ that equals a conditional expectation with respect to $\prod_{l>k} Q_{O(l)}$. It is of interest to note that $H^*_{O(k)}(Q)$ only depends on Q through the "future" factors $Q_{O(l)}$, $l > k$; This monotonicity property of H^* allows a particular convenient closed-form implementation of the TMLE, presented in detail in next section (van der Laan 2010a,b).

A.8 Factorization in Terms of Binary Conditional Distributions

Summary. The efficient influence curve allows one to construct an efficient estimator of the target parameter. The TMLE uses the efficient influence curve to define a parametric submodel through an initial estimator of the data-generating distribution, whose parametric maximum likelihood estimator defines the targeted update of the initial estimator, and the iterative application of this updating step defines the TMLE. We present such a TMLE for general longitudinal data structures, based on a factorization of the observed data density in terms of conditional distributions of binary random variables. The targeted updates can be computed based on standard logistic regression software.

The TMLE is defined by a choice of loss function $L(Q)$ and a submodel $\{Q(\epsilon) : \epsilon\}$ through Q at $\epsilon = 0$, where we will require that $\langle D^*(Q,g)\rangle \subset \langle < \frac{d}{d\epsilon} L(Q(\epsilon))\big|_{\epsilon=0}\rangle >$, where $D^*(Q,g)$ is the efficient influence curve at $P = Qg$, and, for a function $f = (f_1, \ldots, f_K)$, $\langle f\rangle$ denotes the linear span of the components of the function f in $L_0^2(P)$. We consider two such choices and thereby two types of TMLE that will be asymptotically equivalent, since both will solve the efficient influence curve estimating equation.

TMLE I. Let

$$P(\epsilon) = \prod_{j\in\mathcal{I}^c} Q(\epsilon)_{O(j)} \prod_{j\in\mathcal{I}} g_{O(j)},$$

where for $j \geq 1$

$$\text{logit}Q(\epsilon)_{O(j)}(1) = \text{logit}Q_{O(j)}(1) + \epsilon_j H^*_{O(j)}(Q,g)$$

is a logistic regression model using the logit of $P_{O(j)}(1 \mid Pa(O(j)))$ as offset, and $H^*_{O(j)} = H^*_{O(j)}(Q,g)$ as d-dimensional covariate of the same dimension as the target parameter ψ_0. Here ϵ_j is a subvector of ϵ. In addition, the fluctuation model $Q(\epsilon)_{O(0)}$ for the distribution of the baseline covariates $O(0)$ is chosen to have a score of $D^*_{O(0)}(Q)$ with respect to ϵ_0. Let $L(Q) = -\log Q$ be the log-likelihood loss function. Indeed, the score $\frac{d}{d\epsilon}\log P(\epsilon)$ of $P(\epsilon)$ at $\epsilon = 0$ equals or spans (if ϵ is multivariate) $D^*(P)$, and the score of $Q_{O(j)}(\epsilon_j)$ at $\epsilon_j = 0$ equals $D^*_{O(j)}(P)$. Thus, $\langle D^*(Q,g)\rangle \subset \langle < \frac{d}{d\epsilon} L(Q(\epsilon))\big|_{\epsilon=0}\rangle$.

Note that the maximum likelihood estimator of ϵ_j for a given initial $P = Qg$ can be determined with univariate logistic regression software regressing the binary $O(j)$ on the clever covariate $H^*_{O(j)}(Q,g)$, using the initial as offset. If one uses a common ϵ, i.e., $\epsilon_j = \epsilon$ for $j > 0$, then one can fit this single ϵ by regressing the binary outcome $O(j)$ on the clever covariate $H^*_{O(j)}(Q,g)$ based on a *pooled* data set, so that all j-specific logistic regressions with common parameter ϵ are fit in one run.

Consider an initial estimator $P_n^0 = Q_n^0 g_n^0$ of P_0, where $Q^0_{O(0),n}$ is the empirical distribution of the baseline covariates $O_i(0)$, $i = 1, \ldots, n$. We will use a separate ϵ_0 for the fluctutation of $Q^0_{O(0),n}$, and it will always equal 0, so that this empirical distribution will not be updated. Given the loss function $L(P) = -\log Q(P)$, we determine

$$\epsilon_n^1 = \arg\min_\epsilon P_n L(P_n^0(\epsilon)).$$

This results in the first-step TMLE $P_n^1 = P_n^0(\epsilon_n^1)$. This updating process $P_n^k = P_n^{k-1}(\epsilon_n^k)$, $k = 1, \ldots, K$, is iterated to convergence defined by $\epsilon_n^k \approx 0$. The final update is the TMLE of P_0 and is denoted by $P_n^* = Q_n^* g_n^0$. We note that g_n^0 is not updated in this process due to the fluctuation working model only allowing fluctuations of Q_n^0. The TMLE of ψ_0 is now defined as the substitution estimator $\Psi(P_n^*) = \Psi(Q_n^*)$.

One may use a separate ϵ_j for each factor $Q^0_{O(j),n}$, $j \geq 1$. These maximum likelihood estimators of ϵ_j can again be determined with logistic linear regression software, as remarked above. Importantly, one may determine the maximum likelihood estimators of these fluctuation parameters recursively, starting with the last factor and working backward to the first factor, always using the most recent update of the estimator of Q_0. In principle, one would start over at the last factor after having finished the update of the first factor and iterate this updating process until convergence. However, it follows that, with this recursive algorithm, the TMLE requires only one update per factor, and thereby converges in one step (representing one round from the last factor to the first factor, always using the most recent update for Q_0) and exists in analytic form. This algorithm is introduced and presented in detail in van der Laan (2010a). The convergence in one round is due to the above-mentioned monotonicity property of $H^*_{O(k)}(Q)$ with respect to its dependence on the Q-factors $Q_{O(k)}$ (van der Laan 2010a,b).

TMLE II. Let

$$P(\epsilon) = \prod_{j\in\mathcal{I}^c} Q(\epsilon)_{O(j)} \prod_{j\in\mathcal{I}} g_{O(j)},$$

where for $j \geq 1$

$$\text{logit}Q(\epsilon)_{O(j)}(1) = \text{logit}Q_{O(j)}(1) + \epsilon_j H_{O(j)}(Q)$$

is a logistic regression model using the logit of $P_{O(j)}(1 \mid Pa(O(j)))$ as offset, and $H_{O(j)}(Q)$ as d-dimensional covariate of the same dimension as the target parameter ψ_0. Recall that $H_{O(j)}(Q, g) = H_{O(j)}(Q)H_{O(j)}(g)$ and that we now only use the $H_{O(j)}(Q)$-factor. Here ϵ_j is a subvector of ϵ. In addition, the fluctuation model $Q(\epsilon)_{O(0)}$ for the distribution of the baseline covariates $O(0)$ is chosen to have a score of $D^*_{O(0)}(Q)$ with respect to ϵ_0.

Let $L_g(Q) = -\log Q_{O(0)} + \sum_{j\in\mathcal{I}^c, j\geq 1}\{\log Q_{O(j)}\}H_{O(j)}(g)$ be the *weighted* log-likelihood loss function. Since $H_{O(j)}(g)$ is only a function of O through $Pa(O(j))$, it follows that $\arg\min_Q P_0 L_g(Q) = Q_0$ and is thus always a valid loss function (even if g is misspecified). Indeed, the score $\frac{d}{d\epsilon}L_g(Q(\epsilon))$ of $Q(\epsilon)$ at $\epsilon = 0$ equals or spans (if ϵ is multivariate) $D^*(Q, g)$, and the score of $Q_{O(j)}(\epsilon_j)$ at $\epsilon_j = 0$ equals $D^*_{O(j)}(P)$. Thus, $\langle D^*(Q, g)\rangle \subset \langle < \frac{d}{d\epsilon}L_g(Q(\epsilon))\big|_{\epsilon=0}\rangle$.

Note that the weighted maximum likelihood estimator $\epsilon_{jn} = \arg\min_{\epsilon_j} P_n L_g(Q(\epsilon))$ of ϵ_j for a given initial $P = Qg$ can be determined with univariate logistic regression software regressing the binary $O(j)$ on the clever covariate $H^*_{O(j)}(Q)$, using the initial as offset, and using as weights $H^*_{O(j)}(g)(O_i)$, $i = 1, \ldots, n$. If one uses a common ϵ, i.e., $\epsilon_j = \epsilon$ for $j > 0$, then one can fit this single ϵ by regressing the binary outcome $O(j)$ on the clever covariate $H^*_{O(j)}(Q)$ based on a *pooled* data set, using corresponding weights $H^*_{O(j)}(g)(O_i)$, so that all j-specific logistic regressions with common parameter ϵ are fit in one run.

Consider an initial estimator $P_n^0 = Q_n^0 g_n^0$ of P_0, where $Q^0_{n,O(0)}$ is the empirical distribution of the baseline covariates $O_i(0)$, $i = 1, \ldots, n$. We will use a separate ϵ_0 for the fluctuation of $Q^0_{n,O(0)}$, and it will always equal 0, so that this empirical distribution will not be updated. Given the loss function $L(P) = -\log Q(P)$, we determine

$$\epsilon_n^1 = \arg\min_\epsilon P_n L_{g_n^0}(P_n^0(\epsilon)).$$

This results in the first-step TMLE $P_n^1 = P_n^0(\epsilon_n^1)$. This updating process $P_n^k = P_n^{k-1}(\epsilon_n^k)$, $k = 1, \ldots, K$, is iterated to convergence defined by $\epsilon_n^k \approx 0$. The final update is the TMLE of P_0 and is denoted with $P_n^* = Q_n^* g_n^0$. We note that g_n^0 is not updated in this process due to the fluctuation working model only allowing fluctuations of Q_n^0. The TMLE of ψ_0 is now defined as the substitution estimator $\Psi(P_n^*) = \Psi(Q_n^*)$.

One may use a separate ϵ_j for each factor $Q^0_{n,O(j)}$, $j \geq 1$, and determine the weighted maximum likelihood estimators of these fluctuation parameters recursively, starting with the last factor and working backward to the first factor, always using the most recent update. In principle, one would start over at the last factor after having finished the update of the first factor and iterate this updating process until convergence. However, as above for TMLE I, it follows that the TMLE requires only one update per factor and thereby converges in one step (representing one round from the last factor to the first factor) and exists in analytic form. We refer the interested reader to the forthcoming Stitelman and van der Laan (2011a) for implementation of TMLE II.

A.9 Efficient Influence Curve Collaborative Double Robustness

Summary. By definition, the canonical gradient is orthogonal to the scores generated by parametric submodels through the data-generating distribution that do not fluctuate the target parameter of interest. That is, the canonical gradient is orthogonal to the nuisance tangent space. This property implies that the canonical gradient at certain misspecified data-generating distributions will still have a mean of zero under the true data-generating distribution, which is called the robustness of the efficient influence curve with respect to misspecification of nuisance parameters. Robustness of the efficient influence curve translates into robustness of estimators that utilize the efficient influence curve, such as estimating-equation-based estimators and TMLEs. We prove a so-called collaborative double robustness property of the efficient influence curve, which is utilized in the C-TMLE.

Let us denote the intervention nodes by $A(j)$, and the nodes in between two subsequent intervention nodes $A(j-1)$ and $A(j)$ by $L(j)$ so that $O(0), \ldots, O(J)$ is represented as $L(0), A(0), \ldots, A(K), L(K+1)$. Our last representation (A.5) of the canonical gradient is then given by

$$
\begin{aligned}
D^*(P_0)(O) &= E_{Q_0}\left(\textstyle\sum_{\bar{a}} h \mid L(0)\right) - \Psi(Q_0) \\
&+ \textstyle\sum_{j=1}^{K+1} \frac{1}{g_{0,\bar{A}(j-1)}} \left\{ E_{Q_0}\left(\textstyle\sum_{\bar{a}(j,K)} h \mid L(j), Pa(L(j))\right) - E_{Q_0}\left(\textstyle\sum_{\bar{a}(j,K)} h \mid Pa(L(j))\right)\right\}, \quad \text{(A.6)}
\end{aligned}
$$

where $\bar{a}(j,K) = (a(j), \ldots, a(K))$. We will use this last representation (A.6) of the efficient influence curve to explicitly prove and demonstrate its collaborative double robustness property. Collaborative double robustness of $D^*(P_0) = D^*(Q_0, g_0)$ can be formulated as follows. For each $Q \in \mathcal{Q}$, and a corresponding specified set $\mathcal{G}(Q, P_0) \subset \mathcal{G}$, we have that

$$g \to P_0 D^*(Q, g)$$

is constant in $g \in \mathcal{G}(Q, P_0)$, and it equals zero if Q is such that $\Psi(Q) = \Psi(Q_0)$. Firstly, we note that $P_0 D^*(Q, g_0) = \psi_0 - \Psi(Q)$, which also follows from the proof below. This shows that $\mathcal{G}(Q, P_0)$ contains, at least, g_0. However, we wish to determine a richer set $\mathcal{G}(Q, P_0)$ of conditional distributions for which $P_0 D^*(Q, g) = \psi_0 - \Psi(Q)$. We will prove the following result.

Result 1 *We have $O = (A, L_A) \sim P_0 = Q_0 g_0$ is a missing-data structure on full-data $X = (L_a : a)$, where $g_0(A \mid X) = \prod_{j=0}^K g_{A(j),0}(A(j) \mid \bar{A}(j-1), X)$ satisfies SRA. We define a reduced collection of counterfactual random variables $X^{r*} = X^{r*}_{Q-Q_0} = (\bar{X}^{r*}_{Q-Q_0}(j) : j)$ (i.e., X^{r*} is a function of X), where*

$$\bar{X}^{r*}_{Q-Q_0}(j) = \Big\{E_{Q-Q_0}\Big(\textstyle\sum_{\bar{a}(j,K)} h \mid \bar{L}_{\bar{a}(j-1)}(j), \bar{A}(j-1) = \bar{a}(j-1)\Big) \\ -E_{Q-Q_0}\Big(\textstyle\sum_{\bar{a}(j,K)} h \mid \bar{L}_{\bar{a}(j-2)}(j-1), \bar{A}(j-1) = \bar{a}(j-1)\Big) : \bar{a}(j-1)\Big\}.$$

Let $\mathcal{G}(Q, P_0)$ be all true (i.e., under P_0) conditional distributions of $\bar{A}$, given a reduction X^r that implies X^{r*}; such true conditional probability distributions are related to g_0 by the relation $g_0(\bar{a} \mid X^r) = E_0(g_0(\bar{a} \mid X) \mid X^r)$. Then, for any Q and $g \in \mathcal{G}(Q, P_0)$, we have

$$P_0 D^*(Q, g) = \psi_0 - \Psi(Q).$$

Proof. Firstly, we note that for any g, $P_0 D^*(Q_0, g) = 0$, by simply conditioning on $Pa(L(j))$ for each j-specific term. Therefore, it suffices to determine the set of g for which $P_0\{D^*(Q, g) - D^*(Q_0, g)\} - \{\psi_0 - \Psi(Q)\} = 0$. The left-hand side equals

$$P_0 E_{Q-Q_0}\left(\textstyle\sum_{\bar{a}} h \mid L(0)\right) \\ + \textstyle\sum_{j=1}^{K+1} P_0 \frac{1}{g_{\bar{A}(j-1)}} \Big\{E_{Q-Q_0}\Big(\sum_{\bar{a}(j,K)} h \mid L(j), Pa(L(j))\Big) - E_{Q-Q_0}\Big(\sum_{\bar{a}(j,K)} h \mid Pa(L(j))\Big)\Big\}.$$

We now utilize the missing-data-structure representation of the observed data $O = (A, L_A)$ as a function of A and the collection of counterfactuals $X = (L_a : a)$, so that, for example, $L(j), Pa(L(j))$ is a function of $(\bar{L}_a(j) : a)$ and $\bar{A}(j-1)$. Thus, the conditional expectations with respect to $Q - Q_0$ are functions of $(\bar{L}_a(j) : a)$ and $\bar{A}(j-1)$. Specifically, at $\bar{A}(j-1) = \bar{a}(j-1)$, the first term of the j-th term equals $E_{Q-Q_0}(\sum_{\bar{a}(j,K)} h \mid \bar{L}_{\bar{a}(j-1)}(j), \bar{A}(j-1) = \bar{a}(j-1))$, and is thus indeed a function of the counterfactual $\bar{L}_{\bar{a}(j-1)}(j)$. Suppose that $g \in \mathcal{G}(Q, P_0)$. Consider now the expectation under P_0 for the jth term, and first take the conditional expectation of $\bar{A}(j-1)$ under g, thereby conditioning on a reduction X^r of X that is rich enough to make the E_{Q-Q_0} terms fixed. This yields

$$P_0 E_{Q-Q_0}\left(\textstyle\sum_{\bar{a}} h \mid L(0)\right) + \textstyle\sum_{j=1}^{K+1} P_0 \sum_{\bar{a}(j-1)} E_{Q-Q_0}\Big(\sum_{\bar{a}(j,K)} h \mid \bar{L}_a(j), \bar{a}(j-1)\Big) \\ - \textstyle\sum_{j=1}^{K+1} P_0 \sum_{\bar{a}(j-1)} E_{Q-Q_0}\Big(\sum_{\bar{a}(j,K)} h \mid \bar{L}_a(j-1), \bar{a}(j-1)\Big).$$

Note that this no longer depends on g. The jth term of the first sum and the $j+1$-th term of the second sum gives the following difference:

$$P_0 \sum_{\bar{a}(j-1)} \left\{ E_{Q-Q_0}\left(\sum_{\bar{a}(j,K)} h \mid \bar{L}_a(j), \bar{a}(j-1) \right) - \sum_{a(j)} E_{Q-Q_0}\left(\sum_{\bar{a}(j+1,K)} h \mid \bar{L}_a(j), \bar{a}(j) \right) \right\}.$$

By SRA we have that

$$E_{Q-Q_0}\left(\sum_{\bar{a}(j+1,K)} h \mid \bar{L}_a(j), \bar{a}(j) \right) = E_{Q-Q_0}\left(\sum_{\bar{a}(j+1,K)} h \mid \bar{L}_a(j), \bar{a}(j-1) \right).$$

We can now bring in the sum over $a(j)$:

$$\sum_{a(j)} E_{Q-Q_0}\left(\sum_{\bar{a}(j+1,K)} h \mid \bar{L}_a(j), \bar{a}(j-1) \right) = E_{Q-Q_0}\left(\sum_{\bar{a}(j,K)} h \mid \bar{L}_a(j), \bar{a}(j-1) \right).$$

This proves that the first term of the jth term and the second term of the $j+1$-th term cancel out. In particular, the very first term $P_0 E_{Q-Q_0}(\sum_{\bar{a}} h \mid L(0))$ cancels out with the second term for $j = 1$. This shows that we are left with a single term, namely, the $j = K+1$-th term of the first sum: $P_0 \sum_{\bar{a}(K)} E_{Q-Q_0}(h \mid \bar{L}_a(K+1), \bar{a}(K))$. However, the conditioning event (both under Q and Q_0) implies the value of h so that this conditional expectation E_{Q-Q_0} equals $h - h = 0$. This proves the desired collaborative double robustness. □

A.10 Example: TMLE with the Outcome Subject to Missingness

Suppose $O = (W, A, \Delta, Y^* = \Delta Y) \sim P_0$. The model for the probability distribution of (W, A, Y) is nonparametric so that the model for P_0 is nonparametric beyond the special structure that Y^* equals 0 when $\Delta = 0$. We have that the likelihood of O under P factorizes as $P = P_W P_A P_\Delta P_{Y^*}^{\Delta}$, using our notation for conditional distributions, where each of these conditional distributions is unspecified, which defines the statistical model $\mathcal{M}$ for P_0. Let $\Psi(P) = E_P[E_P(Y^* \mid W, A = 1, \Delta = 1) - E_P(Y^* \mid W, A = 0, \Delta = 1)]$ be the target parameter of P defined on this model $\mathcal{M}$. We wish to determine the efficient influence curve $D^*(P)$ of $\Psi : \mathcal{M} \to \mathbb{R}$ at a P, and subsequently a TMLE of ψ_0. We note that $P = Q \times g$, with g being the conditional distribution of (A, Δ), given W, $Q = Q_W Q_{Y^*}$, is a product of the other two factors of P, and we also note that $\Psi(P) = \Psi(Q)$.

As the initial gradient of the pathwise derivative of Ψ at $P = Q \times g$ in the model with g known, we can choose $D_{IPCW}(P) = H(g)Y - \Psi(P)$, where $H(g) = I(A = 1, \Delta = 1)/g(A, \Delta \mid W) - I(A = 0, \Delta = 1)/g(A, \Delta \mid W)$. This is a gradient in the model with g known, but its projection onto the tangent space of Q will yield the efficient influence curve in our model. One way to verify that D_{IPCW} is a valid IPCW gradient is to use a missing-data-structure representation of $O = (W, A, \Delta, \Delta Y_A)$ on full-data $X = (W, Y_0, Y_1)$, use the theory for CAR censored-data models as presented in van der Laan and Robins (2003) for determining IPCW gradients, and apply the invariance principle presented in Appendix A.7. That is, (1) assume CAR, $P(A, \Delta \mid X) = P(A, \Delta \mid W)$, (2) note that $\Psi(P) = EY_1 - EY_0$ is a parameter of full-data distribution, (3) note that the gradient of the full-data parameter $EY_1 - EY_0$ in the full-data model for X is given by $D^F(X) = (Y_1 - Y_0 - \psi)$, and (4) show that $E(D_{IPCW} \mid X) = D^F(X)$. We refer to van der Laan and Robins (2003) for detailed theory on determining gradients for censored-data models in terms of the gradients of the underlying full-data model.

The efficient influence curve $D^*(P)$ equals the projection of D_{IPCW} onto the tangent space of Q. The projection onto the tangent space of Q_W is given by $E(D_{IPCW} \mid W)$, and the projection onto the tangent space of $Q_{Y^*|W,A,\Delta}$ is given by $\Delta\{D_{IPCW} - E(D_{IPCW} \mid W, A, \Delta = 1)\}$. Since the sum of these two projections yields the efficient influence curve $D^*(P)$, we have

$$D^*(P) = H(g)(Y^* - \bar{Q}(W, A)) + \bar{Q}(W, 1) - \bar{Q}(W, 0) - \Psi(Q),$$

where $\bar{Q}(W, a) = E_P(Y^* \mid W, A = a, \Delta = 1)$.

The TMLE. If Y, and thereby Y^*, is binary, then we use the fluctuation working model $\text{logit}\bar{Q}(\epsilon) = \text{logit}\bar{Q} + \epsilon H(g)$ and use as loss function for $\bar{Q}$ the log-likelihood for a binary distribution given by $L(\bar{Q}) = \bar{Q}^{Y^*\Delta}(1 - \bar{Q})^{(1-Y^*)\Delta}$. We can also propose a fluctuation working model for Q_W with score $D_W = \Pi(D^* \mid T_W)$, but since we will use as initial estimator of $Q_{W,0}$ the empirical distribution, the maximum likelihood estimator of the fluctuation parameter will be zero, so that no updates of $Q_{W,n}$ will occur. Let $\bar{Q}_n^0$ be an initial estimator of $\bar{Q}_0$. One now computes $\epsilon_n = \arg\max_\epsilon P_n L(\bar{Q}_n^0(\epsilon))$, and one defines the TMLE update as $\bar{Q}_n^1 = \bar{Q}_n^0(\epsilon_n)$. Further iteration does not result in further updates, so that the TMLE Q_n^* is defined as $Q_n^* = (Q_{W,n}, \bar{Q}_n^1)$. The TMLE of ψ_0 is thus given by $\Psi(Q_n^*)$. If Y is continuous with values in $(0, 1)$, one can use the same loss function $L(\bar{Q})$ and fluctuation function for the conditional mean $\bar{Q}$. If Y is bounded in (a, b), then one can transform the outcome into $Y^* = (Y - a)/(b - a) \in (0, 1)$ and apply this same TMLE. For continuous Y, one can also use the squared error loss function and the linear fluctuation function, but such a fluctuation function is not guaranteed to respect known bounds on Y and is thus not generally recommended.

A.11 Example: TMLE of Causal Effect in a Two-Stage RCT

Let us denote the observed data structure on a randomly sampled patient from the target population with $O = (L(0), A(0), L(1), A(1), Y = L(2)) \sim P_0$. Let $Pa(L(j)) = (\bar{A}(j-1), \bar{L}(j-1))$ and $Pa(A(j)) = (\bar{L}(j), \bar{A}(j-1))$, where we make the convention that for $j = 0$, $\bar{A}(j-1)$ and $\bar{L}(j-1)$ are empty. The likelihood of O can be factorized as $P = P_{L(0)} \prod_{l=1}^{L} P_{L(1,l)} P_Y \prod_{j=0}^{1} P_{A(j)}$, where the first factors will be denoted by $Q_{L(0)}$, $Q_{L(1,l)}$, Q_Y, and the latter two factors denote the treatment mechanism and are denoted by $g_{A(j)}$, $j = 0, 1$.

Suppose our parameter of interest is the treatment-specific mean EY_d for a certain treatment rule d that assigns treatment $d_0(L(0))$ at time 0 and treatment $d_1(\bar{L}(1), A(0))$ at time 1. For example, $d_0(L(0)) = 1$ is a static treatment assignment, $L(1)$ is binary, and $d_1(\bar{L}(1), A(0)) = I(L(1) = 1)\times 1 + I(L(1) = 0)\times 0$ assigns treatment 1 if the patients responds well to the first line treatment (i.e., $L(1) = 1$) and treatment 0 if the patient does not respond well to the first line treatment. We note that any treatment rule can be viewed as a function of $\bar{L} = (L(0), L(1))$ only, and therefore we will use the shorter notation $d(\bar{L}) = (d_0(L(0)), d_1(\bar{L}))$ for the two rules at times 0 and 1.

Note that $EY_d = \Psi(Q)$ for a well-defined mapping Ψ. Specifically, we have $\Psi(Q) = E_{P_d}Y$, where the postintervention distribution P_d of $(L(0), L(1), L(2))$ is defined by the g-computation formula: $P_d(\bar{L}) = \prod_{j=0}^{2} Q_{L(j),d}(\bar{L}(j))$, where, for notational convenience, we used the notation $Q_{L(j),d}(\bar{L}(j)) = Q_{L(j)}(L(j) \mid \bar{L}(j-1), \bar{A}(j-1) = d(\bar{L}(j-1)))$. From this analytic expression it also follows that, even if Y is continuous, $\Psi(Q)$ only depends on the conditional distribution of Y through its mean. Using the techniques given above we obtain the following representation of the efficient influence curve.

Theorem A.2. *The efficient influence curve for* $\psi = EY_d$ *at the distribution* $P = Qg$ *of* O *can be represented as* $D^* = \Pi(D_{IPCW} \mid T_Q)$, *where* $D_{IPWC}(O) = \frac{I(\bar{A}=d(\bar{L}))}{\prod_{j=0}^{1} g_{A(j)}} Y - \psi$, T_Q *is the tangent space of* Q *in the nonparametric model, and* Π *denotes the projection operator onto* T_Q *in the Hilbert space* $L_0^2(P)$ *of square* P*-integrable functions of* O*, endowed with inner product* $\langle h_1, h_2 \rangle = E_P h_1 h_2(O)$. *We have that* $T_Q = \sum_{j=0}^{2} T_{Q_{L(j)}}$ *is the orthogonal sum of the tangent spaces* $T_{Q_{L(j)}}$ *of the* $Q_{L(j)}$*-factors, which consists of functions of* $(L(j), Pa(L(j)))$ *with conditional mean zero, given the parents* $Pa(L(j))$ *of* $L(j)$, $j = 0, 1, 2$. *Recall that we also denote* $L(2)$ *by* Y. *Let* $D_{L(j)} = \Pi(D^* \mid T_{Q_{L(j)}})$, $j = 0, 1, 2$. *We have* $D_{L(1)} = \sum_{l=1}^{L} D_{L(1),l}$, *where* $D_{L(1),l} = \Pi(D \mid T_{Q_{L(1,l)}})$, *and*

$$D_{L(0)}(O) = E(Y_d \mid L(0)) - \psi,$$

$$D_{L(1,l)}(O)) = \frac{I(A(0) = d_0(L(0)))}{g_{A(0)}} \{C_{L(1,l)}(1) - C_{L(1,l)}(0)\} \{L(1,l) - Q_{L(1,l)}(1)\},$$

$$D_{L(2)}(O) = \frac{I\left(\bar{A} = d(\bar{L})\right)}{\prod_{j=0}^{1} g_{A(j)}} \left\{L(2) - E(L(2) \mid \bar{L}(1), \bar{A}(1))\right\},$$

where, for $\delta \in \{0, 1\}$, $C_{L(1,l)}(\delta) = E(Y_d \mid Pa(L(1,l)), L(1,l) = \delta)$. *We also note that:* $E(Y_d \mid L(0), A(0) = d_0(L(0)), L(1)) = E(Y \mid \bar{L}(1), \bar{A} = d(\bar{L}))$.

The TMLE. Consider now an initial estimator $Q_{L(j),n}$ of each $Q_{L(j)}$, $j = 0, 1, 2$. We will estimate the first marginal probability distribution $Q_{L(0)}$ of $L(0)$ with the empirical distribution of $L_i(0)$, $i = 1, \ldots, n$. We use the log-likelihood loss function $L(Q_{L(0)}) = -\log Q_{L(0)}$ and consider a submodel $Q_{L(0)}(\epsilon_0)$ with score $D_{L(0)}(Q)$ defined above.

We can estimate the conditional distributions of the binary $L(1,l)$ with loss-based learning based on the loss function $L(Q_{L(1)}) = -\sum_l \log Q_{L(1,l)}$. For example, one could use logistic regression machine learning algorithms, $l = 1, \ldots, L$, where one could also smooth in l. Similarly, we can estimate the conditional mean of $Y = L(2)$ with loss-based learning using the log-likelihood or squared error loss function. We will now define fluctuations of this initial estimator $Q_{L(1),n}$ and $Q_{L(2),n}$. Firstly, let

$$\text{logit}\bar{Q}_{L(1,l),n}(\epsilon_1) = \text{logit}\bar{Q}_{L(1,l),n} + \epsilon_1 H^*_{L(1,l)}(Q_n, g_n)$$

be the fluctuation function of the conditional probability $\bar{Q}_{L(1,l),n} = Q_{L(1,l),n}(1)$ of $L(1,l) = 1$ with fluctuation parameter ϵ_1, where we added the covariate $H^*_{L(1,l)}(Q,g) = \{I(A(0) = d(L(0)))/g_{A(0)}\}(C_{L(1,l)}(1) - C_{L(1,l)}(0))$ defined above in Theorem A.2. This defines a fluctuation working model $Q_{L(1),n}(\epsilon_1)$, and we can use the log-likelihood $-\log Q_{L(1)}$ as loss function. In the special case where $L(1)$ is itself already a binary variable, we have

$$H^*_{L(1)}(L(0), A(0)) = \frac{I(A(0)=d_0(L(0)))}{g_{A(0)}(d_0(L(0))|L(0))}\{C_{L(1)}(Q)(1) - C_{L(1)}(Q)(0)\},$$

where $C_{L(1)}(Q)(\delta) = E_Q(Y_d \mid L(0), A(0), L(1) = \delta)$. We refer to these covariate choices as *clever* covariates, since they represent a covariate choice that identifies a least favorable fluctuation model, thereby providing the desired targeted bias reduction. Similarly, if $Y = L(2)$ is binary, then let $\text{logit}\bar{Q}_{L(2)n}(\epsilon_2) = \text{logit}\bar{Q}_{L(2)n} + \epsilon_2 H^*_{L(2)}(Q_n, g_n)$, where the added clever covariate $H^*_{L(2)}(Q,g)(\bar{L}(1), \bar{A}(1)) = I(\bar{A} = d(\bar{L}))/\prod_{j=0}^{1} g_{A(j)}$. If Y is continuous with values in $(0,1)$, then we can use the same "log-likelihood" loss function $L(\bar{Q}_Y) = -\{Y \log \bar{Q}_Y + (1-Y)\log(1-\bar{Q}_Y)\}$, and fluctuation working model as we use for binary Y, and this yields then also a TMLE for Y bounded in (a,b). As a side remark, one may also select the squared error loss function for $\bar{Q}_Y$ and linear fluctuation working model $\bar{Q}_{L(2),n} + \epsilon H_{L(2)}(Q_n, g_n)$. We note that the above fluctuation function and use of the loss function $L(Q) = L(Q_{L(0)}) - \sum_l \log Q_{L(1,l)} + L(\bar{Q}_Y)$ indeed satisfies that the score of $\epsilon = (\epsilon_0, \epsilon_1, \epsilon_2)$ at $\epsilon = 0$ spans the efficient influence curve $D^*(Q_n, g_n)$, as presented in Theorem A.2 above.

Let $\epsilon_n = \arg\max_\epsilon \prod_{j=1}^{2} \prod_{i=1}^{n} Q_{L(j),n}(\epsilon)(O_i)$ be the maximum likelihood estimator of ϵ according to the working fluctuation model. If one uses separate ϵ for different factors of Q, then one could also obtain a separate maximum likelihood estimator of ϵ_j for each factor $j = 1, 2$, or even an $\epsilon_{1,l}$ for each factor $Q_{L(1,l)}$ indexed by l. This process is now iterated to convergence, which defines the TMLE (Q^*_n, g_n), starting at initial estimator (Q_n, g_n). Note that this does not involve updating of g_n. The TMLE of ψ is now given by $\Psi(Q^*_n)$.

If Y is binary or continuous in $(0,1)$, then a single/common ϵ_n defined above requires applying a single logistic regression applied to a repeated measures data set with one line of data for each of the factors of the likelihood, creating a clever covariate column that alternates the clever covariates $H_{L(1,l)}$ and $H_{L(2)}$, and uses the corresponding offsets. Thus, in both cases (separate or common ϵ), the update step can be carried out with a simple univariate logistic regression maximum likelihood estimator. Computing a MLE of a common ϵ in the case where we use the linear fluctuation working model and squared error loss function for Q_Y requires some programming.

A one-step closed-form TMLE. For the sake of illustration, suppose $L(1)$ is itself binary. If one uses a separate $\epsilon_{L(j)}$ for $j = 0, 1, 2$, first carry out the TMLE update for $Q_{L(2),n}$ and use this updated $Q^*_{L(2),n}$ in the clever covariate required to compute the targeted update of $Q_{L(1),n}$. Then we obtain a TMLE algorithm that converges in these two simple updating steps, representing a single-step update of Q^*_n and

TMLE $\Psi(Q_n^*)$. Similarly, this particular one-step TMLE involving iterative updating (starting with the last factor of the likelihood and ending with the update of the first factor) generalizes to general $L(1)$ and general longitudinal data structures (van der Laan 2010a), and was presented above.

A.12 Example: TMLE with Right-Censored Survival Time

Let $O = (W, A, dN(t), dA_c(t), t = 1, \ldots, \tau) \sim P_0$, where $dN(t) = I(\tilde{T} = t, \Delta = 1)$ and $dA_c(t) = I(\tilde{T} = t, \Delta = 0)$, are indicators of an observed failure and observed censoring event at time t, respectively. The likelihood of O under P factorizes as $P = Q_W g_A \prod_t Q_{dN(t)} \prod_t g_{dA_c(t)}$, using our short-hand notation, where $Pa(dN(t)) = (W, A, \bar{N}(t-1), \bar{A}_c(t-1))$, $Pa(A) = W$, and $Pa(dA_c(t)) = (W, A, \bar{A}_c(t-1), \bar{N}(t))$. The model for P_0 is nonparametric on the Q_0-factor but may incorporate assumptions about $g_0 = g_{0,A} \prod_t g_{0,dA_c(t)}$. The efficient influence curve of a parameter of Q is the same in any such a model. Let $\Psi(P) = E_P[S(t_0 \mid A = 1, W) - S(t_0 \mid A = 0, W)]$, where $S(t_0 \mid A = a, W) = \prod_{t=0}^{t_0}(1 - \bar{Q}_{dN(t)}(t \mid W, A = a))$, and $\bar{Q}_{dN(t)}(t \mid W, A) = E_P(dN(t) \mid \tilde{T} \geq t, W, A)$ would be equal to the conditional hazard of an underlying time-to-event T under a CAR-model (see below). We wish to determine the efficient influence curve $D^*(P)$ of this target parameter at P and define a TMLE.

As initial gradient in the model in which g is known, we can choose

$$D_{IPCW} = \frac{I(A=1, \bar{A}_c(t_0)=\bar{0}(t_0)) - I(A=0, \bar{A}_c(t_0)=\bar{0}(t_0))}{g_A \prod_{t \leq t_0} g_{dA_c(t)}} I(\tilde{T} > t_0) - \Psi(Q).$$

One way to show that this is indeed a gradient in the model with g known is (based on van der Laan and Robins 2003) (1) to represent O as a missing-data structure on full data structure $X = (W, T_0, T_1)$ with censoring process $(A, I(C = t) : t = 1, \ldots, \tau)$, so that $T = T_A$, $dN(t) = I(T_A = t, C \geq t)$, and $dA_c(t) = I(C = t, T_A > t)$; (2) assuming CAR on the conditional distribution of (A, A_c), given X, so that $P(A \mid X) = P(A \mid W)$ and $P(dA_c(t) \mid X, \bar{A}_c(t-1), A) = P(dA_c(t) \mid \bar{A}_c(t-1), \bar{N}(t), W, A)$; (3) noting that $\Psi(P) = P(T_1 > t_0) - P(T_0 > t_0)$ and that the gradient of this full-data parameter in the full data model equals $D^F(X) = I(T_1 > t_0) - I(T_0 > t_0) - \Psi(P)$; and (4) showing that $E(D_{IPCW} \mid X) = D^F(X)$. Such a CAR censored-data representation of the observed data model provides no restrictions on the statistical model, so that its only role is to provide a working model for carrying out calculations, such as the calculation of an efficient influence curve (Appendix A.7).

The efficient influence curve $D^*(P)$ equals the projection of $D_{IPCW}(P)$ onto the tangent space of $Q = Q(P)$. The projection onto the tangent space $T_W(P)$ of Q_W equals $E_P(D_{IPCW} \mid W)$, which equals $S(t_0 \mid A = 1, W) - S(t_0 \mid A = 0, W) - \Psi(Q)$. The projection onto the tangent space $T_{dN(t)}(P)$ of $Q_{dN(t)}$ is given by $H^*_{dN(t)}(dN(t) - \bar{Q}_{dN(t)}(t \mid W, A))$, where

$$H^*_{dN(t)} = E_P(D_{IPCW} \mid dN(t) = 1, Pa(dN(t))) - E_P(D_{IPCW} \mid dN(t) = 0, Pa(dN(t))).$$

Since $Pa(dN(t)) = (W, A, \bar{N}(t-1), \bar{A}_c(t-1))$ and the projection onto $T_{dN(t)}$ equals zero if $\tilde{T} \leq t-1$, it follows that we can condition on $\tilde{T} \geq t$ in these two conditional expectations. For $t \leq t_0$ we have $E_P(D_{IPCW} \mid W, A, dN(t) = 1, \tilde{T} \geq t) = 0$, since $dN(t) = 1$ implies $\tilde{T} \leq t_0$ so that $D_{IPCW} = 0$. For $t > t_0$, this same conditional expectation reduces to $(I(A=1) - I(A=0)) / \left(g_A \prod_{s \leq t_0} g_{dA_c(s)}(0)\right)$. Regarding the first conditional expectation in the expression for $H_{dN(t)}$, we conclude

$$E_P(D_{IPCW} \mid W, A, dN(t) = 1, \tilde{T} \geq t) = I(t > t_0) \frac{I(A=1) - I(A=0)}{g_A \prod_{s \leq t_0} g_{dA_c(s)}(0)}.$$

Let us now consider the second conditional expectation in $H_{dN(t)}$. If $t > t_0$, then this term equals the first term we just displayed. For $t \leq t_0$, we obtain

$$\begin{aligned} &E_P(D_{IPCW} \mid W, A, dN(t) = 0, \tilde{T} \geq t) \\ &\quad = \frac{I(A=1)-I(A=0)}{g_A \prod_{s \leq t-1} g_{dA_C(s)}(0)} E_P\left(\frac{I(\bar{A}_c(t,t_0)=0, \tilde{T} > t_0)}{\prod_{s \in [t,t_0]} g_{dA_C(s)}} \mid W, A, \tilde{T} \geq t, dN(t) = 0 \right). \end{aligned}$$

In the CAR censored-data model representation, the latter conditional expectation equals $E_P(I(T > t_0) \mid W, A, T > t)$. Regarding the second term, we conclude:

$$\begin{aligned} &E_P(D_{IPCW} \mid W, A, dN(t) = 0, \tilde{T} \geq t) \\ &\quad = I(t > t_0) \frac{I(A=1)-I(A=0)}{g_A \prod_{s \leq t_0} g_{dA_C(s)}(0)} + I(t \leq t_0) \frac{I(A=1)-I(A=0)}{g_A \prod_{s \leq t-1} g_{dA_C(s)}(0)} \frac{S(t_0 \mid W,A)}{S(t \mid W,A)}. \end{aligned}$$

Thus, we have shown that

$$H^*_{dN(t)} = -I(t \leq t_0) \frac{I(A=1)-I(A=0)}{g_A \prod_{s \leq t-1} g_{dA_C(s)}(0)} \frac{S(t_0 \mid W,A)}{S(t \mid W,A)}$$

and that the efficient influence curve can be represented as

$$D^*(P) = \sum_{t=1}^{\tau} H_{dN(t)}(dN(t) - \bar{Q}_{dN(t)}) + S(t_0 \mid A = 1, W) - S(t_0 \mid A = 0, W) - \Psi(Q).$$

The TMLE. In our chapters on TMLE for time-to-event outcomes, we presented the TMLE based on this representation of the efficient influence curve, involving TMLE updates of an estimator of the conditional hazard $\bar{Q}_{dN(t)}$ using a logistic regression working fluctuation model with a time-dependent clever covariate $H^*_{dN(t)}$.

A.13 Example: TMLE of a Causal Effect Among the Treated

Suppose we observe n i.i.d. observations of $O = (W, A, Y) \sim P_0$, W baseline covariates, subsequently assigned binary treatment A, and final outcome Y of interest. Suppose the statistical model is nonparametric and we wish to estimate the following parameter of the data-generating distribution P_0 of $O = (W, A, Y)$:

$$\Psi(P_0) = E_0 \left[E_0(Y \mid A = 1, W) - E_0(Y \mid A = 0, W) \mid A = 0 \right].$$

Another way of representing this parameter is $\Psi(P_0) = -E_0(Y - E(Y \mid A = 1, W) \mid A = 0)$, i.e., among the nontreated in the population, one evaluates the outcome minus the predicted outcome if, contrary to fact, one would have been treated, and one takes the population average of all these differences over all nontreated subjects. Under an SCM, $W = f_W(U_W)$, $A = f_A(W, U_A)$, $Y = f_Y(W, A, U_Y)$, and the randomization assumption stating that U_A is independent of U_Y, one can interpret this parameter as a causal effect among the nontreated $E(Y_1 - Y_0 \mid A = 0)$. Suppose one wants to estimate the effect among the treated, given by

$$\Psi_1(P_0) = E_0[E_0(Y \mid A = 1, W) - E_0(Y \mid A = 0, W) \mid A = 1],$$

which under the above-mentioned SCM can be represented as $E(Y_1 - Y_0 \mid A = 1)$. Switching the roles of $A = 1$ and $A = 0$ in the formulas below provides the efficient influence curve and TMLE of $-\Psi_1(P_0)$. We make this explicit below.

Note that a probability distribution P is determined by the marginal distribution P_W of W, the conditional distribution $P_{A|W}$ of A, given W, and the conditional distribution $P_{Y|A,W}$ of Y, given A, W. The parameter $\Psi(P)$ depends on P through both $P_W, P_{Y|A,W}$ as well as the treatment mechanism $P_{A|W}$. We will denote the treatment mechanism by $g = g(P)$ and the other two factors of the likelihood by Q_W and $Q_{Y|A,W}$. We will use the notation $\bar{Q}(A, W) = E_P(Y \mid A, W)$ and $\bar{Q}_0$ for this conditional mean of Y under P_0.

Efficient influence curve of target parameter. Firstly, consider the parameter $P \to \Psi(P)(1) = E_P(E_P(Y \mid A = 1, W) \mid A = 0)$. Using the functional delta method technique presented in Appendix A.3, it follows that the efficient influence curve of this parameter at P is given by

$$D_1^*(P) = \frac{I(A=1)}{P(A=0)} \frac{g(0|W)}{g(1|W)}(Y - \bar{Q}(1, W)) + \frac{I(A=0)}{P(A=0)}(\bar{Q}(1, W) - \Psi(P)(1)).$$

Similarly, the efficient influence curve of $\Psi(P)(0) = E_P(E_P(Y \mid A = 0, W) \mid A = 0)$ at P is given by

$$D_0^*(P) = \frac{I(A=0)}{P(A=0)}(Y - \bar{Q}(0, W)) + \frac{I(A=0)}{P(A=0)}(\bar{Q}(0, W) - \Psi(P)(0)).$$

Thus the efficient influence curve of $\Psi(P) = \Psi(P)(1) - \Psi(P)(0)$ is given by

$$D^*(P) = \left\{\frac{I(A=1)}{P(A=0)} \frac{g(0|W)}{g(1|W)} - \frac{I(A=0)}{P(A=0)}\right\}(Y - \bar{Q}(A, W)) + \frac{I(A=0)}{P(A=0)}\left\{\bar{Q}(1, W) - \bar{Q}(0, W) - \Psi(P)\right\}.$$

The efficient influence curve of $\Psi(P) = E_P(E_P(Y \mid A = 1, W) - E_P(Y \mid A = 0, W) \mid A = 1)$ is obtained by changing the roles of $A = 1$ and $A = 0$, and assigning a minus sign, giving

$$D^*(P) = \left\{\frac{I(A=1)}{P(A=1)} - \frac{I(A=0)}{P(A=1)} \frac{g(1|W)}{g(0|W)}\right\}(Y - \bar{Q}(A, W)) + \frac{I(A=1)}{P(A=1)}\left\{\bar{Q}(1, W) - \bar{Q}(0, W) - \Psi(P)\right\}.$$

Collaborative double robustness of efficient influence curve. This efficient influence curve of $\Psi(P)$ can be represented as an estimating function $D^*(Q, g, \psi)$, where we suppress the dependence on the scalar $P(A = 0)$ and use notation $Q = (Q_W, \bar{Q})$.

We note that this estimating function is double robust in the sense that it is an unbiased estimating function for ψ_0, if either Q is correctly specified or g is correctly specified. Formally, this is stated as

$$P_0 D^*(Q, g, \psi_0) = 0 \text{ if } Q = Q_0 \text{ or } g = g_0,$$

and $g(1 \mid W) > 0$, a.e. This double robustness result can be explicitly verified.

In fact, we can establish a stronger collaborative double robustness, defined as follows. Let $W(Q)$ be a subset/reduction of W so that conditioning on $W(Q)$ also fixes $(\bar{Q} - \bar{Q}_0)(a, W)$ for $a \in \{0, 1\}$. Then, for all Q and corresponding $g_0(Q) = P(A = \cdot \mid W(Q))$ for such a $W(Q) \subset W$, we have

$$P_0 D^*(Q, g_0(Q), \psi_0) = 0.$$

Note that this implies, in particular, $P_0 D^*(Q_0, g) = 0$ for all g, since, if $Q = Q_0$, then we can select $W(Q)$ as the empty set. Thus, g_0 only needs to adjust for the covariates that still play a role in $\bar{Q} - \bar{Q}_0$. This can also be stated as the following collaborative double robustness of the efficient influence curve $D^*(P) = D^*(Q, g)$. For a given Q, let $\mathcal{G}(Q, P_0)$ be the set of conditional distributions under P_0 of A, given $W(Q)$ as defined above. For each Q, and for each $g \in \mathcal{G}(Q, P_0)$, we have that $P_0 D^*(Q, g) = 0$ implies $\Psi(Q, g) = \psi_0$.

Implications for double robust efficient estimation. One could define a closed-form asymptotically efficient double robust estimator $\psi_{DR,n}$ as the solution of the efficient influence curve estimating equation

$$0 = P_n D^*(Q_n, g_n, \psi),$$

given estimators Q_n of Q_0 and g_n of g_0. We can also compute a collaborative double robust asymptotically efficient TMLE that has various previously presented advantages. In particular, it is guaranteed to be a substitution estimator, and it will only pursue adjustment in g_n that remains helpful after the adjustment carried out by Q_n, thereby resulting in more effective adjustment sets and bias reduction.

A TMLE is a substitution estimator $\Psi(P_n^*)$, where the estimated data-generating distribution P_n^* is such that it solves the efficient influence curve estimating equation

$$0 = P_n D^*(Q(P_n^*), g(P_n^*), \Psi(P_n^*)).$$

As a consequence, the substitution estimator (TMLE) $\Psi(P_n^*)$ is double robust and efficient, and collaborative double robust if one uses the C-TMLE that builds g_n based on the loss function for $\bar{Q}_0$.

The TMLE. Let us now present the TMLE that maps an initial estimator P_n^0 into a targeted fit P_n^*. Suppose Y is binary. Given an initial estimator $\bar{Q}_n^0$ of $\bar{Q}_0$, an initial estimator g_n^0 of g_0, and empirical distribution $Q_{W,n}$ of W, we define the parametric working model for fluctuating the initial estimator: $\text{logit}\bar{Q}_n^0(\epsilon_1) = \text{logit}\, \bar{Q}_n^0 + \epsilon_1 C_1(g_n^0)$, and $\text{logit}(g_n^0(\epsilon_2)(0 \mid W)) = \text{logit}(g_n^0(0 \mid W)) + \epsilon_2 C_2(P_n^0)(W)$, where these two clever covariates are defined as

$$C_1(g) = \left\{ \frac{I(A=1)}{P(A=0)} \frac{g(0 \mid W)}{g(1 \mid W)} - \frac{I(A=0)}{P(A=0)} \right\},$$

$$C_2(P) = \frac{1}{P(A=0)} \left\{ \bar{Q}(P)(1,W) - \bar{Q}(P)(0,W) - \Psi(P) \right\}.$$

Let $Q_{W,n}(\epsilon_0)$ be a parametric working model with score $D_W^* = g(0 \mid W)(\bar{Q}(1,W) - \bar{Q}(0,W) - \Psi(P))$. These three one-dimensional working models represent a parametric working model $\{P_n^0(\epsilon) : \epsilon\}$ for fluctuating P_n^0. We use the log-likelihood loss function $L(P) = -\log P$. We estimate ϵ with maximum likelihood. Note that $\epsilon_{0n} = 0$, ϵ_1 is estimated with standard linear logistic regression fixing $\bar{Q}_n$ as an offset, and ϵ_2 is estimated with standard linear logistic regression fixing $g_n(0 \mid W)$ as offset in the logistic regression model for $P(A = 0 \mid W)$.

This maximum likelihood estimator $\epsilon_n^1 = (\epsilon_{0n}, \epsilon_{1n}, \epsilon_{2n})$ now defines an update $P_n^1 = P_n^0(\epsilon_n^1)$. The targeted maximum likelihood updating is iterated to convergence, and the final P_n^*, identified by a $\bar{Q}_n^*, g_n^*$ and the empirical distribution $Q_{W,n}$, is called the TMLE of the distribution P_0, while $\Psi(P_n^*)$ is called the TMLE of ψ_0. We have that the TMLE $\Psi(P_n^*)$ solves the efficient influence curve estimating equation, as presented above. We can use machine learning/super learning to obtain the initial P_n^0 (i.e., $\bar{Q}_n^0$ and g_n^0).

Since P_n^* solves, in particular,

$$0 = \tfrac{1}{n} \textstyle\sum_{i=1}^n \tfrac{I(A_i=0)}{P(A=0)} \left\{ \bar{Q}_n^*(1,W_i) - \bar{Q}_n^*(0,W_i) - \Psi(P_n^*) \right\},$$

it follows that the TMLE $\Psi(P_n^*)$ can also be evaluated as

$$\Psi(P_n^*) = \tfrac{1}{\sum_i I(A_i=0)} \textstyle\sum_i I(A_i = 0) \left\{ \bar{Q}_n^*(1,W_i) - \bar{Q}_n^*(0,W_i) \right\},$$

i.e., as the empirical mean of $\bar{Q}_n^*(1,W) - \bar{Q}_n^*(0,W)$ among the observations with $A_i = 0$. Apparently, in this evaluation of $\Psi(P_n^*)$, g_n^* can be ignored.

Collaborative TMLE. The collaborative double robustness of the efficient influence curve allows us to also implement the C-TMLE as presented in Chap. 19. A TMLE requires iterative estimation of $\bar{Q}_0$ and g_0, so that other parts of the probability distribution can be ignored. In this case, given the initial estimator Q_n^0 (thus $\bar{Q}_n^0$ and empirical distribution $Q_{W,n}$ of W), one starts with a g_n^0 as an intercept model, and one selects the main term extension g_n^1 of g_n^0 whose TMLE yields the best fit of $\bar{Q}_0$ as measured by the loss function for $\bar{Q}_0$ used by the TMLE. This process is iterated, thereby building a sequence of main term regression fits for g_0 and corresponding TMLEs P_n^k, $k = 1, \ldots, K$. If at a certain k, the loss-function-specific fit of the corresponding TMLE of $\bar{Q}_0$ is not increasing relative to the $k-1$-th TMLE, then we accept the previously selected TMLE, reject the kth TMLE, and proceed as before but now use the $k-1$-th TMLE as initial estimator in the next TMLEs. These subsequent TMLEs will still keep updating the previous g_0 fit by adding main terms.

In this manner, the algorithm generates a sequence of candidate TMLEs indexed by the number of main terms that were included in the g_0 fit. The empirical risk (with respect to the $\bar{Q}_0$ loss function) of these TMLEs decreases with the number of main terms. This number of main terms, and thereby the TMLE, is selected with ($\bar{Q}_0$-) loss-function-specific cross-validation, possibly penalizing the cross-validated risk, as proposed in van der Laan and Gruber (2010) and presented in Chap. 19. The main terms can include propensity score dimension reductions indexed by different adjustment sets, so that the above algorithm is still arbitrarily nonparametric in fitting g_0. We refer the reader to Appendix A.17 for a detailed understanding of the C-TMLE.

A.14 Example: TMLE Based on an Instrumental Variable

Suppose we observe $O = (W, R, A, Y) \sim P_0$. Consider the following SCM: $W = f_W(U_W)$, $R = f(W, U_R)$, $A = f(W, R, U_A)$, $Y = f_Y(W, R, A, U_Y)$. This SCM allows us to define counterfactuals corresponding with setting R and setting simultaneously (R, A), and corresponding postintervention distributions. It is assumed that U_R is independent of U_Y, given W, which means that R is randomized, conditional on W. R plays the role of an instrumental variable that can be used to estimate the causal effect of a treatment A on Y, even if there are unmeasured variables that affect both A and Y (i.e., not captured by W). We consider the following causal parameter of the distribution of counterfactuals corresponding with interventions on R:

$$\Psi_r^F(P_{X,0}) = \frac{E_0 Y(R = r) - EY(R = 0)}{E_0 A(R = r) - E_0 A(R = 0)}. \tag{A.7}$$

By the randomization assumption, this parameter is identifiable from P_0 through the following statistical parameter:

$$\Psi_r(P_0) = \frac{E_0(E_0(Y \mid W, R = r) - E_0(Y \mid W, R = 0))}{E_0(E_0(A \mid W, R = r) - E_0(A \mid W, R = 0))}.$$

We will use the following notation: $\bar{Q}_0(W, r) = E_0(Y \mid W, R = r)$, $\bar{g}_0(W, r) = E_0(A \mid W, R = r)$, $Q_{W,0}(w) = P_0(W = w)$, and $Q_0 = (Q_{W,0}, \bar{Q}_0)$.

Causal interpretation of $\psi_{r,0}$. If the exclusion restriction given by $f_Y(W, R, A, U_Y) = f_Y(W, A, U_Y)$ holds, and $f_Y(W, A, U_Y) = f_Y(W, 0, U_Y) + \beta_0 A$, then it follows that $\beta_0 = \Psi_{r,1}^F(P_{X,0})$. Since the causal interpretation of $\psi_{r,0}$ is constant in r, we can define as estimand a weighted average of the r-specific parameters $\Psi_r(P_0)$, such as $\Psi(P_0) = \sum_{r>0} h(r)\Psi_r(P_0)$, where $\sum_{r>0} h(r) = 1$.

Efficient influence curve. Since $\Psi_r(P_0)$ is a simple function of $E_0 Y(r)$, $E_0 Y(0)$, $E_0 A(r)$, and $E_0 A(0)$, and we know the efficient influence curves of these parameters, the delta method provides us with the efficient influence curve of Ψ_r at P:

$$
\begin{aligned}
D_r^*(P) = & \frac{1}{E\{A(r)-A(0)\}} \frac{I(R=r)-I(R=0)}{g(R \mid W)}(Y-\bar{Q}(W,R)) \\
& -\frac{E(Y(r)-Y(0))}{E^2(A(r)-A(0))} \frac{I(R=r)-I(R=0)}{g(R \mid W)}(A-\bar{g}(W,R)) \\
& +\frac{1}{E\{A(r)-A(0)\}}\left\{\bar{Q}(W,r)-\bar{Q}(W,0)-E(Y(r)-Y(0))\right\} \\
& -\frac{E(Y(r)-Y(0))}{E^2(A(r)-A(0))}\{\bar{g}(W,1)-\bar{g}(W,0)-E(A(r)-A(0))\}.
\end{aligned}
$$

Again, by the δ-method, the efficient influence curve of Ψ is given by $D^* = \sum_{r>0} h(r) D_r^*$.

Double robustness of r-specific efficient influence curve. The solution of the equation $P_0 D_r^*(\bar{Q}, \bar{g}, g_{R,0}, \psi_r) = 0$ in ψ_r equals

$$
\begin{aligned}
\psi_r &= \frac{P_0\left\{\frac{I(R=r)-I(R=0)}{g_0(R|W)}(Y-\bar{Q}(W,R))+\bar{Q}(W,r)-\bar{Q}(W,0)\right\}}{P_0\left\{\frac{I(R=r)-I(R=0)}{g_0(R|W)}(A-\bar{g}(W,R))+\bar{g}(W,r)-\bar{g}(W,0)\right\}} \\
&= \frac{P_0\left\{\bar{Q}_0(W,r)-\bar{Q}_0(W,0)\right\}}{P_0\left\{\bar{g}_0(W,r)-\bar{g}_0(W,0)\right\}} \\
&= \psi_{r,0}.
\end{aligned}
$$

Thus this solution is correct even if both $\bar{Q}$ and $\bar{g}$ are misspecified. This result also implies a robustness for $D^* = \sum_{r>0} h(r) D_r^*$.

TMLE of Ψ. Define

$$
\begin{aligned}
C_{Y,r}(P) &= \frac{1}{E\{A(r)-A(0)\}} \frac{I(R=r)-I(R=0)}{g(R \mid W)} \\
C_{A,r}(P) &= \frac{E(Y(r)-Y(0))}{E^2(A(r)-A(0))} \frac{I(R=r)-I(R=0)}{g(R \mid W)}.
\end{aligned}
$$

If Y is continuous in $(0,1)$ or binary in $\{0,1\}$, then we can use the quasi-log-likelihood loss function $L_Y(\bar{Q})(O) = Y \log \bar{Q}(W,R) + (1-Y)\log(1-\bar{Q}(W,R))$ for $\bar{Q}_0$. Regarding parametric submodel $\bar{Q}(\epsilon)$, we use the logistic regression $\text{logit}\bar{Q}(\epsilon) = \text{logit}\bar{Q} + \epsilon C_Y$ with clever covariate $C_Y = \sum_{r>0} h(r) C_{Y,r}$.

Similarly, if A is continuous in $(0,1)$ or binary in $\{0,1\}$, then we can use the quasi-log-likelihood loss function $L_A(\bar{g})(O) = A \log \bar{g}(W,R) + (1-A)\log(1-\bar{g}(W,R))$ for $\bar{g}_0$. Regarding parametric submodel $\bar{g}(\epsilon)$, we use the logistic regression $\text{logit}\bar{g}(\epsilon) = \text{logit}\bar{g} + \epsilon C_A$ with clever covariate $C_A = \sum_{r>0} h(r) C_{A,r}$. For the marginal distribution of W, we use the log-likelihood loss function $L_W(Q_W) = -\log Q_W$, and as submodel we select $(1+\epsilon D_W^*)Q_W$, where $D_W^* = \Pi(D^* \mid T_W)$. We can now define the loss function $L(Q_W, \bar{Q}, \bar{g}) = L_W(Q_W) + L_Y(\bar{Q}) + L_A(\bar{g})$ for the combined $(Q, \bar{g})$, and the submodel above was selected so that $\frac{d}{d\epsilon} L(Q_W(\epsilon_1), \bar{Q}(\epsilon_2), \bar{g}(\epsilon_2))$ at $\epsilon = 0$ spans the efficient influence curve $D^*(Q, \bar{g})$. Here $Q = (Q_W, \bar{Q})$.

The initial estimator of Q_W is the empirical distribution function. We can obtain initial estimators of $\bar{Q}_0$, $\bar{g}_0$, and $g_{R,0}$ with loss-based learning. Let $(Q_n^0, \bar{g}_n^0, g_{n,R})$ represent this initial estimator of $(Q_{W,0}, \bar{Q}_0, \bar{g}_0, g_{0,R})$. The TMLE is now defined: $\epsilon_n^1 = \arg\min_\epsilon P_n L(Q_n^0(\epsilon), \bar{g}_n^0(\epsilon))$, set $Q_n^1 = Q_n^0(\epsilon_n^1)$, $\bar{g}_n^1 = \bar{g}_n^0(\epsilon_n^1)$, and iterate this updating process to convergence. We note that ϵ_1 is estimated at zero so that the empirical distribution of W will not be updated, and $g_{n,R}$ is not updated either. Let $Q_n^*, \bar{g}_n^*$ denote the limit. Then the TMLE of ψ_0 is given by $\psi_{1n}^* = \Psi_1(Q_n^*, \bar{g}_n^*)$.

In this formulation of the TMLE, we are not providing a guarantee that ψ_n^* is a completely valid substitution estimator since the conditional means $\bar{Q}_n^*(W, R)$ and $\bar{g}_n^*(W, R)$ are not variation independent. The formal recipe of TMLE can be based on the orthogonal factorization of the density $P(O) = P(W)P(R \mid W)P(A \mid W, R)P(Y \mid W, R, A)$ in variation-independent conditional distributions, providing a loss function for $\bar{Q}(W, R, A)$ (instead of $\bar{Q}(W, R)$), the required parts of the conditional distribution of A, given W, R, and for the marginal distribution of W, and choosing working submodels based on the corresponding orthogonal decomposition of the efficient influence curve. We leave this exercise to the reader.

A.15 Example: TMLE of the Conditional Relative Risk

We consider n i.i.d. observations of $O = (W, A, Y) \sim P_0 \in \mathcal{M}$, where W is a vector of baseline covariates, A is an exposure of interest, and $Y = \{0, 1\}$ is a binary outcome. We define the statistical model $\mathcal{M}$ as all probability distributions P_0 satisfying

$$\bar{Q}_0(A, W) = e^{m_{\beta_0}(A,V)} \theta_0(W),$$

where $\bar{Q}_0(A, W) \equiv P_0(Y = 1 \mid A, W)$, $m_{\beta_0}(A, V)$ is a specified function of A and effect modifiers $V \subset W$, and $\theta_0(W) \equiv P_0(Y = 1 \mid A = 0, W)$. We will also use the notation $\bar{Q}_{\beta_0,\eta_0}$ for $\bar{Q}_0$. For simplicity, we first consider the case where $m_{\beta_0}(A, V) = \beta_0 A$, but we also provide the general formulas below.

Constructing the efficient score. The probability distribution of O in this semiparametric model is indexed by a finite-dimensional parameter β and infinite-dimensional nuisance parameter η consisting of θ, the marginal distribution of W, and the conditional distribution of A, given W. Let g_0 denote the conditional distribution of A, given W. The efficient influence curve $D^*(P_0)$ at P_0 happens to only depend on P_0 through β_0, θ_0, and g_0, so that we will also denote it by $D^*(\beta_0, \eta_0)$ or $D^*(\beta_0, \theta_0, g_0)$. We have

$$D^*(\beta_0, \eta_0) = -\left[\frac{d}{d\beta_0} P_0 S^*(\beta_0, \eta_0)\right]^{-1} S^*(\beta_0, \eta_0), \tag{A.8}$$

where $S^*(\beta_0, \eta_0)$ denotes the efficient score given by $S(\beta_0, \eta_0) - \Pi(S(\beta_0, \eta_0) \mid T_{nuis})$. Here $S(\beta_0, \eta_0)(Y \mid A, W) = \frac{d}{d\beta_0} \log P_{\beta_0,\theta_0}(Y \mid A, W)$ is the score of the parameter of interest β_0, and T_{nuis} is the nuisance tangent space, viewed as a subspace of the Hilbert space $L_0^2(P_0)$ endowed with the inner product $\langle h_1, h_2 \rangle = E_0 h_1 h_2(O)$. Recall that a projection of a function S on a subspace T_{nuis} of a Hilbert space is uniquely defined as follows: (1) the projection is an element of the subspace T_{nuis}, and (2) $S - \Pi(S \mid T_{nuis}) \perp T_{nuis}$. T_{nuis} is the direct sum of the three orthogonal spaces involving each of the nuisance parameters: $T_{nuis} = T_W \bigoplus T_{A|W} \bigoplus T_\theta$. Specifically, T_W consists of all functions in $L_0^2(P_0)$ of W with mean zero, $T_{A|W}$ consists of all functions in $L_0^2(P_0)$ of (A, W) with conditional mean zero, given W, and T_θ is the tangent space spanned by all the scores of parametric submodels through P_0 that only fluctuate θ. Thus,

$$S^*(\beta_0, \eta_0) = S(\beta_0, \eta_0) - \left[\Pi(S(\beta_0, \eta_0) \mid T_W) + \Pi(S(\beta_0, \eta_0) \mid T_{A|W}) + \Pi(S(\beta_0, \eta_0) \mid T_\theta)\right].$$

We have $\log P_{\beta,\theta}(Y = 1 \mid A, W) = \log \theta(W) + \beta A$. It follows that

$$S(\beta_0, \eta_0)(O) = \frac{d}{d\beta_0} \log P_{\beta_0,\theta_0}(Y \mid A, W) = \frac{A}{1-\bar{Q}_{\beta_0,\theta_0}}(Y - \bar{Q}_{\beta_0,\theta_0}(A, W)).$$

Since $S(\beta_0, \eta_0)$ has a conditional mean, given (A, W), equal to zero, it follows that it is orthogonal to T_W and $T_{A|W}$, so that its projection onto $T_W + T_{A|W}$ equals zero.

To calculate the tangent space T_θ, we consider submodels $P_0(\epsilon)(Y \mid A, W)$ implied by $\log \bar{Q}_0(\epsilon)(A, W) = \log \theta_0(W) + \beta_0 A + \epsilon h_3(W)$ for an arbitrary function h_3. Notice that this indeed implies a submodel in our semiparametric regression model. It is straightforward to show that the score of this submodel at $\epsilon = 0$ equals $1/(1 - \bar{Q}_0(A, W))h_3(W)(Y - \bar{Q}_0(A, W))$. This shows that $T_\theta = \{1/(1 - \bar{Q}_0(A, W))h_3(W)(Y - \bar{Q}_0(A, W)) : h_3\}$.

It remains to determine $\Pi(S(\beta_0, \eta_0) \mid T_\theta)$. As repeatedly used and shown in van der Laan and Robins (2003), any function $S(B, Pa(B))$ of a binary variable B and other variables $Pa(B)$ that has a conditional mean of zero, given $Pa(B)$, can be written as $(S(1, Pa(B)) - S(0, Pa(B))(B - P(B = 1 \mid Pa(B)))$. For a function V, let $h_V(A, W) = (V(1, A, W) - V(0, A, W))$, so that $V - E_0(V \mid A, W) = h_V(A, W)(Y - \bar{Q}_0)$. Thus,

$$\begin{aligned}
\Pi(V \mid T_\theta) &= \Pi(V - E_0(V \mid A, W) \mid T_\theta) \\
&= \Pi(h_V(Y - \bar{Q}_0) \mid T_\theta).
\end{aligned}$$

We need to find h_3^* such that

$$\begin{aligned}
E_0\left[\left\{h_V(A, W)(Y - \bar{Q}_0) - \frac{h_3^*(W)}{1 - \bar{Q}_0}(Y - \bar{Q}_0)\right\} \frac{h_3(W)}{1 - \bar{Q}_0}(Y - \bar{Q}_0)\right] &= 0 \text{ for all } h_3(W), \\
E_0\left[\left(h_V(A, W) - \frac{h_3^*(W)}{1 - \bar{Q}_0}\right) \frac{h_3(W)}{1 - \bar{Q}_0}(Y - \bar{Q}_0)^2\right] &= 0 \text{ for all } h_3(W), \\
E_0\left[\left(h_V(A, W) - \frac{h_3^*(W)}{1 - \bar{Q}_0}\right) \frac{h_3(W)}{1 - \bar{Q}_0}\sigma^2(A, W)\right] &= 0 \text{ for all } h_3(W), \\
E_0\left[\left(h_V(A, W)\frac{\sigma^2}{1 - \bar{Q}_0} - \frac{h_3^*(W)}{(1 - \bar{Q}_0)^2}\sigma^2\right) h_3(W)\right] &= 0 \text{ for all } h_3(W),
\end{aligned}$$

$$E_0\left[\left(E_0\left[\frac{h_V(A,W)}{1-\bar{Q}_0}\sigma^2 \mid W\right] - h_3^*(W)E_0\left[\frac{\sigma^2}{(1-\bar{Q}_0)^2} \mid W\right]\right)h_3(W)\right] = 0 \text{ for all } h_3(W),$$

where $\sigma^2(A, W) = \mathrm{VAR}_0(Y \mid A, W) = \bar{Q}_0(1 - \bar{Q}_0)$. Therefore

$$h_3^*(W) = \frac{E_0\left(\frac{h_V(A,W)\sigma^2}{1-\bar{Q}_0} \mid W\right)}{E_0\left(\frac{\sigma^2}{(1-\bar{Q}_0)^2} \mid W\right)}.$$

This provides us with the projection of V onto the nuisance tangent space T_{nuis}. In particular, if $V = S(\beta_0, \eta_0)$, we have $V = A/(1-\bar{Q}_0)(Y-\bar{Q}_0)$, so that $h_V = A/(1-\bar{Q}_0)$. This yields

$$\Pi(S(\beta_0, \eta_0) \mid T_\theta) = \frac{E_0\left[\frac{A\bar{Q}_0}{1-\bar{Q}_0} \mid W\right]}{E_0\left[\frac{\bar{Q}_0}{1-\bar{Q}_0} \mid W\right]}\frac{(Y-\bar{Q}_0)}{1-\bar{Q}_0}.$$

It follows that the efficient score is given by

$$S^*(\beta_0, \eta_0) = \left(A - \frac{E_0\left[\frac{A\bar{Q}_0}{(1-\bar{Q}_0)} \mid W\right]}{E_0\left[\frac{\bar{Q}_0}{1-\bar{Q}_0} \mid W\right]}\right)\frac{(Y-\bar{Q}_0)}{1-\bar{Q}_0}. \tag{A.9}$$

Double robustness of efficient score. It is of interest to note that the efficient score can also be represented as:

$$S^*(\beta_0, \eta_0) = h^*(A \mid W)\left(Y\frac{\bar{Q}_0(0,W)}{\bar{Q}_0(A,W)} - \bar{Q}_0(0, W)\right),$$

where

$$h^*(A \mid W) \equiv \frac{\bar{Q}_0}{\bar{Q}_0(0,W)(1-\bar{Q}_0)}\left(A - \frac{E_0\left[\frac{A\bar{Q}_0}{(1-\bar{Q}_0)} \| W\right]}{E_0\left[\frac{\bar{Q}_0}{1-\bar{Q}_0} | W\right]}\right)$$

is a function satisfying $E_0(h^*(A \mid W) \mid W) = 0$. This representation shows that $P_0S^*(\beta_0, \theta, g) = 0$ if either $\theta = \theta_0$ or $g = g_0$, thereby establishing the double robustness of the efficient score as the estimating function for β_0.

The derivation above assumes that $m_{\beta_0}(A, V) = \beta_0 A$. In general, the efficient score is given by

$$S^*(\beta_0, \eta_0)(O) = \frac{1}{1-\bar{Q}_0}\left(\frac{d}{d\beta_0}m_{\beta_0} - \frac{E_0\left[\frac{d}{d\beta_0}m_{\beta_0}\frac{\bar{Q}_0}{(1-\bar{Q}_0)} \mid W\right]}{E_0\left[\frac{\bar{Q}_0}{1-\bar{Q}_0} \mid W\right]}\right)(Y - \bar{Q}_0).$$

The efficient influence curve is defined as the standardized version $c_0^{-1}S^*(\beta_0, \eta_0)$, where $c_0 = -\frac{d}{d\beta_0}P_0S^*(\beta_0, \eta_0)$.

Constructing a parametric submodel having a score that spans the efficient score. If we assume $\bar{Q}_0 = \exp(m_{\beta_0}(A, W))\theta_0(W)$, and we use as submodel $\log \bar{Q}_0(\epsilon) = m_{\beta_0+\epsilon} + \log\theta_0 + \epsilon r$, then the score equals $(d/d\beta_0 m_{\beta_0} + r)(Y - \bar{Q}_0)/(1 - \bar{Q}_0)$. Thus, to arrange that this score equals the efficient score we set r equal to

$$r^*(\bar{Q}_0, g_0) = -\frac{E_0\left[d/d\beta_0 m_{\beta_0} \frac{\bar{Q}_0}{(1-\bar{Q}_0)} \mid W\right]}{E_0\left[\frac{\bar{Q}_0}{1-\bar{Q}_0} \mid W\right]}.$$

The iterative TMLE. This defines the desired ϵ-extension $\bar{Q}_n^0(\epsilon)$ of an initial fit $\bar{Q}_n^0$. We use the log-likelihood loss function for $\bar{Q}_0$: $L(\bar{Q}) = -\{Y \log \bar{Q} + (1-Y)\log(1-\bar{Q})\}$. For example, if $m_\beta(W, A) = \beta A$, then this ϵ-fluctuation corresponds with adding $\epsilon C(A, W)$ to the initial fit $\log \bar{Q}_n^0(A, W) = \beta_n^0 A + r_n^0(W)$, where the clever covariate is given by

$$C(Q_n^0, g_n^0)(A, W) = A - \frac{E_{g_n^0}\left(\frac{Q_n^0(A,W)}{1-Q_n^0(A,W)} A \mid W\right)}{E_{g_n^0}\left(\frac{Q_n^0(A,W)}{(1-Q_n^0)(A,W)} \mid W\right)}.$$

Let ϵ_n^0 be the maximum likelihood estimator over ϵ for this parametric submodel $\{Q_n^0(\epsilon) : \epsilon\}$. This requires fitting a log-binomial regression model. Let $\bar{Q}_n^1 = \bar{Q}_n^0(\epsilon_n^0)$ be the updated estimate of $\bar{Q}_0$, which corresponds with an updated β_n^1 and θ_n^1. We iterate this updating process until the corresponding sequence β_n^k is such that $\beta_n^k - \beta_n^{k-1}$ no longer significantly change. We denote the selected final update by $\bar{Q}_n^*$ and let β_n^* be the corresponding TMLE of β_0.

A.16 IPCW Reduced-Data TMLE

Summary. IPCW estimators have gained popularity due to their simplicity. However, this gain in simplicity comes at a severe cost in terms of bias and variance. We show that by inverse probability of censoring weighting a TMLE based on a reduction of the original observed data structure, one obtains a valid substitution estimator of the target parameter. This estimator is a special case of the TMLE presented in Appendix A.6, corresponding with a particular IPCW loss function and parametric fluctuation function. These estimators are relatively easy-to-implement substitution estimators with good efficiency and robustness properties.

The TMLE of a target parameter ψ_0 is characterized by two ingredients: a choice of loss function for Q_0 and a parametric fluctuation working model to fluctuate Q. These two choices combined determine the estimating function $D(Q, \eta) \equiv \frac{d}{d\epsilon} L(Q_\eta(\epsilon))\big|_{\epsilon=0}$ whose estimating equation $P_n D(Q_n^*, \eta_n) = 0$ will be solved by the resulting TMLE Q_n^*. If D is the efficient influence curve, then we will refer to this TMLE as an efficient TMLE. The efficient TMLE, based on, e.g., the log-likelihood loss function $L(Q)$ and efficient influence curve estimating function $D^*()$, can be quite involved for complex longitudinal data structures with time-dependent covariates, since Q_0 may be a very high-dimensional function. Therefore, it is of interest to also provide TMLE for which Q_0 is chosen to be of lower dimension, at the cost of having to work with a loss function $L_{\eta_0}(Q)$ that is indexed by an unknown nuisance parameter, and fluctuation model that generates an inefficient estimating function $D()$. For that purpose we propose a general class of so-called inverse probability of censoring-weighted reduced-data TMLEs, which modify the efficient TMLE for a user-supplied reduced (simplified-)data structure by weighting the loss function with inverse probability of censoring weights.

Let $O = (L(0), A(0), \ldots, L(K), A(K), L(K + 1)) \sim P_0$. Assume an SCM $A(t) = f_{A(t)}(Pa(A(t)), U_{A(t)})$, $t = 1, \ldots, K$, $L(t) = f_{L(t)}(Pa(L(t)), U_{L(t)})$, $t = 1 \ldots, K + 1$, where $Pa(A(t)) = (\bar{A}(t - 1), \bar{L}(t))$, and $Pa(L(t)) = (\bar{A}(t - 1), \bar{L}(t - 1))$. Here $A(t)$, $t = 0, \ldots, K$ denote the intervention nodes, which can include both treatment and censoring actions. This SCM allows us to define counterfactuals L_a and L_d indexed by static interventions a and dynamic treatments d, respectively. We assume the SRA about the error nodes U in the SCM so that the g-computation formula provides us with the identifiability of any parameter of the distribution of a counterfactual L_d for a given rule d, possibly a static rule. Specifically, under this SRA, the probability distribution of the observed data random variable $O = (A, L = L_A)$ factorizes into a factor Q_0 implied by the full-data distribution of the counterfactuals $X = (L_a : a)$ and a factor $g_0(\cdot \mid X) = \prod_{t=0}^{K} g_{A(t),0}(A(t) \mid Pa(A(t)))$ that corresponds with the conditional distribution of A, given X:

$$P_{Q_0,g_0}(O) = \prod_{t=0}^{K+1} Q_{L(t),0}(L(t) \mid Pa(L(t))) \prod_{t=0}^{K} g_{A(t),0}(A(t) \mid Pa(A(t))).$$

By SRA (which implies coarsening at random), we have $Q_{L(t),0}(l(t) \mid \bar{l}(t - 1), \bar{a}(t - 1)) = P(L_a(t) = l(t) \mid \bar{L}_a(t-1) = \bar{l}(t-1))$ so that indeed Q_0 represents the identifiable part of the full-data distribution of the counterfactuals X.

A statistical model $\mathcal{M}$ for P_0 can be represented as all probability distributions $P_{Q,g}$ with $Q \in \mathcal{Q}$ and $g \in \mathcal{G}$ for some specified models $\mathcal{Q}$ and SRA model $\mathcal{G}$ for Q_0 and g_0, respectively. Given a parameter $\Psi : \mathcal{Q} \to \mathbb{R}^d$, our goal is to estimate $\Psi(Q_0)$.

The basic idea of IPCW-R-TMLE is as follows. Our target parameter can also be written as a function of the distribution of a reduction L_a^r of the counterfactual L_a, obtained by removing a number of the time-dependent components of $L_a(t)$. Thus, we can write our parameter as $\Psi(Q_0) = \Psi^r(Q_0^r)$, where $Q_0^r(a, l^r)$ represents the distribution of L_a^r: $Q^r_{L^r(t),0}(l^r(t) \mid \bar{l}^r(t - 1), \bar{a}(t - 1)) = P(L_a^r(t) = l^r(t) \mid \bar{L}_a^r(t - 1) = \bar{l}^r(t - 1))$. Now, we note that the inverse-weighted log-likelihood loss function, for any marginal probability distribution g^r of A, $L_{g_0}(Q^r) \equiv -g^r/g_0 \log Q^r$, is a valid loss function for Q_0^r, since

$$Q^r \to P_0 \log Q^r \frac{g^r}{g_0} = P_{Q_0,g^r} \log Q^r = P_{Q_0^r,g^r} \log Q^r,$$

is maximized at Q_0^r. To see the last equality, use the representation $O = (A, L_A)$ and that $Q_0(a, l) = P_0(L_a = l)$ so that

$$E_{Q_0,g^r} \log Q^r(A, L_A^r) = E_{Q_0^r} \sum_a \log Q^r(a, L_a^r) g^r(a),$$

which is indeed maximized at Q_0^r. In addition, the inverse-probability-weighted reduced-data efficient influence curve, $D(Q^r, g^r, g_0) \equiv D^{*r}(Q^r, g^r)g^r/g_0$, is a targeted estimating function for the target parameter $\Psi(Q_0^r)$, as discussed in detail below. We can now apply TMLE, as described in the Appendix A.6, with this inverse-weighted log-likelihood loss function, a fluctuation working model $\{Q_{g^r}^r(\epsilon) : \epsilon\}$ with score at $\epsilon = 0$ equal to the reduced-data efficient influence curve $D^{r*}(Q^r, g^r)$, so that the TMLE will solve $P_n D(Q_n^{r*}, g^r, g_n) = 0$. Our proposal below refines the choice of IPCW log-likelihood loss function by inverse weighting each factor $Q_{L^r(t),0}$ of Q_0^r separately with more stable weights $g^r(\bar{A}(t-1) \mid X^r)/g_0(\bar{A}(t-1) \mid X)$, as described in the procedure below.

We will use the notation $\mathcal{M}(g) = \{P_{Q,g} : Q \in \mathcal{Q}\}$ for the statistical model implied by a model $\mathcal{Q}$ for Q_0 and a treatment mechanism g contained in the set $\mathcal{G}$ of all SRA-conditional distributions of A, given X. We note that, since Q_0 is identifiable based on i.i.d. sampling from an element in $\mathcal{M}(g)$, one can also view Ψ as a parameter on the model $\mathcal{M}(g)$. The IPCW-R-TMLE is defined by the following steps.

(Optional) specify reduced-data structure. Determine a reduction $O^r = (A, L^r)$ of $O = (A, L)$, where L^r is a function of L and where the reduction is such that it is still possible to identify the parameter of interest ψ_0 from the probability distribution of $O^r = (A, L^r = L_A^r)$ under the SRA for the reduced full-data structure $X^r = (L_a^r : a \in \mathcal{A})$. In other words, $\Psi(Q_0)$ needs to depend on the distribution of $X = (L_a : a)$ only through the distribution of $X^r = (L_a^r : a)$. For example, $O = (W = L(0), A, \bar{L}(K), Y = L(K+1))$ consists of baseline covariates W, treatment regimen $A = (A(0), \ldots, A(K))$, time-dependent covariate process $\bar{L}(K)$, and a final outcome Y, one is concerned with the estimation of EY_a for some static regimen a, and one defines $O^r = (W, A, Y)$, which is obtained from O by deleting all time-dependent covariates.

Reduced-data model. Let $O^r = (A, L_A^r)$, $X^r = (L_a^r : a)$, g^r a conditional distribution of A, given X^r, satisfying SRA with respect to reduced-data O^r. Let $\mathcal{M}^r(g^r) = \{P_{Q^r,g^r}^r = Q^r g^r : Q^r \in \mathcal{Q}^r\}$ be a statistical model for O^r, where the model $\mathcal{Q}^r = \{Q^r : Q \in \mathcal{Q}\}$ for Q_0^r is implied by the model $\mathcal{Q}$ for Q_0. Let $\Psi^r : \mathcal{Q}^r \to \mathbb{R}^d$ be such that $\Psi^r(Q^r) = \Psi(Q)$ for all $Q^r \in \mathcal{Q}^r$, and, in particular, $\Psi^r(Q_0^r) = \Psi(Q_0)$. In the example with $O^r = (W, A, Y)$, g^r is a conditional distribution of A, given W, Q^r is the distribution of $(W, (Y_a : a))$ implied by the distribution of L_a under Q, and $\Psi^r(Q^r) = E_{Q^r} Y_a$. In particular, if the data are not reduced in the previous step, then $O^r = O$, $Q^r = Q$, $g^r = g$, $\mathcal{M}^r(g^r) = \mathcal{M}(g)$, $\Psi^r = \Psi$.

Factorization of Q^r. Suppose $P_{Q_0^r, g_0^r} = \prod_j Q_{0j}^r g_0^r$ factors into various terms Q_{0j}^r, $j = 1, \ldots, J$ (e.g., $J = K+1$). Suppose that $Q_{0j}^r(O^r)$ depends on O^r only through $(A(0), \ldots, A(j^r - 1), \bar{L}^r(j^r))$, $j = 1, \ldots, J$. In a typical scenario, we have that Q_{0j}^r denotes the conditional distribution of $L^r(j^r)$, given $(A(0), \ldots, A(j^r - 1))$ and $\bar{L}^r(j^r - 1)$. For notational convenience, we used the short-hand notation $j^r = j^r(j)$, suppressing its deterministic dependence on j. In the example with $O^r = (W, A, Y)$, Q_0^r factors as $Q_0^r(w, a, y) = Q_{0w}(w) Q_0^r(y \mid w, a)$, where $Q_0^r(y \mid w, a) = P_0(Y(a) = y \mid W = w)$, giving us factorization $Q^r(w, a, y) = Q_1^r(w) Q_2^r(y \mid w, a)$. In particular, if the data are not reduced, then $P_{Q_0,g_0} = \prod_t Q_{t0}g_0$, $t = 1, \ldots, K+1$, where $Q_{t,0}$ denotes the conditional distribution of $L(t)$, given $\bar{L}(t-1), \bar{A}(t-1)$, so that $Q_{t,0}(O)$ depends on O only through $(A(0), \ldots, A(t-1))$, $t = 1, \ldots, K+1$.

Determine Q^r_j-components of efficient influence curve for reduced-data model. Let $D^r(P^r)$ be the efficient influence curve at $P^r = P^r_{Q^r,g^r} = Q^r g^r$ for the parameter Ψ^r in the model $\mathcal{M}^r(g^r)$ for the reduced-data structure O^r. This efficient influence curve can be decomposed orthogonally as $D^r(P^r) = D^r(Q^r, g^r) = \sum_{j=1}^J D^r_j(P^r)$, where $D^r_j(P^r)$ is an element of the tangent space generated by the jth factor Q^r_j of $Q^r = \prod_j Q^r_j$ at P^r, $j = 1, \ldots, J$. In the example with $O^r = (W, A, Y)$, this efficient influence curve for the reduced data is given by (and decomposed as):

$$D^r(Q^r, g^r)(W, A, Y) = \{I(A = a)/g^r(a \mid W)(Y - \bar{Q}^r(A, w))\} + \{\bar{Q}^r(a, W) - \Psi^r(Q^r)\},$$

where $\bar{Q}^r(a, w) = E_{Q^r}(Y_a \mid W)$. This defines D^r_1 and D^r_2. In particular, if the data were not reduced and the model for Q_0 is nonparametric, then the efficient influence curve $D(P) = \sum_{t=1}^{K+1} D_t(P)$, with

$$D_t(P) = E_P(D(P)(O) \mid \bar{A}(t-1), \bar{L}(t)) - E_P(D(P)(O) \mid \bar{A}(t-1), \bar{L}(t-1))$$

being the projection of $D(P)$ on the tangent space generated by the conditional distribution Q_t of $L(t)$, given $\bar{L}(t-1), \bar{A}(t-1)$.

Determine hardest Q^r_j-fluctuation working models. Given a Q^r, construct submodels $\{Q^r_j(\epsilon) : \epsilon\}$ through Q^r_j and loss functions $L(Q^r_j)$, such as $L(Q^r_j) = -\log Q^r_j$, so that

$$\frac{d}{d\epsilon} L(Q^r_j(\epsilon))\Big|_{\epsilon=0} = D^r_j(Q^r, g^r),\ j = 1, \ldots, J.$$

In the example, [say Y is binary or bounded in (0, 1)] we can fluctuate Q^r_2 using a logistic fluctuation working model with clever covariate $I(A = a)/g^r(A \mid W)$ and employ the binary-outcome log-likelihood loss function for the conditional mean (or probability) $\bar{Q}^r_2(w, a) = E_{Q^r_2}(Y_a \mid W = w)$. In particular, if the data are not reduced, then, given a $Q \in \mathcal{Q}$ construct submodels $\{Q_t(\epsilon) : \epsilon\}$ through Q_t at $\epsilon = 0$, with score at $\epsilon = 0$ equal to $D_t(Q, g)$,

$$\frac{d}{d\epsilon} L(Q_t(\epsilon))\Big|_{\epsilon=0} = D_t(Q, g),\ t = 1, \ldots, K+1.$$

Construct IPCW weights for each j-specific Q^r_j-factor. For each j, construct the weight function

$$w_{j,0} = \frac{g^r_0(\bar{A}(j^r - 1) \mid X^r)}{g_0(\bar{A}(j^r - 1) \mid X)},\ j = 1, \ldots, J.$$

We will often denote the weights $g^r_0(\bar{A}(j^r-1) \mid X^r)/g_0(\bar{A}(j^r-1) \mid X)$ by $g^r_{j,0}/g_{j,0}$. We note that for each $j = 1, \ldots, J$

$$Q^r_{j,0} = \arg\min_{Q^r_j \in \mathcal{Q}^r_j} P_{Q_0,g_0} w_{j,0} L(Q^r_j) = \arg\min_{Q^r_j \in \mathcal{Q}^r_j} P_{Q^r_0,g^r_0} L(Q^r_j),$$

such that, for each choice g_0^r (can be any function), the IPCW-R loss function $L_{w_0}(Q^r) \equiv \sum_j w_{j,0} L(Q_j^r)$ is a valid loss function for Q_0^r [i.e., for the true distribution of $(L_a^r : a)$], indexed by nuisance parameter (g_0^r, g_0). In our example we have $w_{1,0} = 1$ (no weighting for marginal distribution of W) and $w_{2,0} = g_0^r(A \mid W)/g_0(A \mid X)$, and the IPTW-R loss function for Q^r is $\sum_{j=1}^2 L(Q_j^r) w_{j,0}$. Note that $g_0^r(A \mid W) = \prod_{t=0}^K g_0^r(A(t) \mid \bar{A}(t-1), W)$. If the data are not reduced, then $w_{t,0} = 1$, and one could select $L(Q) = -\log Q$ as the log-likelihood loss function.

Estimate the weights. Construct estimators g_n^r and g_n of g_0^r and g_0, respectively, and construct the corresponding estimator w_n of the weight function w_0. In our example, this requires fitting the conditional distribution of the time-dependent treatments $A(t)$, given past treatment, and baseline covariates (thus ignoring the time-dependent covariates), as well as the true treatment mechanism.

IPCW-R-TMLE at specified weights. We will now compute the TMLE under i.i.d. sampling $O_1^r, \ldots, O_n^r$ from $P^r_{Q_0^r, g^r}$, but assigning the above IPCW weights w_n, as follows. Let $Q^{r,0}$ be an initial estimator of Q_0^r. For example, let $Q_j^{r,0} = \arg\min_{Q_j^r \in \mathcal{Q}_j^r} \sum_i L(Q_j^r)(O_i^r) w_{j,i,n}$ be a weighted maximum likelihood estimator of Q_{0j}^r according to a working model $\mathcal{Q}_j^r$. In general, we can use a weighted-ML-based estimator, such as the super learner, based on this weighted log-likelihood loss function $L_{w_0}(Q^r) = \sum_{j=1}^J L(Q_j^r) w_{j,0}$. Subsequently, we compute the overall amount of fluctuation with an IPCW loss-based estimation,

$$\epsilon_n^1 = \arg\min_\epsilon \sum_i \sum_j L(Q_j^{r,0}(\epsilon))(O_i^r) w_{j,i,n},$$

and compute the corresponding first-step targeted update $Q_j^{r,1} = Q_j^{r,0}(\epsilon_n^1)$, $j = 1, \ldots, J$, and thereby the overall update $Q^{r,1} = Q^{r,0}(\epsilon_n^1)$. Iterate this process till convergence (i.e., $\epsilon_n^k \approx 0$) and denote the final update by $Q_n^{r*} = (Q_{j,n}^{r*} : j = 1, \ldots, J)$. Let $D(Q^r, g^r, g) = \sum_j D_j^r(Q^r, g^r) \frac{g_j^r}{g_j}$ be the IPCW efficient influence curve estimating function for the reduced-data structure O^r. We have that Q_n^{r*}, in conjunction with an estimate of the weights, solves the corresponding estimating equation:

$$0 = \sum_i D(Q_n^{r*}, g_n^r, g_n)(O_i) = \sum_i \sum_j D_j^r(Q_n^{r*}, g_n^r)(O_i^r) w_{j,i,n}. \tag{A.10}$$

In our example, the marginal empirical distribution of W would not be updated (we would use separate ϵ for fluctuation of the marginal distribution of W), so that only $Q_2^{r,0}$ is updated, and the IPCW-R efficient influence curve is given by $D_1^r(W) + D_2^r(W, A, Y) g_0^r(A \mid W)/g_0(A \mid X)$. In particular, if the data are not reduced, then Q_n^*, g_n solves the efficient influence curve equation $0 = \sum_i \sum_t D_t(Q_n^*, g_n)(O_i)$.

Substitution estimator. Our estimator of ψ_0 is given by $\Psi^r(Q_n^{r*})$. In our example, EY_a is estimated as $\Psi^r(Q_n^{r*}) = \sum_w Q_{1,n}^r(w) \sum_y y Q_{2,n}^{r*}(y \mid w, a)$. In particular, if the data are not reduced, then ψ_0 is estimated with $\Psi(Q_n^*)$.

The IPCW-R-TMLE is an estimator Q_n^{r*} of Q_0^r (i.e., of the true distribution of L_a^r for each a), solving an IPCW reduced-data efficient influence curve equation (A.10).

Firstly, we establish that this IPCW reduced-data efficient influence curve is an "estimating function" for the target parameter $\Psi^r(Q_0^r)$ with nice robustness properties with respect to its nuisance parameters Q_0^r and g_0 (for each choice of g_0^r). Subsequently, we discuss the corresponding implications for the statistical properties of the IPCW-R-TMLE.

Robustness properties of IPCW reduced-data efficient influence function. Recall that $D^r(Q^r, g^r)$ denotes the efficient influence curve for the reduced-data $O^r \sim P_{Q^r,g^r}$ for model $\mathcal{M}^r$ and parameter Ψ^r. It follows from the general results in van der Laan and Robins (2003) that $P_{Q_0^r,g_0^r} D^r(Q^r, g^r) = 0$ if either $Q^r = Q_0^r$ or $\Psi(Q^r) = \Psi(Q_0^r)$ and $g^r = g_0^r$. This double robustness result for D^r is exploited/inherited by the estimating function $D(Q^r, g^r, g_0) \equiv \sum_j D_j^r(Q^r, g^r) g_j^r / g_{0j}$, whose corresponding estimating equation is solved by our IPCW-R-TMLE, in the following manner. If the denominator of the weights $g = g_0$ is correctly specified, then we have

$$P_{Q_0,g_0} D(Q^r, g^r, g_0) = P_{Q_0,g_0} \sum_j D_j^r(Q^r, g^r) \frac{g_j^r}{g_{j,0}} = P_{Q_0,g^r} \sum_j D_j^r(Q^r, g^r).$$

This implies that if $g = g_0$ (i.e., the action mechanism is correctly specified), then $P_{Q_0,g_0} D(Q^r, g^r, g_0) = 0$ for all choices of Q^r, g^r with $\Psi(Q^r) = \Psi(Q_0^r)$. That is, $D(Q^r, g^r, g_0)$ represents an unbiased estimating function in ψ for each choice of g^r.

In a typical scenario, we have that $Q_{j,0}^r$ denotes the conditional distribution of $L^r(j^r)$, given $A(0), \ldots, A(j^r - 1)$ and $\bar{L}^r(j^r - 1)$. In this case, if $g_{j,0}$ is only a function of O^r, then if $Q^r = Q_0^r$, it follows that $P_{Q_0,g^r} D_j^r(Q_0^r, g^r) \frac{g_j^r}{g_j} = 0$ for all g_j only being a function of O^r [by using that the conditional expectation of a score $D_j^r(Q_0^r, g^r)$ of Q_{j0}^r, given $(A(0), \ldots, A(j^r - 1)$ and $\bar{L}^r(j^r - 1)$, equals zero], and as a consequence, $P_{Q_0,g_0} D(Q_0^r, g^r, g) = 0$ for such misspecified g. That is, in the case that the true g_0 and its asymptotic (possibly misspecified) fit are only functions of the reduced-data structure O^r, we have the double robustness of the estimating function $D(Q^r, g^r, g)$ in the sense that, for any choice g^r, $P_{Q_0,g_0} D(Q^r, g^r, g) = 0$ if $\Psi(Q^r) = \Psi(Q_0^r)$ and, either $Q^r = Q_0^r$ or $g = g_0$. In particular, if the data are not reduced, then we have $P_{Q_0,g_0} D(Q, g) = 0$ if $\Psi(Q) = \psi_0$ and either $Q = Q_0$ or $g = g_0$. In fact, the efficient influence curve satisfies a stronger collaborative double robustness property presented above.

Statistical properties of IPCW-R-TMLE. The above-mentioned robustness property of the estimating function $D(Q^r, g^r, g)$ has immediate implications for the statistical properties of a solution $\Psi(Q_n^{r*})$ such that $\sum_i D(Q_n^{r*}, g_n^r, g_n) = 0$. Firstly, under appropriate regularity conditions, if g_n consistently estimates g_0, then ψ_n will be a consistent and asymptotically linear estimator of ψ_0. In addition, if $g_n(A \mid X)$ and its target $g_0(A \mid X)$ are only functions of the reduced-data structure O^r so that g_n^r / g_n converges to 1, then ψ_n is consistent and asymptotically linear if either Q_n^{r*} consistently estimates Q_0^r, or g_n consistently estimates g_0, and if both estimates are consistent, then the estimator ψ_n is more efficient than an efficient estimator based on n i.i.d.

observations of the reduced-data structure $O^r \sim P^r_{Q^r_0,g^r_0}$ only. In our example with $O^r = (W, A, Y)$, if g_0 is consistently estimated, the IPCW-R-TMLE is asymptotically more efficient and less biased than the R-TMLE (which will be biased if there is time-dependent confounding), and if there is no time-dependent confounding so that $g^r_0/g_0 = 1$ and the estimated weights converge to 1, then the IPCW-R-TMLE is double robust with respect to misspecification of either g^r_0 or Q^r_0, just like the R-TMLE.

A.17 Collaborative Double Robust TMLE

Summary. A TMLE of a causal effect of an intervention requires an estimator of the conditional distribution of an intervention node, given its parents, across all intervention nodes, where this combined set of intervention-node-specific conditional distributions is called the intervention assignment mechanism (such as treatment mechanism). If the estimator of the intervention-assignment mechanism converges to the truth, then the TMLE will be asymptotically unbiased. However, including correct parent nodes for an intervention node that play no role in the g-computation formula for the target parameter only hurts the finite sample bias reduction and can dramatically increase the variance of the TMLE. This suggests that the goal should not be to estimate the true intervention-assignment mechanism but the true conditional distributions of the intervention nodes that condition on sufficient reduction of the true parent nodes so that the desired bias reduction of the TMLE is achieved. The collaborative double robustness of the efficient influence curve and the TMLE formalizes this concept of a sufficient adjustment set for the intervention assignment mechanism, showing that only functions of parent nodes that explain the residual bias of the initial estimator of the g-computation factor of the data-generating distributions need to be included. This collaborative double robustness of the efficient influence curve implies another fundamental invariance property of the TMLE when applied to an infinite sample of the true probability distribution: If the initial estimator is already targeted with a sufficient intervention-assignment mechanism, then the TMLE will not further modify the initial estimator, even when it uses another sufficient intervention-assignment mechanism besides that used by the initial estimator. These fundamental insights yield the theoretical underpinnings of the C-TMLE. The C-TMLE at infinite sample size (i.e., $P_n = P_0$) and its properties are presented.

Let $O = \Phi(C, X) \sim P_0$ for some many-to-one mapping Φ, and consider a CAR censored-data model that assumes some model $\mathcal{Q}$ on the distribution of X, and assumes, minimally, that the conditional distribution g_0 of C, given X, satisfies CAR. Let $\mathcal{G}$ be the model for g_0. Let $\Psi(Q_0)$ be a target parameter for some $Q_0 = Q(P_0)$.

Firstly, we will consider the TMLE algorithm at infinite sample size, so that the empirical probability distribution function P_n is replaced by P_0. In the TMLE, we require that $\frac{d}{d\epsilon}L(Q_g(\epsilon))\big|_{\epsilon=0} = D(Q,g)$ for some loss function L, fluctuation working model $\{Q_g(\epsilon) : \epsilon\}$ through an initial Q, and estimating function D. As a consequence, if we apply the TMLE to an initial Q using a certain g, then we obtain a solution Q^* (indexed by g used in the working fluctuation model) so that $P_0D(Q^*, g) = 0$. These functions D are chosen such that $P_0D(Q, g_0) = 0$ implies $\Psi(Q) = \Psi(Q_0)$ [or, minimally, are such that $P_0D(Q, g_0) = 0$ if $\Psi(Q) = \psi_0$], even if Q itself is misspecified. In this way, using the true g_0 in the TMLE, we obtain a Q^* with $\Psi(Q^*) = \psi_0$ that has thereby removed all the bias of the initial $\Psi(Q^0)$ with respect to the true target ψ_0. However, the estimating functions we will use satisfy a stronger collaborative robustness property in terms of a specified subset $\mathcal{G}(Q, P_0)$ of the parameter space $\mathcal{G}$ for g_0, which includes the true g_0. If $g \in \mathcal{G}(Q, P_0)$, then

$$P_0D(Q, g) = 0 \text{ implies } \Psi(Q) = \Psi(Q_0).$$

In a coarsening at random censored-data model, this set $\mathcal{G}(Q, P_0)$ includes any true conditional distribution of the censoring variable, conditioning on a reduction of the full data that captures a specified difference defined in terms of $Q - Q_0$ (Appendix A.8). In particular, if Q converges to Q_0, then the set $\mathcal{G}(Q, P_0)$ grows to the set $\mathcal{G}$ of all distributions. In particular, by applying this result at $Q = 0$, it follows that $\mathcal{G}(Q, P_0)$ includes distributions that do not condition on variables used by the true g_0 that Q_0 does not depend on.

Suppose now that the TMLE Q_n^* uses an estimator g_n that converges to a $g_0(Q^*) \in \mathcal{G}(Q^*, P_0)$. In that case, the corresponding TMLE Q_n^* that solves $P_nD(Q_n^*, g_n) = 0$ will asymptotically solve $P_0D^*(Q^*, g_0(Q^*)) = 0$, which implies $\Psi(Q^*) = \psi_0$. That is, the desired asymptotic bias reduction can be obtained by using an estimator g_n that is inconsistent for the true g_0 but that converges to an element $g_0(Q^*) \in \mathcal{G}(Q^*, P_0)$. This suggests that we should be using collaborative estimators g_n in TMLE that aim to converge to such a $g_0(Q^*)$ that takes into account the residual bias of the initial estimator. We state the following theorem laying out two properties of the TMLE algorithm when applied to P_0 (instead of finite data set P_n).

Theorem A.3. *For a given Q and P_0, let $\mathcal{G}(Q, P_0) \subset \mathcal{G}$ be such that $g \rightarrow P_0D(Q, g)$ is constant in $\mathcal{G}(Q, P_0)$, and that for each $g \in \mathcal{G}(Q, P_0)$ $P_0D(Q, g) = 0$ implies $\Psi(Q) = \psi_0$. Define $f(\epsilon) = P_0L(Q_g(\epsilon))$ and assume $\frac{d}{d\epsilon}L(Q_g(\epsilon))\big|_{\epsilon=0} = D(Q, g)$. Assume f has a unique local minimum satisfying $f'(\epsilon) = 0$. For a TMLE Q that used $g^0 \in \mathcal{G}(Q, P_0)$ to fluctuate an initial Q^0, we have $P_0D(Q, g^0) = 0$ and thereby $\Psi(Q) = \psi_0$. Consider a TMLE Q^* that uses this TMLE Q as initial estimator, and uses another $g \in \mathcal{G}(Q, P_0)$. Then $Q^* = Q$, and thus $\Psi(Q^*) = \psi_0$.*

Proof. By the constant property, $P_0D(Q, g) = P_0D(Q, g^0)$, and since $P_0D(Q, g^0) = 0$, we also have that $P_0D(Q, g) = 0$. Recall that the TMLE update will calculate: $\epsilon^1 = \arg\min_\epsilon P_0L(Q_g(\epsilon))$. By being a minimum of $f(\epsilon) \equiv P_0L(Q_g(\epsilon))$ at an interior point, we have that ϵ^1 solves the derivative equation $0 = f'(\epsilon) \equiv \frac{d}{d\epsilon}f(\epsilon)$. By assumption, the derivative $f'(\epsilon)$ has only one solution with $f'(\epsilon) = 0$: For example, the fluctuation $f(\epsilon)$ has only one local maximum. However, $\epsilon = 0$ is a solution since

$f'(0) = P_0D(Q, g)$, which equals zero since $g \in \mathcal{G}(Q, P_0)$, as shown above. Thus, the TMLE algorithm will set $\epsilon_n^1 = 0$ and thus not update the initial Q. □

This proves that, not only does the TMLE algorithm only require a $g_0(Q) \in \mathcal{G}(Q, P_0)$ in order to achieve the full asymptotic bias reduction, but, in addition, the TMLE algorithm using such a $g_0(Q)$ will not update an initial Q that already solves a $P_0D(Q, g) = 0$ for a $g \in \mathcal{G}(Q, P_0)$. That is, TMLE is "smart enough" to keep an unbiased initial (TMLE) unbiased. This motivates the following C-TMLE at P_0.

Theorem A.4. *Suppose that we are given a sequence $g^1, \ldots, g^K$ of candidates satisfying the following property: For any Q, there exists a $k \in \{1, \ldots, K\}$ so that $g^k \in \mathcal{G}(Q, P_0)$ (e.g., $g^K = g_0$). Consider the following C-TMLE algorithm. Start with Q^0, g^1; as the first step, compute TMLE Q^{1*} based on initial Q^0 using g^1; as the second step, compute TMLE Q^{2*} based on initial Q^{1*} using g^2, and, in general, at the kth step, compute TMLE Q^{k*} updating Q^{k-1*} using g^k, $k = 1, \ldots, K$. Select $k_0 = \arg\min_k P_0L(Q^{k*})$, where we select the smallest among the minima. The output of the C-TMLE is now $(Q^* \equiv Q^{k_0*}, g^{k_0*})$ and the corresponding C-TMLE $\Psi(Q^*)$ of ψ_0. Assume that, for each k, if $g^k \in \mathcal{G}(Q^{k*}, P_0)$, then $g^{k+1} \in \mathcal{G}(Q^{k*}, P_0)$.*

Properties. *This procedure generates K TMLEs $(Q^{1^*}, g^1), \ldots, (Q^{K^*}, g^K)$. This sequence of candidate TMLEs has the following properties. (1) There exists a smallest $k_0 \in \{1, \ldots, K\}$ so that $\Psi(Q^{k_0*}) = \psi_0$; (2) for $k \geq k_0$, $Q^{k^*} = Q^{k_0*}$, and, in particular, $\Psi(Q^{k^*}) = \psi_0$; and (3) $P_0L(Q^{k^*})$ is decreasing in $k \in \{1, \ldots, k_0\}$ and constant for $k \geq k_0$. The C-TMLE selects this smallest k_0 and thus satisfies $\Psi(Q^*) = \psi_0$.*

The existence of a $g_k \in \mathcal{G}(Q, P_0)$ is guaranteed by making $g_K = g_0$. The conservation part of this property can typically be arranged by, for each k, making g^{k+1} a more nonparametric fit of g_0 than g^k. For example, g^{k+1} could be a conditional distribution of C, adjusting for an extra binary variable beyond the k variables that g^k adjusted for. This extra binary variable could be selected from among a set of candidates as the one that yields the maximal decrease in risk for the resulting Q^{k*}, thereby allowing for algorithms that build sequences $(g^k : k)$ that are maximally effective in bias reduction. In this way, the elements g^k also approximate the true g_0 when k increases. We wish to select this smallest k_0 since it corresponds with a TMLE that uses the smallest sufficient approximation of g_0. The additional efforts in bias reduction for steps $k > k_0$ in the C-TMLE algorithm are useless at P_0, and will induce unnecessary variance and bias for finite samples.

In the above C-TMLE algorithm the next TMLE in the sequence used the previous TMLE as initial estimator, thereby guaranteeing that the risk $P_0L(Q)$ (i.e., the expectation of the loss function) of the candidate TMLEs decreases in k. If, just by virtue of using the next g^{k+1}, the next TMLE $Q^{k+1,*}$ already decreases the risk, i.e., $P_0L(Q^{k+1,*}) < P_0L(Q^{k,*})$, when using the same initial estimator as $Q^{k,*}$ uses, then we do not have to update the initial estimator. With this modification of the above C-TMLE algorithm, the updating of the initial estimator, which involves extra fitting of the data, is preserved for when it is necessary. As a consequence, the resulting C-TMLE algorithm can be applied with long sequences $(g^k : k)$ that slowly approximate g_0 in k and only now and then update the initial estimator for the TMLEs.

The empirical counterpart of this algorithm represents the C-TMLE algorithm one applies to a data set. That is, in the above description of C-TMLE, Q plays the role of an initial estimator $\hat{Q}^0(P_n)$, g^k plays role of the kth estimator $\hat{g}^k(P_n)$ of g_0, and P_0 is replaced by P_n. In addition, minimizing the risk $P_0 L(Q^{k*})$ over the candidates indexed by k to select the desired TMLE among the sequence of TMLEs is replaced by minimizing the cross-validated risk of the estimator $P_n \rightarrow \hat{Q}^{k*}(P_n)$, so that k_0 is replaced by the optimal cross-validation selector for which oracle results are available.

A.18 Asymptotic Linearity of (C-)TMLE

Summary. We provide a template for proving the asymptotic linearity of the C-TMLE and explain the conditions.

Consider a TMLE or C-TMLE Q_n^* with corresponding g_n, which solves the efficient influence curve estimating equation or some other estimating equation:

$$0 = P_n D^*(Q_n^*, g_n).$$

It is a reasonable assumption that Q_n^* converges to some element Q^* in the model for Q_0, where Q^* is not necessarily equal to the true Q_0. We assume that consistency has been established in the sense that g_n converges to a $g_0 \in \mathcal{G}(Q^*, P_0)$, so that $\Psi(Q^*) = \Psi(Q_0) = \psi_0$. Recall that $\mathcal{G}(Q^*, P_0)$ is such that for each $g \in \mathcal{G}(Q^*, P_0)$ $P_0 D^*(Q^*, g) = 0$ implies $\Psi(Q^*) = \psi_0$. For notational convenience, we will also denote the limit of g_n by g_0 even though it does not need to represent the actual censoring mechanism of the data-generating experiment. Given the consistency of Q_n^* and g_n, we will also have that $P_0 D^*(Q^*, g_0) = 0$.

To derive the influence curve of $\Psi(Q_n^*)$, the asymptotic linearity theorem below assumes that the limit g_0 of the selected censoring mechanism estimator satisfies:

$$P_0 D^*(Q_n^*, g_0) = \psi_0 - \Psi(Q_n^*) + (P_n - P_0) IC_Q + o_P(1/\sqrt{n}) \tag{A.11}$$

for some $IC_Q \in L_0^2(P_0)$. The $o_P(1/\sqrt{n})$ can be replaced by $O\left(\left\|\Psi(Q_n^*) - \psi_0\right\|^2\right)$ as well. In the special case where $IC_Q = 0$, the influence curve does not involve a contribution requiring the analysis of a function of Q_n^*. This potential important simplification of the influence curve allows straightforward calculation of standard errors for the C-TMLE. This assumption is best illustrated with an example, which we provide after the theorem below.

Theorem A.5. *Let $(Q, g) \rightarrow D^*(Q, g)$ be a well-defined function that maps any possible (Q, g) into a function of O. Let $O_1, \ldots, O_n \sim P_0$ be i.i.d. and let P_n be the empirical probability distribution. Let $Q \rightarrow \Psi(Q)$ be a d-dimensional parameter, where $\psi_0 = \Psi(Q_0)$ is the parameter value of interest. In the following template* *for proving the asymptotic linearity of $\Psi(Q_n^*)$ as an estimator of $\Psi(Q_0)$, Q_n^* and g_n represent a (C-)TMLE of Q_0, coupled with an estimator g_n used in the TMLE step, but it can be any estimator. Let Q^* and g_0 denote the limits of Q_n^* and g_n. Make the following assumptions.*

Efficient influence curve estimating equation. $0 = P_n D^*(Q_n^*, g_n)$.

Censoring mechanism estimator is nonparametric *enough*. $P_0 D^*(Q^*, g_0) = 0$ *and* $\Psi(Q^*) = \psi_0$.

Consistent estimation of D^*. $P_0(D^*(Q_n^*, g_n) - D^*(Q^*, g_0))^2 \to 0$ *in probability, as* $n \to \infty$. *The same is assumed if one component of* (Q_n^*, g_n) *is replaced by its limit* (Q^*, g_0).

Donsker class. $\{D^*(Q, g) : Q, g\}$ *is* P_0*-Donsker, where* (Q, g) *vary over sets that contain* (Q_n^*, g_n), (Q^*, g_n), (Q_n^*, g) *with probability tending to 1.*

Asymptotic linearity condition for censoring mechanism estimator. *Define the mapping* $g \to \Phi(g) \equiv P_0 D^*(Q^*, g)$. *Assume* $\Phi(g_n) - \Phi(g_0) = (P_n - P_0)IC_{g_0} + o_P(1/\sqrt{n})$ *for some mean-zero function* $IC_{g_0} \in L_0^2(P_0)$.

Asymptotic linearity of Q_0-estimator.

$$P_0 D^*(Q_n^*, g_0) = \psi_0 - \Psi(Q_n^*) + (P_n - P_0)IC_{Q^*} + o_P(1/\sqrt{n}). \tag{A.12}$$

Second-order term. *Define also the second-order term*

$$R_n = P_0\{D^*(Q_n^*, g_n) - D^*(Q_n^*, g_0)\} - P_0\{D^*(Q^*, g_n) - D^*(Q^*, g_0)\},$$

and assume $R_n = o_P(1/\sqrt{n})$. *Note* R_n *is a second-order term involving the product of the differences* $Q_n^* - Q^*$ *and* $g_n - g_0$.

Then ψ_n *is an asymptotically linear estimator of* ψ_0 *at* P_0 *with the influence curve*

$$IC(P_0) = D^*(Q^*, g_0, \psi_0) + IC_{Q^*} + IC_{g_0}.$$

In particular, $\sqrt{n}(\psi_n - \psi_0)$ *converges in distribution to a multivariate normal distribution with mean zero and covariance matrix* $\Sigma_0 = E_0 IC(P_0) IC(P_0)^\top$.

Proof. The principal equations are $0 = P_n D^*(Q_n^*, g_n) = P_0 D^*(Q^*, g_0)$, and the first second-order-term condition $P_0 D^*(Q_n^*, g_0) = \psi_0 - \Psi(Q_n^*) + (P_n - P_0)IC_{Q^*} + o_P(1/\sqrt{n})$. This yields

$$\Psi(Q_n^*) - \psi_0 = (P_n - P_0)\{D^*(Q_n^*, g_n) + IC_{Q^*}\} + P_0\{D^*(Q_n^*, g_n) - D^*(Q_n^*, g_0)\} + o_P(1/\sqrt{n}).$$

By the consistency condition and Donsker condition, the first term on the right-hand side equals $(P_n - P_0)D^*(Q^*, g_0) + o_P(1/\sqrt{n})$ (van der Vaart and Wellner 1996). The second term on the right-hand-side equals R_n plus the term $\Phi(g_n) - \Phi(g) = P_0\{D^*(Q^*, g_n) - D^*(Q^*, g_0)\}$. The asymptotic linearity condition on the censoring mechanism estimator shows that this equals $(P_n - P_0)IC_{g_0} + o_P(1/\sqrt{n})$. This completes the proof. □

Illustration of condition (A.12). Suppose $O = (W, A, Y) \sim P_0$, the model for P_0 is nonparametric, and the target parameter is $\psi_0 = E_0[E_0(Y \mid A = 1, W)]$. Suppose g_n converges to some true conditional distribution of A, given W^s, for some reduction W^s of W, and we will denote the latter by g_0. For any g_0, we have

$$P_0 D^*(Q_n^*, g_0) = P_0 \frac{A}{g_0(A \mid W^s)}(\bar{Q}_0(1, W) - \bar{Q}_n^*(1, W)) + \bar{Q}_n^*(1, W) - \Psi(Q_n^*)$$
$$= P_0 \left\{ \frac{A}{g_0(A \mid W^s)} - 1 \right\} (\bar{Q}_0(1, W) - \bar{Q}_n^*(1, W)) + \psi_0 - \Psi(Q_n^*).$$

Verification of condition (A.12) requires showing that the first term involving the expectation with respect to P_0 is asymptotically linear with some influence curve IC_{Q^*}. Firstly, consider the case that g_0 is the true conditional distribution of A, given W, i.e., $W^s = W$. In that case, by conditioning on W, and noting that $E_0(A/g_0(A \mid W) - 1) = 0$, it follows that this term equals zero, so that (A.12) holds with $IC_{Q^*} = 0$. Secondly, consider the case where $\bar{Q}_0(A, W) = E_0(Y \mid A, W)$ only depends on W through W^s, and that $\bar{Q}_n^*$ is only a function of W^s. In this case, the residual bias $\bar{Q}_0(1, W) - \bar{Q}_n^*(1, W)$ is only a function of W^s. As a consequence, by conditioning on W^s, it follows again that this first term equals zero, so that (A.12) holds with $IC_{Q^*} = 0$. However, if we only know that $\bar{Q}_n^*$ converges to a $\bar{Q}^*$ for which the asymptotic residual bias $\bar{Q}^*(1, W) - \bar{Q}_0(1, W)$ is only a function of W^s, then this first term equals $P_0 \left\{ \frac{A}{g_0(A|W^s)} - 1 \right\} (\bar{Q}^* - \bar{Q}_n^*)(1, W)$, which might potentially contribute an influence curve term IC_{Q^*}. The latter term would require showing that this integrated difference $\bar{Q}_n^* - \bar{Q}^*$ is asymptotically linear. In practice, one might consider adjusting for $\bar{Q}_n^0$ or, using an iterative procedure, for $\bar{Q}_n^*$, in g_n, so that W^s will include this potential dependence of $\bar{Q}_n^*$ on covariates that do not theoretically affect Y.

To summarize, (1) if g_n converges to a true conditional distribution $g_0(A \mid W^s)$ that conditions minimally on all relevant confounders (i.e., all variables that the conditional mean of Y depends on), and the estimator $\bar{Q}_n^*$ is a function of W^s only with probability tending to 1, then it follows that condition (A.12) holds with $IC_{Q^*} = 0$; (2) if, on the other hand, g_n is a collaborative estimator that converges to the true conditional distribution $g_0(A \mid W^s)$ that conditions on a rich enough reduction W^s of W that captures the asymptotic residual bias $\bar{Q}^*(1, W) - \bar{Q}_0(1, W)$ (which is sufficient for the consistency of the C-TMLE), then the estimator $\bar{Q}_n^*$ will contribute an IC_{Q^*} to the influence curve of $\Psi(Q_n^*)$ through $P_0 \left\{ \frac{A}{g_0(A|W^s)} - 1 \right\} (\bar{Q}^* - \bar{Q}_n^*)(1, W) \approx (P_n - P_0) IC_{Q^*}$.

A.19 Efficiency Maximization and TMLE

Summary. Consider estimating a pathwise differentiable parameter on a semi-parametric model based on n i.i.d. observations. The TMLE is a consistent, asymptotically linear, locally efficient substitution estimator of the target parameter under appropriate regularity conditions. The asymptotic efficiency corresponds with asymptotic optimal estimation [usually implying remarkable robustness such as double robustness in censored-data models that satisfy the CAR assumption, van der Laan and Robins (2003)], while being a substitution estimator guarantees that the estimator respects the global constraints on the target parameter imposed by the statistical model and the target parameter mapping. The latter allows the estimator to be robust under sparsity. Another property of interest of an estimator is that it is guaranteed to asymptotically outperform a user supplied class of asymptotically linear estimators, i.e., even when it is not asymptotically efficient, but still asymptotically linear, it will outperform each of the estimators in this class. That is, the estimator is guaranteed to asymptotically dominate a certain user-supplied class of asymptotically linear estimators. This can be achieved with empirical efficiency maximization (EEM) as introduced in Rubin and van der Laan (2008) for empirical efficiency over parametric models, refined by Tan (2008) to preserve double robustness, and presented in terms of cross-validation to select among candidate C-TMLE in van der Laan and Gruber (2010). In the next sections we demonstrate in great generality how EEM and TMLE can be combined into a TMLE that also satisfies this dominance property. It involves an application of loss-based super learning with the squared-efficient-influence-curve loss function and a library of candidate TMLEs. For RCTs it guarantees that the resulting TMLE dominates a user-supplied class of asymptotically linear estimators.

Super learner with squared efficient influence curve loss. Let $O \sim P_0 \in \mathcal{M}$, and let $\Psi : \mathcal{M} \rightarrow \mathbb{R}$ be the target parameter of interest. Let $O_1, \ldots, O_n$ be i.i.d. copies of O. Suppose that $\Psi(P_0)$ only depends on P_0 through a parameter Q_0. We will also use the notation $\Psi(Q_0)$. Let L be a loss function for Q_0 so that $Q_0 = \arg\min_{Q \in Q} P_0 L(Q)$. Let $D^*(P)$ be the efficient influence curve at P of the parameter $\Psi : \mathcal{M} \rightarrow \mathbb{R}$, and suppose that it depends on $Q(P)$ and $g(P)$ for some other (nuisance) parameter g. In addition, for given values Q, g, let $\{Q_g(\epsilon) : \epsilon\} \subset \mathcal{M}$ be a submodel with $Q_g(\epsilon = 0) = Q$ satisfying $D^*(Q, g) \in \langle \frac{d}{d\epsilon} L(Q_g(\epsilon))\big|_{\epsilon=0} \rangle$. A TMLE can now be defined in terms of an initial estimator $Q_n^0 = \hat{Q}^0(P_n)$ of Q_0, an estimator $g_n = \hat{g}(P_n)$ of g_0, and an iterative TMLE-updating algorithm resulting in a TMLE $Q_n^* = \hat{Q}^*(P_n)$ solving $P_n D^*(Q_n^*, g_n) = 0$.

Consider a collection of initial estimators $\hat{Q}_j : \mathcal{M}_{NP} \rightarrow Q$, $j = 1, \ldots, J$, of Q_0. This provides us with a collection of candidate TMLEs $\hat{Q}_j^*$, $j = 1, \ldots, J$. Let $\hat{Q}_\alpha = f_\alpha(\hat{Q}_j : j)$ be a combination of the J initial estimators indexed by a weight-vector α. For example, $\hat{Q}_\alpha = \sum_j \alpha(j)\hat{Q}_j$. Note that $\hat{Q}_\alpha$ is just another initial estimator indexed by a vector of weights α. This family of candidate initial estimators $\hat{Q}_\alpha$ indexed by a choice α includes the discrete choices $\hat{Q}_j$, $j = 1, \ldots, J$. This family of candidate initial estimators $\hat{Q}_\alpha$ generates a corresponding family of TMLEs given by $\hat{Q}_\alpha^*$ indexed by α. We wish to select among these candidate TMLEs. (The method below also applies for selection among candidate C-TMLEs $\hat{Q}^*_\alpha$ involving a collaborative estimator $g_{n,\alpha}$ of g_0.) For that purpose, we need a loss function for Q_0 so that we can use the cross-validation selector. We wish to choose a loss function that selects the estimator with the best asymptotic efficiency among all the α-specific candidate TMLEs of ψ_0. A related goal (and equivalent goal if g_0 is known) is to choose a loss function that selects the estimator $\hat{Q}^*_\alpha$ that yields the best estimator $D^*(\hat{Q}^*_\alpha, g_0)$ of the true efficient influence curve $D^*(Q_0, g_0)$. We demonstrate how both goals can be achieved.

This is a sensible goal if one believes that all candidate TMLEs are considered asymptotically linear estimators of ψ_0. We will first consider the case where we have available a consistent estimator g_n of g_0, and, in this case, we wish to make sure that the proposed selector achieves its goal. For example, g_0 might be known, such as in an RCT, or the design provides enough knowledge about g_0 (e.g., it is known that censoring is independent) such that a good consistent estimator of g_0 will be available. Either way, g_0 is typically a much easier to estimate parameter than Q_0, so that utilizing an estimator of g_0 in order to improve the estimation of Q_0 is sensible.

We could now apply loss-based super learning, with this library of candidate estimators $\hat{Q}^*_\alpha$ indexed by α, to estimate Q_0 with the following targeted loss function:

$$L_{g_0}(Q) = \{D^*(Q, g_0)\}^2.$$

Since our candidate estimators are supposedly consistent for ψ_0, this is a valid loss function if $P_0\{D^*(Q, g_0)\}^2$ is minimized at $Q = Q_0$ among all Qs with $\Psi(Q) = \psi_0$. We now explain why this is indeed a valid loss function. The basic point is that as long as Q correctly specifies ψ_0 (and in some models one needs to correctly specify a larger parameter of Q_0), then $D^*(Q, g_0)$ is typically a gradient of the target parameter mapping $\Psi : \mathcal{M}(g_0) \rightarrow \mathbb{R}$ for the model $\mathcal{M}(g_0) \subset \mathcal{M}$ where g_0 is known. As a consequence, $D^*(Q_0, g_0) = \Pi(D^*(Q, g_0) \mid T_{Q_0}(P_0))$, where $T_{Q_0}(P_0)$ is the tangent space of model $\mathcal{M}(g_0)$ and Π is the projection operator in the Hilbert space $L^2_0(P_0)$. This proves that $\| D^*(Q_0, g_0) \|^2_{P_0} \leq \| D^*(Q, g_0) \|^2_{P_0}$. More importantly, by the theorem of Pythagoras, this proves that for a Q that correctly specifies the desired part of Q_0 (including ψ_0), we have

$$\| D^*(Q, g_0 \|^2_{P_0} - \| D^*(Q_0, g_0) \|^2_{P_0} = \| D^*(Q, g_0) - D^*(g_0, Q_0) \|^2 .$$

The left-hand side equals the loss-based dissimilarity $P_0\{L_{g_0}(Q) - L_{g_0}(Q_0)\}$. This proves that indeed the loss function L_{g_0} is a valid loss function with a loss-based dissimilarity equal to a squared $L^2(P_0)$-norm of $D^*(Q, g_0) - D^*(Q_0, g_0)$!

This argument relies on $D^*(Q, g_0)$ being a gradient in the model where g_0 is known and Q correctly specifies ψ_0. This can be further supported as follows. By Theorem 1.3 in van der Laan and Robins (2003) for CAR censored-data models for $O = \Phi(C, X) \sim P_0$ with the censoring mechanism $g_0(C \mid X)$ being known, a class of gradients of the pathwise derivative can typically be represented as $D^*(Q, g_0) = D_{IPCW}(\Psi(Q), \theta(Q), g_0) + D_{CAR}(Q, g_0)$ for any Q satisfying $\Psi(Q) = \psi_0$ and $\theta(Q) = \theta_0$, where in many cases the additional nuisance parameter $\theta_0 = \theta(Q_0)$

is not present. Here ψ_0, θ_0 represent the part of Q_0 that need to be consistently estimated, while the remaining part of Q_0 is protected against misspecification in the sense that $P_0 D^*(Q, g_0) = 0$ as long as $\Psi(Q) = \psi_0$ and $\theta(Q) = \theta_0$. Here D_{IPCW} is an IPCW estimating function and $D_{CAR}(Q, g_0) \in T_{CAR}(P_0)$ is an element in the tangent space $T_{CAR}(P_0) = \{V(O) : E_{g_0}(V(O) \mid X) = 0\}$ of g_0 when only assuming CAR on g_0. The optimal choice in this set of gradients is achieved at $Q = Q_0$ so that $D^*(Q_0, g_0) = D_{IPCW}(\psi_0, \theta_0, g_0) + D_{CAR}(Q_0, g_0)$. This shows that $Q \rightarrow P_0\{D^*(Q, g_0)\}^2$ is minimized at Q_0 over all Q with $\Psi(Q) = \psi_0$ and $\theta(Q) = \theta_0$. As a consequence, indeed, $\{D^*(Q, g_0)\}^2$ is a valid loss function to select Q_0 among a class of Q with $\Psi(Q) = \psi_0$ and $\theta(Q) = \theta_0$. For the sake of presentation (and the examples covered in this book do not have a θ_0 due to our observed data models being nonparametric), we consider the case that θ_0 is not present. In particular, if g_0 is known, then the TMLE $\Psi(Q_n^*)$ using the known g_0 is asymptotically linear with influence curve $D^*(Q, g_0)$ with Q being the limit of Q_n^*, so that the optimal influence curve among all these influence curves is the efficient influence curve $D^*(Q_0, g_0)$. In this special case where g_0 is known, the cross-validation selector based on $L_{g_0}(Q)$ corresponds with minimizing the variance of the influence curves of the candidate TMLEs $\hat{Q}_\alpha^*$. We conclude that $Q_0 = \arg\min_Q P_0 L_{g_0}(Q)$, where the minimum is taken over all $Q \in \mathcal{Q}$ with $\Psi(Q) = \psi_0$.

Given a cross-validation scheme $B_n \in \{0, 1\}^n$ with corresponding empirical distributions P_{n,B_n}^1, P_{n,B_n}^0 for the B_n-specific validation and training sample, we select the TMLE indexed by

$$\alpha_n = \arg\min_\alpha E_{B_n} P_{n,B_n}^1 L_{g_0}(\hat{Q}_\alpha^*(P_{n,B_n}^0)).$$

The resulting estimator of ψ_0 is given by

$$\psi_n^* = \Psi(\hat{Q}_{\alpha_n}^*(P_n)).$$

The cross-validation selector needs to be applied to estimators that are consistent for ψ_0 at a faster rate than the rate at which Q_0 can be estimated with respect to the loss-based dissimilarity. For example, if all the candidate estimators $\Psi(\hat{Q}_\alpha^*(P_n))$ are asymptotically linear, then this holds. It is also possible to use the above loss function by plugging in a separate estimator for ψ_0 in a representation $D^*(Q_0, g_0, \psi_0)$ of the efficient influence curve, so that both g_0 and ψ_0 are treated as nuisance parameters of this loss function for Q_0 that need to be estimated once and for all before the selection process starts. In many examples of interest, $D^*(Q, g_0) = D(Q, g_0) - \psi_0$ for some $D(Q, g_0)$, in which case, we can define the loss as

$$L_{g_0}(Q) = D(Q, g_0)^2,$$

which no longer depends on ψ_0. The latter is now a valid loss function over all Q (i.e., no need to restrict to Q with $\Psi(Q) = \psi_0$).

Before we proceed in our discussion of the theoretical properties of this cross-validation selector α_n in the next section, we conclude this section with a few remarks. Firstly, one could decide not to cross-validate the candidate TMLEs, such that

$$\alpha_n^e = \arg\min_{\alpha} P_n L_{g_0}(\hat{Q}_\alpha^*(P_n)).$$

This includes the case where $\hat{Q}_\alpha(P_n)$ is constant in P_n so that $\{\hat{Q}_\alpha : \alpha\}$ represents a parametric model, and $\hat{Q}_\alpha^*$ represents the TMLE that updates this particular nonrandom initial $\hat{Q}_\alpha$. In this special case, the empirical α_n^e corresponds with empirical efficiency as defined in Rubin and van der Laan (2008) for computing the optimal parameter value of a parametric model that maximizes empirical efficiency of the resulting double robust estimator. Even though α_n^e is appropriate for parametric models, we strongly recommend the cross-validation selector α_n when $\hat{Q}_\alpha$ are adaptive estimators. Our oracle result below for the cross-validation selector α_n proves that α_n will be robust against adaptive initial estimators.

We also note that in great generality $D^*(Q, g_0, \psi_0)$ is linear in Q. For a smooth parametric family $\{Q_\alpha : \alpha\}$, this linearity makes $D^*(Q_\alpha, g_0, \psi_0)^2$ a nice smooth function in α, so that the computation of α_n or α_n^e is computationally tractable. For example, if $Q_\alpha = \sum_j \alpha_j Q_j$, then $D^*(Q_\alpha, g_0, \psi_0) = \sum_j \alpha_j D^*(Q_j, g_0, \psi_0)$, so that optimizing $\alpha \rightarrow P_0\{D^*(Q_\alpha, g_0, \psi_0)\}^2$ is equivalent with linear least squares regression, which can be done with simple standard software.

We remark that one could also select among candidate (C)-TMLEs $\hat{Q}_\alpha^*$ by minimizing over α an estimator of the variance of $\Psi(\hat{Q}_\alpha^*(P_n))$. That is, if this estimator has influence curve $IC_\alpha(P_0)$, then we could estimate its variance with $E_{B_n} P_{n,B_n}^1 IC_{\alpha,P_{n,B_n}^0}^2/n$, where IC_{α,P_{n,B_n}^0} is an estimator of the influence curve $IC_\alpha(P_0)$ based on the training sample P_{n,B_n}^0 only. This is slightly different from the above selector α_n since the influence curve of the TMLE $\Psi(\hat{Q}_\alpha^*(P_n))$ equals $D^*(Q_\alpha^*, g_0)$ plus a term due to estimating g_0 with g_n. The latter contribution improves the influence curve relative to using the true g_0. As shown in van der Laan and Robins (2003) the influence curve of $\Psi(\hat{Q}_\alpha^*(P_n))$ can still be represented as $IC_\alpha(P_0) = D_{IPCW}(\psi_0, g_0) + D_{CAR}(Q_\alpha^*, g_0)$, where the element $D_{CAR}(Q_\alpha^*, g_0) \in T_{CAR}(P_0)$ is a sum of the element in $T_{CAR}(P_0)$ it would have been for known g_0 plus another term due to estimation of g_0. As a consequence, minimizing the variance of the influence curve $IC_\alpha(P_0)$ over choices Q_α^* (all satisfying $\Psi(Q_\alpha^*) = \psi_0$) can still be represented as minimizing $P_0 L_{g_0,1}(Q_\alpha^*)$ for a valid loss function $L_{g_0,1}(Q_\alpha^*)$ that equals the square of the influence curve of $IC_\alpha(P_0)$. However, the form of the loss-based dissimilarity of L_{g_0}, as established in the next section, shows that the cross-validation selector α_n drives the estimated efficient influence curve to the actual efficient influence curve $D^*(Q_0, g_0)$, even when g_0 is estimated with a consistent estimator g_n. This suggests that, in practice, if g_0 is estimated, the variance of the influence curve of the cross-validated selected estimator $\Psi(\hat{Q}_{\alpha_n}^*(P_n))$ will still closely approximate the choice that would select the influence curve with the smallest variance. Therefore, we suggest that for practical purposes no modification of the loss function $L_{g_0}(Q)$ is necessary when the TMLE uses an estimator g_n of g_0.

Our proposed cross-validation selector based on the square efficient influence curve $L_{g_0}(Q)$ does rely on the availability of a consistent estimator g_n of g_0. If one does not want to rely on the consistency of g_n as an estimator of g_0 (e.g., g_0 has similar complexity to Q_0), and it is not possible to find a robust version of the loss function L_{g_0} so that L_g remains a valid loss function for Q_0 at misspecified g (as we demonstrate in the example in a later section), then one might still utilize this loss function L_{g_0} that targets the variance, by adding it as a penalty to a loss function L for Q_0 (that is not affected by g_0). For some positive constant a, b, let

$$L_{1,g_0}(Q) = aL(Q) + b\frac{L_{g_0}(Q)}{n}.$$

In this case, even if g_0 is misspecified, the loss function $L_{1,g_0}(Q)$ remains valid. Thus, now (say $a = b = 1$)

$$\alpha_n = \arg\min_\alpha E_{B_n} P^1_{n,B_n} \left\{ L(\hat{Q}^*_\alpha(P^0_{n,B_n})) + L_{g_n}(\hat{Q}^*_\alpha(P^0_{n,B_n})) \right\}.$$

This type of valid targeted loss function was utilized in van der Laan and Gruber (2010) to build C-TMLE and to select among candidate TMLEs, where one should note that $P_0 L_{g_0}(Q)/n$ equals the asymptotic variance of the TMLE $\Psi(Q^*_n)$ of ψ_0, if $g_n = g_0$ and Q denotes the limit of Q^*_n. The first loss function $L(Q)$ drives the selection towards Q_0, regardless of the estimator g_n, while the second loss L_{g_0}/n targets the selection toward minimizing the variance of the resulting TMLE of ψ_0. Such a robust targeted loss function can also be used to select among candidate C-TMLEs $\hat{Q}^*_\alpha$, involving a collaborative estimation procedure of g_0 (van der Laan and Gruber 2010).

A.20 Oracle Inequality of Cross-Validation Selector

Let us now present the oracle inequality for this cross-validation selector α_n, as presented originally in van der Laan and Dudoit (2003). Let $d_{g_0}(Q, Q_0) = P_0\{L_{g_0}(Q) - L_{g_0}(Q_0)\}$ denote the loss-function based dissimilarity. Assume that the loss function is bounded: $M_1 \equiv \sup_Q \mid L_{g_0}(Q) - L_{g_0}(Q_0) \mid < \infty$. In addition, we assume that

$$P_0 \left\{ L_{g_0}(Q) - L_{g_0}(Q_0) \right\}^2 \leq M_2 P_0\{L_{g_0}(Q) - L_{g_0}(Q_0)\}.$$

As explained in van der Laan and Dudoit (2003), the latter assumption corresponds with the loss-based dissimilarity being quadratic in the difference between Q and Q_0. Below, we show that indeed, in great generality, $P_0 L_{g_0}(Q) - P_0 L_{g_0}(Q_0) \leq P_0\{D^*(Q, g_0) - D^*(Q_0, g_0)\}^2$. Thus, to prove the second property of the loss function L_{g_0}, it remains to show that $P_0\{D^{*2}(Q, g_0) - D^{*2}(Q_0, g_0)\}^2 \leq M_2 P_0\{D^*(Q, g_0) - D^*(Q_0, g_0)\}^2$ for some $M_2 < \infty$. The latter trivially holds for bounded D^*:

$$\begin{aligned}
&P_0\{D^{*2}(Q, g_0) - D^{*2}(Q_0, g_0)\}^2 \\
&\quad = P_0\{D^*(Q, g_0) - D^*(Q_0, g_0)\}^2\{D^*(Q, g_0) + D^*(Q_0, g_0)\}^2 \\
&\quad \leq \sup_o \mid \{D^*(Q, g_0) + D^*(Q_0, g_0)\}^2 \mid (o) P_0\{D^*(Q, g_0) - D^*(Q_0, g_0)\}^2,
\end{aligned}$$

which completes the proof. This allows us to apply the oracle inequality for the cross-validation selector as presented in van der Laan and Dudoit (2003) providing us with the following result. If the cross-validation selector α_n is defined as a minimizer over a grid with $K(n)$ α-values, then for any $\delta > 0$,

$$Ed_{g_0}(\hat{Q}_{\alpha_n}(P^0_{n,B_n}), Q_0) \leq (1 + 2\delta) E \min_{\alpha} E_{B_n} d_{g_0}(\hat{Q}_\alpha(P^0_{n,B_n}), Q_0) + C(M_1, M_2, \delta) \frac{\log K(n)}{n},$$

where $C(M_1, M_2, \delta)$ is a specified constant. The $\tilde{\alpha}_n$ that attains the minimum on the right-hand side is referred to as the oracle selector that selects the α that minimizes the dissimilarity with Q_0 for the given sample P_n. By choosing a grid with width $1/n$, we obtain a grid such that no precision is lost. In that case, the $\log K(n)$ is bounded by a constant times $\log n$. Theorem 1 of van der Laan and Dudoit (2003) also present a finite sample oracle inequality for the case where g_0 in the loss function L_{g_0} is estimated with g_n. From this finite sample inequality it follows that, if g_n converges faster to g_0 than $Q^*_{\alpha_n,n}$ converges to Q_0, then the finite sample oracle inequality is asymptotically equivalent to the above inequality (i.e., the estimation of g_n has an asymptotically negligible effect).

A.21 Loss-Based Dissimilarity

We now want to understand the loss-based dissimilarity $d_{g_0}(Q, Q_0) = P_0\{L_{g_0}(Q) - L_{g_0}(Q_0)\}$ implied by this loss function, so that the oracle result for the cross-validation selector can be interpreted accordingly. Above, we showed that this loss-based dissimilarity is the $L^2_0(P_0)$-norm of $D^*(Q, g_0) - D^*(Q_0, g_0)$, but we provide some additional detail here. Suppose $\Psi(Q) = \psi_0$. As remarked earlier, by Theorem 1.3 in van der Laan and Robins (2003) for CAR censored-data models for the observed data structure $O = \Phi(C, X)$ for some mapping Φ, full-data structure X, and censoring variable C, it follows that $D^*(Q, g_0) = D(\psi_0, g_0) - D_{CAR}(Q, g_0)$, where $D_{CAR}(Q, g_0)$ is an element of $T_{CAR}(P_0)$, $T_{CAR}(P_0) = \{V \in L^2_0(P_0) : E_{g_0}(V(O) \mid X) = 0\}$ is the tangent space of the conditional distribution g_0 of C, given X, when only assuming CAR, $D(\psi_0, g_0)$ is an IPCW function (i.e., a gradient in the model in which g_0 is known), and $D_{CAR}(Q_0, g_0)$ is the projection of $D(\psi_0, g_0)$ onto $T_{CAR}(P_0)$ in $L^2_0(P_0)$. Thus, $D^*(Q_0, g_0) = D(\psi_0, g_0) - \Pi(D(\psi_0, g_0) \mid T_{CAR}(P_0))$, while $D^*(Q, g_0) = D(\psi_0, g_0) - D_{CAR}(Q, g_0)$ with $D_{CAR}(Q, g_0) \in T_{CAR}(P_0)$. Recall $L_{g_0}(Q) = D^{*2}(Q, g_0)$. The risk $P_0 L_{g_0}(Q)$ equals the variance of $D^{*2}(Q, g_0)$ and can be denoted by $\| D^*(Q, g_0) \|^2$, where $\| \cdot \|$ is the inner-product norm in $L^2_0(P_0)$. By the theorem of Pythagoras, we have that

$$\begin{aligned} P_0 L_{g_0}(Q) - P_0 L_{g_0}(Q_0) &= \| D^*(Q, g_0) \|^2 - \| D^*(Q_0, g_0) \|^2 \\ &= \| D_{CAR}(Q, g_0) - D_{CAR}(Q_0, g_0) \|^2 \\ &= \| D^*(Q, g_0) - D^*(Q_0, g_0) \|^2 . \end{aligned}$$

This shows that L_{g_0} is a valid loss function for Q_0 and that its loss-based dissimilarity is a quadratic dissimilarity between Q and Q_0. Moreover, it shows that the loss-based dissimilarity is a direct $L^2(P_0)$ distance between the candidate efficient influence curve $D^*(Q, g_0)$ and the efficient influence curve $D^*(Q_0, g_0)$, or equivalently, between $D_{CAR}(Q, g_0)$ and $D_{CAR}(Q_0, g_0)$.

Thus, the oracle selector $\tilde{\alpha}_n$ selects, for the given sample $O_1, \ldots, O_n$, the estimator among $\{Q^*_\alpha : \alpha\}$ that yields the best estimator of the efficient influence curve $D^*(Q_0, g_0)$ with respect to the $L^2(P_0)$-norm. Since the finite sample and asymptotic behavior of a TMLE is driven by how well the efficient influence curve is estimated (see our asymptotic linearity theorem), this is essentially the best possible (i.e., most targeted) dissimilarity measure, and thereby loss function, for selecting among the candidate TMLEs.

In particular, this result teaches us that, if g_0 is known, the selected TMLE $\Psi(\hat{Q}^*_{\alpha_n}(P_n))$ will be asymptotically at least as efficient as any of the TMLEs $\Psi(\hat{Q}^*_\alpha(P_n))$, and, in case there are several candidate TMLEs that are asymptotically efficient, it is expected to achieve the efficiency bound at a faster rate in sample size than other asymptotically efficient candidate TMLEs. In addition, even if g_0 is estimated and the estimator g_n approaches g_0 faster than Q_n approaches Q_0, the selected TMLE $\Psi(\hat{Q}^*_{\alpha_n}(P_n))$ will be asymptotically equivalent to the oracle selected TMLE $\Psi(\hat{Q}^*_{\tilde{\alpha}_n}(P_n))$ (where the oracle uses the true g_0!), and thereby will yield the best selection with respect to the approximation of the true efficient influence curve $D^*(Q_0, g_0)$. As mentioned earlier, if g_0 is estimated, the selector α_n is not directly concerned with selecting the α-specific TMLE of ψ_0 whose influence curve is optimal, since it ignores that the true influence curve of the α-specific TMLE involves a possible contribution due to estimating g_n (where this contribution equals zero if $\hat{Q}_\alpha$ is consistent for Q_0). However, the oracle inequality shows that, indirectly, it will still get very close to minimizing the actual asymptotic variance.

Since, typically, an element $D_{CAR}(Q, g_0)$ factorizes as $D_{CAR}(Q, g_0) - D_{CAR}(Q_0, g_0) = H_{1,g_0} H_{2,Q-Q_0}$, the loss-based dissimilarity can be represented as a weighted L^2-norm, $P_0 H^2_{1,g_0} H^2_{2,Q-Q_0}$ (which is also a valid norm at misspecified g_0!). The latter also suggests that it might be possible to find an alternative weighted-squared-error-type loss function with the same or similar dissimilarity so that it remains a valid loss function for Q_0 at misspecified g. Such a loss function preserves the double robustness of the resulting TMLE $\Psi(\hat{Q}^*_{\alpha_n}(P_n))$. Indeed, as in the example below, it appears that this is sometimes possible.

A.22 Examples: Loss-Based Dissimilarity

Let us consider an example to demonstrate this last point. Consider the missing-data example $O = (W, \Delta, \Delta Y) \sim P_0$, a nonparametric statistical model, and target parameter $\psi_0 = E_0 Y$. Let $g_0(\delta \mid W) = P_0(\Delta = \delta \mid W)$ and $\bar{Q}_0(W) = E_0(Y \mid W, \Delta = 1)$. In this case, $D^*(Q_0, g_0) = D_{IPCW}(g_0, \psi_0) - D_{CAR}(\bar{Q}_0, g_0)$, where $D_{IPCW}(g_0, \psi_0) = Y\Delta / g_0(1 \mid W) - \psi_0$ and $D_{CAR}(\bar{Q}_0, g_0) = \bar{Q}_0(W)\left(\frac{\Delta}{g_0(1 \mid W)} - 1\right)$, so that by our general result

$$P_0 L_{g_0}(Q) - P_0 L_{g_0}(Q_0) = E_0(\bar{Q} - \bar{Q}_0)^2 \frac{g_0(0 \mid W)}{g_0(1 \mid W)}$$
$$= E_0(Y - \bar{Q}(W))^2 \frac{g_0(0 \mid W)}{g_0(1 \mid W)} - E_0(Y - \bar{Q}_0(W))^2 \frac{g_0(0 \mid W)}{g_0(1 \mid W)}.$$

This shows that the loss function L_{g_0} has a dissimilarity that is equivalent to the dissimilarity implied by the weighted-least-squares *full-data* loss function

$$L_{2,g_0}(\bar{Q}) = (Y - \bar{Q}(W))^2 \frac{g_0(0 \mid W)}{g_0(1 \mid W)}.$$

This full-data loss function could be mapped into an observed-data IPCW version of L_{2,g_0}:

$$L_{IPCW,g_0}(\bar{Q}) = (Y - \bar{Q}_0(W))^2 \Delta \frac{g_0(0 \mid W)}{g_0^2(1 \mid W)}.$$

Note that this loss function $L_{IPCW,g_0}(\bar{Q})$ has the same risk, and thereby loss-based dissimilarity, as L_{g_0}. However, this IPCW loss function has the property that it remains a valid loss function if g_0 is misspecified, so that the resulting TMLE $\Psi(Q^*_{\alpha_n,n})$ remains double robust.

Let us now consider a more complex example. Consider a right-censored data structure $O = (C, \bar{X}(C))$, where $X = (X(t) : t \in (0, \tau])$ is a time-dependent process representing the full-data structure, C is a right-censoring time, and $\bar{X}(t) = (X(s) : s \leq t)$. Let $R(t) = I(T \leq t)$ be a component of $X(t)$, where T denotes a time to final event of interest, at which time $X()$ is truncated: $X(t) = X(\min(t, T))$. Assume the CAR assumption: $g_0(c \mid X)$ is a function of $(c, \bar{X}(c))$, or equivalently, $\lambda_{g_0}(t \mid X)$ is only a function of $(t, \bar{X}(t))$, where λ_{g_0} is the conditional hazard of censoring, given X. Let Q_0 represent the factor of the density of O under P_0 that only depends on the full-data distribution: $P_0 = Q_0 g_0$, where $Q_0(c, \bar{x}(c)) = P_0(\bar{X}(c) = \bar{x}(c))$.

Consider a particular pathwise differentiable parameter, such as a survival function $\psi_0 = P_0(T > t_0)$ at time t_0. Chapter 3 in van der Laan and Robins (2003) teaches us that the efficient influence curve $D^*(Q_0, g_0)$ can be represented as $D_{IPCW}(g_0, \psi_0) - D_{CAR}(Q_0, g_0)$, where $D_{IPCW}(g_0, \psi_0) = I(T > t_0)I(C > T)/\bar{G}_0(T \mid X) - \psi_0$, $\bar{G}_0(t \mid X) = P_0(C > t \mid X)$, $D_{CAR}(Q_0, g_0) = \int H_{Q_0,g_0}(u) dM_{g_0}(u)$ for a specified function $H_{Q_0,g_0}(u, \bar{X}(u)) = E_0(D_{IPCW}(g_0, \psi_0) \mid \bar{X}(u), C > u)$, and $dM_{g_0}(u) = I(C = u) - I(C \geq u)\lambda_{g_0}(u \mid X)$. Note that $D^*(Q_0, g_0) = D(Q_0, g_0) - \psi_0$ so that we can define the loss function as $L_{g_0}(Q) = D^2(Q, g_0)$. By our general result, we have that the loss-based dissimilarity for Q is given by

$$P_0 D^2(Q, g_0) - P_0 D^2(Q_0, g_0) = P_0 \{D_{CAR}(Q, g_0) - D_{CAR}(Q_0, g_0)\}^2$$
$$= E_0 \int \{H_{Q-Q_0,g_0}(u, \bar{X}(u))\}^2 \lambda_{g_0}(1 - \lambda_{g_0})(du \mid X).$$

Here we essentially used that $T_{CAR}(P_0)$ allows an orthogonal decomposition in $L_0^2(P_0)$ according to the factorization of $g_0(C \mid X) = \prod_t g_0(A(t) \mid \bar{A}(t-), X)$ as a product of conditional distributions of Bernoulli random variables $A(t) = I(C = t)$, given $(X, \bar{A}(t-) = (I(C = s), s < t))$, and thereby that the variance (i.e., the square of the norm) of an element $D_{CAR}(Q - Q_0, g_0)$ in $T_{CAR}(P_0)$ is a sum of variances. This formula also applies to continuous C through the well-known results for martingales of counting processes (Andersen et al. 1993). Thus, the loss-based dissimilarity is an L^2-norm of $(H_{Q,g_0} - H_{Q_0,g_0})$, where H_{Q_0,g_0} is the principle element that makes up the efficient influence curve. This shows that the super learner $\hat{Q}^*_{\alpha_n}$ will select an estimator that is the best for the purpose of estimating H_{Q_0,g_0}, and thereby the efficient influence curve $D^*(Q_0, g_0)$.

The above result for the loss-based dissimilarity for the loss function L_{g_0} generalizes immediately to causal inference data structures (A, L_A), with A a time-dependent process representing censoring and treatment actions (i.e., the intervention nodes), L_A a time-dependent process including time-dependent covariates and outcomes, and L_a the counterfactual corresponding with a multiple-time-point intervention that sets A equal to the treatment profile a.

A.23 Example: EEM and TMLE

Let us revisit the missing outcome example with $O = (W, \Delta, \Delta Y) \sim P_0 \in \mathcal{M}$, $\mathcal{M}$ the nonparametric model, and $\psi_0 = E_0 Y$. Let $\Pi_0(W) = P_0(\Delta = 1 \mid W) = g_0(1 \mid W)$. The efficient influence curve is given by

$$D^*(Q_0, \Pi_0)(O) = \Delta/\Pi_0(W)(Y - \bar{Q}_0(W)) + \bar{Q}_0(W) - \Psi(Q_0),$$

where $\bar{Q}_0(W) = E_0(Y \mid W, \Delta = 1)$, $Q_0 = (Q_{W,0}, \bar{Q}_0 = E_0(Y \mid W, \Delta = 1))$. Note $D^*(Q_0, \Pi_0) = D(\bar{Q}_0, \Pi_0) - \psi_0$, . Given a parametric family Q^w for $\bar{Q}_0$, as shown in Rubin and van der Laan (2008) and above, minimizing $E_0 D^2(\bar{Q}, g_0)$ over $\bar{Q} \in Q^w$ corresponds with

$$\arg\min_{\bar{Q} \in Q^w} E_0 \frac{\Delta(1 - \Pi_0)}{\Pi_0^2}(Y - \bar{Q}(W))^2.$$

TMLE is a substitution estimator and thus has advantages over other asymptotically efficient estimators. We now want to combine TMLE with EEM, so that we can also claim that TMLE is asymptotically linear with influence curve that is optimal among a given class of influence curves $D^*(\bar{Q}, \Pi_0, \psi_0)$ with $\bar{Q} \in Q^w$. We consider EEM for the linear and logistic TMLE with respect to a parametric family $\{\bar{Q}_\alpha : \alpha\}$. The linear TMLE provides a closed-form algebraic demonstration, but does not respect known bounds, so that the preferred TMLE is the logistic TMLE, which follows. Let $Y \in [0, 1]$. Let $H_{\Pi_0} = H_0 = \frac{\Delta}{\Pi_0}$.

TMLE, squared error loss, linear fluctuation. Consider the linear fluctuation $\bar{Q}_\alpha(\epsilon) = \bar{Q}_\alpha + \epsilon H_{\Pi_0}$. Define

$$\epsilon_n(\alpha) = \arg\min_{\epsilon} P_n L_2(\bar{Q}_\alpha(\epsilon)),$$

where $L_2(\bar{Q})(O) = \Delta(Y - \bar{Q}(W))^2$. Note $\epsilon_n(\alpha)$ is the univariate linear regression coefficient (no intercept) of $(Y - \bar{Q}_\alpha)$ on H_{Π_0}. Thus

$$\epsilon_n(\alpha) = \frac{E_{P_n}\Delta(Y - \bar{Q}_\alpha)H_{\Pi_0}}{E_{P_n}\Delta H^2_{\Pi_0}}.$$

The candidate TMLEs are defined as $\bar{Q}^*_{\alpha,n} = \bar{Q}_\alpha + \epsilon_n(\alpha)H_{\Pi_0}$. We wish to determine α so that

$$\alpha \to E_0 D^2(\bar{Q}^*_{\alpha,n}, \Pi_0)$$

is minimized. Directly minimizing the empirical counterpart

$$\alpha \to P_n D(Q_\alpha, g_0)^2 = E_{P_n}\left\{Y\frac{\Delta}{\Pi_0} - \bar{Q}^*_{\alpha,n}(W)\left(\frac{\Delta}{\Pi_0} - 1\right)\right\}^2$$

corresponds with an unweighted least squares regression of an inverse-weighted outcome on an inverse-weighted corrected covariate. By the above result, this choice can also be estimated as

$$\alpha_n = \arg\min_\alpha E_{P_n}\frac{\Delta(1 - \Pi_0)}{\Pi_0^2}(Y - \bar{Q}^*_{\alpha,n}(W))^2.$$

The resulting TMLE is given by $\bar{Q}^*_{\alpha_n,n} = \bar{Q}_{\alpha_n} + \epsilon_n(\alpha_n)H_{\Pi_0}$. Note,

$$\begin{aligned}
\alpha_n &= \arg\min_\alpha E_{P_n}\frac{\Delta(1 - \Pi_0)}{\Pi_0^2}(Y - \bar{Q}_\alpha - \epsilon_n(\alpha)H_0)^2 \\
&= \arg\min_\alpha E_{P_n}\frac{\Delta(1 - \Pi_0)}{\Pi_0^2}\left(Y - \bar{Q}_\alpha - \frac{E_{P_n}\Delta(Y - \bar{Q}_\alpha)H_0}{E_{P_n}\Delta H_0^2}H_0\right)^2 \\
&= \arg\min_\alpha E_{P_n}\frac{\Delta(1 - \Pi_0)}{\Pi_0^2}\left(Y - \frac{E_{P_n}\Delta Y H_0}{E_{P_n}\Delta H_0^2}H_0 - \bar{Q}_\alpha + \frac{E_{P_n}\Delta\bar{Q}_\alpha H_0}{E_{P_n}\Delta H_0^2}H_0\right)^2.
\end{aligned}$$

If $\bar{Q}_\alpha = \alpha W$ is linear, then it follows that α_n is a weighted-linear-least-squares estimator regressing $Y - \frac{E_{P_n}\Delta Y H_0}{E_{P_n}\Delta H_0^2}H_0$ on the covariate

$$W' \equiv W - \frac{E_{P_n}\Delta W H_0}{E_{P_n}\Delta H_0^2}H_0$$

according to a linear model $\alpha W'$.

TMLE, quasi-log-likelihood loss, logistic fluctuation. The above TMLE behaves poorly under violations of the positivity assumption, since the linear fluctuation does not respect bounds, for example, $Y \in [a, b]$ for some values $[a, b]$. Therefore, we proposed an alternative TMLE based on the binary-log-likelihood loss function and logistic fluctuation. Let $\{\bar{Q}_\alpha : \alpha\}$ be a logistic regression family. Consider $\text{logit}\bar{Q}_\alpha(\epsilon) = \text{logit}\bar{Q}_\alpha + \epsilon H_0$. Define

$$\epsilon_n(\alpha) = \arg\min_\epsilon P_n L(\bar{Q}_\alpha(\epsilon)),$$

where $L(\bar{Q})(O) = \Delta\left\{Y \log \bar{Q}_\alpha + (1-Y)\log(1-\bar{Q}_\alpha)\right\}$. Note $\epsilon_n(\alpha)$ is the univariate linear logistic regression coefficient Y on H_0 using logit$\bar{Q}_\alpha$ as intercept. We have that $\epsilon_n(\alpha)$ solves

$$0 = \textstyle\sum_i \Delta_i H_0(W_i)(Y_i - \bar{Q}_\alpha(\epsilon)(W_i)).$$

Even though $\epsilon_n(\alpha)$ is not a closed form function of α, this equation allows us to determine closed-form expressions for first-order derivatives $\frac{d}{d\alpha}\epsilon_n(\alpha)$. If $\epsilon(\alpha)$ is defined as $U(\alpha, \epsilon(\alpha)) = 0$ for an equation U, then

$$\frac{d}{d\alpha}\epsilon(\alpha) = -\left\{\frac{d}{d\epsilon}U(\alpha,\epsilon)\Big|_{\epsilon=\epsilon(\alpha)}\right\}^{-1}\frac{d}{d\alpha}U(\alpha,\epsilon).$$

The candidate TMLEs are defined as logit$\bar{Q}^*_{\alpha,n}$ = logit$\bar{Q}_\alpha + \epsilon_n(\alpha)H_0$. We want to determine the minimizer of

$$\alpha \rightarrow P_0 D^2(\bar{Q}^*_{\alpha,n}, \Pi_0).$$

This choice can be estimated as

$$\alpha_n = \arg\min_\alpha E_{P_n}\frac{\Delta(1-\Pi_0)}{\Pi_0^2}(Y - \bar{Q}^*_{\alpha,n}(W))^2.$$

The desired TMLE is given by $\bar{Q}^*_{\alpha_n,n} = \bar{Q}_{\alpha_n}(\epsilon_n(\alpha_n))$. Solving for α_n corresponds with a nonlinear least squares problem. Fast algorithms for solving for this α_n will require (1) fast evaluation of $\epsilon_n(\alpha)$ and (2) closed-form expression for the derivatives in α. Since we have closed-form derivatives of $\alpha \rightarrow \epsilon_n(\alpha)$ this can be carried out with available software.

TMLE logistic with linear regression family. Suppose that we want to optimize efficiency over a linear regression model $\bar{Q}_\alpha = \alpha W$ instead of the logistic linear regression model above. We could use the optimal α_n as defined for the linear TMLE. This now defines an initial linear-least-squares estimator $\bar{Q}_{\alpha_n}$. We can truncate this fit between (0, 1) and compute the logistic TMLE update.

Appendix B
Introduction to R Code Implementation

This appendix includes a brief introduction to the implementation of super learning and the TMLE in R. Packages and supplementary code are posted online at http://www.targetedlearningbook.com. We conclude with a few coding guides for data structures and research questions presented in Parts II–IX. The book's Web site will be a continually updated resource for new code, demonstrations, and packages.

Suppose you want to implement super learning. In order to include user-specified regressions in parametric statistical models (default specification is main terms), you must write additional wrappers for the super learner function. A sample wrapper is included below, and more information on writing wrappers is on our Web site.

```
SL.glm.2 <- function(Y.temp, X.temp, newX.temp,
      family, obsWeights, ...){
fit.glm <- glm(Y.temp ~ A+W1, data=X.temp,
      family=family, weights = obsWeights)
out <- predict(fit.glm, newdata=newX.temp,
      type="response")
fit <- list(object=fit.glm)
foo <- list(out=out, fit=fit)
class(foo$fit) <- c("SL.glm")
return(foo)}
```

Sample code to run the SuperLearner package in a simulated data set called "samp," including a small proposed collection of algorithms, is included below. (Package author: Eric C. Polley.)

```
library(SuperLearner)
SL.library <- list("SL.glm.2", "SL.bayesglm",
      "SL.glmnet", "SL.glmnet.alpha50", "SL.gam",
      "SL.gam.3", "SL.nnet", "SL.nnet.4")
fit.SL <- SuperLearner(Y=samp$Y,X=samp[,c(1:3,5:6)],
      SL.library=SL.library, family=binomial,
      method="NNLS", verbose=TRUE, V=10)
```

Note that there are several options available beyond the selection of the algorithms in the super learner function. Familiarize yourself with these options in the help file. In order to obtain the *cross-validated* risk of the super learner, one must run CV.SuperLearner. Sample code is given below.

```
fit.SL.CV <- CV.SuperLearner(Y=samp$Y,
      X=samp[,c(1:3,5:6)],SL.library=SL.library,
      family=binomial,method="NNLS",
      verbose=TRUE, outside.V=10, inside.V=10)
QSL.risk <- mean((samp$Y-fit.SL.CV$pred.SL)^2)
```

Now we give sample code to implement the R package tmle (Gruber and van der Laan 2011) to estimate the parameter $\Psi(P_0) = E_{W,0}[E_0(Y \mid A = 1, W) - E_0(Y \mid A = 0, W)]$ in simulated data. We refer interested readers to Gruber and van der Laan (2011) and the supplemental materials on our Web site for additional code, explanations, and options.

```
run1 <- tmle(Y, A, W, family="binomial",
      Q.SL.library = c("SL.glm", "SL.step",
      "SL.DSA.2"), gform = A ~ W1 + W2 + W3,)
```

Implementation notes for other data structures and parameters of interest presented throughout the book for selected chapters are given below. This is not a comprehensive tutorial. As noted, additional materials are available online.

Chapters 13–15: Case-control implementation. Implementation of super learning and TMLE for case-control studies and other biased study designs is straightforward. Using weights requires a simple weight statement within the functions, for example, in Chapter 15, we call

```
fit.SL <- SuperLearner(Y=ccData$death_yn,
      X=ccData[,2:167],SL.library=SL.library,
      family=binomial,method="NNLS",obsWeights=weight,
      verbose=TRUE, V=10)
```

when generating the function for risk score using super learner.

Chapter 16: Super learning for censored data structures. Required wrappers to run super learning in censored data structures are available on our Web site. Below we present an example of hazard estimation in the publicly available lung cancer data set studied in Chapter 16 using these wrappers and the collection of algorithms discussed in the chapter. (Author: Eric C. Polley.)

```
data(lung)
subLung <- subset(lung, select = c(time, status, age,
      ph.ecog, ph.karno, pat.karno))
subLung$female <- (lung$sex - 1)
subLung <- subLung[complete.cases(subLung), ]
```

```
## Expand subLung to Long Format
longData <- SuperLearner:::createDiscrete(time =
    subLung$time, event = (subLung$status == 2),
    dataX = subset(subLung, select =
    -c(time, status)), n.delta = 30)

## Super Learner
fit.SL <- SuperLearner(Y = longData$N.delta,
    X = data.frame(age = longData$age, ph.ecog =
    longData$ph.ecog, female = longData$female,
    ph.karno = longData$ph.karno, pat.karno =
    longData$pat.karno, time = longData$delta.upper),
    V = 10, SL.library = SL.library, shuffle = FALSE,
    verbose = TRUE, id = longData$ID, family =
    binomial(), method = "NNLS")

## CV Super Learner
fit.SL.CV <- CV.SuperLearner(Y = longData$N.delta,
    X = data.frame(age = longData$age, ph.ecog =
    longData$ph.ecog, female = longData$female,
    ph.karno = longData$ph.karno, pat.karno =
    longData$pat.karno, time = longData$delta.upper),
    outside.V = 10, inside.V = 10, SL.library =
    SL.library, shuffle = FALSE, verbose = TRUE, id =
    longData$ID, family = binomial(), method = "NNLS")
```

Chapters 19–21: C-TMLE. A simple example using the C-TMLE code available on our Web site is included below. (Author: Susan Gruber.)

```
set.seed(10)
n <-1000
W <- matrix(rnorm(n*5), ncol=5)
colnames(W) <- paste("W",1:5,sep="")
logitA <- .3*W[,1]+.2*W[,2]-3*W[,3]
pA <- plogis(logitA)
Wstar <- rbinom(n,1,pA)
pA3 <- plogis(.15*logitA)
A3 <- rbinom(n,1,pA3)
Y3 <- A3+.5*W[,1]-8*W[,2]+W[,3]+8*W[,3]^2
      -2*W[,5] +rnorm(n)
d.sim3 <- data.frame(Y=Y3, A=A3, W, Wstar)
ctmle.sim3 <- ctmle(Y=d.sim3$Y, A=d.sim3$A,
      W=d.sim3[,-c(1:2)])
summary(ctmle.sim3)
```

Chapter 25: Longitudinal data. We include code that uses the DAIFI data and related functions (available on our Web site) to run the analysis presented in the corresponding chapter. (Author: Antoine Chambaz.)

```
source("DAIFI.extract_fun.R")
true <- 0.652187 ## based on 1e6 simulated data
obs <- getSample(3001, FALSE)
fit0 <- getInitialFit(obs, whole = TRUE, V = 10)
gcomp <- getEstimate(obs, fit0)
gcomp <- gcomp[1:4]
fit1 <- updateFit(obs, fit0)
tmle <- getEstimate(obs, fit1)
tmle <- tmle[1:4]
```

Chapter 29: Bayesian TMLE. We include code to run an example of Bayesian targeted learning. A uniform prior on the interval $(-1, 1)$ is used, logistic regressions are used as initial estimators of $\bar{Q}_0(A, W)$ and $g_0(A \mid W)$, and 1000 posterior observations are drawn by using the function BTL. The simulated data and required functions are available on our Web site. (Author: Iván Díaz Muñoz.)

```
data <- read.csv("data.csv")
prior.psi <- list(func = debeta, args = list(a = -1,
      b = 1, shape1 = 1, shape2 = 1))
Y <- data$Y
A <- data$A
W <- data.frame(W1 = data$W1, W2 = data$W2)
Q <- Y ~ A*W1*W2
g_A <- A ~ W1*W2
family <- "binomial"
output <- BTL(Y, A, W, prior.psi , Q, g_A, family)
```

References

A. Abadie and G.W. Imbens. Large sample properties of matching estimators for average treatment effects. *Econometrica*, 74:235–267, 2006.

G.D. Adamson, J. de Mouzon, P. Lancaster, K.-G. Nygren, E. Sullivan, and F. Zegers-Hochschild. World collaborative report on in vitro fertilization, 2000. *Fertil Steril*, 85:1586–1622, 2006.

A. Afifi and S. Azen. *Statistical Analysis: A Computer Oriented Approach.* Academic, New York, 2nd edition, 1979.

H. Akaike. Information theory and an extension of the maximum likelihood principle. In B.N. Petrov and F. Csaki, editors, *Second International Symposium on Information Theory*, Budapest, 1973. Academiai Kiado.

K. Akazawa, T. Nakamura, and Y. Palesch. Power of logrank test and Cox regression model in clinical trials with heterogenous samples. *Stat Med*, 16(5):583–597, 1997.

C. Ambroise and G.J. McLachlan. Selection bias in gene extraction on the basis of microarray gene-expression data. *Proc Natl Acad Sci*, 99(10):6562–6566, 2002.

P.K. Andersen, O. Borgan, R.D. Gill, and N. Keiding. *Statistical Models Based on Counting Processes.* Springer, Berlin Heidelberg New York, 1993.

J.A. Anderson. Separate sample logistic discrimination. *Biometrika*, 59:19–35, 1972.

K.M. Anderson, P.W.F. Wilson, P.M. Odell, and W.B. Kannel. An updated coronary risk profile. a statement for health professionals. *Circulation*, 83:356–362, 1991.

A.C. Atkinson and A. Biswas. Adaptive biased-coin designs for skewing the allocation proportion in clinical trials with normal responses. *Stat Med*, 24(16): 2477–2492, 2005.

E. Balciunaite, A. Spektor, N.H. Lents, H. Cam, H. Te Riele, A. Scime, M.A. Rudnicki, R. Young, and B.D. Dynlacht. Pocket protein complexes are recruited to distinct targets in quiescent and proliferating cells. *Mol Cell Biol*, 25(18):8166–78, 2005.

U. Bandyopadhyay and A. Biswas. Adaptive designs for normal responses with prognostic factors. *Biometrika*, 88(2):409–419, 2001.

D.R. Bangsberg, F. Hecht, E.D. Charlebois, M. Chesney, and A.R. Moss. Comparing objectives measures of adherence to hiv antiretroviral therapy: Electronic medication monitors and unannounced pill counts. *AIDS Behav*, 5:275–281, 2001.

W.E. Barlow, E. White, R. Ballard-Barbash, P.M. Vacek, L. Titus-Ernstoff, P.A. Carney, J.A. Tice, D.S. Buist, B.M. Geller, R. Rosenberg, B.C. Yankaskas, and K. Kerlikowske. Prospective breats cancer risk prediction model for women undergoing screening mammography. *J Natl Cancer Inst*, 98(17):1204–1214, 2006.

R. Baron and D. Kenny. The moderator-mediator variable distinction in social psychological research: Conceptual, strategic, and statistical considerations. *J Personal Soc Psychol*, 51:1173–1182, 1986.

J. Baselga. Herceptin alone or in combination with chemotherapy in the treatment of HER2-positive metastatic breast cancer: Pivotal trials. *Oncology*, 61(S2):14–21, 2001.

C.J. Basten, B.S. Weir, and Z.B. Zeng. *QTL Cartographer*, 2001. URL http://statgen.ncsu.edu/qtlcart/.

O. Bembom and M.J. van der Laan. A practical illustration of the importance of realistic individualized treatment rules in causal inference. *Electron J Stat*, 1: 574–596, 2007a.

O. Bembom and M.J. van der Laan. Comment: Statistical methods for analyzing sequentially randomized trials. *J Natl Cancer Inst*, 99(21):1577–1582, 2007b.

O. Bembom and M.J. van der Laan. Data-adaptive selection of the truncation level for inverse-probability-of-treatment-weighted estimators. Technical Report 230, Division of Biostatistics, University of California, Berkeley, 2008.

O. Bembom, W.J. Fessel, R.W. Shafer, and M.J. van der Laan. Data-adaptive selection of the adjustment set in variable importance estimation. 231, Division of Biostatistics, University of California, Berkeley, 2008.

O. Bembom, M.L. Petersen, S.-Y. Rhee, W.J. Fessel, S.E. Sinisi, R.W. Shafer, and M.J. van der Laan. Biomarker discovery using targeted maximum likelihood estimation: Application to the treatment of antiretroviral resistant HIV infection. *Stat Med*, 28:152–72, 2009.

Y. Benjamini and Y. Hochberg. Controlling the false discovery rate: A practical and powerful approach to multiple testing. *J R Stat Soc Ser B*, 57:289–300, 1995.

E.R. Berndt. *The Practice of Econometrics*. Addison–Wesley, New York, 1991.

J. Bhattacharya and W. Vogt. Do instrumental variables belong in propensity scores? Technical Report 343, National Bureau of Economic Research, 2007.

P.J. Bickel, C.A.J. Klaassen, Y. Ritov, and J. Wellner. *Efficient and adaptive estimation for semiparametric models*. Springer, Berlin Heidelberg New York, 1997.

W.Z. Billewicz. The efficiency of matched samples: An empirical investigation. *Biometrics*, 21(3):623–644, 1965.

M.D. Birkner, A.E. Hubbard, and M.J. van der Laan. Data adaptive pathway testing. Technical Report 197, Division of Biostatistics, University of California, Berkeley, 2005.

J. Boivin, L. Bunting, J.A. Collins, and K.G. Nygren. International estimates of infertility prevalence and treatment-seeking: Potential need and demand for infertility medical care. *Hum Reproduct*, 22:1506–1512, 2007.

G.E.P. Box and N.R. Draper. *Empirical Model-Building and Response Surfaces*. Wiley, Hoboken, 1987.

V.L. Boyartchuk, K.W. Broman, R.E. Mosher, S.E.F. D'Orazio, M.N. Starnbach, and W.F. Dietrich. Multigenic control of listeria monocytogenes susceptibility in mice. *Nat Genet*, 2001.

H. Bozdogan. Choosing the number of component clusters in the mixture model using a new informational complexity criterion of the inverse fisher information matrix. In O. Opitz, B. Lausen, and R. Klar, editors, *Information and Classification*. Springer, Berlin Heidelberg New York, 1993.

H. Bozdogan. Akaike's information criterion and recent developments in information complexity. *J Math Psychol*, 44:62–91, 2000.

H. Brady. Causation and explanation in social science. In J.M. Box-Steffensmeier, H.E. Brady, and D. Collier, editors, *The Oxford Handbook of Political Methodology*. Oxford, New York, 2008.

L. Breiman. Heuristics of instability and stabilization in model selection. *Ann Stat*, 24(6):2350–2383, 1996a.

L. Breiman. Out-of-bag estimation. Technical Report, Department of Statistics, University of California, Berkeley, 1996b.

L. Breiman. Stacked regressions. *Mach Learn*, 24:49–64, 1996c.

L. Breiman. Bagging predictors. *Mach Learn*, 24(2):123–140, 1996d.

L. Breiman. Arcing classifiers. *Ann Stat*, 26:801–824, 1998.

L. Breiman. Random forests - random features. Technical Report 567, Department of Statistics, University of California, Berkeley, 1999.

L. Breiman. *Notes on setting up, using, and understanding random forests V3.0*, 2001a.

L. Breiman. Random forests. *Mach Learn*, 45:5–32, 2001b.

L. Breiman and P. Spector. Submodel selection and evaluation in regression. The *X* random case. *Int Stat Rev*, 60:291–319, 1992.

L. Breiman, J.H. Friedman, R. Olshen, and C.J. Stone. *Classification and Regression Trees*. Chapman & Hall, Boca Raton, 1984.

N.E. Breslow. Statistics in epidemiology: The case-control study. *J Am Stat Assoc*, 91:14–28, 1996.

N.E. Breslow and N.E. Day. *Statistical Methods in Cancer Research: Volume 1 – The Analysis of Case-Control Studies*. International Agency for Research on Cancer, Lyon, 1980.

N.E. Breslow, N.E. Day, K.T. Halvorsen, R.L. Prentice, and C. Sabal. Estimation of multiple relative risk functions in matched case-control studies. *Am J Epidemiol*, 108(4):299–307, 1978.

K.W. Broman. Mapping quantitative trait loci in the case of a spike in the phenotype distribution. *Genetics*, 2003.

F. Bunea, A.B. Tsybakov, and M.H. Wegkamp. Aggregation and sparsity via L1 penalized least squares. In G. Lugosi and H.-U. Simon, editors, *COLT*, volume

4005 of *Lecture Notes in Computer Science*, Berlin Heidelberg New York, 2006. Springer.

F. Bunea, A.B. Tsybakov, and M.H. Wegkamp. Aggregation for gaussian regression. *Ann Stat*, 35(4):1674–1697, 2007a.

F. Bunea, A.B. Tsybakov, and M.H. Wegkamp. Sparse density estimation with L1 penalties. In N.H. Bshouty and C. Gentile, editors, *COLT*, volume 4539 of *Lecture Notes in Computer Science*, Berlin Heidelberg New York, 2007b. Springer.

Centers for Disease Control and Prevention. 1993 revised classification system for HIV infection and expanded surveillance case definition for AIDS among adolescents and adults. *Morbid Mortal W Rep*, 41:1–19, 1992.

P. Chaffee, A.E. Hubbard, and M.J. van der Laan. Permutation-based pathway testing using the super learner algorithm. Technical Report 263, Division of Biostatistics, University of California, Berkeley, 2010.

A. Chambaz and M.J. van der Laan. Targeting the optimal design in randomized clinical trials with binary outcomes and no covariate. Technical Report 258, Division of Biostatistics, University of California, Berkeley, 2010.

C.-C. Chang and C.-J. Lin. *LIBSVM: A library for support vector machines*, 2001. URL http://www.csie.ntu.edu.tw/ cjlin/libsvm.

H.A. Chipman and R.E. McCulloch. *BayesTree: Bayesian methods for tree-based models*, 2009. URL http://CRAN.R-project.org/package=BayesTree. R package version 0.3-1.

H.A. Chipman, E.I. George, and R.E. McCulloch. BART: Bayesian additive regression trees. *Ann Appl Stat*, 4(1):266–298, 2010.

N.A. Christakis and T.I. Iwashyna. The health impact of health care on families: A matched cohort study of hospice use by decedents and mortality outcomes in surviving, widowed spouses. *Soc Sci Med*, 57(3):465–475, 2003.

S. Chu. Pricing the C's of diamond stones. *J Stat Educ*, 9(2), 2001.

E. Clappier, W. Cuccuini, A. Kalota, A. Crinquette, J.M. Cayuela, W.A. Dik, A.W. Langerak, B. Montpellier, B. Nadel, P. Walrafen, O. Delattre, A. Aurias, T. Leblanc, H. Dombret, A.M. Gewirtz, A. Baruchel, F. Sigaux, and J. Soulier. The C-MYB locus is involved in chromosomal translocation and genomic duplications in human t-cell acute leukemia (T-ALL), the translocation defining a new T-ALL subtype in very young children. *Blood*, 110(4):1251–61, 2007.

W.S. Cleveland, E. Groose, and W.M. Shyu. Local regression models. In J.M. Chambers and T.J. Hastie, editors, *Statistical Models in S*. Chapman & Hall, Boca Raton, 1992.

W.G. Cochran. Matching in analytical studies. *Am J Public Health*, 43:684–691, 1953.

W.G. Cochran. Analysis of covariance: Its nature and uses. *Biometrics*, 13:261–281, 1957.

W.G. Cochran. The planning of observational studies of human populations. *J R Stat Soc Ser A Gen*, 128(2):234–266, 1965.

W.G. Cochran. *Planning and Analysis of Observational Studies*. Wiley, New York, 1983. Edited posthumously by L.E. Moses and F. Mosteller.

W.G. Cochran and Donald B. Rubin. Controlling bias in observational studies: A review. *Sankhya Ser A*, 35:417–446, 1973.

S.R. Cole and M.A. Hernan. Constructing inverse probability weights for marginal structural models. *Am J Epidemiol*, 168:656–664, 2008.

D. Cook. *Regression Graphics: Ideas for Studying Regression Through Graphics.* Wiley, New York, 1998.

D. Cook and S. Weisberg. *An Introduction to Regression Graphics.* Wiley, New York, 1994.

J. Cornfield. A method of estimating comparative rates from clinical data. applications to cancer of the lung, breast, and cervix. *J Nat Cancer Inst*, 11:1269–1275, 1951.

J. Cornfield. A statistical problem arising from retrospective studies. In J. Neyman, editor, *Proceedings of the 3rd Berkeley symposium, Vol IV*, Berkeley, 1956. University of California Press.

C. Cortes and V. Vapnik. Support-vector networks. *Mach Learn*, 20:273–297, December 1995.

J.P. Costantino, M.H. Gail, D. Pee, S. Anderson, C.K. Redmond, J. Benichou, and H.S. Wieand. Validation studies for models projecting the risk of invasive and total breast cancer incidence. *J Natl Cancer Inst*, 91(18):1541–1548, 1999.

M.C. Costanza. Matching. *Prev Med*, 24:425–433, 1995.

D.R. Cox. *Planning of Experiments.* Wiley, New York, 1958.

R.K. Crump, V.J. Hotz, G.W. Imbens, and O.A. Mitnik. Moving the goalposts: Addressing limited overlap in the estimation of average treatment effects by changing the estimand. Technical Report 330, National Bureau of Economic Research, 2006.

A.S. Dalalyan and A.B. Tsybakov. Aggregation by exponential weighting and sharp oracle inequalities. In N.H. Bshouty and C. Gentile, editors, *COLT*, volume 4539 of *Lecture Notes in Computer Science*, Berlin Heidelberg New York, 2007. Springer.

A.S. Dalalyan and A.B. Tsybakov. Aggregation by exponential weighting, sharp pac-Bayesian bounds and sparsity. *Mach Learn*, 72(1–2):39–61, 2008.

E. de la Rochebrochard, N. Soullier, R. Peikrishvili, J. Guibert, and J. Bouyer. High in vitro fertilization discontinuation rate in France. *Int J Gynecol Obstet*, 103: 74–75, 2008.

E. de la Rochebrochard, C. Quelen, R. Peikrishvili, J. Guibert, and J. Bouyer. Long-term outcome of parenthood project during in vitro fertilization and after discontinuation of unscuccessful in vitro fertilization. *Fertil Steril*, 92:149–156, 2009.

R. Dehejia and S. Wahba. Causal effects in nonexperimental studies: Reevaluating the evaluation of training programs. *J Am Stat Assoc*, 94:1053–1062, 1999.

R. Dehejia and S. Wahba. Propensity score matching methods for nonexperimental causal studies. *Rev Econ Stat*, 84(1):151–161, 2002.

Department of Health and Human Services. Guidelines for the use of antiretroviral agents in HIV-1 infected adults and adolescents. Technical Report, Panel on Clinical Practices for Treatment of HIV Infection, 2004.

E. Dimitriadou, K. Hornik, F. Leisch, D. Meyer, and A. Weingessel. *e1071: Misc functions of the Department of Statistics (e1071)*, 2009. URL http://CRAN.R-project.org/package=e1071. R package version 1.5-22.

T.A. Diprete and H. Engelhardt. Estimating causal effects with matching methods in the presence and absence of bias cancellation. *Sociol Meth Res*, 32(4):501–528, 2004.

S. Dudoit and M.J. van der Laan. Asymptotics of cross-validated risk estimation in estimator selection and performance assessment. *Stat Methodol*, 2(2):131–154, 2005.

S. Dudoit and M.J. van der Laan. *Resampling Based Multiple Testing with Applications to Genomics*. Springer, Berlin Heidelberg New York, 2008.

S. Dudoit, J. Fridlyand, and T. P. Speed. Comparison of discrimination methods for the classification of tumors using gene expression data. *J Am Stat Assoc*, 97(457): 77–87, 2002.

B. Efron. Better bootstrap confidence intervals. *J Am Stat Assoc*, 82(397):171–185, 1987.

B. Efron and T. Hastie. lars. R package, 2007.

B. Efron and R. J. Tibshirani. *An Introduction to the Bootstrap*. Chapman & Hall, Boca Raton, 1993.

B. Efron, T. Hastie, I. Johnstone, and R. Tibshirani. Least angle regression. *Ann Stat (with discussion)*, 32(2):407–499, 2004.

S.S. Emerson. Issues in the use of adaptive clinical trial designs. *Stat Med*, 25: 3270–3296, 2006.

Food and Drug Administration. Critical path opportunities list. Technical Report, U.S. Department of Health and Human Services, Food and Drug Administration, 2006.

D.A. Freedman. *Statistical Models: Theory and Practice*. Cambridge, New York, 2005.

D.A. Freedman. Statistical models for causation: What inferential leverage do they provide? *Eval Rev*, 30:691–713, 2006.

D.A. Freedman. On regression adjustments to experimental data. *Adv Appl Math*, 40:180–193, 2008a.

D.A. Freedman. On regression adjustments to experiments with several treatments. *Ann Appl Stat*, 2:176–96, 2008b.

D.A. Freedman. Randomization does not justify logistic regression. *Stat Sci*, 23: 237–249, 2008c.

D.A. Freedman and R.A. Berk. Weighting regressions by propensity scores. *Eval Rev*, 3:392–409, 2008.

D.A. Freedman, D.B. Petitti, and J.M. Robins. On the efficacy of screening for breast cancer. *Int J Epidemiol*, 33:43–55, 2004.

D.H. Freedman. *Wrong: Why Experts Keep Failing Us—And How to Know When Not to Trust Them*. Little, Brown and Company, New York, 2010.

R. Freedman. Incomplete matching in ex post facto studies. *Am J of Soc*, 55(5): 485–487, 1950.

J.H. Friedman. Multivariate adaptive regression splines. *Ann Stat*, 19(1):1–141, 1991.

J.H. Friedman. Flexible metric nearest neighbor classification. Technical Report, Department of Statistics, Stanford University, 1994.

J.H. Friedman. Greedy function approximation: A gradient boosting machine. *Ann Stat*, 29:1189–1232, 2001.

J.H. Friedman, T.J. Hastie, and R.J. Tibshirani. Regularization paths for generalized linear models via coordinate descent. *J Stat Softw*, 33(1), 2010a.

J.H. Friedman, T.J. Hastie, and R.J. Tibshirani. *glmnet: Lasso and elastic-net regularized generalized linear models*, 2010b. URL http://CRAN.R-project.org/package=glmnet. R package version 1.1-5.

D.A. Fruman, S.B. Snapper, C.M. Yballe, L. Davidson, J.Y. Yu, F.W. Alt, and L.C. Cantley. Impaired B cell development and proliferation in absence of phosphoinositide 3-kinase p85-alpha. *Science*, 283:393–397, 1999.

T. Fujii, S. Nomoto, K. Koshikawa, Y.Yatabe, O. Teshigawara, T. Mori, S. Inoue, S. Takeda, and A. Nakao. Overexpression of pituitary tumor transforming gene 1 in HCC is associated with angiogenesis and poor prognosis. *Hepatology*, 43: 1267–1275, 2006.

M.H. Gail. Adjusting for covariates that have the same distribution in exposed and unexposed cohorts. In S. H. Moolvankar and R. L. Prentice, editors, *Modern Statistical Methods in Chronic Disease Epidemiology*. Wiley, New York, 1986.

M.H. Gail, L.A. Brinton, D.P. Byar, D.K. Corle, S.B. Green, C. Schairer, and J.J. Mulvihill. Projecting individualized probabilities of developing breast cancer for white females who are being examined annually. *J Natl Cancer Inst*, 81(24): 1879–1886, 1989.

S. Galiani, P. Gertler, and E. Schargrodsky. Water for life: The impact of the privatization of water services on child mortality. *J Polit Econ*, 113(1):83–120, 2005.

Y. Ge and S. Dudoit. Multiple testing procedures, multtest. R package, 2002. URL www.bioconductor.org.

S. Geisser. The predictive sample reuse method with applications. *J Am Stat Assoc*, 70(350):320–328, 1975.

A. Gelman, A. Jakulin, M.G. Pittau, and Y.-S. Su. A weakly informative default prior distribution for logistic and other regression models. *Ann Appl Stat*, 2(3): 1360–1383, 2009.

A. Gelman, Y.-S. Su, M. Yajima, J. Hill, M.G. Pittau, J. Kerman, and T. Zheng. *arm: Data analysis using regression and multilevel/hierarchical models*, 2010. URL http://CRAN.R-project.org/package=arm. R package version 1.3-02.

R.D. Gill. Non- and semiparametric maximum likelihood estimators and the von mises method (part 1). *Scand J Stat*, 1989.

R.D. Gill and J.M. Robins. Causal inference in complex longitudinal studies: Continuous case. *Ann Stat*, 29(6):1785–1811, 2001.

H.L. Golub. The need for more efficient trial designs. *Stat Med*, 25:3231–3235, 2006.

T.R. Golub, D.K. Slonim, P. Tamayo, C. Huard, M. Gaasenbeek, J.P. Mesirov, H. Coller, M.L. Loh, J.R. Downing, M.A. Caligiuri, C.D. Bloomfield, and E.S.

Lander. Molecular classification of cancer: Class discovery and class prediction by gene expression monitoring. *Science*, 286:531–537, 1999.

S. Greenland. Multivariate estimation of exposure-specific incidence from case-control studies. *J Chron Dis*, 34:445–453, 1981.

S. Greenland. Model-based estimation of relative risks and other epidemiologic measures in studies of common outcomes and in case-control studies. *Am J Epidemiol*, 160(4):301–305, 2004.

S. Gruber and M.J. van der Laan. An application of collaborative targeted maximum likelihood estimation in causal inference and genomics. *Int J Biostat*, 6(1), 2010a.

S. Gruber and M.J. van der Laan. A targeted maximum likelihood estimator of a causal effect on a bounded continuous outcome. *Int J Biostat*, 6(1):Article 26, 2010b.

S. Gruber and M.J. van der Laan. tmle: An R package for targeted maximum likelihood estimation. Technical Report 275, Division of Biostatistics, University of California, Berkeley, 2011.

L. Györfi, M. Kohler, A. Krzyżak, and H. Walk. *A Distribution-Free Theory of Nonparametric Regression*. Springer, Berlin Heidelberg New York, 2002.

L. Haignere. *Paychecks: A Guide to Conducting Salary-Equity Studies for Higher Education Faculty*. American Association of University Professors, Washington, DC, 2nd edition, 2002.

C.S. Haley and S.A. Knott. A simple regression method for mapping quantitative trait loci in line crosses using flanking markers. *Heredity*, 1992.

S.M. Hammer, J.J. Eron, P. Reiss, R.T. Schooley, M.A. Thompson, S. Walmsley, P. Cahn, M.A. Fischl, J.M. Gatell, M.S. Hirsch, D.M. Jacobsen, J.S.G. Montaner, D.D. Richman, P.G. Yeni, and P.A. Volberding. Antiretroviral treatment of adult HIV infection: 2008 recommendations of the International AIDS Society-USA panel. *J Am Med Asoc*, 300(5):555–70, 2008.

F.R. Hampel, E.M. Ronchetti, P.J. Rousseeuw, and W.A. Stahel. *Robust Statistics: The Approach Based on Influence Functions*. Wiley, New York, 1986.

B.B. Hansen. The prognostic analogue of the propensity score. *Biometrika*, 95: 481–8, 2008.

F.E. Harrell, Jr. *Regression Modeling Strategies with Applications to Linear models, Logistic Regression, and Survival Analysis*. Springer, Berlin Heidelberg New York, 2001.

T.J. Hastie. Generalized additive models. In J.M. Chambers and T.J. Hastie, editors, *Statistical Models in S*. Chapman & Hall, Boca Raton, 1992.

T.J. Hastie and R.J. Tibshirani. *Generalized Additive Models*. Chapman & Hall, Boca Raton, 1990.

T.J. Hastie, R.J. Tibshirani, and J.H. Friedman. *The Elements of Statistical Learning: Data Mining, Inference, and Prediction*. Springer, Berlin Heidelberg New York, 2001.

S.C. Heath. Markov chain Monte Carlo segregation and linkage analysis of oligogenic models. *Am J Hum Genet*, 1997.

J. Heckman. Causal parameters and policy analysis in economics: A twentieth century retrospective. *Q J Econ*, 115:45–97, 2000.

J. Heckman. Building bridges between structural and program evaluation approaches to evaluating policy. *J Econ Lit*, 48:356–398, 2010.

J. Heckman, H. Ichimura, and R. Todd. Matching as an econometric evaluation estimator: Evidence from evaluating a job training programme. *Rev of Econ Stud*, 64:605–654, 1997.

M.A. Hernan, B. Brumback, and J.M. Robins. Marginal structural models to estimate the causal effect of zidovudine on the survival of HIV-positive men. *Epidemiol*, 11(5):561–570, 2000.

M.A. Hernan, E. Lanoy, D. Costagliola, and J.M. Robins. Comparison of dynamic treatment regimes via inverse probability weighting. *Basic Clin Pharmacol*, 98: 237–242, 2006.

A.V. Hernández, M.J. Eijkemans, and E.W. Steyerberg. Randomized controlled trials with time-to-event outcomes: How much does prespecified covariate adjustment increase power? *Ann Epidemiol*, 16(1):41–48, 2006.

M.C. Herron and J. Wand. Assessing partisan bias in voting technology: The case of the 2004 New Hampshire recount. *Elect Stud*, 26(2):247–261, 2007.

T.R. Holford, C. White, and J.L. Kelsey. Multivariate analysis for matched case-control studies. *Am J Epidemiol*, 107(3):245–255, 1978.

J.H. Holland and J.S. Reitman. Cognitive systems based on adaptive algorithms. *SIGART Bull*, 63:49–49, 1977.

P.W. Holland. Statistics and causal inference. *J Am Stat Assoc*, 81(396):945–960, 1986.

P.W. Holland. Comment: Causal mechanism or causal effect: Which is best for statistical science? *Stat Sci*, 3(2):186–188., 1988.

P.W. Holland and Donald B. Rubin. Causal inference in retrospective studies. In Donald B. Rubin, editor, *Matched Sampling for Causal Effects*. Cambridge, Cambridge, MA, 1988.

T. Hothorn, P. Buhlmann, S. Dudoit, A.M. Molinaro, and M.J. van der Laan. Survival ensembles. *Biostatistics*, 7:355–373, 2006.

F. Hu and W.F. Rosenberger. *The Theory of Response Adaptive Randomization in Clinical Trials*. Wiley, New York, 2006.

A.E. Hubbard, M.J. van der Laan, and J.M. Robins. Nonparametric locally efficient estimation of the treatment specific survival distributions with right censored data and covariates in observational studies. In D. Berry E. Halloran, editor, *Statistical Models in Epidemiology: The Environment and Clinical Trials*. Springer, Berlin Heidelberg New York, 1999.

S.P. Hunger. Chromosomal translocations involving the E2A gene in acute lymphoblastic leukemia: Clinical features and molecular pathogenesis. *Blood*, 87: 1211–1224, 1996.

K. Imai. Do get-out-the-vote calls reduce turnout? the importance of statistical methods for field experiments. *Am Polit Sci Rev*, 99(2):283–300, 2005.

J.P.A. Ioannidis. Why most published research findings are false. *Neonatal Intensive Care J Perinatol Neonatol*, 19(3), 2006.

H. Ishwaran, U.B. Kogalur, E.H. Blackstone, and M.S. Lauer. Random survival forests. *Ann Appl Stat*, 2(3):841–860, 2008.

R. Jackson. Updated new zealand cardiovascular disease risk-benefit prediction guide. *Br Med J*, 320(7236):709–710, 2000.

R.C. Jansen. Interval mapping of multiple quantitative trait loci. *Genetics*, 1993.

C. Jennison and B.W. Turnbull. *Group Sequential Methods with Applications to Clinical Trials*. Chapman & Hall, Boca Raton, 2000.

N.P. Jewell. *Statistics for Epidemiology*. Chapman & Hall, Boca Raton, 2004.

H. Jiang, J. Symanowski, S. Paul, Y. Qu, A. Zagar, and S. Hong. The type I error and power of nonparametric logrank and Wilcoxon tests with adjustment for covariates – a simulation study. *Stat Med*, 27(28):5850–5860, 2008.

C. Jin, J.P. Fine, and B.S. Yandell. A unified semiparametric framework for quantitative trait loci analysis, with application to spike phenotypes. *J Am Stat Assoc*, 2007.

V.A. Johnson, F. Brun-Vezinet, B. Clotet, H.F. Gunthard, D.R. Kuritzkes, D. Pillay, J.M. Schapiro, and D.D. Richman. Update of the drug resistance mutations in HIV-1: December 2009. *Top HIV Med*, 17(5):138–45, 2009.

A. Juditsky, A.V. Nazin, A.B. Tsybakov, and N. Vayatis. Generalization error bounds for aggregation by mirror descent with averaging. In *NIPS*, 2005.

J. Kang and J.L. Schafer. Demystifying double robustness: A comparison of alternative strategies for estimating a population mean from incomplete data (with discussion). *Stat Sci*, 22:523–39, 2007.

W.B. Kannel, D. McGee, and T. Gordon. A general cardiovascular risk profile: The Framingham study. *Am J Cardiol*, 38:46–51, 1976.

C.H. Kao, Z.B. Zeng, and R.D. Teasdale. Multiple interval mapping for quantitative trait loci. *Genetics*, 1999.

S.H. Kaufmann, S.D. Gore, C.B. Miller, R.J. Jones, L.A. Zwelling, E. Schneider, P.J. Burke, and J.E. Karp. Topoisomerase II and the response to antileukemic therapy. *Leukemia Lymphoma*, 29(3-4):217–237, Apr 1998a.

S.H. Kaufmann, J.E. Karp, P.A. Svingen, S. Krajewski, P.J. Burke, S.D. Gore, and J.C. Reed. Elevated expression of the apoptotic regulator Mcl-1 at the time of leukemic relapse. *Blood*, 91(3):991–1000, 1998b.

N. Keiding, C. Hols, and A. Green. Retrospective estimation of diabetes incidence from information in a current prevalent population and historical mortality. *Am J Epidemiol*, 130:588–600, 1989.

S. Keleş, M.J. van der Laan, and S. Dudoit. Asymptotically optimal model selection method for regression on censored outcomes. Technical Report 124, Division of Biostatistics, University of California, Berkeley, 2002.

D. Kibler, D.W. Aha, and M.K. Albert. Instance-based prediction of real-valued attributes. *Comput Intell*, 5:51, 1989.

I. Kirsch, B.J. Deacon, T.B. Huedo-Medina, A. Scoboria, T.J. Moore, and B.T. Johnson. Initial severity and antidepressant benefits: A meta-analysis of data submitted to the Food and Drug Administration. *PLoS Med*, 5(2):e45. doi:10.1371/journal.pmed.0050045, 2008.

L. Kish. Weighting for unequal p_i. *J Off Stat*, 8:183–200, 1992.

G.G. Koch, C.M. Tangen, J.W. Jung, and I.A. Amara. Issues for covariance analysis of dichotomous and ordered categorical data from randomized clinical trials and nonparametric strategies for addressing them. *Stat Med*, 17:1863–1892, 1998.

I. Komuro, T. Yasuda, A. Iwamoto, and K.S. Akagawa. Catalase plays a critical role in the CSF-independent survival of human macrophages via regulation of the expression of BCL-2 family. *J Biol Chem*, 280(50):41137–45, 2005.

C. Kooperberg. *polspline: Polynomial spline routines*, 2009. URL http://CRAN.R-project.org/package=polspline. R package version 1.1.4.

C. Kooperberg, C.J. Stone, and Y.K. Truong. Hazard regression. *J Am Stat Assoc*, 90(429):78–94, 1995.

J. Kos and T.T. Lah. Cysteine proteinases and their endogenous inhibitors: Target proteins for prognosis, diagnosis and therapy in cancer (review). *Oncol Rep*, 5 (6):1349–61, 1998.

H. Koul, V. Susarla, and J. van Ryzin. Regression analysis with randomly right censored data. *Ann Stat*, 9:1276–88, 1981.

K. Kozar, M.A. Ciemerych, V.I. Rebel, H. Shigematsu, A. Zagozdzon, E. Sicinska, Y. Geng, Q. Yu, S. Bhattacharya, R.T. Bronson, K. Akashi, and P. Sicinski. Mouse development and cell proliferation in the absence of D-cyclins. *Cell*, 118:477–491, 2004.

L.L. Kupper, J.M. Karon, D.G. Kleinbaum, H. Morgenstern, and D.K. Lewis. Matching in epidemiologic studies: Validity and efficiency considerations. *Biometrics*, 37:271–291, 1981.

R.J. LaLonde. Evaluating the econometric evaluations of training programs with experimental data. *Am Econ Rev*, 76:604–620, 1986.

E.S. Lander and D. Botstein. Mapping Mendelian factors underlying quantitative traits using RFLP linkage maps. *Genetics*, 1989.

A.A. Lane and T.J. Ley. Neutrophil elastase cleaves PML-RAR-alpha and is important for the development of acute promyelocytic leukemia in mice. *Cell*, 115 (305-318), 2003.

M. LeBlanc and J. Crowley. Relative risk trees for censored data. *Biometrics*, 48: 411–425, 1992.

M. LeBlanc and R.J. Tibshirani. Combining estimates in regression and classification. *J Am Stat Assoc*, 91:1641–1650, 1996.

S.S.F. Lee, L. Sun, R. Kustra, and S.B. Bull. EM-random forest and new measures of variable importance for multi-locus quantitative trait linkage analysis. *Bioinformatics*, 2008.

E.L. Lehmann. *Testing Statistical Hypotheses*. Springer, Berlin Heidelberg New York, 2nd edition, 1986.

S. Leon, A.A. Tsiatis, and M. Davidian. Semiparametric estimation of treatment effect in a pretest-posttest study. *Biometrics*, 59:1046–1055, 2003.

G. Leone, R. Sears, E. Huang, R. Rempel, F. Nuckolls, C.H. Park, P. Giangrande, L. Wu, H.I. Saavedra, S.J. Field, M.A. Thompson, H. Yang, Y. Fujiwara, M.E. Greenberg, S. Orkin, C. Smith, and J.R. Nevins. Myc requires distinct E2F activities to induce S phase and apoptosis. *Mol Cell*, 8:105–113, 2001.

A. Liaw and M. Wiener. Classification and regression by randomforest. *R News*, 2 (3):18–22, 2002. URL http://CRAN.R-project.org/package=randomForest.

D.V. Lindley. *Introduction to Probability and Statistics from a Bayesian Point of View, Part 2*. Cambridge, Cambridge, MA, 1980.

R.J.A. Little and Donald B. Rubin. *Statistical Analysis with Missing Data*. Wiley, Hoboken, 2nd edition, 2002.

Z. Liu and T. Stengos. Nonlinearities in cross country growth regressions: A semi-parametric approach. *J of Appl Econom*, 14:527–538, 1999.

C.L. Loprinzi, J.A. Laurie, H.S. Wieand, J.E. Krook, P.J. Novotny, J.W. Kugler, J. Bartel, M. Law, M. Bateman, and N.E. Klatt. Prospective evaluation of prognostic variables from patient-completed questionnaires, North Central Cancer Treatment Group. *J Clin Oncol*, 12(3):601–607, 1994.

X. Lu and A.A Tsiatis. Improving the efficiency of the log-rank test using auxiliary covariates. *Biometrika*, 95(3):679–694, 2008.

D. MacKinnon. *Introduction to Statistical Mediation Analysis*. Erlbaum, New York, 2008.

D. MacKinnon, C. Lockwood, C. Brown, W. Wang, and J. Hoffman. The intermediate endpoint effect in logistic and probit regression. *Clin Trials*, 4:499–513, 2007.

R. Mansson, M.M. Joffe, W. Sun, and S. Hennessy. On the estimation and use of propensity scores in case-control and case-cohort studies. *Am J Epidemiol*, 166 (3):332–339, 2007.

J. Marschak. Studies in econometric method. In W. C. Hood and T. C. Koopmans, editors, *Economic Measurements for Policy and Prediction*. Wiley, New York, 1953.

J.I. Martin-Subero, R. Ibbotson, W. Klapper, L. Michaux, E. Callet-Bauchu, F. Berger, M.J. Calasanz, C. De Wolf-Peeters, M.J. Dyer, P. Felman, A. Gardiner, R.D. Gascoyne, S. Gesk, L. Harder, D.E. Horsman, M. Kneba, R. Kuppers, A. Majid, N. Parry-Jones, M. Ritgen, M. Salido, F. Sole, G. Thiel, H.H. Wacker, D. Oscier, I. Wlodarska, and R. Siebert. A comprehensive genetic and histopathologic analysis identifies two subgroups of B-cell malignancies carrying a t(14;19)(q32;q13) or variant BCL3-translocation. *Leukemia*, 21(7):1532–1544, 2007.

G.L. Masinde, X. Li, W. Gu, H. Davidson, S. Mohan, and D.J. Baylink. Identification of wound healing/regeneration quantitative trait loci (QTL) at multiple time points that explain seventy percent of variance in (MRL/MpJ and SJL/J) mice F2 population. *Genome Res*, 2001.

P. McCullagh. Quasi-likelihood functions. *Ann Stat*, 11:59–67, 1983.

P. McCullagh and J.A. Nelder. *Generalized Linear Models*. Chapman & Hall, Boca Raton, 2nd edition, 1989.

S.M. McKinlay. Pair-matching – a reappraisal of a popular technique. *Biometrics*, 33(4):725–735, 1977.

K.L. Moore and M.J. van der Laan. Covariate adjustment in randomized trials with binary outcomes. Technical Report 215, Division of Biostatistics, University of California, Berkeley, April 2007.

K.L. Moore and M.J. van der Laan. Application of time-to-event methods in the assessment of safety in clinical trials. In Karl E. Peace, editor, *Design, Summarization, Analysis & Interpretation of Clinical Trials with Time-to-Event Endpoints*, Boca Raton, 2009a. Chapman & Hall.

K.L. Moore and M.J. van der Laan. Covariate adjustment in randomized trials with binary outcomes: Targeted maximum likelihood estimation. *Stat Med*, 28(1):39–64, 2009b.

K.L. Moore and M.J. van der Laan. Increasing power in randomized trials with right censored outcomes through covariate adjustment. *J Biopharm Stat*, 19(6): 1099–1131, 2009c.

K.L. Moore, R.S. Neugebauer, M.J. van der Laan, and I.B. Tager. Causal inference in epidemiological studies with strong confounding. Technical Report 255, Division of Biostatistics, University of California, Berkeley, 2009.

S.L. Morgan and D.J. Harding. Matching estimators of causal effects: Prospects and pitfalls in theory and practice. *Sociol Meth Res*, 35(1):3–60, 2006.

A.P. Morise, G.A. Diamon, R. Detrano, M. Bobbio, and Erdogan Gunel. The effect of disease-prevalence adjustments on the accuracy of a logistic prediction model. *Med Decis Making*, 16:133–142, 1996.

K.M. Mortimer, R. Neugebauer, M.J. van der Laan, and I.B. Tager. An application of model-fitting procedures for marginal structural models. *Am J Epidemiol*, 162 (4):382–388, 2005.

A.R. Moss, J.A. Hahn, S. Perry, E.D. Charlebois, D. Guzman, R.A. Clark, and D.R. Bangsberg. Adherence to highly active antiretroviral therapy in the homeless population in San Francisco: A prospective study. *Clin Infect Dis*, 39(8):1190–1198, 2004.

K. Nebral, H.H. Schmidt, O.A. Haas, and S. Strehl. NUP98 is fused to topoisomerase (DNA) IIbeta 180 kDa (TOP2B) in a patient with acute myeloid leukemia with a new t(3;11)(p24;p15). *Clin Cancer Res*, 11(18):6489–6494, 2005.

R. Neugebauer and J. Bullard. *DSA: Data-adaptive estimation with cross-validation and the D/S/A algorithm*, 2009. URL http://www.stat.berkeley.edu/ laan/Software/. R package version 3.1.3.

R. Neugebauer and M. J. van der Laan. Nonparametric causal effects based on marginal structural models. *J Stat Plan Infer*, 137(2):419–434, 2007.

R. Neugebauer and M.J. van der Laan. Why prefer double robust estimates. *J Stat Plan Infer*, 129(1-2):405–26, 2005.

R. Neugebauer, M.J. Silverberg, and M.J. van der Laan. Observational study and individualized antiretroviral therapy initiation rules for reducing cancer incidence in HIV-infected patients. 272, Division of Biostatistics, University of California, Berkeley, 2010.

D.J. Newman, S. Hettich, C.L. Blake, and C.J. Merz. UCI Repository of Machine Learning Databases, 1998.

S. Newman. Causal analysis of case-control data. *Epid Persp Innov*, 3:2, 2006.

J. Neyman. Sur les applications de la theorie des probabilites aux experiences agricoles: Essai des principes (In Polish). English translation by D.M. Dabrowska and T.P. Speed (1990). *Stat Sci*, 5:465–480, 1923.

T. Palomero, D.T. Odom, J. O'Neil, A.A. Ferrando, A. Margolin, D.S. Neuberg, S.S. Winter, R.S. Larson, W. Li, X.S. Liu, R.A. Young, and A.T. Look. Transcriptional regulatory networks downstream of TAL1/SCL in T-cell acute lymphoblastic leukemia. *Blood*, 108(3):986–992, 2006.

M. Pavlic and M.J. van der Laan. Fitting of mixtures with unspecified number of components using cross validation distance estimate. *Comput Stat Data An*, 41: 413–428, 2003.

J. Pearl. Causal diagrams for empirical research. *Biometrika*, 82:669–710, 1995.

J. Pearl. Direct and indirect effects. In *Uncertainty in Artificial Intelligence, Proceedings of the 17th Conference*, San Francisco, 2001. Morgan Kaufmann.

J. Pearl. *Causality: Models, Reasoning, and Inference*. Cambridge, New York, 2nd edition, 2009.

J. Pearl. On a class of bias-amplifying variables that endanger effect estimates. *Proceedings of Uncertainty in Artificial Intelligence*, 2010a.

J. Pearl. An introduction to causal inference. *Int J Biostat*, 6(2):Article 7, 2010b.

J. Pearl. The mediation formula: A guide to the assessment of causal pathways in nonlinear models. In C. Berzuini, P. Dawid, and L. Bernardinelli, editors, *Statistical Causality*. 2011.

K. Pearson. *Grammar of Science*. Black, London, 3rd edition, 1911.

K. Penrose, A. Nelson, and A. Fisher. Generalized body composition prediction equation for men using simple measurement techniques. *Med Sci Sport Exer*, 17: 189, 1985.

A. Peters and T. Hothorn. *ipred: Improved Predictors*, 2009. URL http://CRAN.R-project.org/package=ipred. R package version 0.8-8.

M.L Petersen, S.G. Deeks, J.N. Martin, and M.J. van der Laan. History-adjusted marginal structural models to estimate time-varying effect modification. *Am J Epidemiol*, 166(9):985–993, 2007a.

M.L. Petersen, S.G. Deeks, and M.J. van der Laan. Individualized treatment rules: Generating candidate clinical trials. *Stat Med*, 26(25):4578–601, 2007b.

M.L. Petersen, M.J. van der Laan, S. Napravnik, J.J. Eron, R.D. Moore, and S.G. Deeks. Long-term consequences of the delay between virologic failure of highly active antiretroviral therapy and regimen modification. *AIDS*, 22(16):2097–106, 2008.

M.L. Petersen, K.E. Porter, S. Gruber, Y. Wang, and M.J. van der Laan. Diagnosing and responding to violations in the positivity assumption. *Stat Meth Med Res*, published online 28 Oct (doi: 10.1177/0962280210386207), 2010.

S.J. Pocock, S.E. Assmann, L.E. Enos, and L.E. Kasten. Subgroup analysis, covariate adjustment, and baseline comparisons in clinical trial reporting: Current practice and problems. *Stat Med*, 21:2917–2930, 2002.

E.C. Polley and M.J. van der Laan. Predicting optimal treatment assignment based on prognostic factors in cancer patients. In K.E. Peace, editor, *Design, Summarization, Analysis & Interpretation of Clinical Trials with Time-to-Event Endpoints*, Boca Raton, 2009. Chapman & Hall.

E.C. Polley and M.J. van der Laan. Super learner in prediction. Technical Report 266, Division of Biostatistics, University of California, Berkeley, 2010.

R.L. Prentice and N.E. Breslow. Retrospective studies and failure time models. *Biometrika*, 65(1):153–158, 1978.

R.L. Prentice and R. Pyke. Logistic disease incidence models and case-control studies. *Biometrika*, 66:403–411, 1979.

R. Puri, A. Tousson, L. Chen, and S.S. Kakar. Molecular cloning of pituitary tumor transforming gene 1 from ovarian tumors and its expression in tumors. *Cancer Lett*, 163:131–139, 2001.

R Development Core Team. *R: A language and environment for statistical computing*. R Foundation for Statistical Computing, Vienna, 2010. URL http://www.R-project.org.

S. Ramaswamy, K.N. Ross, E.S. Lander, and T.R. Golub. A molecular signature of metastasis in primary solid tumors. *Nat Genet*, 33:49–54, 2003.

L.E. Ramsay, I.U. Haq, P.R. Jackson, and W.W. Yeo. Sheffield risk and treatment table for cholesterol lowering for primary prevention of coronary heart disease. *Lancet*, 346(8988):1467–1471, 1995.

L.E. Ramsay, I.U. Haq, P.R. Jackson, and W.W. Yeo. The Sheffield table for primary prevention of coronary heart disease: Corrected. *Lancet*, 348(9036):1251, 1996.

S.J. Reynolds, G. Nakigozi, K. Newell, A. Ndyanabo, R. Galiwongo, I. Boaz, T.C. Quinn, R. Gray, M. Wawer, and D. Serwadda. Failure of immunologic criteria to appropriately identify antiretroviral treatment failure in Uganda. *AIDS*, 23(6): 697–700, 2009.

G. Ridgeway. *gbm: Generalized boosted regression models*, 2007. R package version 1.6-3.

B.D. Ripley. *Pattern Recognition and Neural Networks*. Cambridge, New York, 1996.

J. Rissanen. Modelling by shortest data description. *Automatica*, 14:465–471, 1978.

P.C. Robert. *The Bayesian Choice: From Decision-Theoretic Foundations to Computational Implementation*. Springer, Berlin Heidelberg New York, 2007.

J.M. Robins. A new approach to causal inference in mortality studies with sustained exposure periods–application to control of the healthy worker survivor effect. *Math Mod*, 7:1393–1512, 1986.

J.M. Robins. Addendum to: "A new approach to causal inference in mortality studies with a sustained exposure period—application to control of the healthy worker survivor effect". *Comput Math Appl*, 14(9–12):923–945, 1987a.

J.M. Robins. A graphical approach to the identification and estimation of causal parameters in mortality studies with sustained exposure periods. *J Chron Dis (40, Supplement)*, 2:139s–161s, 1987b.

J.M. Robins. Information recovery and bias adjustment in proportional hazards regression analysis of randomized trials using surrogate markers. In *Proceedings of the Biopharmaceutical Section*. American Statistical Association, 1993.

J.M. Robins. Correcting for noncompliance in randomized trials using structural nested mean models. *Commun Stat*, 23:2379–2412, 1994.

J.M. Robins. Marginal structural models. *1997 Proceedings of the American Statistical Association. Section on Bayesian Statistical Science*, pages 1–10, 1998.

J.M. Robins. [Choice as an alternative to control in observational studies]: Comment. *Stat Sci*, 14(3):281–293, 1999a.

J.M. Robins. Marginal structural models versus structural nested models as tools for causal inference. In *Statistical Models in Epidemiology: The Environment and Clinical Trials*. Springer, Berlin Heidelberg New York, 1999b.

J.M. Robins. Robust estimation in sequentially ignorable missing data and causal inference models. In *Proceedings of the American Statistical Association*, 2000.

J.M. Robins and S. Greenland. Identifiability and exchangeability for direct and indirect effects. *Epidemiol*, 3:143–155, 1992.

J.M. Robins and A. Rotnitzky. Recovery of information and adjustment for dependent censoring using surrogate markers. In *AIDS Epidemiology*. Birkhäuser, Basel, 1992.

J.M. Robins and A. Rotnitzky. Semiparametric efficiency in multivariate regression models with missing data. *J Am Stat Assoc*, 90:122–129, 1995.

J.M. Robins and A. Rotnitzky. Comment on the Bickel and Kwon article, "Inference for semiparametric models: Some questions and an answer". *Stat Sinica*, 11(4): 920–936, 2001.

J.M. Robins and N. Wang. Inference for imputation estimators. *Biometrika*, 87: 113–124, 2000.

J.M. Robins, S.D. Mark, and W.K. Newey. Estimating exposure effects by modelling the expectation of exposure conditional on confounders. *Biometrics*, 48(479–495), 1992.

J.M. Robins, A. Rotnitzky, and L.P. Zhao. Estimation of regression coefficients when some regressors are not always observed. *J Am Stat Assoc*, 89(427):846–866, 1994.

J.M. Robins, A. Rotnitzky, and L.P. Zhao. Analysis of semiparametric regression models for repeated outcomes in the presence of missing data. *J Am Stat Assoc*, 90:106–121, 1995.

J.M. Robins, M.A. Hernan, and B. Brumback. Marginal structural models and causal inference in epidemiology. *Epidemiol*, 11(5):550–560, 2000a.

J.M. Robins, A. Rotnitzky, and M.J. van der Laan. Comment on "On profile likelihood". *J Am Stat Assoc*, 450:431–435, 2000b.

J.M. Robins, M.A. Hernan, and A. Rotnitzky. Effect modification by time-varying covariates. *Am J Epidemiol*, 166(9):994–1002, 2007a.

J.M. Robins, M. Sued, Q. Lei-Gomez, and A. Rotnitzky. Comment: Performance of double-robust estimators when "inverse probability" weights are highly variable. *Stat Sci*, 22:544–559, 2007b.

J.M. Robins, L. Orellana, and A. Rotnitzky. Estimation and extrapolation of optimal treatment and testing strategies. *Stat Med*, 27:4678–4721, 2008.

A.J. Rodger, Z. Fox, J.D. Lundgren, J.L. Kuller, C. Boesecke, D. Gey, A. Skoutelis, M.B. Goetz, A.N. Phillips, and INSIGHT Strategies for Management of Antiretroviral Therapy (SMART) Study Group. Activation and coagulation biomarkers are independent predictors of the development of opportunistic disease in patients with HIV infection. *J Infect Dis*, 200(6):973–83, 2009.

S. Rose and M.J. van der Laan. Simple optimal weighting of cases and controls in case-control studies. *Int J Biostat*, 4(1):Article 19, 2008.

S. Rose and M.J. van der Laan. Why match? Investigating matched case-control study designs with causal effect estimation. *Int J Biostat*, 5(1):Article 1, 2009.

S. Rose and M.J. van der Laan. A targeted maximum likelihood estimator for two-stage designs. *Int J Biostat*, 7(1):Article 17, 2011.

S. Rose, J.M. Snowden, and K.M. Mortimer. Rose et al. respond to "G-computation and standardization in epidemiology". *Am J Epidemiol*, 173(00):000–000, 2011.

P.R. Rosenbaum. *Observational Studies*. Springer, Berlin Heidelberg New York, 2nd edition, 2002.

P.R. Rosenbaum and Donald B. Rubin. The central role of the propensity score in observational studies for causal effects. *Biometrika*, 70:41–55, 1983.

W.F. Rosenberger. New directions in adaptive designs. *Stat Sci*, 11:137–149, 1996.

W.F. Rosenberger, A.N. Vidyashankar, and D.K. Agarwal. Covariate-adjusted response-adaptive designs for binary response. *J Biopharm Stat*, 11(227–236), 2001.

M. Rosenblum and M.J. van der Laan. Using regression models to analyze randomized trials: Asymptotically valid hypothesis tests despite incorrectly specified models. *Biometrics*, 65(3):937–945, 2009a.

M. Rosenblum and M.J. van der Laan. Confidence intervals for the population mean tailored to small sample sizes, with applications to survey sampling. *Int J Biostat*, 1:Article 4, 2009b.

M. Rosenblum and M.J. van der Laan. Targeted maximum likelihood estimation of the parameter of a marginal structural model. *Int J Biostat*, 6(2):Article 19, 2010a.

M. Rosenblum and M.J. van der Laan. Simple, efficient estimators of treatment effects in randomized trials using generalized linear models to leverage baseline variables. *Int J Biostat*, 6(1):Article 13, 2010b.

M. Rosenblum, S.G. Deeks, M.J. van der Laan, and D.R. Bangsberg. The risk of virologic failure decreases with duration of HIV suppression, at greater than 50% adherence to antiretroviral therapy. *PLoS ONE*, 4(9): e7196.doi:10.1371/journal.pone.0007196, 2009.

B. Rosner. *Fundamentals of Biostatistics*. Duxbury, Pacific Grove, 5th edition, 1999.

K.J. Rothman and S. Greenland. *Modern Epidemiology*. Lippincott, Williams & Wilkins, Philadelphia, 2nd edition, 1998.

Daniel B. Rubin and M.J. van der Laan. Empirical efficiency maximization: Improved locally efficient covariate adjustment in randomized experiments and survival analysis. *Int J Biostat*, 4(1):Article 5, 2008.

Donald B. Rubin. Estimating causal effects of treatments in randomized and non-randomized studies. *J Educ Psychol*, 66:688–701, 1974.

Donald B. Rubin. Bayesian inference for causality: The importance of randomization. In *The Proceedings of the Social Statistics Section of the American Statistical Association*. American Statistical Association, Alexandria, 1975.

Donald B. Rubin. Multivariate matching methods that are equal percent bias reducing, II: Maximums on bias reduction for fixed sample sizes. *Biometrics*, 32(1): 121–132, 1976.

Donald B. Rubin. Bayesian inference for causal effects: The role of randomization. *Ann Stat*, 6:34–58, 1978.

Donald B. Rubin. Comment: Neyman (1923) and causal inference in experiments and observational studies. *Stat Sci*, 5(4):472–480, 1990.

Donald B. Rubin. Estimating causal effects from large data sets using propensity scores. *Ann of Intern Med*, 127(8S):757–763, 1997.

Donald B. Rubin. Using propensity scores to help design observational studies: Application to the tobacco litigation. *Health Serv Outcome Res Meth*, 2(1):169–188, 2002.

Donald B. Rubin. *Matched Sampling for Causal Effects.* Cambridge, Cambridge, MA, 2006.

Donald B. Rubin. For objective causal inference, design trumps analysis. *Ann of Appl Stat*, 2(3):808–840, 2008.

I. Ruczinski, C. Kooperberg, and M. LeBlanc. Logic regression – methods and software. In D. Denison, M. Hansen, C. Holmes, B. Mallick, and B. Yu, editors, *Proceedings of the MSRI workshop on Nonlinear Estimation and Classification*, pages 333–344, 2002.

K. Rudser, M. LeBlanc, and S.S. Emerson. Estimation for arbitrary functionals of survival. Technical Report 335, Department of Biostatistics, University of Washington, 2008.

J.M. Satagopan, B.S. Yandell, M.A. Newton, and T.C. Osborn. A Bayesian approach to detect quantitative trait loci using Markov chain Monte Carlo. *Genetics*, 1996.

K. Sax. The association of size difference with seed-coat pattern and pigmentation in *Phaseolus vulgaris*. *Genetics*, 1923.

J.L. Schafer. *Analysis of Incomplete Multivariate Data.* Chapman & Hall, London, 1997.

D.O. Scharfstein, A. Rotnitzky, and J.M. Robins. Adjusting for nonignorable drop-out using semiparametric nonresponse models, (with discussion and rejoinder). *J Am Stat Assoc*, 94:1096–1120 (1121–1146), 1999.

J.J. Schlesselman. *Case-Control Studies: Design, Conduct, Analysis.* Oxford, Oxford, 1982.

G. Schwartz. Estimating the dimension of a model. *Ann Stat*, 6:461–464, 1978.

M.R. Segal. Regression trees for censored data. *Biometrics*, 44:35–47, 1988.

J.S. Sekhon. Alternative balance metrics for bias reduction in matching methods for causal inference. Technical Report, University of California, Berkeley, 2006.

J.S. Sekhon. Multivariate and propensity score matching software with automated balance optimization: The matching package for R. *J Stat Softw*, 2008a.

J.S. Sekhon. The Neyman-Rubin model of causal inference and estimation via matching methods. In J.M. Box-Steffensmeier, H.E. Brady, and D. Collier, editors, *The Oxford Handbook of Political Methodology*. Oxford, New York, 2008b.

J.S. Sekhon. Opiates for the matches: Matching methods for causal inference. *Annu Rev of Polit Sci*, 12:487–508, 2010.

J.V. Selby, D.H. Smith, E.S. Johnson, M.A. Raebel, G.D. Friedman, and B.H. McFarland. Kaiser Permanente medical care program. In B.L. Strom, editor, *Pharmacoepidemiology*. Wiley, 2005.

S. Senturker, B. Karahalil, M. Inal, H. Yilmaz, H. Muslumanoglu, G. Gedikoglu, and M. Dizdaroglu. Oxidative DNA base damage and antioxidant enzyme levels in childhood acute lymphoblastic leukemia. *FEBS Letters*, 416(3):286–290, 1997.

J. Shao, X. Yu, and B. Bob Zhong. A theory for testing hypotheses under covariate-adaptive randomization. *Biometrika*, 2010.

M.J. Sillanpaa and E. Arjas. Bayesian mapping of multiple quantitative trait loci from incomplete inbred line cross data. *Genetics*, 1998.

S.E. Sinisi and M.J. van der Laan. Deletion/Substitution/Addition algorithm in learning with applications in genomics. *Stat Appl Genet Mol*, 3(1), 2004. Article 18.

H.L. Smith. Matching with multiple controls to estimate treatment effects in observational studies. *Sociol Meth*, 27:305–353, 1997.

J.M. Snowden, S. Rose, and K.M. Mortimer. Implementation of g-computation on a simulated data set: Demonstration of a causal inference technique. *Am J Epidemiol*, 173(00):000–000, 2011.

N. Soullier, J. Bouyer, Pouly J-L., J. Guibert, and de la Rochebrochard. Estimating the success of an in vitro fertilization programme using multiple imputation. *Hum Reproduct*, 23:187–192, 2008.

T.P. Speed. Introductory remarks on Neyman (1923). *Stat Sci*, 5(4):463–464, 1990.

O.M. Stitelman and M.J. van der Laan. Collaborative targeted maximum likelihood for time-to-event data. *Int J Biostat*, 6(1):Article 21, 2010.

O.M. Stitelman and M.J. van der Laan. Targeted maximum likelihood estimation of time-to-event parameters with time-dependent covariates. Technical Report, Division of Biostatistics, University of California, Berkeley, 2011a.

O.M. Stitelman and M.J. van der Laan. Targeted maximum likelihood estimation of effect modification parameters in survival analysis. *Int J Biostat*, 7(1), 2011b.

M. Stone. Cross-validatory choice and assessment of statistical predictions. *J R Stat Soc Ser B*, 36(2):111–147, 1974.

M. Stone. Asymptotics for and against cross-validation. *Biometrika*, 64(1):29–35, 1977.

J.S. Stringer, I. Zulu, J. Levy, E.M. Stringer, A. Mwango, B.H. Chi, V. Mtonga, S. Reid, R.A. Cantrell, M. Bulterys, M.S. Saag, R.G. Marlink, A. Mwinga, T.V. Ellerbrock, and M. Sinkala. Rapid scale-up of antiretroviral therapy at primary care sites in Zambia: Feasibility and early outcomes. *J Am Med Asoc*, 296(7): 782–93, 2006.

I. Tager, M. Hollenberg, and W. Satariano. Self-reported leisure-time physical activity and measures of cardiorespiratory fitness in an elderly population. *Am J Epidemiol*, 147:921–931, 1998.

Z. Tan. A distributional approach for causal inference using propensity scores. *J Am Stat Assoc*, 101:1619–1637, 2006.

Z. Tan. Comment: Improved local efficiency and double robustness. *Int J Biostat*, 4 (1):Article 10, 2008.

C.M. Tangen and G.G. Koch. On-parametric analysis of covariance for hypothesis testing with logrank and Wilcoxon scores and survival-rate estimation in a randomized clinical trial. *J Biopharm Stat*, 9(2):307–338, 1999.

G. Taubes. Do we really know what makes us healthy? *The New York Times*, 2007.

P.F. Thall, C. Logothetis, L.C. Pagliaro, S. Wen, M.A. Brown, D. Williams, and R.E. Millikan. Adaptive therapy for androgen-independent prostate cancer: A randomized selection trial of four regimens. *J Natl Cancer Inst*, 99:1613–22, 2007.

T. Therneau and T. Lumley. *survival: Survival analysis, including penalised likelihood*, 2009. URL http://CRAN.R-project.org/package=survival. R package version 2.35-8.

J.M. Thoday. Location of polygenes. *Nature*, 1960.

R. Tibshirani. Regression shrinkage and selection via the lasso. *J R Stat Soc Ser B*, 58(1):267–288, 1996.

R.J. Tibshirani. The lasso method for variable selection in the Cox model. *Stat Med*, 16:385–395, 1997.

R.M. Tombes and G.W. Krystal. Identification of novel human tumor cell-specific CaMK-II variants. *Biochim Biophys Acta*, 1355:281–292, 1997.

A.A. Tsiatis. *Semiparametric Theory and Missing Data*. Springer, Berlin Heidelberg New York, 2006.

A.A. Tsiatis, M. Davidian, M. Zhang, and X. Lu. Covariate adjustment for two-sample treatment comparisons in randomized clinical trials: A principled yet flexible approach. *Stat Med*, 27:4658–4677, 2008.

A.B. Tsybakov. Optimal rates of aggregation. In B. Schölkopf and M.K. Warmuth, editors, *COLT*, volume 2777 of *Lecture Notes in Computer Science*, Berlin Heidelberg New York, 2003. Springer.

C. Tuglus and M.J. van der Laan. Targeted methods for biomarker discovery, the search for a standard. Technical Report 233, Division of Biostatistics, University of California, Berkeley, 2008.

C. Tuglus and M.J. van der Laan. Modified FDR controlling procedure for multi-stage analyses. *Stat Appl Genet Mol*, 8(1):Article 12, 2009.

J. Tyrer, S.W. Duffy, and J. Cuzick. A breast cancer prediction model incorporating familial and personal risk factors. *Stat Med*, 23(7):1111–1130, 2004.

U.S. Preventive Services Task Force. Screening for breast cancer: U.S. Preventive Services Task Force recommendation statement. *Ann Intern Med*, 151(10):716–726, 2009.

M.J. van der Laan. Statistical inference for variable importance. *Int J Biostat*, 2(1): Article 2, 2006.

M.J. van der Laan. Estimation based on case-control designs with known prevalance probability. *Int J Biostat*, 4(1):Article 17, 2008a.

M.J. van der Laan. The construction and analysis of adaptive group sequential designs. Technical Report 232, Division of Biostatistics, University of California, Berkeley, 2008b.

M.J. van der Laan. Targeted maximum likelihood based causal inference: Part I. *Int J Biostat*, 6(2):Article 2, 2010a.

M.J. van der Laan. Targeted maximum likelihood based causal inference: Part II. *Int J Biostat*, 6(2):Article 3, 2010b.
M.J. van der Laan. Estimation of causal effects of community-based interventions. Technical Report 268, Division of Biostatistics, University of California, Berkeley, 2010c.
M.J. van der Laan and S. Dudoit. Unified cross-validation methodology for selection among estimators and a general cross-validated adaptive epsilon-net estimator: Finite sample oracle inequalities and examples. Technical Report 130, Division of Biostatistics, University of California, Berkeley, 2003.
M.J. van der Laan and S. Gruber. Collaborative double robust penalized targeted maximum likelihood estimation. *Int J Biostat*, 6(1):Article 17, 2010.
M.J. van der Laan and M.L. Petersen. Causal effect models for realistic individualized treatment and intention to treat rules. *Int J Biostat*, 3(1):Article 3, 2007a.
M.J. van der Laan and M.L. Petersen. Statistical learning of origin-specific statically optimal individualized treatment rules. *Int J Biostat*, 3(1):Article 6, 2007b.
M.J. van der Laan and M.L. Petersen. Direct effect models. *Int J Biostat*, 4(1): Article 23, 2008.
M.J. van der Laan and J.M. Robins. *Unified Methods for Censored Longitudinal Data and Causality*. Springer, Berlin Heidelberg New York, 2003.
M.J. van der Laan and S. Rose. Statistics ready for a revolution: Next generation of statisticians must build tools for massive data sets. *Amstat News*, 399:38–39, 2010.
M.J. van der Laan and Daniel B. Rubin. Targeted maximum likelihood learning. *Int J Biostat*, 2(1):Article 11, 2006.
M.J. van der Laan and Daniel B. Rubin. A note on targeted maximum likelihood and right-censored data. Technical Report 226, Division of Biostatistics, University of California, Berkeley, 2007.
M.J. van der Laan, S. Dudoit, and S. Keleş. Asymptotic optimality of likelihood-based cross-validation. *Stat Appl Genet Mol*, 3(1):Article 4, 2004.
M.J. van der Laan, M.L. Petersen, and M.M. Joffe. History-adjusted marginal structural models and statically-optimal dynamic treatment regimens. *Int J Biostat*, 1 (1):10–20, 2005.
M.J. van der Laan, S. Dudoit, and A.W. van der Vaart. The cross-validated adaptive epsilon-net estimator. *Stat Decis*, 24(3):373–395, 2006.
M.J. van der Laan, M.L. Petersen, and M.M. Joffe. Response to invited commentary: Petersen et. al. respond to "Effect modification by time-varying covariates". *Am J Epidemiol*, 166(9):1003–1004, 2007a.
M.J. van der Laan, E.C. Polley, and A.E. Hubbard. Super learner. *Stat Appl Genet Mol*, 6(1):Article 25, 2007b.
A.W. van der Vaart. *Asymptotic Statistics*. Cambridge, New York, 1998.
A.W. van der Vaart and J.A. Wellner. *Weak Convergence and Empirical Processes*. Springer, Berlin Heidelberg New York, 1996.
A.W. van der Vaart, S. Dudoit, and M.J. van der Laan. Oracle inequalities for multi-fold cross-validation. *Stat Decis*, 24(3):351–371, 2006.

H.C. van Houwelingen, T. Bruinsma, A.A.M. Hart, L.J. van't Veer, and L.F.A. Wessels. Cross-validated Cox regression on microarray gene expression data. *Stat Med*, 25:3201–3216, 2006.

J.P. Vandenbrouke, E. von Elm, D.G. Altman, P.C. Gotzsche, C.D. Mulrow, S.J. Pocock, C. Poole, J.J. Schlesselman, and M. Egger for the STROBE Initiative. Strengthening the reporting of observational studies in epidemiology (STROBE): Explanation and elaboration. *PLoS Med*, 4(10):1628–1654, 2007.

L.J. van't Veer, H. Dal, M.J. van de Vijver, Y.D. He, A.A.M. Hart, M. Mao, H.L. Peterse, K. van der Kooy, M.J. Marton, A.T. Witteveen, G.J. Schreiber, R.M. Kerkhoven, C. Roberts, P.S. Linsley, R. Bernards, and S.H. Friend. Gene expression profiling predicts clinical outcome of breast cancer. *Nature*, 415:530–536, 2002.

W.N. Venables and B.D. Ripley. *Modern Applied Statistics with S*. Springer, Berlin Heidelberg New York, 4th edition, 2002.

C. Vitale, C. Romagnani, A. Puccetti, D. Olive, R. Costello, L. Chiossone, A. Pitto, A. Bacigalupo, L. Moretta, and M.C. Mingari. Surface expression and function of p75/AIRM-1 or CD33 in acute myeloid leukemias: Engagement of CD33 induces apoptosis of leukemic cells. *Proc Natl Acad Sci*, 98:5764–5769, 2001.

S. Wacholder. The case-control study as data missing by design: Estimating risk differences. *Epidemiology*, 7(2):144–150, 1996.

H. Wang, S. Rose, and M.J. van der Laan. Finding quantitative trait loci genes with collaborative targeted maximum likelihood learning. *Stat Prob Lett*, published online 11 Nov (doi: 10.1016/j.spl.2010.11.001), 2010.

H. Wang, S. Rose, and M.J. van der Laan. Targeted methods for finding quantitative trait loci. Technical Report, Division of Biostatistics, University of California, Berkeley, 2011.

Y. Wang, M.L. Petersen, D.R. Bangsberg, and M.J. van der Laan. Diagnosing bias in the inverse probability of treatment weighted estimator resulting from violation of experimental treatment assignment. Technical Report 211, Division of Biostatistics, University of California, Berkeley, 2006.

R.W.M. Wedderburn. Quasi-likelihood functions, generalized linear models, and the gauss-newton method. *Biometrika*, 61(3):439–447, 1974.

C.W. Wester, A.M. Thomas, H. Bussmann, S. Moyo, J.M. Gaolathe, V. Novitsky, M. Essex, V. De Gruttola, and R.G. Marlink. Nonnucleoside reverse transcriptase inhibitor outcomes among combination antiretroviral therapy-treated adults in Botswana. *AIDS*, 24:S27–S36, 2010.

P.W.F. Wilson, R.B. D'Agostino, D. Levy, A.M. Belanger, H. Silbershatz, and W.B. Kannel. Prediction of coronary heart disease using risk factor categories. *Circulation*, 97:1837–1847, 1998.

C. Winship and S.L. Morgan. The estimation of causal effects from observational data. *Annu Rev Sociol*, 25:659–707, 1999.

D. H. Wolpert. Stacked generalization. *Neural Networks*, 5:241–259, 1992.

H.P. Wong, L. Yu, E.K. Lam, E.K. Tai, W.K. Wu, and C.H. Cho. Nicotine promotes cell proliferation via alpha7-nicotinic acetylcholine receptor and catecholamine-synthesizing enzymes-mediated pathway in human colon adenocarcinoma HT-29 cells. *Toxicol Appl Pharm*, 221(3):261–267, 2007.

J. Wooldridge. Should instrumental variables be used as matching variables? Technical Report, Michigan State University, 2009.

World Health Organization. Antiretroviral therapy for HIV infection in adults and adoloescents: Recommendations for a public health approach, 2006.

L. Yang and A.A. Tsiatis. Efficiency study for a treatment effect in a pretest-posttest trial. *Am Stat*, 56:29–38, 2001.

Z. Yu and M.J. van der Laan. Construction of counterfactuals and the g-computation formula. Technical Report 122, Division of Biostatistics, University of California, Berkeley, 2002.

Z. Yu and M.J. van der Laan. Measuring treatment effects using semiparametric models. Technical Report 136, Division of Biostatistics, University of California, Berkeley, 2003.

Z.B. Zeng. Precision mapping of quantitative trait loci. *Genetics*, 1994.

H.H. Zhang and W. Lu. Adaptive lasso for Cox's proportional hazards model. *Biometrika*, 94(3):691–703, 2007.

L.-X. Zhang and F.-F. Hu. A new family of covariate-adjusted response adaptive designs and their properties. *Appl Math J Chinese Univ Ser B*, 24(1):1–13, 2009.

L.-X. Zhang, F.-F. Hu, S.H. Cheung, and W.S. Chan. Asymptotic properties of covariate-adjusted response-adaptive designs. *Ann Stat*, 35(3):1166–1182, 2007.

M. Zhang, A.A. Tsiatis, and M. Davidian. Improving efficiency of inferences in randomized clinical trials using auxiliary covariates. *Biometrics*, 64(3):707–715, 2008.

W. Zheng and M.J. van der Laan. Asymptotic theory for cross-validated targeted maximum likelihood estimation. Technical Report 273, Division of Biostatistics, University of California, Berkeley, 2010.

X. Zhu, Z. Mao, Y. Na, Y. Guo, X. Wang, and D. Xin. Significance of pituitary tumor transforming gene 1 (PTTG1) in prostate cancer. *Anticancer Res*, 26:1253–1259, 2006.

Index

Author Index

CPSIA information can be obtained at www.ICGtesting.com
Printed in the USA
LVOW02*2359220813

349257LV00007B/105/P

9 781441 997814